T0314044

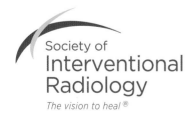

Society of
Interventional
Radiology
The vision to heal ®

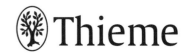

Portal Hypertension

Imaging, Diagnosis, and Endovascular Management

Third Edition

Wael E.A. Saad, MBBCh, FSIR
Professor of Radiology
Director, Vascular & Interventional Radiology and
  Neuro-Interventional Radiology
Department of Radiology
University of Michigan Health System
Ann Arbor, Michigan

Thieme
New York • Stuttgart • Delhi • Rio de Janeiro

Executive Editor: William Lamsback
Managing Editor: J. Owen Zurhellen
Production Editors: Jeri Litteral, Naamah Schwartz
Director, Editorial Services: Mary Jo Casey
International Production Director: Andreas Schabert
International Marketing Director: Fiona Henderson
International Sales Director: Louisa Turrell
Director of Sales, North America: Mike Roseman
Senior Vice President and Chief Operating
   Officer: Sarah Vanderbilt
President: Brian D. Scanlan

Library of Congress Cataloging-in-Publication Data

Names: Saad, Wael E. A., editor.
Title: Portal hypertension : imaging, diagnosis, and endovascular
   management / [edited by] Wael E.A. Saad.
Other titles: Portal hypertension (Saad)
Description: Third edition. | New York : Thieme, [2018] | Includes
   bibliographical references and index.
Identifiers: LCCN 2016043179 (print) | LCCN 2016044313 (ebook) |
   ISBN 978-1-62623-326-3 (eBook) | ISBN 978-1-62623-327-0
   (hardcover : alk. paper) | ISBN 978-1-62623-326-3 (e-book)
Subjects: | MESH: Hypertension, Portal–diagnosis | Diagnostic
   Imaging | Hypertension, Portal–surgery | Endovascular Procedures
Classification: LCC RC685.H8 (ebook) | LCC RC685.H8 (print) | NLM
   WI 720 | DDC 616.1/32075–dc23
LC record available at https://lccn.loc.gov/2016043179

© 2018 Thieme Medical Publishers, Inc.

Thieme Publishers New York
333 Seventh Avenue, New York, NY 10001 USA
+1 800 782 3488, customerservice@thieme.com

Thieme Publishers Stuttgart
Rüdigerstrasse 14, 70469 Stuttgart, Germany
+49 [0]711 8931 421, customerservice@thieme.de

Thieme Publishers Delhi
A-12, Second Floor, Sector-2, Noida-201301
Uttar Pradesh, India
+91 120 45 566 00, customerservice@thieme.in

Thieme Publishers Rio de Janeiro, Thieme Publicações Ltda.
Edifício Rodolpho de Paoli, 25º andar
Av. Nilo Peçanha, 50 – Sala 2508,
Rio de Janeiro 20020-906 Brasil
+55 21 3172-2297 / +55 21 3172-1896

Cover design: Thieme Publishing Group
Typesetting by Aptara, Inc.

Printed in India by Replika Press Pvt. Ltd.   5 4 3 2 1

ISBN 978-1-62623-327-0

Also available as an e-book:
eISBN 978-1-62623-326-3

Important note: Medicine is an ever-changing science undergoing continual development. Research and clinical experience are continually expanding our knowledge, in particular our knowledge of proper treatment and drug therapy. Insofar as this book mentions any dosage or application, readers may rest assured that the authors, editors, and publishers have made every effort to ensure that such references are in accordance with **the state of knowledge at the time of production of the book.**

Nevertheless, this does not involve, imply, or express any guarantee or responsibility on the part of the publishers in respect to any dosage instructions and forms of applications stated in the book. **Every user is requested to examine carefully** the manufacturers' leaflets accompanying each drug and to check, if necessary in consultation with a physician or specialist, whether the dosage schedules mentioned therein or the contraindications stated by the manufacturers differ from the statements made in the present book. Such examination is particularly important with drugs that are either rarely used or have been newly released on the market. Every dosage schedule or every form of application used is entirely at the user's own risk and responsibility. The authors and publishers request every user to report to the publishers any discrepancies or inaccuracies noticed. If errors in this work are found after publication, errata will be posted at www.thieme.com on the product description page.

Some of the product names, patents, and registered designs referred to in this book are in fact registered trademarks or proprietary names even though specific reference to this fact is not always made in the text. Therefore, the appearance of a name without designation as proprietary is not to be construed as a representation by the publisher that it is in the public domain.

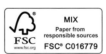

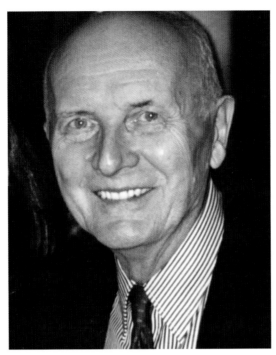

Josef Rösch
1925–2016

It is only fitting that this book on the transjugular intrahepatic portosystemic shunt (TIPS) be dedicated to the noted Josef Rösch. Josef died in January 2016 following an extraordinary clinical, academic, and research career in interventional radiology. His most significant interventional discovery, TIPS, was serendipitous. Having already spent a year with Charles Dotter, Josef was primed to constantly be considering new interventional possibilities. Thus, in 1969, his occasional inadvertent portal vein entry during clinical transjugular cholangiography aroused his research curiosity. This led to the logical next step: a transjugular intrahepatic portosystemic shunt. It took until the mid-1990s, however, with the development of metallic stents, to make TIPS a viable clinical procedure. Today, three decades after its clinical introduction, TIPS has become widely accepted as a minimally invasive treatment for portal hypertension, benefiting millions of patients and essentially replacing surgical portosystemic shunting.

In addition to TIPS, Josef Rösch was the first person to use embolotherapy to control acute gastrointestinal hemorrhage. He pioneered both the use of self-expandable metallic stents to treat stenoses and occlusions of the major veins, trachea, and esophagus, and the technique of fallopian tube recanalization. Josef was the driving force in establishing the Dotter Interventional Institute. It is the first free-standing interventional radiology department in an academic medical center. During his career, Josef received the gold medal from five prestigious interventional radiology societies, in addition to lifetime achievement awards from the Cardiovascular and Interventional Society of Europe (CIRSE) and the American Heart Association. The "Josef Rösch Endowed Chair of Interventional Radiology Research" was established at Oregon Health & Science University in his honor.

Josef was a pioneer and distinguished leader in the development of interventional radiology. He was a great friend and colleague to interventional radiologists around the world and an inspirational mentor to scores of young trainees. Those who had the opportunity to work with him or know him were truly fortunate.

Frederick S. Keller, MD

In addition to the late Josef Rösch (who co-wrote Chapter 13 before his death), this book is dedicated to my mother and father, who taught me beyond medicine; to my wife Aya; to my daughters Luna and Solara; and to my brother Nael (who has co-written Chapter 12), a talented interventional radiologist dedicated to his patients.

Wael E.A. Saad, MBBCh, FSIR

Contents

Section IV Percutaneous and Endovascular Management: Transvenous Obliteration

Foreword

Over the past few decades, advances in imaging and image-guided intervention have transformed the management of patients with portal hypertension. Today, the cause and severity of portal hypertension can be assessed noninvasively, and treatments can be based on individual parameters and tailored to the needs of each patient. Progress in the management of patients with portal hypertension is due in no small measure to the efforts of interventional radiologists. Pioneers in the field like Dr. Josef Rösch, to whom this book is dedicated, made transformative contributions to both the diagnostic imaging of portal hypertension and to the minimally invasive approaches to management. The transjugular intrahepatic portosystemic shunt (TIPS) procedure, which Dr. Rösch developed in the 1980s and 1990s, is now a standard treatment for patients with refractory ascites and variceal bleeding.

Dr. Wael E.A. Saad follows in the footsteps of Dr. Rösch and is today one of the leading clinical researchers in the field of portal hypertension. Dr. Saad has pioneered advances such as balloon-occluded retrograde transvenous obliteration (BRTO) and endovascular approaches to the management of encephalopathy, and he has gathered evidence to prove the value of these techniques. As was the case with Dr. Rösch, Dr. Saad's enthusiasm and zeal for understanding the nature of portal hypertension and devising new and better treatments is infectious. He is not only a leading researcher in this area but is also the preeminent interventional radiology educator in the field.

In this third edition of *Portal Hypertension: Imaging, Diagnosis, and Endovascular Management*, Dr. Saad has created an up-to-date and authoritative text. He has brought together noted experts from around the world to explain state-of-the-art developments in the endovascular management of patients with portal hypertension. Recent advances in transvenous obliteration are highlighted. In-depth discussions of difficult TIPS situations are presented. Special situations such as portal hypertension in the pediatric patient and management of patients with portal thrombosis are elucidated.

Anyone interested in being in on the cutting edge of developments in minimally invasive portal interventions should read this book. It showcases the value of innovation and creativity in medicine and provides inspiration and direction for young researchers in the field.

Jeanne M. LaBerge, MD, FSIR
Professor of Radiology
University of California San Francisco
San Francisco, California

Preface

In 1969, Josef Rösch serendipitously came across and described the concept of the transjugular intrahepatic portosystemic shunt (TIPS), igniting the era of endovascular management of portal hypertension. TIPS was clinically realized with the advent of stent technology in the mid-1980s. Ernest J. Ring, and later Jeanne LaBerge, popularized the clinical use of stent-lined TIPS in the 1990s. With the advent of the broad utilization of commercially available purpose-built stent-grafts in the early to mid-2000s, a new era of stent-graft TIPS started with its superior patency.

In the past decade, however, the endovascular management of portal hypertension has expanded in its clinical practice to a broad number of procedures, performed alone or in combination. The field is no longer confined to TIPS decompression but now includes a multitude of other procedures, including portal vein recanalization and/or angioplasty, splenic embolization, transvenous obliteration (including BRTO and BATO), and peritoneal shunt creation. This does not take away from the TIPS procedure, which remains the mainstay procedure. TIPS itself has also seen advances in the last decade, with the introduction and broad use of ePTFE covered stents improving TIPS patency and resultant clinical outcomes.

This book is the third edition of the Society of Interventional Radiology (SIR) book series of Management of Portal Hypertension (originally called SIR Syllabus) and is the first publication of this series by Thieme Publishers. The book is a contemporary approach to endovascular management of portal hypertension; its publication occurs in interesting times, where outcomes of various techniques have matured to stimulate a healthy addition to the field of portal hypertension management. I hope and expect you will find it useful to your practice.

Wael E.A. Saad, MBBCh, FSIR

Acknowledgments

I thank all the contributors to this book. I thank my family, whose members have endured the length and vigors of my work. I thank my interventional radiology mentors in the order they appeared in my life: Tony Venbrux, Dave Waldman, Mike Darcy, Dan Picus, Tom Vesely, Suresh Vedantham, Alan Matsumoto, and Dave Williams. I thank my life-mentors: my father and Magdy Omar, Mark Davies, Francis Beurgener, Matt Mauro, John Cardella, and Vickie Marx.

Many persons have significantly contributed to patient care and to the science of endovascular management of portal hypertension and liver transplantation, and of those I would especially like to acknowledge the late Josef Rösch, as well as Ernest J. Ring, Jeanne LaBerge, Albert Zajko, David Waldman, Ziv J. Haskal, Hector Ferral, Timothy Clark, Dan Sze, and Brian Funaki.

Contributors

Abdullah M.S. Al-Osaimi, MD, FACP, FACG, AGAF, FAASLD
Professor of Medicine
Division Chief, Hepatology
Medical Director, Liver Transplantation
Department of Medicine
Temple University
Philadelphia, Pennsylvania

David M. Arner, MD
Major, United States Air Force
Director of Endoscopy
Department of Gastroenterology/Hepatology
Landstuhl Regional Medical Center
Landstuhl, Germany

Deddeh Ballah, MD
Department of Radiology and Biomedical Imaging
University of California San Francisco
San Francisco, California

George Behrens, MD
Vascular and Interventional Partners (VIR Chicago)
Advocate Sherman Hospital
Elgin, Illinois

Wissam Bleibel, MD, FACG
Clinical Assistant Professor
University of Kentucky
Owensboro, Kentucky

Jeffrey Forris Beecham Chick, MD, MPH
Assistant Professor of Radiology
Division of Vascular and Interventional Radiology
University of Michigan Health System
Ann Arbor, Michigan

Timothy W.I. Clark, MD, FSIR
Associate Professor of Clinical Radiology and Surgery
University of Pennsylvania Perelman School of Medicine
Director, Interventional Radiology
Penn Presbyterian Medical Center
Philadelphia, Pennsylvania

Celia P. Corona-Villalobos, MD
Research Associate
Division of Nephrology
Department of Medicine
The Johns Hopkins University School of Medicine
Baltimore, Maryland

Nirvikar Dahiya, MD
Chair, Division of Ultrasound
Department of Radiology
Mayo Clinic
Phoenix, Arizona

Michael D. Darcy, MD, FSIR
Professor of Radiology
Chief, Interventional Radiology
Mallinckrodt Institute of Radiology
Washington University
St. Louis, Missouri

Narasimham L. Dasika, MD
Department of Radiology
University of Michigan Health System
Ann Arbor, Michigan

Hector Ferral, MD
Senior Medical Educator
North Shore University Health System
Evanston, Illinois

Kathryn J. Fowler, MD
Assistant Professor
Department of Radiology
Washington University
St. Louis, Missouri

Ron C. Gaba, MD, FSIR
Associate Professor
Vice Chair for Research
Department of Radiology
Division of Interventional Radiology
University of Illinois Hospital & Health Sciences System
Chicago, Illinois

Ziv J. Haskal, MD, FSIR, FAHA, FACR, FCIRSE
Professor of Radiology
Dept. of Radiology and Medical Imaging/Interventional
   Radiology
University of Virginia School of Medicine
Charlottesville, Virginia

Shozo Hirota, MD
Professor and Chairman
Department of Radiology
Hyōgo College of Medicine
Nishinomiya, Japan

Bogdan Iliescu, MD
Vascular and Interventional Radiology
Atlanta Veterans Administration Medical Center
Atlanta, Georgia

Mona H. Ismail, MD
Consultant of Hepatology
Associate Professor of Medicine
King Fahad Hospital of the University (KFHU)
University of Dammam
Al-Khobar, Saudi Arabia

Raj A. Jain, MD
Vascular and Interventional Radiology
Pueblo Radiological Group
Pueblo, Colorado

Alexandria Jo, MD
Department of Radiology
University of Michigan Health Systems
Ann Arbor, Michigan

Kaj H. Johansen, MD, PhD, FACS
Vascular and Endovascular Surgery
Swedish Medical Center
Clinical Professor of Surgery
University of Washington School of Medicine
Seattle, Washington

Ihab R. Kamel, MD, PhD
Professor of Radiology and Oncology
Clinical Director, MRI
Johns Hopkins Hospital
Baltimore, Maryland

John A. Kaufman, MD
Director, Dotter Interventional Institute
The Frederick S. Keller Professor of Interventional Radiology
Oregon Health and Science University
Portland, Oregon

Frederick S. Keller, MD, FSIR, FACR, FRCR(Hon)
The Cook Professor of Interventional Therapy
Professor of Interventional Radiology, Diagnostic Radiology, Surgery, and Cardiovascular Medicine
Dotter Interventional Institute
Oregon Health & Science University
Portland, Oregon

Robert K. Kerlan Jr., MD, FSIR
Professor of Clinical Radiology and Surgery
Chief of Interventional Radiology
Department of Radiology and Biomedical Imaging
University of California–San Francisco
San Francisco, California

Minhaj S. Khaja, MD, MBA
Assistant Professor of Radiology
Program Director, Interventional Radiology Residency
Associate Program Director, Diagnostic Radiology Residency
University of Michigan Health System
Ann Arbor, Michigan

Kaoru Kobayashi, MD
Research Associate
Department of Radiology
Hyōgo College of Medicine
Nishinomiya, Japan

Kanti Pallav Kolli, MD
Assistant Professor of Clinical Radiology
Department of Radiology and Biomedical Imaging
University of California San Francisco
San Francisco, California

Jeanne M. LaBerge, MD
Professor
Department of Radiology and Biomedical Imaging
University of California San Francisco
San Francisco, California

Michael F. Lin, MD
Assistant Professor of Radiology
Abdominal Imaging Section
Mallinckrodt Institute of Radiology
Washington University School of Medicine
St. Louis, Missouri

David C. Madoff, MD, FSIR, FACR
Professor of Radiology
Vice Chairman for Academic Affairs
Department of Radiology
Weill Cornell Medical College
New York, New York

Bill S. Majdalany, MD
Assistant Professor of Radiology
Department of Radiology
University of Michigan Health System
Ann Arbor, Michigan

Louis G. Martin, MD, FSIR, FACR
Professor of Radiology
Vascular and Interventional Radiology Section
Emory University School of Medicine
Atlanta, Georgia

Luciana G. Matteoni-Athayde, MD
Postdoctoral Research Fellowship
Russell H. Morgan Department of Radiology and Radiological Sciences
The Johns Hopkins Hospital
Baltimore, Maryland

Christine O. Menias, MD
Professor of Radiology
Mayo Clinic
Scottsdale, Arizona
Adjunct Professor of Radiology
Washington University
St. Louis, Missouri

Paula M. Novelli, MD
Visiting Associate Professor of Radiology
Department of Radiology
University of Pittsburgh Medical Center
Pittsburgh, Pennsylvania

Bertrand Janne d'Othée, MD, MPH, MBA, FSIR
Chief of Interventional Radiology
Baystate Health
Springfield, Massachusetts

Bryan D. Petersen, MD
Associate Professor
Interventional Radiology
Interventional Neuroradiology
Dotter Institute of Interventional Therapy
Oregon Health & Science University
Portland, Oregon

Sundeep Punamiya, MD, FAMS, FSIR
Senior Consultant and Head, Vascular and Interventional
   Radiology
Department of Radiology
Tan Tock Seng Hospital
Singapore

Neda Rastegar, MD
Department of Radiology
Rutgers, The State University of New Jersey
Newark, New Jersey

Charles E. Ray Jr., MD, PhD
Professor and Chair
Department of Radiology
University of Illinois Hospital and College of Medicine
Chicago, Illinois

Sue J. Rhee, MD
Clinical Professor of Pediatrics
Interim Chief, Pediatric Gastroenterology, Hepatology,
   and Nutrition
Medical Director, Pediatric Liver Transplant Program
UCSF Benioff Children's Hospital
San Francisco, California

Josef Rösch, MD, Dr Sc, FSIR [deceased]
Professor of Interventional Radiology and Diagnostic Radiology
Dotter Interventional Institute
Oregon Health & Science University
Portland, Oregon

Nael E. Saad, MD
Associate Professor
Department of Radiology
Washington University
St. Louis, Missouri

Wael E.A. Saad, MBBCh, FSIR
Professor of Radiology
Director, Vascular & Interventional Radiology and
   Neuro-Interventional Radiology
Department of Radiology
University of Michigan Health System
Ann Arbor, Michigan

Faisal M. Sanai, ABIM, SBG
Consultant Hepatologist
Gastroenterology Unit
Department of Medicine
King Abdulaziz Medical City
Jeddah, Saudi Arabia

Kunal V. Shah, MD
Cardiology Fellow
University of Texas Health
Houston, Texas

Ravi N. Srinivasa, MD, DABR
Assistant Professor of Radiology
Quality Assurance & Safety Officer, Vascular and Interventional
   Radiology
Department of Radiology
University of Michigan Health System
Ann Arbor, Michigan

Adam D. Talenfeld, MD
Assistant Professor of Radiology
Division of Interventional Radiology
Weill Cornell Medical College
New York, New York

Satoshi Yamamoto, MD, PhD
Assistant Professor
Department of Radiology
Hyōgo College of Medicine
Nishinomiya, Japan

Section I

Pathogenesis and Diagnosis

Chapter 1: Pathophysiology and Classification of Liver Cirrhosis and Portal Hypertension

Faisal M. Sanai, Mona H. Ismail, and Abdullah M.S. Al-Osaimi

Introduction

Liver cirrhosis and portal hypertension (PHT) are common clinical encounters. Chronic liver disease and cirrhosis is the 12th leading cause of death in the United States, according to the Centers for Disease Control and Prevention (CDC). Deaths related to chronic liver disease and cirrhosis have increased 3.3% between 2009 and 2010.[1,2] Liver disease continues to account for a substantial portion of health-care utilization in the United States and worldwide and is a significant cause of morbidity.[3] Understanding the pathophysiology of cirrhosis and PHT is imperative to identify patients at highest risk for complications. Such knowledge would enable early intervention and potentially alter the clinical course of patients with chronic liver disease toward a favorable outcome. This chapter discusses the definition, pathophysiology, and classification of cirrhosis and PHT.

Liver Anatomy and Function

The liver is a wedge-shaped organ located in the upper right quadrant of the abdomen nestled just beneath the diaphragm. It is the largest organ in the body, weighing approximately 1400 g in women and 1800 g in men. The liver attaches to the diaphragm and anterior abdominal wall, via a series of ligaments. Its posterior and inferior surfaces lie over the kidney, adrenal glands, stomach, gallbladder, and colon. A fibrous sheath known as Glisson's capsule encases the entire organ.[4,5]

"Cantlie's" imaginary line, extending from the gallbladder fossa to the inferior vena cava (IVC), grossly separates the liver into its right and left lobes. The right lobe makes up about 70% of the liver's mass with the left lobe accounting for the remainder. In the 1950s, a French surgeon named Couinard further subdivided the liver into eight independently functioning segments based on the branching patterns of the portal triads and hepatic veins. Dr. Couinard numbered the segments clockwise beginning with the caudate lobe now designated as segment I (► Fig. 1.1).[4] The left lobe contains the left lateral segment (segments II and III) and the left medial segment (segment IV) in addition to segment I. Four other segments make up the right lobe, with segments V and VIII comprising the right anterior lobe and segments VI and VII the right posterior lobe. Segment IV further subdivides into IVA and IVB. Segment IVA is cephalad and sits just below the diaphragm while IVB sits caudally and adjacent to the gallbladder fossa.

The liver forms the interface between the digestive system and the blood. It is the site where nutrients, drugs, and other substances entering the gastrointestinal tract undergo a first round of processing. In this sense, the liver acts as the gatekeeper by allowing passage of useful substances while eliminating others.[6] Blood flows into the liver through a dual supply system that includes the hepatic artery and portal vein (PV). The PV delivers most of the hepatic blood (75%–80%) and provides the main route of entry for all materials absorbed by the intestine except for chylomicrons (► Fig. 1.1; ► Fig. 1.2).

The PV originates from the stomach, intestine, and spleen and terminates in the porta hepatis, where it divides into right and left branches carrying with it nutrient-rich but oxygen-poor blood to the liver.[7] The hepatic artery arises from the celiac trunk and supplies the remaining 25% of the 1500-mL blood volume entering the liver each minute, which unlike portal blood is high in oxygen (► Fig. 1.1). Because of the dual blood supply, most patients can tolerate some obstruction of the PV or hepatic artery. In rare cases, thrombosis or some other type of occlusion caused, for example, by Banti's syndrome or hepatocellular carcinoma (HCC), may create potentially lethal complications.[6]

Splenic and superior mesenteric veins unite to form the PV at the second lumbar vertebra from where it travels 6 to 9 cm before reaching the liver hilum, subsequently branching off into the left and right branches. From the celiac axis, the common hepatic artery ascends to the hepatoduodenal ligament and gives rise to the gastric, gastroduodenal, and proper hepatic artery, which then divides into left and right arterial branches at the liver hilum.[5,6] Intrahepatic branching from the PV, hepatic artery, and bile duct run together within the portal tract and terminate at the corners of the liver lobules. Within the lobules, interconnected plates of hepatocytes branch and join together rather freely to form a spongelike structure. Spaces between these plates contain the sinusoids, which are lined by endothelial and Kupffer cells.[7] The Kupffer cells break down aged erythrocytes and recycle them, remove unwanted material entering from the portal system, and act as antigen-presenting cells in adaptive immunity. Other fat-storing cells called stellates reside in the perisinusoidal space and help maintain the extracellular matrix (ECM) of this compartment, which is composed of collagens (types I, II, and IV), among other molecules.[8] The stellate cells store much of the body's vitamin A and assist with local immunity. After cell injury,

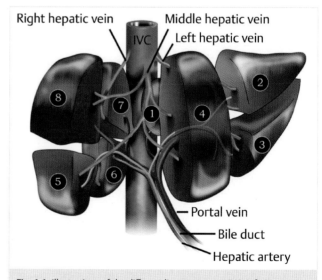

Fig. 1.1 Illustrations of the different liver segments. IVC: inferior vena cava.

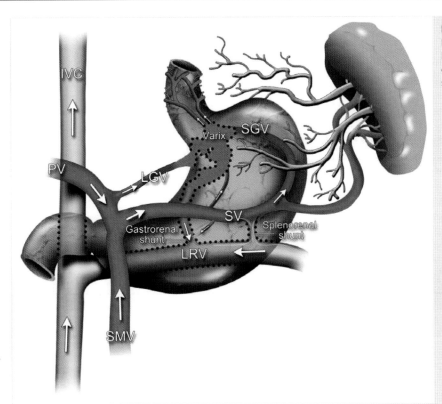

Fig. 1.2 Anatomy of the portal circulation. IVC: inferior vena cava; LGV: left gastric vein; LRV: left renal vein; PV: portal vein; SGV: short gastric veins; SMV: superior mesenteric vein; SV: splenic vein.

they become activated and induce collagen production, resulting in hepatic fibrosis.

Blood flows from the periphery to the center of each lobule, carrying essential oxygen and nutrients with it. Distributing venules running within the lobules lead into the sinusoids and converge into veins at the lobule center and then eventually merge into hepatic veins, which empty into the IVC (▶ Fig. 1.1). Hepatocytes located near the lobule's periphery and close to its blood supply carry out the more aerobic tasks such as protein synthesis; those less exposed to oxygen and nutrients at the lobular center play a larger role in detoxification and glycogen metabolism. Contrary to blood flow, bile drains from the center of the lobule to its periphery through the tubular canaliculi located at the interface of adjoining hepatocytes.[5] At the periphery, the bile empties into special ductules composed of cholangiocytes and eventually reaches the intrahepatic bile ducts in the portal spaces. These ducts subsequently enlarge and unite to form the right and left hepatic ducts for transporting bile away from the liver (▶ Fig. 1.1).

The liver serves many functions.[9] It plays a critical role in carbohydrate metabolism by storing glycogen, converting fructose and galactose to glucose, carrying out gluconeogenesis, and removing excess glucose from the blood as needed. Because of the glucose buffering action provided by the liver, hypoglycemia commonly occurs in individuals with liver failure. The liver also supports fat metabolism, manufactures lipoproteins and all major plasma proteins, except for the immunoglobulins, and preserves cholesterol homeostasis. Blood originating from the gut or elsewhere in the body is mostly detoxified by the liver. Kupffer cells trap and break down bacteria and other particulates, and the cytochrome p450 enzymes biochemically transform drugs and other foreign chemicals into metabolites, which

are then excreted into the bile for elimination via the digestive tract. Bile secreted by the liver aids in the absorption of lipids and fat-soluble vitamins (A, D, E, and K) and serves as the vehicle for removing bilirubin.

Liver Cirrhosis: Definition, Classification, and Epidemiology

Definition of Cirrhosis

Cirrhosis is the end result of the common histologic pathway for a multitude of chronic liver diseases. The term *cirrhosis* was first introduced by Laennec in 1826, being derived from the Greek term *scirrhus*. It was used to describe the orange or tawny surface of the liver observed at autopsy.

Hepatic fibrosis is defined as an excess deposition of the components of ECM (i.e., collagens, glycoproteins, proteoglycans) within the liver. Fibrosis is the wound-healing response of organ systems, which in the liver can progress to the different stages of liver fibrosis and eventually cirrhosis. Sustained signals of inflammation associated with chronic liver disease are required for significant fibrosis to accumulate. Inflammation acts as the driving force for the ever-expanding accumulation of ECM components, eventually leading to cirrhosis and hepatic failure.[8] A variety of factors, including infection, drugs, metabolic disorders, and immune-mediated liver injury, can stimulate the fibrogenic process, in turn marked by excessive synthesis and deposition of collagen in the ECM. Myofibroblasts drive matrix production in response to cytokines and growth factors released by activated Kupffer cells. At the early stage of fibrogenesis, certain proteolytic enzymes, such as the matrix metalloproteinases, can usually remove the excess matrix material, thereby reversing the process.[8]

Liver fibrosis is a dynamic process, resulting from the equilibrium between fibrogenesis and altered matrix degradation, and may be reversible before the establishment of advanced architectural changes in the liver. The excess deposition of ECM proteins disrupts the normal architecture of the liver, which alters the normal functioning of the organ, ultimately leading to PHT. This resultant PHT is the earliest and most important consequence of cirrhosis and underlies most of the clinical complications of the disease. Cirrhosis is defined histologically as a diffuse alteration in the liver architecture with the concomitant development of regenerative nodules. Clinicians consider cirrhosis as the end stage of a chronic condition, which becomes irreversible when presenting in advanced stages. Liver transplantation represents the only cure for patients who have reached this disease stage, with the expected 1- and 8-year survival rates set at 83% and 61%, respectively.[10] Achieving cirrhosis reversibility depends on the stage of the disease and the level of which Kupffer cells and macrophages can retard progression. Reversing fibrosis therapeutically can be manifested by 2 different approaches. One approach involves treating the underlying disease such as autoimmune hepatitis, hepatitis B or C virus, or abstaining from alcohol. The second approach demands developing antifibrotic agents, which to date have shown success only in animal models.[8,11] There are challenges in defining validated endpoints, recruiting sufficient numbers of patients, and overcoming high risk of failure because clinical trials involving these agents have hampered antifibrotic drug development.

The etiology of cirrhosis (▶ Table 1.1) varies according to the region with hepatitis C and alcoholism predominating in Western countries and hepatitis B in parts of East Asia and Africa. Although the exact worldwide prevalence of cirrhosis is unknown, mortality rates from the disease show favorable trends in most areas of the world, especially in North America, Australia, and part of Southern Europe, likely because of declines in alcohol consumption in these regions.[12,13]

Table 1.1 The Most Common Etiologies of Cirrhosis[8,13]

Etiology	Associating Physical Conditions
Alcohol	Dementia, peripheral neuropathy, oral or esophageal cancer
HCV	Cryoglobulinemia (arthritis, vasculitis)
HBV	Arthritis, PAN
PBC	Sicca syndrome, xanthelasma, hyperlipidemia
PSC	IBD, UC
NAFLD, NASH	Obesity, metabolic syndrome, type II diabetes
Wilson's disease	Neurologic symptoms (Parkinson-like)
Hemochromatosis	Arthritis, myocarditis, diabetes
Autoimmune hepatitis	Autoimmune hemolytic anemia, IBD, celiac disease, autoimmune thyroiditis

HBV: hepatitis B virus; HCV: hepatitis C virus; IBD: inflammatory bowel disease; NAFLD: nonalcoholic fatty liver disease; NASH: nonalcoholic steatohepatitis; PAN: polyarteritis nodosa; PBC: primary biliary cirrhosis; PSC: primary sclerosing cholangitis; UC: ulcerative colitis.

A poor correlation frequently exists between hepatic histologic findings and the clinical picture. Some patients with cirrhosis are completely asymptomatic and have a reasonably normal life expectancy. On the other hand, individuals may manifest a variety of severe symptoms of end-stage liver disease and have a poor survival. Common clinical features may stem from decreased hepatic synthetic function (e.g., coagulopathy), decreased detoxification capacity (e.g., portosystemic encephalopathy), or PHT (e.g., ascites).

Classification of Cirrhosis

Cirrhosis had been historically classified on the basis of a mixture of pathogenesis, morphologic appearances, and etiology. However, since then there has been a general recognition that such mixtures are confusing and unwarranted and that any one classification should be restricted to a specific base or axis. Hence, morphologic and etiologic classifications are considered as complementary rather than as alternatives. As such, the complete characterization of cirrhosis in an individual study would have to take into account the morphology, etiology, stage of evolution, disease activity, and complications of the disease.[14] Based on this, the subdivision of cirrhosis is better described as a characterization rather than a classification. Historically, this morphologic categorization has been made as micronodular, macronodular, or mixed type determined to some extent by the underlying disease process. This may allow for the different patterns to be studied epidemiologically, in turn allowing for their correlation with various etiologies.[14]

1. **Micronodular pattern:** This describes a cirrhotic liver in which the vast majority of nodules are smaller than 3 mm in size. The nodules in such cirrhotic livers rarely contain portal tracts or central veins. Early in the course of disease evolution, micronodules tend to predominate; in a later stage, larger nodules may develop. Examples of cirrhosis with this type of nodular pattern include those related to steatosis (alcoholic or otherwise), bile ductal and venous outflow obstruction, and hemochromatosis. These livers are usually normal in size or even enlarged.[14]

2. **Macronodular pattern:** Most nodules in this type of cirrhosis are larger than 3 mm in size, with the size varying considerably, and some nodules being several centimeters in size. Nodules in this type of cirrhosis may contain portal tracts and central veins, although their relationship to each other is not maintained architecturally. The separating fibrous septae may be of the fine, reticulate type or the broad, thickened variety. Examples of this cirrhosis with this type of nodularity include that related to hepatotropic viruses (hepatitis B and C), Wilson's disease, and autoimmune hepatitis. These livers are usually shrunken but may be normal in size.[14]

3. **Mixed pattern:** The nodules in this type are both micronodular and macronodular, approximately in equal proportions.[14]

Epidemiology of Cirrhosis

The estimated prevalence of cirrhosis, as identified from autopsy studies, ranges from 4.5% to 9.5% of the general population, reflecting hundreds of millions of patients affected with cirrhosis worldwide.[15,16] However, the precise incidence or prevalence of cirrhosis is difficult to ascertain because cirrhosis is often clinically silent.[17]

Up to 40% of patients with cirrhosis are asymptomatic and may remain so for more than a decade.[18,19] Currently, a liver biopsy is required to establish the diagnosis of cirrhosis. However, the recent availability of accurate, validated, noninvasive diagnostic tools such as FibroScan and FibroTest may make the specter of population screening in the near future a feasible option.[20]

Nonetheless, in the absence of comprehensive and measurable indices for measuring the incidence and prevalence of cirrhosis in the general population, much of the epidemiologic data for this condition have been derived from disease-related mortality. Understandably, though, for a variety of reasons, the death rate is not always a valid surrogate for measuring the prevalence of cirrhosis, making it difficult to estimate the true prevalence and burden of the disease, especially in the absence of hepatic decompensation.[21]

In 2001, 771,000 people were estimated to have died from cirrhosis, ranking it 14th and 10th as leading cause of death in the world and in developed countries, respectively.[22] Worldwide, deaths from cirrhosis have been projected to increase, making it the 12th leading cause of death in 2020.[23] According to a World Health Organization (WHO) database that incorporates mortality data from 41 countries, age-adjusted mortality rates from cirrhosis were the highest in some countries in Central and South America and in southern Europe in the early 1980s.[24] In southern European countries, mortality rates in the early 2000s decreased by more than 50% compared with earlier decades, but rates in Northern European countries reportedly show a gradual yet continued increase.[25,26] Chronic liver disease and cirrhosis is the 12th leading cause of death in the United States, according to the CDC. Deaths related to chronic liver disease and cirrhosis increased 3.3% between 2009 and 2010.[1,2] Liver disease continues to account for a substantial portion of health-care utilization in the United States and worldwide and is a significant cause of morbidity.[3]

Hepatitis B Virus

Hepatitis B virus (HBV) infection is a global health problem, affecting approximately 2 billion people (i.e., one third of the world's population) based on serologic evidence of past or present HBV infection, including 360 million people with chronic HBV infection.[27,28] Although the development of cirrhosis is dependent on a variety of host and viral factors such as age at infection and viremia level, cirrhosis develops in about 30% of individuals with active disease during their lifetime. After cirrhosis is established, 23% are expected to undergo decompensation, and 10% to 15% are expected to develop HCC at 5 years.[29,30] Although HBV is globally present, it is endemic in China, Southeast Asia, Pacific Islands, sub-Saharan Africa, Alaska, Peru, and northwestern Brazil.[31,32] In developed countries, HBV infection tends to be more prevalent in certain population groups such as immigrants from endemic areas and drug abusers.[33] Because HBV-associated cirrhosis usually does not manifest until the fifth decade in life or later, it is expected to remain a major public health problem worldwide until the cohort of vaccinated children reach adulthood.[34]

Hepatitis C Virus

The hepatitis C virus (HCV) epidemic affects about 2.3% of the worldwide population, that is, an estimated 160 million individuals.[35] An estimated 1.8% of the U.S. population has chronic HCV infection. Northern European countries have a low HCV prevalence (<1%), and southern and eastern European countries such as Romania and rural areas in Greece, Italy, and Russia, exhibit higher (>2%) prevalence.[36] A recent systematic review of the epidemiology of HCV in Asia, Australia, and Egypt estimated that 49.3 to 64.0 million adults of this geographical area were anti-HCV positive.[37] Although most countries of these regions have prevalence rates from 1% to 2%, countries such as Egypt (15%), Pakistan (4.7%), and Taiwan (4.4%) have relatively high prevalence rates.[37]

As with HBV, chronic HCV-related cirrhosis is also modulated by a number of host and viral factors, including age, host genetic factors, presence of steatosis, and alcohol consumption.[38,39] After being infected, the lifetime risk of an individual to develop cirrhosis is about 20% over a period of 2 or 3 decades. With the establishment of cirrhosis, roughly 3% to 5% will decompensate, and 1% to 4% will develop HCC on a yearly basis.[40] Because of the aging of the currently HCV-infected population, the burden of HCV-related cirrhosis is expected to increase in the medium term. A study from United States has shown that aging of the HCV-infected population has already resulted in a significant increase in the prevalence of cirrhosis during the period 1996 to 2006.[41] According to another report from United States, the number of HCV-associated cirrhosis cases is estimated to rise by 24% and that of decompensated cirrhosis cases by 50%.[42]

Alcohol and HCV are thought to be the most important causes of cirrhosis in the United States. Mortality statistics from 1998 show that of patients dying from chronic liver disease, about 40% of deaths were alcohol related, 15% were HCV related, and about 4% were HBV related.[42] Projections showed that although the prevalence of HCV infection may be decreasing currently because of the decline in incidence in the 1990s, the number of persons infected for 20 years has been projected to increase substantially before reaching a peak in 2015.[43,44]

Alcoholic Liver Disease

Patterns of alcohol intake around the world are constantly evolving and have a strong bearing on the prevalence and incidence of alcoholic liver disease (ALD). The annual per capita change in alcohol consumption in various countries has a direct correlation to cirrhosis mortality rates. This was confirmed in a Canadian study in which per capita alcohol consumption was demonstrated to closely correlate with mortality rates from alcoholic cirrhosis in both men and women.[45] Although the precise incidence of alcoholic hepatitis (AH) is unknown, a prevalence of approximately 20% is estimated based on the liver biopsy findings in a cohort of 1604 patients with alcoholism.[46] Moreover, because up to 35% of those with alcoholism are estimated to have AH, the number of affected patients in the United States may be nearly 5 million.

Alcoholic liver disease is the second most common indication for orthotopic liver transplantation (OLT) for end-stage liver disease in the Western world.[47] According to the United Network for Organ Sharing (UNOS) database, 41,734 cadaveric liver transplants were performed in the United States between 1992 and 2001.[48] Of those, 12.5% were performed on patients with ALD. The probability of developing cirrhosis in patients with AH is approximately 10% to 20% per year, translating to an eventual cirrhosis development rate of approximately 70%.[49] In another study, approximately 40% of patients with documented AH developed cirrhosis within 5 years.[50]

Nonalcoholic Fatty Liver Disease

Nonalcoholic fatty liver disease (NAFLD) comprises a wide spectrum of liver damage, ranging from simple steatosis to steatohepatitis and cirrhosis, occurring in patients who do not consume significant amounts of alcohol.[51] Whereas simple hepatic steatosis is believed to have a generally benign course, fat deposition in the hepatocyte is complicated by liver inflammation and fibrosis (nonalcoholic steatohepatitis [NASH]) and can progress to cirrhosis.

There is a rising prevalence of NAFLD because of an increasing number of individuals at risk in the general population,[52–54] translating to an ever-increasing population progressing to cirrhosis.[55,56] Because of its causal association with metabolic syndrome, NAFLD commonly occurs in individuals with obesity, diabetes, and hyperlipidemia.[51] It is estimated that 90% of people with obesity have some form of fatty liver, ranging from simple steatosis to more severe forms of NASH, including cirrhosis.[57–59] In the past 3 decades, the prevalence of obesity in North America has doubled and continues to rise exponentially.[58] It is currently regarded as the most common form of chronic liver disease in the United States and in many parts of the world.[60] In unselected populations, the estimated prevalence of NAFLD ranges from 3% to 36.9%.[60] A recent study in the United States found that 34% of the population had hepatic steatosis.[59] Additionally, many cases of cryptogenic cirrhosis appear to result from NAFLD, wherein they demonstrate one or more of the classical risk factors for the disease such as obesity, diabetes, and hypertriglyceridemia.

Autoimmune Hepatitis

Although autoimmune hepatitis (AIH) has a global occurrence, it was originally described in white northern Europeans and North Americans. Its incidence among white northern Europeans is 1.9 cases per 100,000 persons per year, with a point prevalence of 16.9 cases per 100,000 persons per year.[61,62] In the United States, this disease affects 100,000 to 200,000 persons and accounts for 5.9% of liver transplants; in Europe, it accounts for 2.6% of the transplants.[63] The frequency of AIH in North America among patients with chronic liver disease is 11% to 23%. Cirrhosis is present in one third of patients at diagnosis, and as many as a quarter of patients initially show signs of decompensated cirrhosis.[64] Cirrhosis is generally more common in black North American patients (85%) than in white North American patients (38%) at initial diagnosis, also reflected by a more frequently diminished synthetic function.[65]

Definition and Classification of Portal Hypertension

Definition of Portal Hypertension

Portal hypertension is the hemodynamic abnormality associated with the most severe complications of cirrhosis, including ascites, bleeding from gastroesophageal varices, and hepatic encephalopathy. PHT may also result from a number of noncirrhotic liver diseases and from nonhepatic diseases (▶ Table 1.2).[66]

The normal portal venous pressure ranges between 5 and 10 mm Hg (equivalent of 7–14 cm H_2O). A wedged hepatic venous pressure or direct portal venous pressure that is more than 5 mm Hg greater than the IVC pressure, a splenic pressure of more than 15 mm Hg, or portal venous pressure, measured at surgery, of greater than 30 cm H_2O is abnormal and indicates the presence of PHT.[67] In the vast majority of patients, PHT is related to increased resistance to flow within the hepatic sinusoids, although it may result from diseases as vastly different as constrictive pericarditis and PV thrombosis.

The pressure gradient between the PV and the IVC represents the real perfusion pressure within the portal and hepatic circulation, which under normal conditions is a high-flow, low-resistance system, considering the high volume of portal blood flow (between 700 and 1000 mL/min). The various causes of an increased portal venous resistance are delineated by changes in the anatomic architecture (fibrous scars delineating nodules, distal venous thrombosis, collagenization of the space of Disse, and loss of the normal elasticity of the sinusoidal endothelium), changes in splanchnic hemodynamics (increased splanchnic blood

Table 1.2 Causes of Noncirrhotic Portal Hypertension

Intrahepatic Presinusoidal PHT	Sinusoidal PHT	Extrahepatic Postsinusoidal PHT
Hepatic schistosomiasis	Cirrhosis	Budd-Chiari syndrome
Congenital hepatic fibrosis	Noncirrhotic alcoholic liver disease	Right heart failure
Noncirrhotic portal fibrosis	Infiltrative disorders:	Constrictive pericarditis
Nodular regenerative hyperplasia	• Amyloidosis	Suprahepatic IVC thrombosis
Primary biliary cirrhosis or primary sclerosing cholangitis	• Systemic mastocytosis • Malignancy • Myeloproliferative disorder	Pulmonary hypertension
		Tricuspid valve regurgitation
Extrahepatic Presinusoidal PHT		**Intrahepatic Postsinusoidal PHT**
Portal vein thrombosis		Veno-occlusive disease
Superior mesenteric vein thrombosis	Peliosis hepatis	
Splenic vein thrombosis	Hypervitaminosis A	

IVC: inferior vena cava; PHT: portal hypertension.
Adapted from Molina et al. with modifications.[66]

flow), and changes in the intrahepatic vascular resistance (vasoconstriction of the sinusoids related to the transformation of stellate cells into myofibroblasts).[68]

Portal pressure is proportional to resistance and flow according to Ohm's law: $\Delta P = Q \leftrightarrow R$, where ΔP is the change in pressure along a vessel, Q is the flow in the vessel, and R is the resistance to that flow. Elevated portal pressure typical of cirrhosis has been postulated to include components of each, increased intrahepatic resistance as well as increased flow through the splanchnic system. The extent of increased resistance to flow varies with the underlying type of liver disease and may occur at presinusoidal or postsinusoidal levels as in schistosomiasis and Budd-Chiari syndrome (BCS), respectively. Many forms of liver injury result in "sinusoidal" PHT. Postulated mechanisms for altered blood flow patterns in this process include regenerative nodules, intrahepatic shunts, and hepatocyte swelling.[69-73] Additionally, extinction of typical vascular units after injury and repair may lead to increased intrahepatic resistance.[74]

Classification of Portal Hypertension

The causes of PHT are usually subcategorized as prehepatic, intrahepatic, and posthepatic (see ▶ Table 1.2). Prehepatic causes of PHT are those affecting the portal venous system before it enters the liver, including portal and splenic vein thrombosis. Posthepatic causes encompass those affecting the hepatic veins and venous drainage to the heart, including BCS, veno-occlusive disease, and chronic right-sided heart failure. Intrahepatic causes account for more than 95% of cases of PHT and are represented by the major forms of cirrhosis. Intrahepatic causes of PHT can be further subdivided into presinusoidal, sinusoidal, and postsinusoidal causes.[66,75] Postsinusoidal causes include veno-occlusive disease, and presinusoidal causes include congenital hepatic fibrosis and schistosomiasis. Sinusoidal causes are related to cirrhosis from various causes. Nonetheless, it is worthy to note that despite this defined nomenclature in stratifying PHT based on the anatomic considerations, there exists a great deal of variation among patients with the same disease as to whether they appear to have sinusoidal, presinusoidal, or a mixed form of PHT, based on the wedged hepatic vein pressure. For instance, patients with nonalcoholic cirrhosis have a portal venous pressure that exceeds the wedged hepatic venous pressure by at least 4 mm Hg (there is a presinusoidal component to their PHT); in the remainder, wedged hepatic venous pressure equals portal venous pressure.

Cirrhosis is the most common cause of PHT in the United States, and clinically significant PHT is present in more than 60% of patients with cirrhosis. PV obstruction may be idiopathic or can occur in association with cirrhosis or with infection, pancreatitis, abdominal trauma, or various hypercoagulable disorders such as polycythemia rubra vera; essential thrombocytosis; or deficiencies in protein C, protein S, antithrombin 3, and factor V Leiden.

Budd-Chiari Syndrome

Budd-Chiari syndrome is characterized by hepatic venous outflow obstruction. Reductions in hepatic venous outflow can occur anywhere, at the level of the small or large hepatic veins, suprahepatic portion of the IVC, or right atrium (▶ Table 1.3).[76] Classically, BCS results from thrombosis of one or more hepatic veins at their points of entry into the IVC. This outflow blockage

Table 1.3 Causes of Budd-Chiari Syndrome

Hypercoagulable States
Antiphospholipid syndrome
Antithrombin deficiency
Factor V Leiden mutation
Lupus anticoagulant
Methylenetetrahydrofolate reductase mutation
Myeloproliferative disorders (including polycythemia vera and essential thrombocytosis)
Oral contraceptives
Paroxysmal nocturnal hemoglobinuria
Postpartum thrombocytopenic purpura
Pregnancy
Prothrombin mutation G20210A
Protein S deficiency
Protein C deficiency
Sickle cell disease

Infections
Aspergillosis
Filariasis
Hydatid cysts
Liver abscess (amebic or pyogenic)
Pelvic cellulitis
Schistosomiasis
Syphilis
Tuberculosis

Malignancies
Adrenal carcinoma
Bronchogenic carcinoma
Hepatocellular carcinoma
Leiomyosarcoma
Leukemia
Renal carcinoma
Rhabdomyosarcoma

Miscellaneous
Behçet's disease
Celiac disease
Dacarbazine therapy
Inflammatory bowel disease
Laparoscopic cholecystectomy
Membranous obstruction of the vena cava
Polycystic liver disease
Sarcoidosis
Trauma to hepatic veins

results in dramatic anatomic and physiologic changes within the liver. These deleterious changes of hepatic venous obstruction are transmitted directly to the hepatic sinusoids, resulting in sinusoidal congestion, PHT, and reduced PV blood flow. The consequent clinical effects are manifested by abdominal pain, hepatomegaly, ascites, and impaired hepatic function. Intensive systematic investigations result in identification of one or several thrombotic risk factors in up to 90% of patients with primary BCS; usually more than one of these factors may be accounted for in at least 25% of patients.[77,78]

In BCS, the liver has a mottled appearance on contrast-enhanced computed tomography (CT). There is delayed enhancement at the margins of the liver and around the hepatic veins.[76,79] The periphery of the liver appears low in density on contrast-enhanced CT because of reversal of portal venous blood flow, related to increased postsinusoidal pressure brought about by hepatic venous obstruction.[76,79] Relative atrophy of the right and left hepatic lobes occurs with compensatory enlargement and increased enhancement of the caudate lobe; the caudate lobe is usually spared because it has a separate venous drainage direct to the IVC. Although the CT findings of BCS are often nonspecific, when thrombosis of the hepatic veins and the IVC is identified in the appropriate clinical setting, the diagnosis of BCS can be established. With magnetic resonance imaging (MRI), the liver appears atrophic and heterogeneous in 64% of patients, and venous thrombosis is identified in 86%.[76,79] The affected areas are low (darker) in signal intensity on T1-weighted images and high (brighter) in signal intensity on T2-weighted images because of the hepatic congestive effects. The liver margin enhances poorly on T1-weighted images after the administration of intravenous gadolinium contrast, especially during the acute phase of the disease. In patients in whom the disease has become chronic, a nodular regenerative hyperplasia may ensue. These nodules have increased signal intensity on T1-weighted images and low to intermediate signal intensity on T2-weighted images. MRI readily demonstrates other features of the disease as well, such as thrombosis, occlusion, and narrowing of the IVC and hepatic veins. Venous collaterals may also be easily identified, including comma-shaped intrahepatic varices, which are a characteristic finding, often not appreciated on other imaging modalities. These collaterals form as means to bypass the level of obstruction.[79] Finally, ultrasonography has a high sensitivity and specificity for the identification of BCS, and can demonstrate the echogenic fibrous cord within the IVC, which is a common cause of chronic BCS. Initially, there may be marked hepatomegaly, often associated with gallbladder wall thickening, ascites, and splenomegaly. Color and Doppler images help demonstrate the underlying vascular abnormality and are able to gauge flow within vessels.[76]

Previously, it was believed that the best management of these patients was portal venous decompression using surgically placed side-to-side portacaval shunts.[80-82] However, more recently it has become obvious that many patients can be managed with anticoagulation alone, but for those with more advanced disease liver transplantation remains the only option.[80] Thus, the number of patients with BCS who require hepatic decompression is limited. Patients with chronic BCS and refractory ascites are reasonable candidates for a transjugular intrahepatic portosystemic shunt (TIPS).[80-83] In contrast, those with a TIPS placement for acute hepatic failure because of BCS fare suboptimally, with the rate of early mortality approaching 50%.[82,83] Generally, TIPS is used in patients with an intermediate prognosis and refractory ascites; those with less advanced disease can be managed with anticoagulation alone, and those with more severe disease are candidates for liver transplantation. For patients with acute hepatic failure caused by BCS, liver transplantation is the best option, and TIPS should only be considered a bridge to transplantation.[82]

Conclusion

The pathophysiology of cirrhosis is complex and intriguing. The etiologies and classifications of cirrhosis and PHT are numerous. Understanding these different etiologies and classifications would yield a better understanding of the disease processes and would allow for a targeted management approach.

Clinical Pearls

- Knowledge of the anatomy and function of the liver, as well as the pathophysiology of cirrhosis and portal hypertension is essential for better understanding of the disease processes associated with cirrhosis and portal hypertension.
- Cirrhosis and portal hypertension have numerous causes, and a thorough history and physical examination with targeted testing is crucial and cost effective.
- Budd-Chiari syndrome is an uncommon disorder but has substantial morbidity and mortality rate if it remains undiagnosed or inadequately managed.

References

1. Murphy SL, Xu J, Kochanek KD. CDC National Vital Statistics Reports. Deaths: Final Data for 2010. May 8, 2013. http://www.cdc.gov/nchs/data/nvsr/nvsr61/nvsr61_04.pdf. Accessed August 26, 2013.
2. US Burden of Disease Collaborators. The State of US Health, 1990–2010 Burden of Diseases, Injuries, and Risk Factors. JAMA 2013;310:591–608.
3. Asrani SK, Kamath PS. Natural history of cirrhosis. Curr Gastroenterol Rep 2013; 15(308):1–6.
4. Brunicardi FC, Anderson D, Billiar D, et al. Schwartz's Principles of Surgery, 9th ed. New York, McGraw-Hill, 2010.
5. Doherty GM. Current Diagnosis and Treatment: Surgery, 13th ed. New York, McGraw-Hill, 2010.
6. Crawford JM. Vascular disorders of the liver. Clin Liver Dis 2010;14:635–650.
7. Mescher AL. Junqueira's Basic Histology, 12th ed. New York, McGraw-Hill, 2010.
8. Schuppan D, Afdhal NH. Liver cirrhosis. Lancet 2008;371:838–851.
9. Barrett KE. Ganong's Review of Medical Physiology, 23rd ed. New York, McGraw-Hill, 2010.
10. Roberts MS, Angus DC, Bryce CL, et al. Survival after liver transplantation in the United States: a disease-specific analysis of the UNOS database. Liver Transpl 2004;10:886–897.
11. Ismail MH, Pinzani M. Reversal of hepatic fibrosis: pathophysiological basis of antifibrotic therapies. Dovepress 2011;3:69–80.
12. Bosetti C, Levi F, Lucchini F, et al. Worldwide mortality from cirrhosis: an update to 2002. J Hepatol 2007;46:827–839.
13. Grattagliano I, Ubaldi E, Bonfrate L, Portincasa P. Management of liver cirrhosis between primary care and specialists. World J Gastroenterol 2011;17:2273–2282.
14. Anthony PP, Ishak KG, Nayak NC, et al. The morphology of cirrhosis: definition, nomenclature, and classification. Bull WHO 1977;55:521–540.
15. Graudal N, Leth P, Marbjerg L, et al. Characteristics of cirrhosis undiagnosed during life: a comparative analysis of 73 undiagnosed cases and 149 diagnosed cases of cirrhosis, detected in 4929 consecutive autopsies. J Intern Med 1991;230:165–171.
16. Melato M, Sasso F, Zanconati F. Liver cirrhosis and liver cancer. A study of their relationship in 2563 autopsies. Zentralbl Pathol 1993;139:25–30.
17. Guha IH, Iredale JP. Clinical and diagnostic aspects of cirrhosis. In: Rodes J, Benhamou JP, Blei AT, et al, editors. Textbook of Hepatology, from Basic Science to Clinical Practice, 3rd ed. Oxford, UK, Oxford: Blackwell, 2007, pp 604–619.
18. Falagas ME, Vardakas KZ, Vergidis PI. Under-diagnosis of common chronic diseases: prevalence and impact on human health. Int J Clin Pract 2007;61:1569–1579.
19. Friedman SL. Liver fibrosis—from bench to bedside. J Hepatol 2003;38(suppl):S38–S53.

20. Poynard T, Morra R, Ingiliz P, et al. Assessment of liver fibrosis: noninvasive means. Saudi J Gastroenterol 2008;14:163–173.

21. Lim YS, Kim WR. The global impact of hepatic fibrosis and end-stage liver disease. Clin Liver Dis 2008;12:733–746.

22. Mathers C, Lopez A, Murray C. The burden of disease and mortality by condition: data, methods, and results for 2001. In: Lopez A, Mathers C, Ezzati M, et al, editors. Global Burden of Disease and Risk Factors. Washington, DC, Oxford University Press and the World Bank, 2006, pp 45–93.

23. Murray CJ, Lopez AD. Alternative projections of mortality and disability by cause 1990–2020: Global Burden of Disease Study. Lancet 1997;349:1498–1504.

24. Bosetti C, Levi F, Lucchini F, et al. Worldwide mortality from cirrhosis: an update to 2002. J Hepatol 2007;46(5):827–839.

25. Singh GK, Hoyert DL. Social epidemiology of chronic liver disease and cirrhosis mortality in the United States, 1935–1997: trends and differentials by ethnicity, socioeconomic status, and alcohol consumption. Hum Biol 2000;72(5):801–820.

26. Ramstedt M. Per capita alcohol consumption and liver cirrhosis mortality in 14 European countries. Addiction 2001;96(suppl):S19–S33.

27. Kane M. Global programme for control of hepatitis B infection. Vaccine 1995; 13(suppl):S47–S49.

28. Lee WM. Hepatitis B virus infection. N Engl J Med 1997;337:1733–1745.

29. Torresi J, Locarnini S. Antiviral chemotherapy for the treatment of hepatitis B virus infections. Gastroenterology 2000;118(suppl):S83–S103.

30. Fattovich G, Giustina G, Schalm SW. Occurrence of hepatocellular carcinoma and decompensation in western European patients with cirrhosis type B. The EURO-HEP Study Group on Hepatitis B Virus and Cirrhosis. Hepatology 1995;21:77–82.

31. Lok AS, McMahon BJ. Chronic hepatitis B. Hepatology 2007;45:507–539.

32. Seeff LB, Hoofnagle JH. Epidemiology of hepatocellular carcinoma in areas of low hepatitis B and hepatitis C endemicity. Oncogene 2006;25:3771–3777.

33. McQuillan GM, Coleman PJ, Kruszon-Moran D, et al. Prevalence of hepatitis B virus infection in the United States: the National Health and Nutrition Examination Surveys, 1976 through 1994. Am J Public Health 1999;89:14–18.

34. Yim HJ, Lok AS. Natural history of chronic hepatitis B virus infection: what we knew in 1981 and what we know in 2005. Hepatology 2006;43(suppl):S173–S181.

35. Lavanchy D. Evolving epidemiology of hepatitis C virus. Clin Microbiol Infect 2011;17:107–115.

36. Shepard CW, Finelli L, Alter MJ. Global epidemiology of hepatitis C virus infection. Lancet Infect Dis 2005;5:558–567.

37. Sievert W, Altraif I, Razavi HA, et al. A systematic review of hepatitis C virus epidemiology in Asia, Australia and Egypt. Liver Int 2011;31(suppl):S61–S80.

38. Massard J, Ratziu V, Thabut D, et al. Natural history and predictors of disease severity in chronic hepatitis C. J Hepatol 2006;44(suppl):S19–S24.

39. Sanai FM, Helmy A, Dale C, et al. Updated thresholds for alanine aminotransferase do not exclude significant histological disease in chronic hepatitis C. Liver Int 2011;31:1039–1046.

40. Lauer GM, Walker BD. Hepatitis C virus infection. N Engl J Med 2001;345:41–52.

41. Kanwal F, Hoang T, Kramer JR, et al. Increasing prevalence of HCC and cirrhosis in patients with chronic hepatitis C virus infection. Gastroenterology 2011;140:1182–1188.

42. Davis GL, Alter MJ, El-Serag H, et al. Aging of hepatitis C virus (HCV)-infected persons in the United States: a multiple cohort model of HCV prevalence and disease progression. Gastroenterology 2010;138:513–521.

43. Vong S, Bell BP. Chronic liver disease mortality in the United States, 1990–1998. Hepatology 2004;39:476–483.

44. Armstrong GL, Alter MJ, McQuillan GM, et al. The past incidence of hepatitis C virus infection: implications for the future burden of chronic liver disease in the United States. Hepatology 2000;31:777–782.

45. Ramstedt M. Alcohol consumption and liver cirrhosis mortality with and without mention of alcohol, the case of Canada. Addiction 2003;98:1267–1276.

46. Naveau S, Giraud V, Borotto E, et al. Excess weight risk factor for alcoholic liver disease. Hepatology 1997;25:108–111.

47. Burra P, Lucey MR. Liver transplantation in alcoholic patients. Transpl Int 2005; 18:491–498.

48. UNOS. Public data from UNOS/OPTN scientific registry, 2002. http://www.srtr.org/national_stats.aspx. Accessed September 3, 2013.

49. Bird GL, Williams R. Factors determining cirrhosis in alcoholic liver disease. Mol Aspects Med 1988;10:97–105.

50. Alexander JF, Lischner MW, Galambos JT. Natural history of alcoholic hepatitis. II. The long-term prognosis. Am J Gastroenterol 1971;56:515–525.

51. Sanyal AJ. AGA technical review on nonalcoholic fatty liver disease. Gastroenterology 2002;123:1705–1725.

52. Flegal KM, Carroll MD, Ogden CL, et al. Prevalence and trends in obesity among US adults, 1999–2000. JAMA 2002;288:1723–1727.

53. Ford ES, Giles WH, Dietz WH. Prevalence of the metabolic syndrome among US adults: findings from the third National Health and Nutrition Examination Survey. JAMA 2002;287:356–359.

54. Mokdad AH, Ford ES, Bowman BA, et al. Prevalence of obesity, diabetes, and obesity-related health risk factors, 2001. JAMA 2003;289:76–79.

55. Bugianesi E. Non-alcoholic steatohepatitis and cancer. Clin Liver Dis 2007;11:191–207.

56. Teli MR, James OF, Burt AD, et al. The natural history of nonalcoholic fatty liver: a follow-up study. Hepatology 1995;22:1714–1719.

57. Neuschwander-Tetri BA, Caldwell SH. Nonalcoholic steatohepatitis: summary of an AASLD Single Topic Conference. Hepatology 2003;37:1202–1219.

58. Klein S. The national obesity crisis: A call for action. Gastroenterology 2004;126:6.

59. Browning JD, Szczepaniak LS, Dobbins R, et al. Prevalence of hepatic steatosis in an urban population in the United States: impact of ethnicity. Hepatology 2004;40:1387–1395.

60. Ong JP, Younossi ZM. Epidemiology and natural history of NAFLD and NASH. Clin Liver Dis 2007;11:1–16.

61. Boberg KM, Aadland E, Jahnsen J, et al. Incidence and prevalence of primary biliary cirrhosis, primary sclerosing cholangitis, and autoimmune hepatitis in a Norwegian population. Scand J Gastroenterol 1998;33:99–103.

62. Boberg KM. Prevalence and epidemiology of autoimmune hepatitis. Clin Liver Dis 2002;6:635–647.

63. Seaberg EC, Belle SH, Beringer KC, et al. Liver transplantation in the United States from 1987–1998: updated results from the Pitt-UNOS Liver Transplant Registry. Clin Transpl 1998:17–37.

64. Czaja AJ, Davis GL, Ludwig J, et al. Autoimmune features as determinants of prognosis in steroid-treated chronic active hepatitis of uncertain etiology. Gastroenterology 1983;85:713–717.

65. Lim KN, Casanova RL, Boyer TD, Bruno CJ. Autoimmune hepatitis in African Americans: presenting features and response to therapy. Am J Gastroenterol 2001;96:3390–3394.

66. Molina E, Reddy KR. Noncirrhotic portal hypertension. Clin Liver Dis 2001;5:769–787.

67. Reynolds TB, Redeker AG, Geller HM. Wedged hepatic vein pressure. Am J Med 1957;22:341–350.

68. Pomier-Layrargues G, Huet P-M. Measurement of hepatic venous pressure gradient: methods, interpretation, and pitfalls. In: Sanyal AJ, Shah VH, editors. Portal Hypertension: Pathobiology, Evaluation, and Treatment. Totowa, NJ, Humana Press, 2005, pp 129–144.

69. Lautt WW, Greenway CV. Conceptual review of the hepatic vascular bed. Hepatology 1987;7:952–963.

70. Sherman IA, Pappas SC, Fisher MM. Hepatic microvascular changes associated with development of liver fibrosis and cirrhosis. Am J Physiol 1990;258: H460–H465.

71. Blendis LM. Hepatocyte swelling and portal hypertension. J Hepatol 1992;15:4–5.

72. Lautt WW. The 1995 Ciba-Geigy Award Lecture. Intrinsic regulation of hepatic blood flow. Can J Physiol Pharmacol 1996;74:223–233.

73. Rockey DC, Weisiger RA. Endothelin induced contractility of stellate cells from normal and cirrhotic rat liver: implications for regulation of portal pressure and resistance. Hepatology 1996;24:233–240.

74. Wanless IR, Wong F, Blendis LM, et al. Hepatic and portal vein thrombosis in cirrhosis: possible role in development of parenchymal extinction and portal hypertension. Hepatology 1995;21:1238–1247.

75. Groszmann RJ, de Franchis R. Portal hypertension. In: Schiff ER, Sorrell MF, Maddrey W, editors. Schiff's Diseases of the Liver. Philadelphia, Lippincott-Raven, 1999, pp 387–442.

76. Ferral H, Behrens G, Lopera J. Budd-Chiari syndrome. AJR Am J Roentgenol 2012;199:737–745.

77. Qi X, Wu F, Ren W, et al. Thrombotic risk factors in Chinese Budd-Chiari syndrome patients. An observational study with a systematic review of the literature. Thromb Haemost 2013;109:878–884.

78. Qi X, De Stefano V, Wang J, et al. Prevalence of inherited antithrombin, protein C, and protein S deficiencies in portal vein system thrombosis and Budd-Chiari syndrome: a systematic review and meta-analysis of observational studies. J Gastroenterol Hepatol 2013;28:432–442.

79. Chundru S, Kalb B, Arif-Tiwari H, et al. MRI of diffuse liver disease: the common and uncommon etiologies. Diagn Interv Radiol 2013;19(6):479–487.

80. Plessier A, Rautou PE, Valla DC. Management of hepatic vascular diseases. J Hepatol 2012;56(suppl):S25–S38.

81. Senzolo M, Riggio O, Primignani M; Italian Association for the Study of the Liver. Vascular disorders of the liver: recommendations from the Italian Association for the Study of the Liver (AISF) ad hoc committee. Dig Liver Dis 2011;43:503–514.

82. DeLeve LD, Valla DC, Garcia-Tsao G; American Association for the Study Liver Diseases. Vascular disorders of the liver. Hepatology 2009;49:1729–1764.

83. Qi X, Yang M, Fan D, Han G. Transjugular intrahepatic portosystemic shunt in the treatment of Budd-Chiari syndrome: a critical review of literatures. Scand J Gastroenterol 2013;48:771–784.

Chapter 2: Clinical Presentation of Portal Hypertension

Mona H. Ismail and Abdullah M.S. Al-Osaimi

Introduction

Liver cirrhosis and portal hypertension (PHT) are common clinical findings, and according to the Centers for Disease Control and Prevention, chronic liver disease and cirrhosis is the 12th leading cause of death in the United States. The recent data suggest that it is the eighth leading cause of death overall and the third leading cause of death in persons 45 to 64 years of age, and deaths related to chronic liver disease and cirrhosis has increased 3.3% between 2009 and 2010. Current studies indicate that the mortality rate related to liver disease over the past 3 decades has remained unchanged.[1,2] Liver disease continues to be a significant cause of morbidity and accounts for a substantial portion of health-care utilization in the United States and worldwide.[3] Understanding the natural history of cirrhosis and PHT is important to identify patients at highest risk for complications of liver disease, including liver cirrhosis. Such knowledge would permit early intervention and potentially alter the clinical course of patients with chronic liver disease toward a favorable outcome. This chapter discusses the clinical presentation of cirrhosis and PHT.

Complications from Cirrhosis and Portal Hypertension

Regardless of the cause of cirrhosis, patients often remain asymptomatic until complications of end-stage liver disease develop (▶ Table 2.1). Diagnosing asymptomatic patients usually follows from noting abnormal laboratory markers during incidental screening tests or from radiologic findings. Diagnosis becomes easier when signs of decompensation, including jaundice, ascites, and asterixis, are present.[4,5] However, these patients are also at the highest risk for developing more serious and potentially life-threatening complications.[5]

Table 2.1 The Most Common Etiologies of Cirrhosis[4,5]

Etiology	Associated Physical Conditions
Alcohol	Dementia, peripheral neuropathy, oral or esophageal cancer
HCV	Cryoglobulinemia (arthritis, vasculitis)
HBV	Arthritis, PAN
Primary biliary cirrhosis	Sicca syndrome, xanthelasma, hyperlipidemia[36]
Primary sclerosing cholangitis	IBD, UC
NAFLD or NASH	Obesity, metabolic syndrome, type II diabetes
Wilson's disease	Neurologic symptoms (Parkinson-like)
Hemochromatosis	Arthritis, myocarditis, diabetes
Autoimmune hepatitis	Autoimmune hemolytic anemia, IBD, celiac disease, autoimmune thyroiditis

HBV: hepatitis B virus; HCV: hepatitis C virus; IBD: inflammatory bowel disease; NAFLD: nonalcoholic fatty liver disease; NASH: nonalcoholic steatohepatitis; PAN: polyarteritis nodosa; UC: ulcerative colitis.

Varices

Patients with cirrhosis often develop esophageal or gastric varices (GVs) caused by the portosystemic shunting that accompanies PHT.[6] GVs usually form in the submucosal layer at the cardia or the fundus of the stomach because the posterior wall in this region of the stomach approaches the portosystemic collateral circulation. GVs receive most of their blood supply from the left, posterior, and short gastric veins and drain mainly through a gastrorenal shunt (▶ Fig. 2.1). About 85% of patients with GVs develop a significant shunt that is able to pass extraordinarily large volumes of blood at high velocities. These GVs and resultant shunts predispose patients to a higher risk of experiencing a massive variceal bleeding or hepatic encephalopathy (HE) (▶ Fig. 2.1; ▶ Fig. 2.2).[7]

Approximately 35% of patients with compensated cirrhosis and 80% of those with decompensated cirrhosis have varices at the time of diagnosis.[8] Bleeding gastroesophageal varices is the most serious complication of cirrhosis (▶ Fig. 2.2; ▶ Fig. 2.3).[9] One third of affected patients will experience a variceal bleed, which accounts for up to 90% of all bleeding episodes seen in these patients. Active bleeding at the time of endoscopy is one of the hallmarks for poor prognosis in patients with varices, particularly when accompanied by bacterial infection, portal vein thrombosis, and a hepatic venous pressure gradient (HVPG) greater than 12 mm Hg.[6] Mortality rates from variceal bleeding have declined in recent years but still remain high. The 6-week mortality rate averages 15% to 20% per bleeding episode and correlates with disease severity.[8] PHT may also lead to portal hypertensive gastropathy (PHG), a serious condition that can cause acute or even massive blood loss. Endoscopic investigation shows abnormalities in the gastric mucosa often described as a mosaic-like pattern that resembles snake skin. Pathologic changes responsible for these lesions originate from vascular ectasia rather than mucosal inflammation as originally thought.[10] The low incidence of PHG, ranging from 2% to 12%, classifies this complication as a less common cause of upper gastrointestinal (GI) bleeding.[10]

Rectal varices, frequently confused with hemorrhoids, develop in about 4% of patients with PHT. Hemorrhoids develop in the submucosa of the anal canal and unlike varices do not communicate with the portal circulation, nor occur with a higher incidence in portal hypertensive patients. A correlation of the thickness of the rectal wall has been suggested by endoscopic studies, but this association remains a topic of debate.[11] Because rectal varices rarely bleed, they are of less clinical importance than either esophageal varices or GVs. Detailed discussions on the medical and endoscopic management of varices are given in other chapters.

Ascites

Ascites develops secondary to PHT when excess fluids accumulate in the peritoneal cavity (▶ Fig. 2.4). It is the most common complication of cirrhosis seen in approximately 60% of compensated patients within 10 years of disease onset.[12] Arterial splanchnic vasodilation leads to arterial hypotension with activation of both sympathetic nervous and renin–angiotensin–aldosterone system (RAAS). Excessive sodium accumulation consequent to the body's

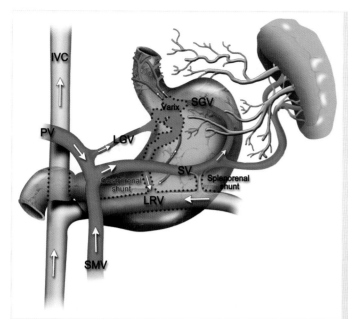

Fig. 2.1 Anatomy of the portal circulation. Gastric varices caused by splenic vein thrombosis (SVT) tend to arise from the short gastric veins running from the hilum of the spleen to the greater curvature aspect of the stomach rather than through splenorenal or gastrorenal shunts common with portal hypertensive fundal varices. IVC: inferior vena cava; LGV: left gastric vein; LRV: left renal vein; PV: portal vein; SGV: short gastric vein; SMV: superior mesenteric vein.

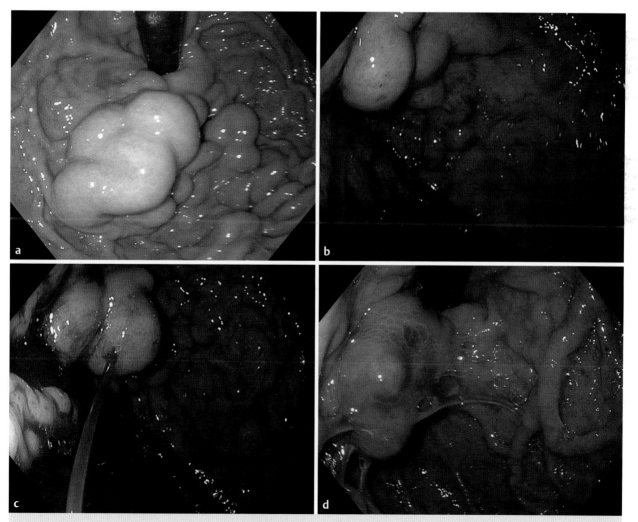

Fig. 2.2 Photographs of gastric varices. (**a**) Large (>3 cm) gastric varices (IGV-1; isolated gastric varices-type 1) with no stigmata of bleeding. (**b**) A large IGV-1 with evidence of recent bleeding (blood in the stomach and a nipple or dimple sign). (**c**) The nipple sign area with active bleeding. (**d**) Mosaic (snake skin–like appearance) pattern of post-BRTO (balloon retrograde transvenous obliteration) findings of a GOV-2 (gastroesophageal varices-type 2).

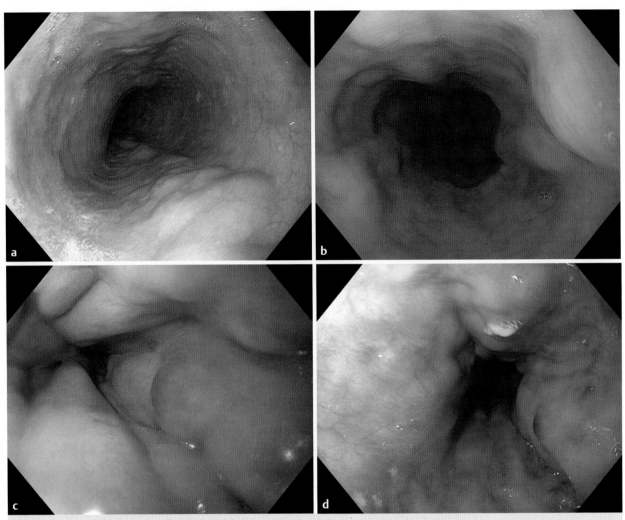

Fig. 2.3 Classifications of esophageal varices. (**a**) Small, low-risk esophageal varices (or F1), almost flattened out with insufflation. (**b**) Medium-sized, low-risk esophageal varices (F2) that did not flatten with insufflation. (**c**) Large esophageal varices greater than one third of the esophageal lumen with some high-risk stigmata (red marks or wheals). (**d**) Esophageal varices with high-risk stigmata for recent bleeding and rebleed with red marks and a nipple sign or fibrin plug.

failure to adequately excrete sodium into urine ultimately results in ascites and edema. Performing a paracentesis and appropriate analysis of the ascitic fluid helps rule out other possible causes of fluid buildup.[12] Cirrhosis accounts for more than 75% of all causes of ascites. The remaining 25% of ascites cases are caused by malignancy (10%), cardiac failure (3%), pancreatitis (1%), tuberculosis (2%), or other factors.[13] Patients who develop ascites tend to have a poor prognosis and diminished quality of life. Thus, they should be considered for liver transplantation upon diagnosis.[12]

Pathogenic alterations responsible for ascites in patients with cirrhosis include 2 separate mechanisms.[14] The first is caused by increased portal flow resistance at the sinusoids, creating sinusoidal PHT and an associated pressure backwash into the splanchnic capillaries. Excess fluid preferentially accumulates in the peritoneal cavity, and blood flow increases to the splanchnic area, leading to further increases in portal pressure. The second mechanism precedes ascites formation and relates to sustained renal sodium retention. The initiating process remains a subject of controversy but may involve hepatorenal baroreflex

from PHT or nominal activation of the RAAS caused by subtle hypovolemia.[14]

The continuous escape of fluids into the interstitial space as a result of these hemodynamic changes is partly compensated by reabsorption into the systemic circulation via the lymphatic system and thoracic duct. When cirrhosis progresses to a point where the lymphatic system can no longer manage the overload, excess fluid progressively accumulates into the peritoneal cavity, which perpetuates sodium and water reabsorption caused by decreased intravascular systemic volume in addition to elevated norepinephrine and other systemic vasoconstrictors. Dietary changes and moderate doses of diuretics can usually manage ascites when presenting at an early stage. However, 10% of patients will become refractory when their condition becomes resistant to diuretics.[14] An appropriate mode of treatment for ascites classified by its severity is shown in ▶ Table 2.2.

Increases in sodium retention (urine sodium <10 mEq/L) is accompanied by a decline in glomerular filtration rate. Patients with more advanced stages of decompensated cirrhosis develop

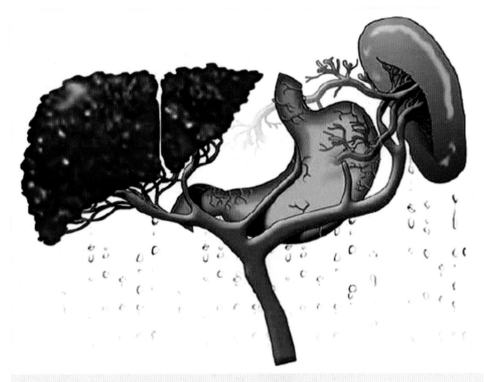

Fig. 2.4 Illustration of ascites caused by cirrhosis and portal hypertension.

low arterial pressure because of a further reduction of the peripheral vascular resistance. Eventually, sodium becomes primarily absorbed at the renal tubules and proximal to the site of diuretic action, explaining why treatment begins to fail in a subset of patients. At this stage, patient prognosis becomes dismal and implies a low 2-year probability of survival.[14]

Refractory ascites typically associates with other serious complications, including spontaneous bacterial peritonitis (SBP), muscle wasting, pleural effusion, and dilutional hyponatremia. The first line of treatment involves large-volume paracentesis and administering albumin if more than 5 L is removed.[12,14] Patients may continue on diuretics if effective and perhaps undergo insertion of a transjugular intrahepatic portosystemic shunt (TIPS) to decompress the portal system (see ▶ Table 2.2).[12] Detailed management of ascites is discussed in a separate chapter.

Spontaneous Bacterial Peritonitis

Patients with cirrhosis have an increased susceptibility to bacterial infections, and development of an infection in cirrhotic patients is often associated with a poor outcome and high mortality rate. SBP is one the commonest infections in cirrhosis. It arises as an acute infection of the ascitic fluid and is defined by an ascitic polymorphonuclear leukocyte (PMN) count of 0.25 $\times 10^9$/L or greater.[15,16] Usually there is no obvious source of infection such as an abscess, hollow viscous perforation, acute pancreatitis, or cholecystitis. SBP infection is precipitated by bacterial translocation of gram-negative bacteria, including *Escherichia coli* and *Klebsiella* spp. from the intestine but may also originate from long-term antibiotic prophylaxis with fluoroquinolones.[15] Most patients with SBP present with symptoms typical of peritoneal infection, especially abdominal pain, fever, and diarrhea, although a small percentage remain asymptomatic.[17] Signs of liver or renal impairment suggestive of SBP include the development of HE and may offer important clues for diagnosis in asymptomatic patients.[18]

Whereas spontaneous bacterial peritonitis almost always develops in patients with cirrhosis who have large-volume ascites, low-volume ascites and ascites from other origins rarely cause concern for infection.[17] Renal dysfunction develops in one third of patients with SBP likely because of a reduced effective circulating volume.[18] Serum creatinine levels greater than 1 mg/dL

Table 2.2 Ascites Severity and Recommended Treatment[12]

Grade of Ascites Defined by Severity	Treatment
Grade 1: Mild (only detectable by ultrasonography)	None; consider dietary sodium restriction
Grade 2: Moderate ascites evidenced by symmetrical distension of abdomen	Dietary sodium restriction and diuretics
Grade 3: Gross ascites marked by abdominal distension	Dietary sodium restriction, diuretics, and large-volume paracenteses; TIPS for persistence/refractory ascites

TIPS: transjugular intrahepatic portosystemic shunt.

Table 2.3 Classification of Ascites Based on the Serum-Ascites Albumin Gradient

Nonportal Hypertensive Ascites SAAG < 1.1 g/dL	Portal Hypertensive Ascites SAAG ≥ 1.1 g/dL
Malignant	Cirrhosis
Infectious	Budd-Chiari syndrome
Nephrogenic	Cardiac congestive heart failure
Pancreatic ascites	Constrictive pericarditis
Bile ascites	Veno-occlusive disease
Myxedema	Portal vein thrombosis
	Polycystic liver disease

SAAG: serum-ascites albumin gradient.

at the time of diagnosis represents an important risk factor for death in these patients, and those at risk may benefit from renal volume expansion with albumin via intravenous infusion.[17,18] Although once considered a highly feared complication of cirrhosis, SBP has become a highly treatable condition, although it has a high recurrence rate.[17]

Serum-Ascites Albumin Gradient

Paracentesis followed by an ascitic fluid analysis provides the most rapid and cost-effective approach for distinguishing portal from nonportal hypertension ascites because the ascitic fluid albumin (and protein) content can readily distinguish the two.[12] Classification of ascites made using the serum-ascites albumin gradient (SAAG) allows reliable assessment of the ascites etiology. This method has largely replaced less reliable techniques that relied on sole measurement of ascitic fluid protein concentration.[13] Calculating the SAAG involves subtracting the concentration of albumin in ascitic fluid from that in serum using samples withdrawn from the patient on the same day. Whereas a SAAG of less than 1.1 g/dL suggests an ascites etiology of nonportal hypertensive origin seen in about 15% of patients (▶ Table 2.3), a SAAG of 1.1 g/dL or greater predicts ascites caused by PHT with more than 97% accuracy.[13,16]

Hepatic Hydrothorax

Hepatic hydrothorax (HH) is defined as serious pleural effusion (>500 mL) that occasionally develops in patients with cirrhosis who otherwise have no underlying pulmonary or cardiac disease.[19,20] This condition appears predominantly right sided in up to 87% of all HH cases but may also affect the left pleural cavity or present bilaterally. HH leads to significant patient morbidity because even modest volumes of pleural fluid can cause serious respiratory problems. Onset occurs when ascitic fluid leaks through small defects in the diaphragm, which is the most plausible explanation. The negative intrathoracic pressure generated by inspiration favors unidirectional passage of fluid from the abdomen to the pleural space that later gets trapped and absorbed. HH occurs when the rate of fluid accumulation exceeds the absorptive capacity of the pleura. Whether patients have clinically detectable ascites at the time HH presents depends on the pleural space leakage caused by the negative thoracic pressures during inspiration.[20]

Hepatorenal Syndrome

Hepatorenal syndrome (HRS) is a type of acute kidney injury and is a serious complication of liver failure and cirrhosis. Its onset follows a severe compromise in renal perfusion, which might reverse with albumin infusion or with administering vasoconstrictors.[21] Two types of HRS exist (types I and II), which may be differentiated based on laboratory findings and clinical features. Whereas renal failure in type II patients progresses slowly (average serum creatinine of 1.5 mg/dL), those with type I HRS experience an acute and rapid onset marked by quickly rising serum creatinine levels that reach above 2.5 mg/dL within 2 weeks.[21] Regardless of the cause of HRS, it is associated with a poor prognosis. The expected survival time of these patients is diminished to weeks after the onset of HRS if left untreated.

Several precipitating events can lead to HRS development, including SBP, but also infections such as pneumonia, cellulitis or urinary tract infection, hepatitis, GI hemorrhage, and major surgical procedures. Type II HRS presents with refractory ascites and likely represents the end result of a complex series of circulatory and renal dysfunctions linked to cirrhosis. The peripheral arterial vasodilation theory best explains the mechanism behind type II onset.[21] Enhanced local release of nitric oxide and other vasodilators during PHT stimulates arterial vasodilation in the splanchnic circulation. A slow deterioration in cardiac function may also precede the onset of HRS.[22] Clinical features seen in individuals with type I HRS include impaired hepatic, renal, cardiovascular, and adrenal function thought to occur as part of a more complex syndrome called acute-on-chronic liver failure (ACLF).[21,23]

Portopulmonary Hypertension and Hepatopulmonary Syndrome

Approximately one third of patients with cirrhosis will develop vascular pulmonary complications broadly categorized into portopulmonary hypertension (PoPH; 4%–8%) and hepatopulmonary syndrome (HPS; 15%–30%).[24] These 2 syndromes constitute opposing responses to the same clinical condition, and neither depends on the underlying cause or severity of PHT. PoPH is a state of pulmonary arterial hypertension defined by a mean pulmonary arterial pressure (mPAP) above 25 mm Hg at rest or above 30 mm Hg while exercising; a pulmonary vascular resistance above 240 dynes.s.cm^{-5}; and a capillary wedge pressure below 15 mm Hg.[24] Dyspnea upon exertion is a sign of PoPH, but patients frequently remain asymptomatic. In fact, PoPH often gets picked up during a routine echocardiogram that shows an elevated right ventricular systolic pressure (RVSP). An RVSP above 40 mm Hg requires following up with right heart catheterization to confirm changes from pulmonary arterial hypertension rather than other causes related to volume overload.[25] Reducing the pulmonary pressure with vasodilators provides an appropriate pharmacotherapy for managing PoPH. Liver transplantation, once contraindicated for patients with PoPH, may now be safely attempted as long as the patient has proper mPAP control and no right heart failure.[25]

The second syndrome is HPS. HPS is due to intrapulmonary microvascular vasodilation and a widened alveolar–arterial oxygen gradient on room air (>15 mm Hg) with or without hypoxemia.[24,25] Although commonly seen in patients with cirrhosis who have PHT, HPS need not associate with either condition. This syndrome has also been described in individuals with acute or chronic hepatitis and no PHT as well as others with PHT and noncirrhotic liver disease such as nodular regenerative hyperplasia.[25] Patients with cirrhosis who have HPS experience increasing pulmonary vasodilation and diminished gas exchange as their condition worsens. HPS is associated with a high mortality rate, but orthotopic liver transplantation (OLT) can successfully reverse the condition.[24] Clinical studies so far have failed to confirm effective medical therapies for HPS; OLT currently provides the only definitive treatment.[25] Supplemental oxygen therapy gives relief when hypoxemia presents.

Hepatic Encephalopathy

Hepatic encephalopathy is the onset of brain dysfunction resulting from metabolic alterations accompanying liver cirrhosis or acute liver failure. The condition arises mainly from reduced clearance of gut-derived neurotoxins, although other substances normally cleared by the liver may also contribute. Initially, patients may appear confused, but if left untreated, this potentially reversible condition can quickly progress to irreversible cognitive dysfunction and coma.[26] Treatment involves identifying and removing precipitating factors and reducing the load of ammonia reaching the liver by giving the patient lactulose.[4] All patients with cirrhosis who present with an altered mental state should be evaluated for focal neurologic signs associated with HE, but these rarely appear and are regressive. After the first HE episode occurs, patient's expected 1- and 3-year survival rates are 42% and 23%, respectively.[26]

Hepatic encephalopathy is divided into 3 nomenclature types. The first, type A, refers to HE in acute liver failure; type B is HE associated with portosystemic bypass and no intrinsic liver disease; and type C describes HE in patients with cirrhosis with PHT.[26] Type C may present persistently, episodically, or minimally depending on the precipitating factors and clinical manifestations. Episodic HE usually occurs secondary to a precipitating event but can also initiate spontaneously. The common precipitating factors for HE are listed in ▶ Table 2.4.

The severity of mental disturbance, ranging from mild cognitive changes to coma, is most often graded by the West Haven Criteria (▶ Table 2.5).[27] Reliable classification in more severe cases relies on using the Glasgow Coma Scale (GCS), which provides a

Table 2.4 Precipitants of Hepatic Encephalopathy[27]

Progressive liver failure
GI bleeding
Infection (e.g., SBP) and SIRS
Constipation
Renal failure or fluid electrolyte disturbance (e.g., dehydration, hypokalemia, and alkalosis)
Excessive protein intake
General anesthesia and psychotropic drugs, including barbiturates, benzodiazepines, and narcotic analgesics
Unknown causes (20%–30% of cases)
GI: gastrointestinal; SBP: spontaneous bacterial peritonitis; SIRS: systemic inflammatory response syndrome.

Table 2.5 Stages of Hepatic Encephalopathy[27]

Stage	Clinical	Neurologic Signs and Symptoms
0	Forgetfulness, mild confusion, and irritability	Abnormalities seen only during psychometric analysis
1	Restlessness, inverted sleep pattern	Tremor, apraxia, small handwriting
2	Lethargic, slowed mentation; disoriented in time and place	Asterixis, dysarthria, ataxia, and hypoactive reflexes
3	Somnolence but arousable; more disoriented in time, place, and person	Asterixis, hyperactive reflexes, muscle rigidity, and Babinski's sign
4	Comatose	Decerebrate posturing, areflexia

more objective and reproducible assessment of mental impairment than West Haven criteria. The portosystemic encephalopathy (PSE) score calculated based on the patient's mental status, electroencephalographic abnormalities, and ammonia levels also objectively describes the clinical severity of HE.[27] The PSE serves primarily as a research tool and has not surpassed West Haven Criteria acceptance for classifying HE in clinical practice.[27]

Despite significant research devoted to understanding the mechanism of HE, controversies still remain regarding its pathophysiology. Most experts believe that nitrogenous toxins originating from the gut adversely influence mental function. In healthy subjects with normal hepatocyte function, 80% to 90% of ammonia derived from the colonic bacteria gets excreted through first-pass metabolism.[27] Buildup of cellular ammonia as a consequence of liver failure may result in cerebral energy failure in addition to altered neurotransmissions by disrupting the GABAergic (gamma-aminobutyric acid) pathway.[28] Astrocyte swelling caused by ammonia detoxification in these cells and a consequent accumulation of glutamine are responsible for the brain edema observed in these patients. Astrocyte swelling may also accompany glutamate uptake or occur in response to extracellular acidosis.[29]

Symptoms and Physical Examination

The majority of patients with cirrhosis are asymptomatic. The onset of symptoms in these patients usually occurs insidiously but can also be abrupt. Cirrhosis may be suspected when the patient presents with mild symptoms, including weakness, fatigue, muscle cramps, weight loss, or sleep disturbances or other symptoms of HE. More telling symptoms usually reflect decompensation, including hematemesis, hematochezia, melena, jaundice, and anorexia with nausea (which can be severe). Patients may complain of abdominal pain related to stretching of Glisson's capsule or the development of ascites. About two thirds of patients will have signs of an enlarged, palpable liver predominantly affecting the left lobe. Women sometimes experience menstrual irregularities, and men might experience erectile dysfunction or sterility.[30,31] Increased estradiol levels in men give rise to proliferation of glandular tissue in the breast, or gynecomastia.[30]

Bulging flank and flank dullness to percussion caused by accumulation of fluid in the abdomen provides the most accurate prediction of ascites. In fact, the absence of flank dullness occurs in only about 10% of patients who have ascites.[30] Examination of whether the dullness shifts with rotation of the patient or it persists when percussed anteriorly can help determine the extent of ascites development. Fever with hypotension, abdominal tenderness, and decreased bowel sound suggests the onset of SBP but can also manifest from alcoholic hepatitis or concurrent infection.

A physical examination may identify changes in the skin apart from jaundice that reveal liver disease. Vascular spider angioma commonly presents on the trunk, face, and upper extremities, and their number and size correlate with disease severity.[30] However, spider angioma can also indicate pregnancy or malnourishment. Palmar erythema characterized by an exaggerated and mottled redness on the thenar and hypothenar eminences develops as a result of changes in metabolism and sex hormones. The nails frequently show discoloration or clubbing and Dupuytren's contractures manifested as thickening and shortening of the palmar fascia commonly occur. Evidence of vitamin deficiency, including glossitis and cheilosis, are frequently present.

Laboratory Evaluation

A positive diagnosis for cirrhosis is made on the basis of laboratory and radiographic findings. Serum albumin and prothrombin time measurements provide clues regarding liver function, and serum bilirubin levels indicate the liver's capacity to conjugate and excrete bilirubin.[4] Elevated aminotransferases with aspartate aminotransferase (AST) greater than alanine aminotransferase (ALT) suggests cirrhosis, but the absence of this finding does not exclude the presence of cirrhosis. A low platelet count is suggestive of PHT and hypersplenism. When SBP is suspected, the patient should be investigated with a full blood count, urinalysis, and ascitic fluid cell count, as well as ascites, blood, and urine cultures.[17] Laboratory tests also help identify the underlying cause of cirrhosis because specific findings can determine the different etiologies of cirrhosis (▶ Table 2.6).

Several laboratory tests, scores, and indices have emerged as noninvasive predictors of cirrhosis.[4,32] The APRI index measures the AST-to-platelet ratio and is able to predict cirrhosis with a high degree of accuracy.[32] Scores generated by the patented FibroTest based on serum biomarkers (haptoglobin, α2-macroglobulin, apolipoprotein A1, γ-glutamyltransferase [γGT], and bilirubin) plus age and gender show a good correlation with PHT severity.[33] Other algorithms include the Hepascore combining hyaluronic acid, total bilirubin, γGT, α2-macroglobulin, age, and sex for predicting the degree of liver fibrosis but with limitations,[34] and the BARD score is composed of 3 variables—body mass index, AST-to-ALT ratio, and presence of diabetes—for identifying nonalcoholic fatty liver disease patients with advanced fibrosis. Despite advances in laboratory testing for evaluating chronic liver disease, liver biopsy remains the gold standard for the diagnosis of liver cirrhosis. However, liver biopsy is an invasive procedure and is costly and not appropriate for all patients (e.g., patients with prolonged prothrombin times or low platelet counts) with potential side effects and risks. Thus, liver biopsy is not necessary in the presence of decompensated cirrhosis or when imaging studies or laboratory tests have confirmed the presence of cirrhosis. The decision on whether to perform a histologic assessment should be reserved for selected patients.[4]

Radiologic Evaluation

Imaging techniques are an attractive method of evaluating cirrhosis because of their noninvasiveness and ability to detect structural changes and determine complications of liver cirrhosis, including ascites, varices, PHT, splenomegaly, and nodular liver or liver masses. Conventional imaging techniques, including ultrasonography, computed tomography (CT), and magnetic resonance imaging (MRI), provide initial evaluation of the hepatic architecture but are not particularly sensitive in detecting cirrhosis and have a low predictive value. Upper GI endoscopy currently sets the bar for reliable identification of esophageal varices, but abdominal CT scanning has shown promise as a reliable tool for identifying varices and is a safer and more cost-effective procedure.[35] Ultrasound color duplex Doppler helps visualize the upper abdominal vasculature changes caused by the development of

Table 2.6 Diagnostic Laboratory Tests for the Most Common Causes of Liver Cirrhosis[4,5]

Cause	Diagnostic Laboratory Parameters
Alcohol	AST/ALT ≥ 2, γGT ($\uparrow$), MCV ($\uparrow$)
HCV	Anti-HCV ELISA antibody, HCV-RNA and genotype
HBV	HBsAg, anti-HBV "s" and "c" antibodies, HBV-DNA
Primary biliary cirrhosis	γGT ($\uparrow$), ALP ($\uparrow$), AMA (+)
Primary sclerosing cholangitis	Anti-pANCA (70%), ALP/γGT; imaging: beaded intra- and extrahepatic bile ducts
NAFLD or NASH	HDL cholesterol ($\downarrow$), glucose ($\uparrow$), triglycerides ($\uparrow$), HbA1C, TSH, insulin resistance
Wilson's disease	Ceruloplasmin ($\downarrow$), 24-hour urinary copper excretion ($\uparrow$), slit-lamp: corneal copper deposits, hepatic copper ($\uparrow$)
Hemochromatosis	Fasting transferrin saturation index >45%, ferritin ($\uparrow$), HFE gene mutation, hepatic iron index/content ($\uparrow$)
Autoimmune hepatitis	ANA (+), ASMA (+), LKM (+), HLA

$\uparrow$: increased; $\downarrow$: decreased; (+): positive test result; ALP: alkaline phosphatase; ALT: alanine aminotransferase; AMA: antimitochondrial antibody; ANA: antinuclear antibody; ASMA: anti–smooth muscle antibody; AST: aspartate aminotransferase; γGT: γ-glutamyltransferase; HbA1C: hemoglobin A1C; HBsAg: hepatitis B surface antigen; HBV: hepatitis B virus; HCV: hepatitis C virus; HDL: high-density lipoprotein; HFE: hemochromatosis; HLA: human leukocyte antigen; LKM: liver-kidney-microsomal; MCV: mean corpuscular volume; NAFLD: nonalcoholic fatty liver disease; NASH: nonalcoholic steatohepatitis; pANCA: perinuclear neutrophils cytoplasmic antigen; TSH: thyroid-stimulating hormone.

Table 2.7 Child-Pugh Classification

	1 point	2 points	3 points
Total bilirubin (mg/dL)	< 2	2–3	> 3
Serum albumin (g/dL)	> 35	28–35	< 28
PT INR	< 1.7	1.71–2.30	> 2.30
Ascites	None	Mild to moderate	Severe
Hepatic encephalopathy	None	Grade I–II	Grade III–IV

INR: international normalized ratio; PT; prothrombin time.

portosystemic collateral circulation and enlarged portal and splanchnic veins from PHT.[35] Supporting information from CT and MRI also helps diagnose PHT by identifying venous structure alterations, particularly portosystemic collaterals.[5] Endosonography, which combines ultrasonography and endoscopy, is the method of choice for identifying deep rectal varices.[11]

Measuring liver stiffness using transient elastography (FibroScan) has shown a reasonable track record for detecting advanced cirrhosis, although its predictive value for moderate disease remains inconclusive.[35] An accurate evaluation of liver stiffness with FibroScan relies on detecting diagnostic patterns in transmitted elastic wave velocities, where increasing degrees of scarring or fibrosis have decreasing elasticity and a shear wave propagating through stiffer material would progress faster than in a more elastic material. Thus, the stiffer the liver, the faster the sheer waves propagates. Thus, FibroScan is a noninvasive, safe, rapid, and reproducible method but has shown some limitations when used for evaluating obese patients and those with ascites and small intercostal spaces. Recent studies have demonstrated good correlations between FibroScan results and HVPG values. However, further studies are needed before recommending this technique as a routine tool for grading PHT.[35]

Severity of Liver Disease Scoring Systems

After a patient has been confirmed to have liver cirrhosis, scoring the severity of disease becomes the next important step. Several predictive scoring systems have been developed and validated to evaluate the severity and prognosis of cirrhosis. Liver-specific scores (Child-Turcotte-Pugh [CTP] and model for end-stage liver disease [MELD]) are the most commonly used. The CTP score assesses liver disease severity and prognosis using a combined evaluation of laboratory (total bilirubin, albumin, and prothrombin time) and clinical (severity and presence of ascites and HE) parameters (▶ Table 2.7). One-year survival rates for patients graded with the CTP scoring system range from 45% (highest) to 100% (lowest score). The MELD score is based on an algorithmic calculation of international normalized ratio, total bilirubin, and creatinine. The MELD score furnishes a more robust assessment of mortality risk from cirrhosis and helps prioritize patients on the transplant waiting list.[4]

A more general prognostic model, referred to as the Acute Physiology and Chronic Health Evaluation (APACHE), was designed for measuring severity of illness in patients admitted to the intensive care unit (ICU). This model and 2 other organ dysfunction models (Organ System Failure [OSF] and Sequential Organ Failure

Assessment [SOFA]) performed very well in ICU patients with cirrhosis perhaps because liver failure contributes only partially to the risk of death in this subpopulation.[35] The fact that the APACHE model contains serum albumin and bilirubin may also bolster its performance in assessing cirrhosis severity specifically.[35]

Conclusion

The clinical presentation of liver cirrhosis and of PHT extends over a wide spectrum and usually involves multiple organs. Each presentation has its potential causes and its different stages and requires specific therapies. The knowledge of the complications, the clinical presentation, and the different stages of liver cirrhosis and PHT is an essential guide to physicians and practitioners to ensure optimal medical care and timely interventions that will lead to successful patient outcomes.

Clinical Pearls

- Knowledge of the appropriate diagnostic criteria and tools of the possible complications of portal hypertension is essential for better outcomes.
- Esophageal and gastric varices are common among patients with cirrhosis.
- The incidence of bleeding varices correlates with Child-Pugh classification and platelet counts below 100,000/mL.
- SBP is common among patients with ascites, and antibiotic-resistant SBP is emerging.
- SAAG is an important indicator for the cause of ascites.

References

1. Murphy SL, XU J, Kochanek KD, et al. CDC National Vital Statistics Reports. Deaths: Final data for 2010. May 8, 2013. http://www.cdc.gov/nchs/data/nvsr/nvsr61/nvsr61_04.pdf. Accessed August 26, 2013.
2. US Burden of Disease Collaborators. The State of US Health, 1990–2010 Burden of Diseases, Injuries, and Risk Factors. JAMA 2013;310:591–608.
3. Asrani SK, Kamath PS. Natural history of cirrhosis. Curr Gastroenterol Rep 2013; 15:308, pp 1–6.
4. Grattagliano I, Ubaldi E, Bonfrate L, Portincasa, P. Management of liver cirrhosis between primary care and specialists. World J Gastroenterol 2011;17: 2273–2282.
5. Schuppan D, Afdhal NH. Liver cirrhosis. Lancet 2008;371:838–851.
6. Hashizume M, Akahoshi T, Tomikawa M. Management of gastric varices. J Gastroenterol Hepatol 2011;26(suppl 1):102–108.
7. Ryan BM, Stockbrugger RW, Ryan JM. A pathophysiologic, gastroenterologic, and radiologic approach to the management of gastric varices. Gastroenterology 2004;126:1175–1189.
8. Cardenas A, Gines P. Management of patients with cirrhosis awaiting liver transplantation. Gut 2011;60:412–421.

9. Garcia-Tsao G, Bosch J. Management of varices and variceal hemorrhage in cirrhosis. N Engl J Med 2010;362:823–832.

10. Cubillas R, Rockey DC. Portal hypertensive gastropathy: a review. Liver Int 2010;30:1094–1102.

11. Wiechowska-Kozlowska A, Bialek A, Milkiewicz P. Prevalence of "deep" rectal varices in patients with cirrhosis: an EUS-based study. Liver Int 2009;29:1202–1205.

12. Pere Ginès P, Angeli P, Lenz K, et al. Clinical practice guidelines: EASL clinical practice guidelines on the management of ascites, spontaneous bacterial peritonitis, and hepatorenal syndrome in cirrhosis. J Hepatol 2010;53:397–417.

13. Moore KP, Wong F, Gines P, et al. The management of ascites in cirrhosis: report on the consensus conference of the International Ascites Club. Hepatology 2003;38:258–266.

14. Salerno F, Guevara M, Bernardi M, et al. Refractory ascites: pathogenesis, definition and therapy of a severe complication in patients with cirrhosis. Liver Int 2010;30:937–947.

15. Bernardi M. Spontaneous bacterial peritonitis: from pathophysiology to prevention. Intern Emerg Med 2010;5(suppl):S37–S44.

16. Kuiper JJ, de Man RA, van Buuren HR. Review article: management of ascites and associated complications in patients with cirrhosis. Aliment Pharmacol Ther 2007;26(suppl 2):183–193.

17. Koulaouzidis A, Bhat S, Saeed AA. Spontaneous bacterial peritonitis. World J Gastroenterol 2009;15:1042–1049.

18. Terg R, Gadano A, Cartier M, et al. Serum creatinine and bilirubin predict renal failure and mortality in patients with spontaneous bacterial peritonitis: a retrospective study. Liver Int 2009;29:415–419.

19. Hemprich U, Papadakos PJ, Lachmann B. Respiratory failure and hypoxemia in the cirrhotic patient including hepatopulmonary syndrome. Curr Opin Anaesthesiol 2010;23:133–138.

20. Roussos A, Philippou N, Mantzaris GJ, Gourgouliannis KI. Hepatic hydrothorax: pathophysiology diagnosis and management. J Gastroenterol Hepatol 2007;22:1388–1393.

21. Guevara M, Arroyo V. Hepatorenal syndrome. Expert Opin Pharmacother 2011;12:1405–1417.

22. Ruiz-del-Arbol L, Monescillo A, Arocena C, et al. Circulatory function and hepatorenal syndrome in cirrhosis. Hepatology 2005;42:439–447.

23. Wasmuth HE, Kunz D, Yagmur E, et al. Patients with acute on chronic liver failure display "sepsis-like" immune paralysis. J Hepatol 2005;42:195–201.

24. Kochar R, Nevah Rubin MI, Fallon MB. Pulmonary complications of cirrhosis. Curr Gastroenterol Rep 2011;13:34–39.

25. Sussman NL, Kochar R, Fallon MB. Pulmonary complications in cirrhosis. Curr Opin Organ Transplant 2011;16:281–288.

26. Bismuth M, Funakoshi N, Cadranel JF, Blanc P. Hepatic encephalopathy: from pathophysiology to therapeutic management. Eur J Gastroenterol Hepatol 2011;23:8–22.

27. Cash WJ, McConville P, McDermott E, et al. Current concepts in the assessment and treatment of hepatic encephalopathy. QJM 2010;103:9–16.

28. Cholongitas E, Senzolo M, Patch D, et al. Review article: scoring systems for assessing prognosis in critically ill adult cirrhotics. Aliment Pharmacol Ther 2006;24:453–464.

29. Zwingmann C, Butterworth R. An update on the role of brain glutamine synthesis and its relation to cell-specific energy metabolism in the hyperammonemic brain: further studies using NMR spectroscopy. Neurochem Int 2005;47:19–30.

30. Heidelbaugh JJ, Bruderly M. Cirrhosis and chronic liver failure: part I. Diagnosis and evaluation. Am Fam Physician 2006;74:756–762.

31. Reshamwala PA. Management of ascites. Crit Care Nurs Clin North Am 2010;22:309–314.

32. Wai CT, Greenson JK, Fontana RJ, et al. A simple noninvasive index can predict both significant fibrosis and cirrhosis in patients with chronic hepatitis C. Hepatology 2003;38:518–526.

33. Thabut D, Imbert-Bismut F, Cazals-Hatem D, et al. Relationship between the Fibrotest and portal hypertension in patients with liver disease. Aliment Pharmacol Ther 2007;26:359–368.

34. Becker L, Salameh W, Sferruzza A, et al. Validation of hepascore, compared with simple indices of fibrosis, in patients with chronic hepatitis C virus infection in United States. Clin Gastroenterol Hepatol 2009;7:696–701.

35. Thabut D, Moreau R, Lebrec D. Noninvasive assessment of portal hypertension in patients with cirrhosis. Hepatology 2011;53:683–694.

36. Sorokin A, Brown JL, Thompson PD. Primary biliary cirrhosis, hyperlipidemia, and atherosclerotic risk: a systematic review. Atherosclerosis 2007;194:293–299.

Chapter 3: Noninvasive Cross-Sectional and Vascular Imaging of Portal Hypertension

Celia P. Corona-Villalobos, Luciana G. Matteoni-Athayde, Neda Rastegar, and Ihab R. Kamel

Introduction

Patients with chronic liver disease, especially those with cirrhosis, are at a higher risk of developing portal hypertension (PHT).[1] PHT is a compromise of the portal venous system as the result of a variety of benign and malignant conditions that cause increase in pressure in the portal venous inflow because of an increase in vascular resistance.[2] It is a major complication in cirrhosis caused by sinusoidal fibrosis and vasoconstriction, which increases intrahepatic resistance, leading to collateral veins and portosystemic shunts.

Portal hypertension has been classified based on the site of increased resistance to portal blood flow. Suprahepatic or prehepatic causes are most commonly caused by thrombosis of the portal or the splenic vein (SV); intrahepatic causes are subdivided into presinusoidal, sinusoidal, and postsinusoidal; and extrahepatic causes (Budd-Chiari syndrome, neoplastic infiltration through the hepatic veins, chronic right ventricular failure, and constrictive pericarditis, among others) overlap often with intrahepatic diseases such as Budd-Chiari syndrome.[3]

Normal portal pressure is between 5 and 10 mm Hg. Portal pressure above 10 mm Hg will diagnose PHT, and if portal pressure exceeds 12 mm Hg (▶ Fig. 3.1), the threshold for variceal rupture is elevated.[4] Hepatic venous pressure gradient (HVPG) and free portal pressure are available methods for accurate evaluation of portal vein (PV) pressure. However, because of their invasiveness, they are not routinely performed. Therefore, there is a need to develop noninvasive and reliable imaging techniques for accurate diagnosis of PHT.

This chapter discusses the anatomy and imaging features of PHT by noninvasive cross-sectional imaging techniques. It also discusses novel cross-sectional techniques that could potentially be applicable to cases of PHT.

Venous Pathways in Portal Hypertension

There are several pathways of collateral circulation that return portal flow to the systemic venous circulation without passing through the liver. Most of the portosystemic collateral veins are preexistent (▶ Fig. 3.2) and simply enlarge in PHT. Despite the formation of collateral circulation, portal pressure usually remains elevated. These facts suggest that other mechanisms besides occlusion are involved in PHT.[5] Noninvasive imaging techniques are used to accurately assess the main PV, diagnose PHT, and detect portosystemic collateral veins. Increased blood flow through collaterals transmitted from portal venous branches results in dilatation of the venous tributaries (▶ Table 3.1). The main pathways for collateral circulation include the following (▶ Fig. 3.3):

1. **Esophageal and paraesophageal varices**
   Esophageal varices are tortuous veins along the distal esophageal wall. These are commonly known as cardiac varices along the submucosa in the lower third of the esophagus (▶ Fig. 3.4). Paraesophageal varices are collaterals in the posterior mediastinum beyond the esophageal wall. They connect with the left gastric vein, azygos, hemiazygos, and vertebral plexus (▶ Fig. 3.5). These varices do not communicate with the esophageal submucosa, which differentiates them from periesophageal veins.[6] Esophageal and paraesophageal varices are the most common causes of upper gastrointestinal bleeding in PHT.[6]

2. **Gastric varices**
   Retrogastric varices are supplied by the left gastric vein (coronary vein), and they drain to the esophageal or paraesophageal vein and then to the azygos system. These veins could present reverse flow direction to form submucosal esophageal and periesophageal varices.

   Gastric veins are primarily supplied by the short gastric vein that connects the gastric fundus and the left side of the greater curvature of the stomach to the SV.[6-8] In most cases, they drain into the superior vena cava (SVC) via the esophageal varices (▶ Fig. 3.6) and remain connected to the inferior vena cava (IVC) via the left renal vein (splenorenal shunt).[7,9,10]

3. **Paraumbilical varices and abdominal wall varices**
   Paraumbilical veins usually are collapsed, forming the falciform ligament. In patients with PHT, they tend to enlarge, arising from the left PV and coursing along the falciform ligament.[9,11] Recanalization of the paraumbilical vein is seen in

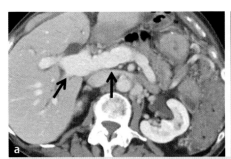
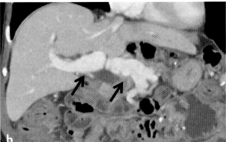
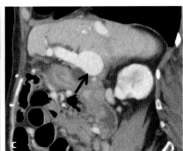

Fig. 3.1 Contrast-enhanced computed tomography scan of a 74-year-old woman. Portal phase in the axial (**a**), coronal (**b**), and sagittal (**c**) planes demonstrating a tortuous and dilated portal vein (*arrows*) measuring approximately 2 cm at the level of the hilum compatible with portal hypertension.

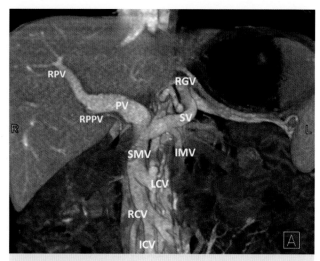

Fig. 3.2 Coronal plane in the portal venous phase showing normal anatomy of the portal vein (PV). ICV: ileocolic vein; IMV: inferior mesenteric vein; LCV: left colic vein; RCV: right colic vein; RGV: right gastric vein; RPPV: right posterior portal vein; RPV: right portal vein; SMV: superior mesenteric vein; SV: splenic vein.

Table 3.1 Portosystemic Collateral Circulation in Portal Hypertension

Collaterals draining to the superior vena cava	Esophageal varices
	Paraesophageal varices
	Left gastric vein
	Short gastric vein
	Posterior gastric vein
	Gastric varices
	Gastrorenal shunt
	Splenorenal shunt
Collaterals draining to the inferior vena cava	Paraumbilical vein
	Abdominal wall vein
	Retroperitoneal shunt
	Mesenteric varices
	Omental collateral vessels
	Rectal varices

43% of the patients with PHT.[12] The majority of paraumbilical veins drain into the SVC through the inferior epigastric veins[9] (▶ Fig. 3.7).

Abdominal varices are commonly described as caput medusa because of their radiating pattern, emerging from the umbilicus and draining into the epigastric veins. Abdominal

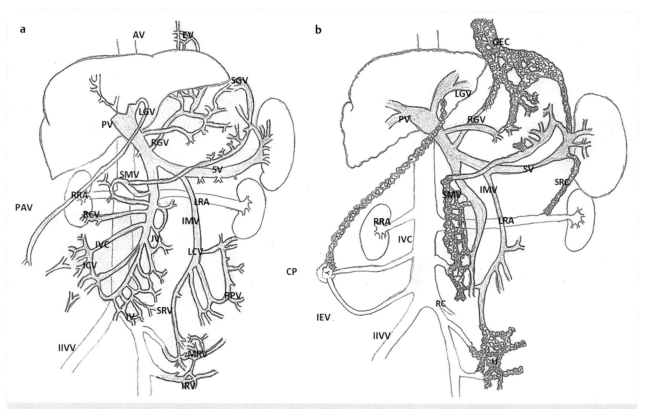

Fig. 3.3 Physiologic portosystemic anastomoses (**a**) and changes in portosystemic anastomoses (**b**) caused by portal hypertension.
    Portal circulation—ICV: ileocolic vein; IMV: inferior mesenteric vein; IRV: inferior rectal vein; IV: ileal veins; JV: jejunal veins; LCV: left colic vein; LGV: left gastric vein; MRV: middle rectal vein; PV: portal vein; RCV: right colic vein; RGV: right gastric vein; RPV: retroperitoneal veins; SGV: short gastric vein; SMV: superior mesenteric vein; SRV: sigmoidal rectal vein; SV: splenic vein.
    Systemic circulation—AV: azygos vein; EV: esophageal vein; IEV: inferior epigastric vein; IIVV: iliac vein; IVC: inferior vena cava; LRA: left renal artery; PAV: paraumbilical vein; RRA: right renal artery.
    Collaterals—CP: caput medusae; GEC: gastroesophageal collaterals; H: hemorrhoids; RC: retroperitoneal collaterals; SRC: splenorenal collaterals.
(Drawing by CP Corona-Villalobos)

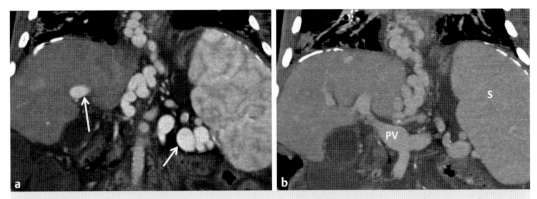

Fig. 3.4 **(a)** Hepatic arterial phase in the coronal plane. Markedly enhancement of the portal vein, splenic vein, and gastroesophageal junction varices caused by shunting (*arrows*). **(b)** Portal venous phase in the coronal plane. The portal vein (PV) is patent. There are retroperitoneal collaterals and splenomegaly (S) of 16 cm.

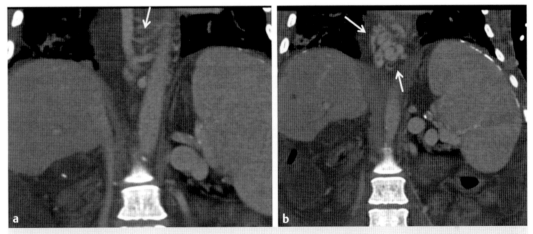

Fig. 3.5 **(a)** Coronal plane contrast-enhanced computed tomography scan in the portal venous phase demonstrating presence of paraesophageal varices arising from the azygos vein (*arrow*). **(b)** Slightly more anterior view better demonstrating paraesophageal varices (*arrows*).

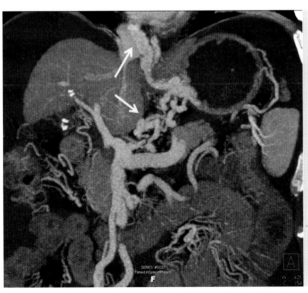

Fig. 3.6 Contrast-enhanced computed tomography scan in the coronal plane demonstrating numerous large collaterals arising from the left gastric vein extending through the gastroesophageal area (*arrows*).

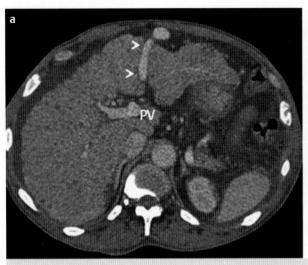 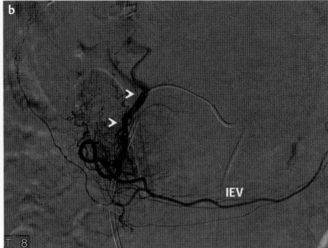

Fig. 3.7 A 55-year-old man with a history of cirrhosis. (**a**) Axial computed tomography scan in the portal venous phase showing a recanalized umbilical vein (*arrowheads*). The portal vein (PV) is patent. (**b**) Left hepatic arteriogram demonstrating recanalization of the umbilical vein (*arrowheads*) extending through the inferior epigastric vein (IEV) forming a caput medusae.

veins are located in the subcutaneous fat and may extent to the pelvis, connecting to the iliac veins (▶ Fig. 3.8).

4. **Perisplenic varices**

   Perisplenic varices usually transverse the splenocolic ligament and are seen as dilated veins in the anterior and posterior aspect of the spleen. Varices at the splenic hilum communicate with retrogastric varices or inferior phrenic veins (▶ Fig. 3.9).

5. **Retroperitoneal varices**

   Retroperitoneal varices may arise from the colic branches, the SV, or the left gastric vein. These veins can form spontaneous shunts that are associated with an increased incidence of encephalopathy (▶ Fig. 3.10).

6. **Rectal varices**

   The rectal plexus drains through the superior hemorrhoidal vein to the inferior mesenteric vein. Reverse flow from the inferior rectal vein forms the rectal and pararectal varices, which drain into the deep pelvic inferior epigastric veins.

7. **Shunts**

   Spontaneous splenorenal shunt in the portosystemic circulation can develop with or without the presence of collateral circulation. Shunts are seen as large, tortuous veins in the region of the splenic and left renal hilum that drain to the left renal vein[9] (▶ Fig. 3.11). Other shunts include gastrorenal shunts, which develop between retrogastric varices and the left renal vein.[11] Formation of a splenorenal or gastrorenal shunt increases the incidence of hepatic encephalopathy.[11]

Noninvasive Imaging Diagnosis

Ultrasonography (US), computed tomography (CT), and magnetic resonance imaging (MRI) are commonly used to evaluate patients with PHT. The choice of imaging modality is probably not as important as strict attention to the imaging features such as detection of collateral circulation and identification of associated abnormalities such as chronic liver disease or cirrhosis, splenomegaly, ascites, thrombosis, or liver neoplasms.

Ultrasonography

Ultrasonography is widely used as the first imaging modality to evaluate patients with PHT. It is well known that US is operator

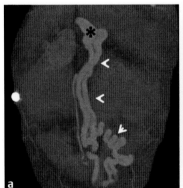 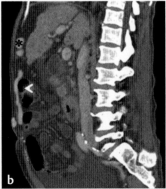 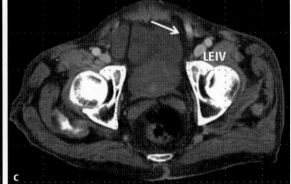

Fig. 3.8 A 55-year-old man with a history of alcoholic cirrhosis. Coronal (**a**) and sagittal (**b**) plane computed tomography scans showing a recanalized paraumbilical vein (*asterisk*) through the subcutaneous tissue and abdominal wall (*arrowheads*) draining to the left external iliac vein (LEIV) (**c**, *arrow*).

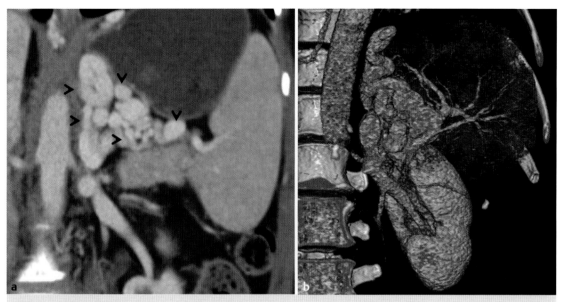

Fig. 3.9 A 61-year-old woman with history of hepatitis C and cirrhosis. (**a**) Arterial phase computed tomography scan in the coronal plane showing multiple splenorenal collaterals (*arrowheads*). Presence of splenomegaly is also noted to be caused by portal hypertension. (**b**) Volume-rendered image showing similar findings.

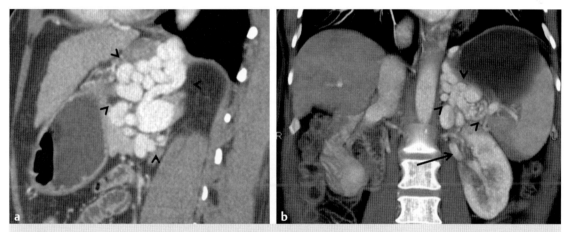

Fig. 3.10 (**a**) Contrast-enhanced computed tomography scan in the sagittal plane demonstrating numerous splenorenal varices extending to the gastroesophageal junction (*arrowheads*). (**b**) Coronal plane showing a dilated left renal vein (*arrow*).

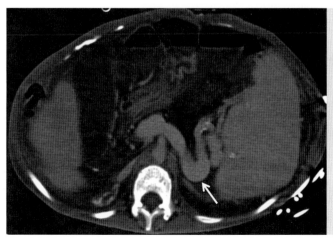

Fig. 3.11 Contrast-enhanced computed tomography scan in the axial plane illustrating dilatation of the splenic vein (*arrow*), which drains to the left renal vein.

and equipment dependent. However, it is a widely available and fast imaging method with low cost and without the added risk of radiation. These advantages should be valued because patients with PHT are imaged not only for diagnosis but also periodically for therapeutic monitoring. US protocols routinely used include gray-scale imaging and color and spectral Doppler (▶ Table 3.2).

Gray-scale images are of great importance in evaluating the splenoportal anatomy. The main PV is present in the hepatoduodenal ligament and is identified by following the SV to the right until its junction with the superior mesenteric vein (SMV).[13] At the crossing point of the PV with the IVC, the PV diameter should be assessed. The PV diameter varies widely according to the site of measurement, fasting state of the patient, and respiratory cycle.[14] Normal diameter of the main PV is considered to be up to 12 mm when measured from the inner anterior to the inner posterior wall and acquired with the patient in a supine position, fasting, and breathing quietly.[15] The SV and SMV should also be measured in the assessment of PHT (▶ Fig. 3.12).

The upper limit diameter of normality for these two vessels is considered 9 mm.[16] An increase in caliber of any of the three vessels that comprise the portal venous system is associated with PHT. A PV caliber over 13 mm acquired with the protocol previously described is indicative of PHT with a specificity of 100% and a sensitivity of 45% to 50%.[17] Patients with known PHT who present with small PV diameters (<8 mm) should be evaluated carefully (▶ Fig. 3.13). Usually in these cases, periportal collaterals are identified in addition to chronic thromboses of the PV, suggesting cavernous transformation.

Patency of the splenoportal venous system is evaluated by gray-scale and Doppler images (▶ Fig. 3.14). The presence of echogenic material within these vessels is highly suspicious for thrombosis (▶ Fig. 3.15). In some cases, however, acute thrombus has low

Table 3.2 List of Features Evaluated by Ultrasonography in Portal Hypertension

Gray-scale imaging	Liver morphology, edge, surface, and parenchymal texture Spleen size and texture Splenoportal anatomy Portal vein diameter Portal systemic collaterals
Doppler imaging	Portal vein flow and velocity Portal vein congestion index Suprahepatic vein flow Hepatic artery flow and velocity Hepatic artery resistance index Portosystemic collaterals

echogenicity or is even anechoic and therefore is difficult to be identified on B-mode imaging. When thrombosis is suspected, Doppler images must be performed. The absence of color and spectral Doppler signal confirms the presence of the suspected thrombus. However, in some situations, flow can be identified, suggesting that the vessel is partially thrombosed. Acute thrombus usually enlarges the caliber of the affected vascular segment, and chronic thrombosis tends to decrease it. Cavernous transformation (▶ Fig. 3.16) is observed in the later phases of chronic thrombosis of the PV when periportal collaterals are identified at the porta hepatis and the main PV is usually no longer visualized. Another tool that can be used while evaluating the patency of a vein by US exam is the manual compression of the vessel with the US probe. In PV thrombosis, the vessel shows reduced or absent compressibility.[18]

The velocity of blood flow in the PV ranges from 15 to 18 cm/s when acquired with the patient breathing quietly.[17] These values

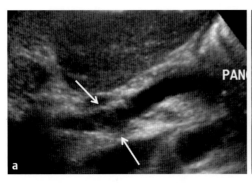
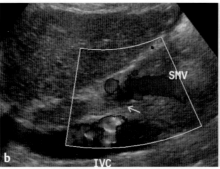

Fig. 3.12 A 59-year-old woman with cirrhosis. Gray-scale ultrasound (a) shows the presence of soft tissue (*arrows*) at the portal vein (PV) confluence extending to the main PV. (b) Doppler ultrasound image demonstrating lack of Doppler signal (*arrow*). IVC: inferior vena cava; PAN: pancreas; SMV: superior mesenteric vein.

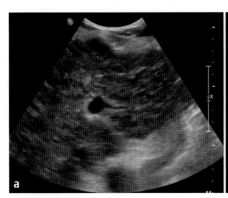
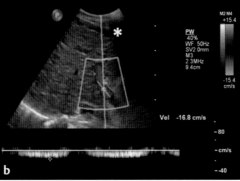

Fig. 3.13 Gray-scale and spectral Doppler ultrasound image of the right upper quadrant. (a) The liver is coarse in echotexture and nodular in appearance. (b) The main portal vein is patent and shows reversed or hepatofugal flow. Note the presence of mild ascites (*asterisk*) caused by portal hypertension.

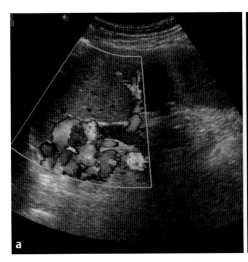
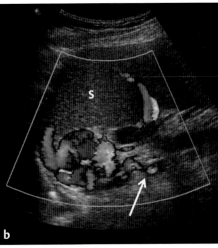

Fig. 3.14 (a) Doppler ultrasound image of the splenic hilum showing an increase in size of the perisplenic vessels with turbulent flow. (b) Notice the presence of a spontaneous portosystemic shunt (*arrow*) and splenomegaly (S).

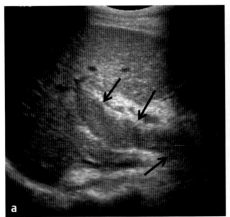
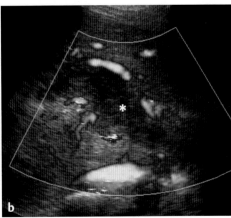

Fig. 3.15 (a) Gray-scale ultrasound image showing an echogenic material (*arrows*) filling the portal vein, which extends to the portal confluence. (b) Doppler ultrasound image showing absence of flow indicative of thrombosis (*asterisk*).

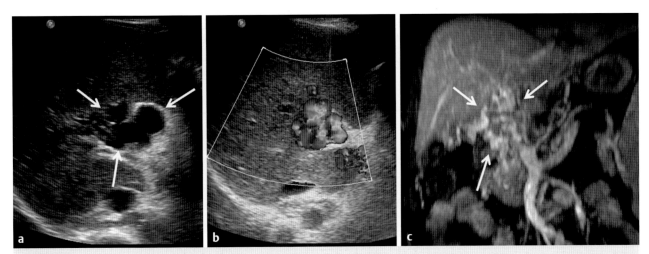

Fig. 3.16 Oblique gray-scale (a) and Doppler (b) ultrasound images showing a mass of tortuous vessels at the porta hepatis caused by cavernous transformation of the portal vein (PV) in a patient with history of cirrhosis. (c) Coronal contrast-enhanced magnetic resonance venogram demonstrating tortuous serpiginous vessels (*arrows*) around the PV with partial thrombosis of the PV.

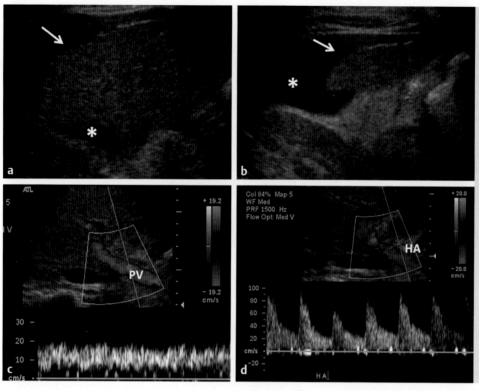

Fig. 3.17 A 65-year-old man with history of hepatitis C and cirrhosis. Gray-scale and spectral Doppler ultrasound image showing coarsened hepatic echotexture with nodular borders (**a**, *arrows*) and the presence of ascites (**b**, *asterisk*). (**c**) Patent portal vein (PV) with turbulent hepatopetal flow. (**d**) Hepatic artery (HA) showing increased velocity caused by portal hypertension.

can vary greatly if the patient is not fasting or has recently exercised.[19] For an accurate measurement of the PV velocity, the angle between the long axis of the vessel and the Doppler beam should be less than 60 degrees (► Fig. 3.17). In the setting of PHT, the PV velocity decreases, and flow direction alters. Normally, the PV flow is toward the liver (hepatopetal) and varies with respiration and heart rate. As PHT increases, flow may become biphasic. Worsening the degree of PH causes reversal of flow, which may even be monophasic and hepatofugal (► Fig. 3.18). When the patient's condition improves or the collateral circulation is set (► Fig. 3.19), hepatopetal flow can recover because of decompression of the portal circulation.[17]

In patients with PHT, when the portal flow starts to be diverted into the collaterals, the portal flow to the liver decreases. This diminished portal venous inflow toward the liver is compensated with an increase in the hepatic arterial flow. The hepatic artery (HA) becomes larger and more tortuous (► Fig. 3.20). With progression of PHT, the HA needs to be "decompressed," and this occurs through arterioportal shunts.[20]

The hepatic veins and the suprahepatic IVC should also be evaluated during the US examination. Posthepatic causes of PHT can be ruled out when the examination shows patency of these vessels. Normally, the hepatic veins waveform (HVW) is triphasic (► Fig. 3.21), consisting of two negative waves and one positive

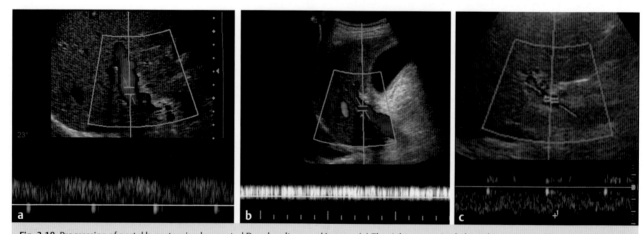

Fig. 3.18 Progression of portal hypertension by spectral Doppler ultrasound images. (**a**) The right parasagittal plane shows a normal hepatopetal triphasic spectrum of the portal vein (PV) with normal velocity (12 cm/s). (**b**) Doppler image shows a monophasic spectrum of the PV with increased portal velocity (18 cm/s). (**c**) Inverted flow of the PV in advanced portal hypertension (portal velocity is 23 cm/s).

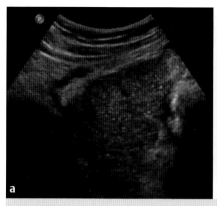 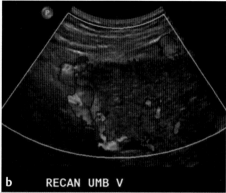 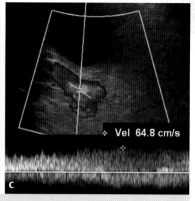

Fig. 3.19 A 49-year-old man with hepatitis C. (**a**) Gray-scale and spectral Doppler ultrasound image of the right upper quadrant of the liver shows nodular contours with coarse echotexture. (**b**) Recanalized umbilical vein is noted. (**c**) The portal vein shows increased velocity (64 cm/s) and turbulent flow.

wave. This waveform is related to the right atrial activity.[19] In the setting of PHT, alteration can be observed in the pattern of the HVW, and it can become either biphasic or monophasic. The exact cause of such changes in the HVW in patients with PHT remains unclear.[21] A correlation between abnormal HVW and HVPG was already described. It was shown that the normal HVW tends to become flat as HVPG increases. Also, a monophasic HVW has a sensitivity and specificity of 74% and 95%, respectively, in the diagnosis of severe PHT.[22]

Several hemodynamic parameters measured with Doppler US are described in ▶ Table 3.3 when the intention is to evaluate PHT. ▶ Table 3.4 summarizes these parameters and their respective sensibility and specificity to diagnose PHT.[23–27]

Although measurement of vessel diameter and Doppler index is useful in patients with PHT, the most reliable and widely used

approach for the diagnosis of PHT is the detection of portal systemic collaterals.[19] During the US examination, it is important to search for collateral veins using gray-scale images in association with color Doppler. Recanalization of the paraumbilical vein (▶ Fig. 3.22) is seen in 43% of patients with PHT, and this is the easiest collateral to assess during the US examination.[12] Also, the coronary vein should be imaged by US. It is the most important portal systemic collateral to focus on, not only because it is the most prevalent, present in about 90% of cases of PHT, but also because its presence implies an increased risk for variceal hemorrhage.[19,28] A coronary vein with diameter larger than 5 mm should be considered abnormal and suggests the presence of PHT.[29] Knowledge of the anatomy of the most common collateral pathways described earlier in this chapter is primordial to visualization of other portosystemic collaterals communications.

Microbubble contrast-enhanced ultrasonography (CEUS) is a new technique with promising preliminary results in the setting of PHT. Microbubble contrast agents developed for US are confined to the intravascular space and were initially used to enhance Doppler US signals. Recent studies have shown that these US contrast agents can also be used for kinetic studies because they enable assessment of the transit time of the microbubbles through the vessels. A recently published study evaluated hepatic vein arrival

Fig. 3.20 Gray-scale and spectral Doppler ultrasound image of the hepatic artery showing a tortuous artery with turbulent flow. There is increased velocity (177 cm/s) and resistance index (0.82) of the hepatic artery.

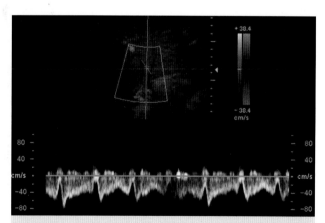

Fig. 3.21 Doppler and spectral ultrasound images of the hepatic vein showing a triphasic waveform commonly seen in normal patients.

Table 3.3 Hemodynamic Parameters Measured by Doppler Ultrasonography to Assess Portal Hypertension

Hemodynamic Parameter	Calculation
Mean portal vein velocity (PVV)	Measured at with angle between the long axis of the vessel and the Doppler beam < 60 degrees
Portal blood flow	Cross-sectional area of portal vein (PV) × Mean PVV
Portal vein congestion index	Cross-sectional area of PV/Mean PVV
Hepatic artery pulsatility index (PI)	(Peak systolic velocity – End-diastolic velocity)/Mean velocity
Hepatic artery resistive index (RI)	(Peak systolic velocity – End-diastolic velocity)/Peak systolic velocity
Liver vascular index	Velocity of blood flow in PV/Hepatic artery PI
Splenic artery pulsatility index	(Peak systolic velocity – End-diastolic velocity)/Mean velocity
Splenic artery resistive index	(Peak systolic velocity – End-diastolic velocity)/Peak systolic velocity
Renal artery pulsatility index	(Peak systolic velocity – End-diastolic velocity)/Mean velocity
Renal artery resistive index	(Peak systolic velocity – End-diastolic velocity)/Peak systolic velocity
Portal hypertension index	Hepatic artery RI 9 × 0.69 × Splenic artery RI × 0.87/PVV
Hepatic buffer index	Hepatic artery PI maximum change/PV blood volume maximum change

PI: pulse index; PV: portal vein; PVV: portal vein velocity; RI: resistive index.
Source: Singal et al.[13]

Table 3.4 Clinical Applications and Changes of Hemodynamic Parameters Assessed by Doppler Ultrasonography in the Setting of Portal Hypertension

Hemodynamic Parameter	Tendency in PHT	Clinical Relevance	Reference
Mean portal vein velocity (PVV)	Decrease	Cut-off of 15 cm/s has a sensibility and specificity of 88% and 96%, respectively, to diagnose PHT.	Zironi et al[23]
Portal vein congestion index	Increase	Values > 0.1 suggest PHT with a sensibility and specificity of 95%.	Haag et al[24]
Hepatic artery resistance indexes (PI and RI)	Increase or no change	PI > 1.05 suggests severe PHT with a sensibility of 86% and specificity of 88%.	Schneider et al[25]
Splenic artery resistance indexes (PI and RI)	Increase or no change	RI > 0.60 has a high accuracy in the diagnosis of relevant PHT (presence of gastroesophageal varices).	Piscaglia et al[26]
Renal artery resistance indexes (PI and RI)	Increase	Abnormal renal impedance has a high positive predictive value for the detection of severe PHT (> 16 mm Hg).	Berzigotti et al[27]

PHT: pulmonary hypertension; PI: pulsatility index; RI: resistive index.

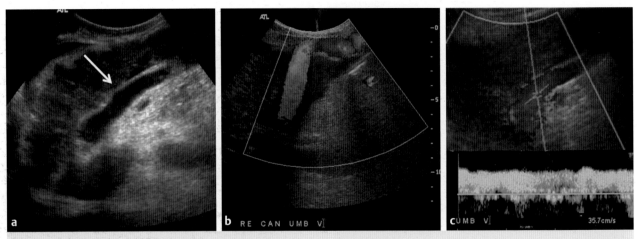

Fig. 3.22 (a,b) Oblique and spectral Doppler ultrasound images of a 61-year-old man with history of cirrhosis. Recanalized umbilical vein (a, *arrow*) arising from the left portal vein. (c) Note the presence of turbulent flow from the umbilical vein.

time (HVAT) as a method of assessing the severity of PHT.[8] Microbubble CEUS is a promising method to assess patients with PHT, but further studies are necessary to show its potential value.

Computed Tomography

Multidetector computed tomography (MDCT) is a powerful imaging method for recognizing PHT complications, illustrating vessel patency (▶ Fig. 3.23) and portosystemic collateral circulation. Three-dimensional CT angiography can aid in understanding the complex variceal anatomy.[30] The main advantage of MDCT over US is its three-dimensional reformatting in maximum intensity projection and volume rendering, which allows creation of vascular maps similar to digital subtraction angiography (▶ Fig. 3.24). Collateral circulation can be evaluated by noncontrast MDCT, but for better visualization and differentiation from adenopathy, bowel loops, and masses, contrast injection is necessary. Enhanced dual-phase CT can be used as a noninvasive tool to demonstrate alterations in the dynamics of the hepatic flow. Dual-CT can also quantify liver perfusion data from the time density curves, calculating the blood flow rate (inflow–outflow) and liver enhancement pattern, useful in liver transplantation.

Contrast-Enhanced Computed Tomography

Abdominal MDCT imaging is acquired with low or iso-osmolality contrast media in the hepatic arterial (20s) and portal-venous (70s) phases followed by a saline flush with thin reconstructions for systematic vascular evaluation. The arterial phase identifies the arterial supply to the liver (originating from the celiac artery). The most common normal variants branching patterns of the PV commonly seen in the PV phase are (i) the trifurcation of the PV (main PV divides into right anterior, right posterior, and left PV) without a right PV, (ii) the right anterior PV arising from the left PV, and (iii) the right posterior PV arising from the main PV (▶ Fig. 3.25). Knowledge of these variants is important during

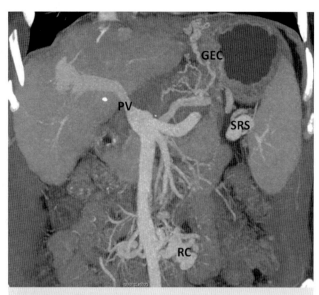

Fig. 3.24 Contrast-enhanced computed tomography scan demonstrating numerous large varices within the abdomen. Notice the presence of splenorenal shunt (SRS). GEC: gastroesophageal collaterals; PV: portal vein; RC: retroperitoneal collaterals.

liver transplantation; the ligation of one of the branches may lead to necrosis of the liver parenchyma.

Variceal Hemorrhage

Bleeding from esophageal varices (▶ Fig. 3.26) is a major cause of death in patients with PHT, which eventually occurs in 30% of cases.[31] The risk of bleeding is associated with varix size because these veins can increase in size and carry up to a half liter of blood per minute.[31] Therefore, it is important to identify collateral vessels and portal thrombosis in the main PV or its branches by CT.

Intrahepatic Shunts

Contrast-enhanced CT will demonstrate the presence of vascular connections between branches of the hepatic artery, PV, and hepatic veins, although these are rare.

Arterioportal Shunts

In the presence of cirrhosis and PHT, arterioportal shunts may occur. However, these shunts are difficult to visualize with cross-sectional imaging. They usually appear as small, subcapsular, wedge-shaped areas of increased attenuation with early enhancement on the arterial phase and normal attenuation during the portal venous phase.[32]

Portosystemic Shunts

These are vascular connections between the PV and the hepatic veins. The most frequent shunts occur between the right PV and the IVC. These shunts are also associated with hepatic encephalopathy.[33] The most clinically important and the frequency of portosystemic shunts are described in ▶ Table 3.5.[34] During the portal venous phase, the communication between the PV and the hepatic veins is well demonstrated (▶ Fig. 3.27).

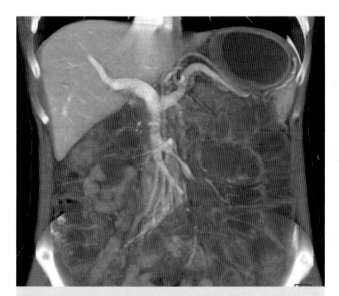

Fig. 3.23 Contrast-enhanced computed tomography scan demonstrating normal portal venous anatomy.

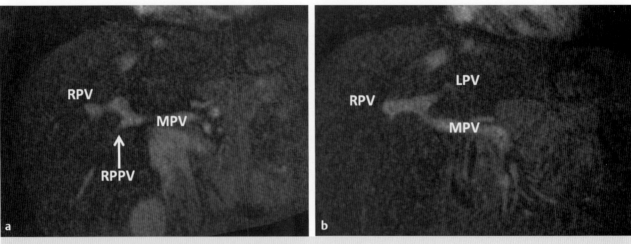

Fig. 3.25 Contrast-enhanced magnetic resonance image demonstrating a normal variation of the main portal vein (PV). (**a**) The right posterior PV (RPPV) arises (*arrow*) from the main PV (MPV). (**b**) Normal bifurcation of the right (RPV) and left (LPV) branches of the PV.

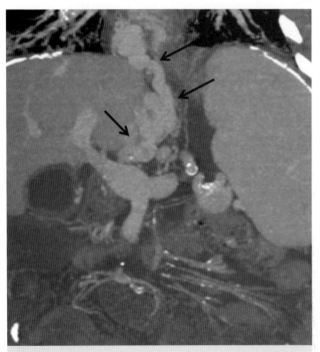

Fig. 3.26 Multiplanar reconstruction in coronal plane of a contrast-enhanced computed tomography scan illustrating multiple tortuous esophageal varices. Note the connection with the left gastric vein (*arrows*).

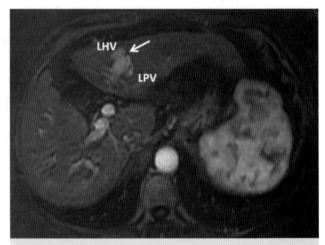

Fig. 3.27 A 63-year-old woman with history of autoimmune cirrhosis. Contrast-enhanced magnetic resonance image showing a dilated left portal vein (LPV) indicative of a portal varix. Early contrast filling extending to the left hepatic vein (LHV) suggesting the presence of a shunt (*arrow*).

Table 3.5 Frequency of Portosystemic Shunts in Portal Hypertension

Varices	% of Presentation	Draining Route	%
Left gastric vein	90	Esophageal varices	88
Short gastric vein	34	Esophageal varices	84
		Left renal vein	12
Paraumbilical vein	24	Left renal vein	18
		Varied	
Splenic vein	7	Left renal vein	100
Inferior mesenteric vein	2	Left renal vein	100

Source: Okuda and Benhamou.[34]

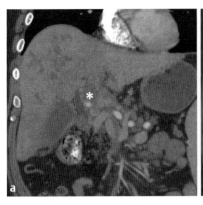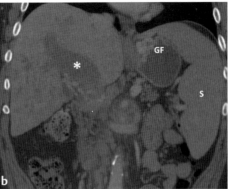

Fig. 3.28 A 53-year-old man with cirrhosis. (a) The portal vein is distended with filling defect (*asterisk*) extending to the superior mesenteric vein representing a thrombus. (b) Large gastric fundus (GF) varices and splenomegaly (S) consistent with portal hypertension.

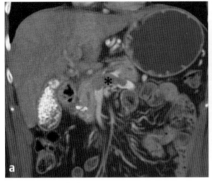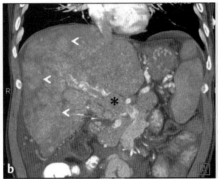

Fig. 3.29 (a) Contrast-enhanced computed tomography scan demonstrating portal thrombosis, which extends to the splenic vein and superior mesenteric vein. (b) Coronal plane in the venous phase showing parenchymal heterogeneity with ill-defined hypervascular masses (*arrowheads*) and portal vein thrombosis (*asterisk*). There is cavernous transformation and collateral circulation.

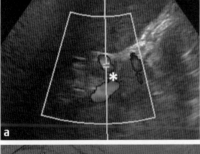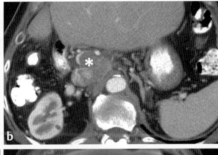
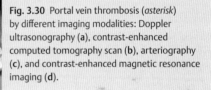
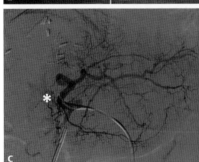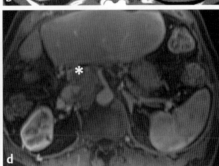

Fig. 3.30 Portal vein thrombosis (*asterisk*) by different imaging modalities: Doppler ultrasonography (a), contrast-enhanced computed tomography scan (b), arteriography (c), and contrast-enhanced magnetic resonance imaging (d).

Thrombosis and Calcifications

Liver cirrhosis is the most common cause of PV thrombosis, although it is not the only one. Thrombosis by nonenhanced CT is defined as focal areas of high attenuation within the portal system and associated vessel enlargement if the thrombosis is acute (▶ Fig. 3.28). Enhanced CT can confirm the site of occlusion, the presence of cavernous transformation, or collateral circulation and shunts (▶ Fig. 3.29; ▶ Fig. 3.30). Perfusion anomalies can be associated with portal thrombosis caused by an increased arterial inflow appearing as increased attenuation of the poorly perfused hepatic segments. Chronic thrombosis shows linear calcifications of the vascular wall within the thrombus.

Cavernous Transformation

Contrast-enhanced CT can determine portal venous patency or location of the collaterals and shunts in patients with cirrhosis

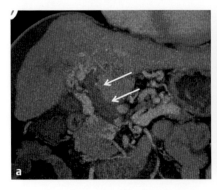
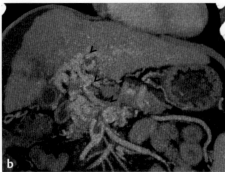

Fig. 3.31 (a,b) A 49-year-old woman with a history of hepatitis C and alcohol use. Complete thrombosis of the main portal vein (*arrows*) showing the presence of multiple collateral veins (*arrowheads*) in the porta hepatis.

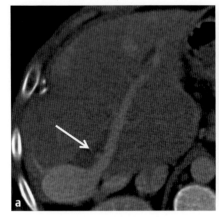
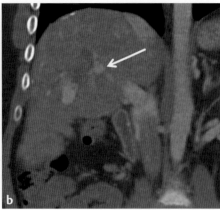

Fig. 3.32 Axial (**a**) and coronal (**b**) plane of a contrast-enhanced computed tomography scan demonstrating a saccular structure along the portal vein (PV) suggesting a PV varix (*arrow*).

or PHT (▶ Fig. 3.31). When the PV is occluded,[35] the venous channels within the occluded PV act as portoportal collaterals called cavernous transformation. Cavernous transformation can occur as early as 6 to 20 days after PV occlusion even if partial recanalization exists.[35] On contrast-enhanced CT, a beaded appearance at the PV is characteristic and is the most frequent finding.[36] Perfusion changes can be seen in the liver parenchyma as inhomogeneous, peripheral, patchy areas of high attenuation caused by a lack of blood supply to the peripheral regions.

Aneurysms and Varices

Aneurysms from the PV are not common, representing only 3% of all aneurysms of the venous system.[37] The most common locations are the splenomesenteric venous confluence, main PV, and intrahepatic PV branches. Less common locations are the splenic, mesenteric, and umbilical veins.[36] Usually, portal venous system aneurysms are asymptomatic. By imaging, aneurysms of the PV are considered if the vessel diameter is significantly larger than the remaining vessels (▶ Fig. 3.32), especially if the morphology is fusiform, saccular, or bilobulated.[36]

Bidimensional and Three-Dimensional Rendering

Image reconstruction can be performed on commercially available consoles; the software allows electronic dissection of selected anatomical structures. Vascular origins can be evaluated with two-dimensional reformation to rule out stenosis and aneurysms. Vascular anatomy requires three-dimensional rendering (▶ Fig. 3.33), allowing better understanding of vascular anatomy

and optimizing perception of the complex course of the vessels. With this tool, radiologists can significantly help patient assessment and treatment.

Volumetrics

Quantitative volumetry of the liver and spleen is useful to determine the severity of PHT[38–40] and provides accurate evaluation in potential donors undergoing living donor liver transplantation.[41]

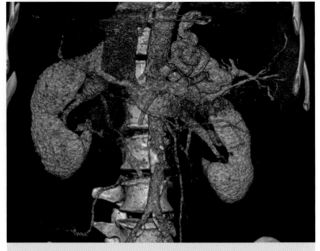

Fig. 3.33 Three-dimensional volume rendering allows a better understanding of vascular anatomy in cases of extensive collateral circulation. Note the presence of perigastric collaterals.

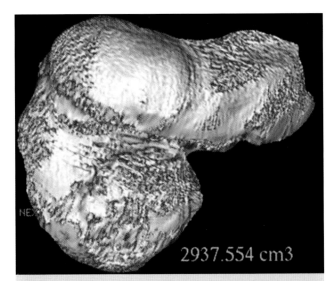

Fig. 3.34 Quantitative total liver volumetry of the liver provides accurate evaluation in potential donors undergoing living liver transplantation.

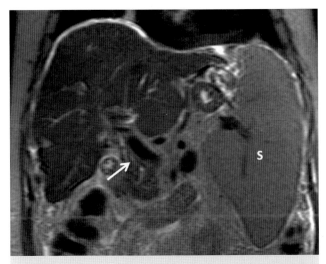

Fig. 3.35 Coronal T2-weighted image showing patency of the portal vein (PV) with the presence of ascites. Patency of the PV is well demonstrated as signal void (*arrow*). Notice the increased dimension of the spleen (S) with a maximal diameter of 20 cm on the longitudinal plane compatible with portal hypertension.

Hepatic volume in patients with PHT decreases, in contrast to the splenic volume which tends to increase, implying congestive splenomegaly. Volumetrics can be performed using CT or MRI images on a commercially available workstation by manually outlining the liver contour on portal-venous phase as described in a previous study,[41] carefully excluding the main vessels, major fissures, and the gallbladder. A three-dimensional model of the liver can be generated for the total liver volume by adding the volume estimated from the area to the thickness of the studied organ on each image (▶ Fig. 3.34).

Magnetic Resonance Imaging

Magnetic resonance imaging is widely used to evaluate patients with PHT without the risk of ionizing radiation. MRI is a reliable noninvasive imaging technique that provides a dedicated study of the liver and is useful in characterizing the liver parenchyma, determining volumetrics, depicting vascular patency (▶ Fig. 3.35), establishing the presence of collateral circulation (▶ Fig. 3.36), and screening for tumors (▶ Fig. 3.37). Other advantages of using MRI are its novel techniques such as flowmetry, T1 mapping, and elastography.

Fast spin-echo (FSE) images are needed to characterize liver parenchyma will help to differentiate liver masses. Pulse sequences by gradient echo images (GRE) help to characterize the PV anatomy and patency. Contrast GRE images can delineate the vascular anatomy, visualizing the portosystemic collateral pathways. They can also distinguish the presence or absence of thrombi and can characterize tumor enhancement pattern. On T1-weighted images, thrombus is hyperintense in the stage phase and isointense to the liver parenchyma in late stages. On T2-weighted images, PV thrombosis appears similar in signal intensity to soft tissue.[42]

Magnetic Resonance Venography

Magnetic resonance venography (MRV) has advantages over other imaging modalities currently used to assess for PHT. MRV can precisely assess the portal venous system in patients with PHT, which is essential before liver transplantation and surgical venous shunting. Time-of-flight (TOF) and phase-contrast (PC) imaging are valuable techniques for assessing vascular anatomy and portosystemic collaterals. TOF angiography is useful in assessing the portal venous system and allows for successful detection of PV thrombosis[43] (▶ Fig. 3.38).

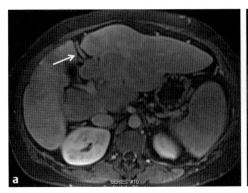
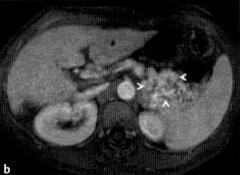

Fig. 3.36 A 32-year-old woman with hepatitis C. (a) Magnetic resonance image (MRI) in the portal venous phase shows a recanalized paraumbilical vein (*arrow*) and cirrhotic background of the liver. (b) Contrast-enhanced MRI demonstrating the presence of multiple perisplenic collaterals (*arrowheads*).

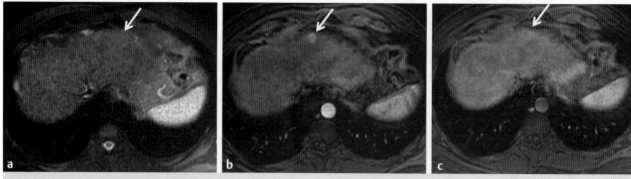

Fig. 3.37 A 50-year-old man with a history of cirrhosis. Irregular borders of the liver with a hyperintense nodule in T2 (**a**, *arrow*). Enhancement (**b**) and washout (**c**) on the delay images are findings that are suspicious for hepatocellular carcinoma (*arrow*).

Usually TOF acquires bidimensional or three-dimensional flow velocity information from the vessel of interest. Whereas patent blood vessels on GRE images are hyperintense, thrombi look like an intraluminal filling defect because of a lack of signal. Contrast administration or PC images are useful to determine the patency of the PV in difficult cases, such as in the presence of calcifications or in slow blood flow that mimics venous thrombosis. The disadvantages of TOF are motion artifacts caused by breathing, long acquisition times, and incomplete coverage of the portal venous system.

Novel Magnetic Resonance Imaging Techniques

Phase Contrast

True fast imaging with steady-state precession and segmented fast GRE MRI sequences with velocity encoding perpendicular to the imaging plane has been used to evaluate vascular flow. The main difference between PC and TOF imaging is the phase shift in transverse magnetization that occurs in blood flowing through the magnetic field gradient. The advantage of PC over TOF imaging is that PC imaging acquires information regarding the flow direction in addition to the information regarding the flow velocity. Therefore, on PC sequences, it is necessary to specify the strength of the flow-encoding gradient of the vessel of interest. Velocity-encoding parameters of 15 to 50 cm/s for the PV have been described in previous studies.[44,45] The disadvantage of PC sequence over TOF imaging is longer times of imaging

acquisition. Flow on PC images depends on its direction; whereas a hyperintense signal ("white" flow) resembles a cephalic direction, caudal flow appears as a hypointense signal ("black" flow) (▶ Fig. 3.39).

Hepatic hemodynamic changes such as increased hepatic vascular resistance influence the degree of hepatic dysfunction and PHT. The presence of collateral circulation in cirrhosis indicates severe PHT. Noninvasive MRI PC measurements overcome operator-dependent difficulties existing from the Doppler US and therefore provide better flow measurements. In one study, PC showed good correlation with Doppler US in predicting intrahepatic or extrahepatic shunting in liver cirrhosis.[46] Another study validated flow parameters with the severity of cirrhosis and PHT.[47] PC imaging of the azygos vein is another promising technique for detecting high-risk esophageal varices in patients with PHT.[48] Mean azygos vein flow measures were significantly higher in subjects with cirrhosis than in subjects with chronic liver disease without cirrhosis.[48] A recent study showed significant correlation between four-dimensional MRI and Doppler US in velocities, flow volume, and vessel area with good image quality and low interobserver variability in patients with liver cirrhosis.[44]

T1 Mapping

Look-Locker imaging technique using GRE MRI sequences with inversion recovery pulse is used to quantify fibrosis. Images are obtained at the level of the porta hepatis (▶ Fig. 3.40). Precontrast prolonged T1 relaxation time in liver cirrhosis has been previously reported. However, T1 relaxation time before contrast is

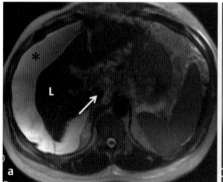

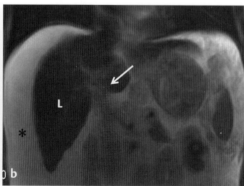

Fig. 3.38 A 62-year-old man with history of pancreatic cancer and cirrhosis. (a) Axial and coronal planes of T2-weighted images showing shrinkage of the liver parenchyma (L) with irregularity of the liver surface and the presence of significant ascites (*asterisk*). (b) The portal vein appears to be occluded because of increased signal, with cavernous transformation (*arrow*).

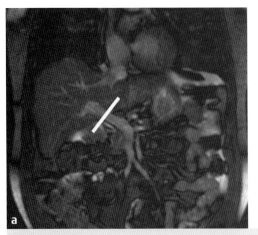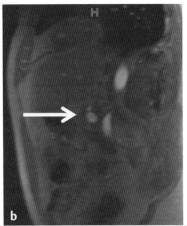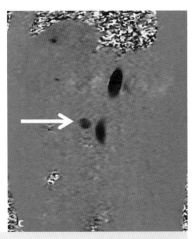

Fig. 3.39 Acquisition of phase contrast images. (**a**) Coronal image for localization of the portal vein (PV) to be obtained 1 cm below the bifurcation (*line*). The diameter of the PV is 13 mm. (**b**) Oblique sagittal image through the PV (*arrow*). (**c**) Phase-contrast image through the same location encoding for flow. A normal PV is demonstrated, with an average flow velocity of 9.5 cm/s.

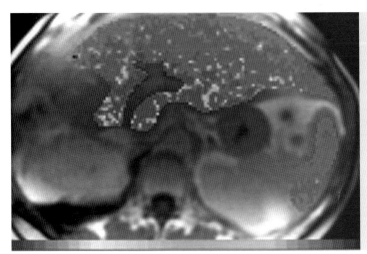

Fig. 3.40 Axial plane in a short modified look-locker inversion recovery (MOLLI) sequence after contrast administration, generating a color-coded T1 mapping in a patient with history of liver cirrhosis. T1 values show inverse correlation with the percentage of hepatic fibrosis.

not specific to liver cirrhosis.[49] A prior study showed that hepatic uptake with gadolinium ethoxybenzyl diethylenetriamine penta-acetic acid (Gd-EOB-DTPA) measuring signal intensity by T1 mapping in liver parenchyma can help to estimate liver function.[50] Quantification and comparison of the signal intensity by MRI needs further investigation with different contrast agents, and the necessity of a correction factor might be useful for different acquisition times. Also, T1 mapping requires further investigation to be compared with liver function test and histologic findings.

Magnetic Resonance Elastography

Magnetic resonance elastography (MRE) is a diagnostic tool used to assess the elasticity properties of the liver or spleen tissues. MRE is a modified PC GRE sequence that propagates shear waves through the liver produced by a piezoelectric device generating elastograms (▶ Fig. 3.41). Several studies have shown that MRE is an excellent tool for diagnosing advanced fibrosis and cirrhosis. Measuring liver stiffness using MRE can predict severe PHT

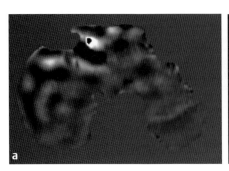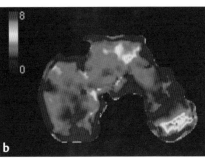

Fig. 3.41 Magnetic resonance elastography measures liver stiffness by acoustic waves (**a**) and a color-coded wave (**b**).

in chronic liver disease, viral hepatitis, or alcoholic cirrhosis in asymptomatic or compensated cirrhosis.[51-53] A previous study established a good correlation between portal pressure, HVPG, and spleen and liver stiffness in animals with PHT.[54] A more recent study showed that MRE of the spleen is a promising quantitative method for predicting the presence of esophageal varices in advanced chronic liver disease.[55] Liver and splenic stiffness measurements are useful new noninvasive techniques for assessing hepatic fibrosis and screening severe PHT. The average mean stiffness number should be reported in kilopascals (KPa); the normal value is less than 2.9 KPa for the liver.

Summary

Knowledge of normal anatomy and anomalies of the portal venous system can help to diagnose and manage PHT. Grayscale, Doppler, and spectral US are useful tools in the diagnosis and evaluation of liver parenchyma and portal circulation. Contrast-enhanced CT and MRI provide a comprehensive assessment of vascular anatomy, liver parenchymal and perfusion disorders, and complications associated with PHT such as portosystemic collateral circulation. In addition, novel MRI techniques can be used as noninvasive routine examination giving promising results and helping treatment decisions for patients with PHT.

Clinical Pearls

- Knowledge of normal portal anatomy and portal anomalies can help with the management of PHT.
- Doppler ultrasound is a useful tool for evaluating portal hemodynamics.
- Contrast-enhanced CT and MR provide a comprehensive assessment of portal vascular anatomy and portosystemic collaterals.
- MRI has the capability of evaluating hepatic parenchyma and its perfusion and compliance.
- Novel MRI techniques can help assess portal hemodynamics and help formulate a management decision.
- Most portosystemic collateral pathways are preexistent (potential connections) but grow in the setting of PHT.

References

1. Garcia-Tsao G. Portal hypertension. Curr Opin Gastroenterol 2003;19(3):250–258.
2. Garcia-Tsao G, Bosch J. Management of varices and variceal hemorrhage in cirrhosis. N Engl J Med 2010;362(9):823–832.
3. Treiber G, Csepregi A, Malfertheiner P. The pathophysiology of portal hypertension. Dig Dis 2005;23(1):6–10.
4. Villanueva C, Lopez-Balaguer JM, Aracil C, et al. Maintenance of hemodynamic response to treatment for portal hypertension and influence on complications of cirrhosis. J Hepatol 2004;40(5):757–765.
5. García-Pagán JC, Gracia-Sancho J, Bosch J. Functional aspects on the pathophysiology of portal hypertension in cirrhosis. J Hepatol 2012;57(2):458–461.
6. Arakawa M, Masuzaki T, Okuda K. Pathomorphology of esophageal and gastric varices. Semin Liver Dis 2002;22(1):73–82.
7. Arakawa M, Masuzaki T, Okuda K. Pathology of fundic varices of the stomach and rupture. J Gastroenterol Hepatol 2002;17(10):1064–1069.
8. Kim M, Mitchell DG, Ito K. Portosystemic collaterals of the upper abdomen: review of anatomy and demonstration on MR imaging. Abdom Imaging 2000; 25(5):462–470.
9. Kang HK, Jeong YY, Choi JH, et al. Three-dimensional multi-detector row CT portal venography in the evaluation of portosystemic collateral vessels in liver cirrhosis. Radiographics 2002;22(5):1053–1061.
10. Balfe DM, Mauro MA, Koehler RE, et al. Gastrohepatic ligament: normal and pathologic CT anatomy. Radiology 1984;150(2):485–490.
11. Moubarak E, Bouvier A, Boursier J, et al. Portosystemic collateral vessels in liver cirrhosis: a three-dimensional MDCT pictorial review. Abdom Imaging 2012;37(5):746–766.
12. Cho KC, Patel YD, Wachsberg RH, Seeff J. Varices in portal hypertension: evaluation with CT. Radiographics 1995;15(3):609–622.
13. Singal AK, Ahmad M, Soloway RD. Duplex Doppler ultrasound examination of the portal venous system: an emerging novel technique for the estimation of portal vein pressure. Dig Dis Sci 2010;55(5):1230–1240.
14. Bellamy EA, Bossi MC, Cosgrove DO. Ultrasound demonstration of changes in the normal portal venous system following a meal. Br J Radiol 1984;57(674): 147–149.
15. De Olivera IRS, Cerri GG. Ultra-Sonografia Abdominal, 2nd ed. São Paulo, Brazil, Revinters, 2002, p 65.
16. Pinto-Silva RA, Abrantes WL, Antunes CM, Lambertucci JR. Sonographic features of portal hypertension in schistosomiasis mansoni. Rev Inst Med Trop Sao Paulo 1994;36(4):355–361.
17. Cokkinos DD, Dourakis SP. Ultrasonographic assessment of cirrhosis and portal hypertension. Curr Med Imaging Rev 2009;5:62–70.
18. Killi RM. Doppler sonography of the native liver. Eur J Radiol 1999;32(1):21–35.
19. Robinson KA, Middleton WD, Al-Sukaiti R, et al. Doppler sonography of portal hypertension. Ultrasound Q 2009;25(1):3–13.
20. Wachsberg RH, Bahramipour P, Sofocleous CT, Barone A. Hepatofugal flow in the portal venous system: pathophysiology, imaging findings, and diagnostic pitfalls. Radiographics 2002;22(1):123–140.
21. Baik SK. Haemodynamic evaluation by Doppler ultrasonography in patients with portal hypertension: a review. 2010;30:1403–1413.
22. Baik SK, Kim JW, Kim HS, et al. Recent variceal bleeding: Doppler US hepatic vein waveform in assessment of severity of portal hypertension and vasoactive drug response. Radiology 2006;240(2):574–580.
23. Zironi G, Gaiani S, Fenyves D, et al. Value of measurement of mean portal flow velocity by Doppler flowmetry in the diagnosis of portal hypertension. J Hepatol 1992;16(3):298–303.
24. Haag K, Rossle M, Ochs A, et al. Correlation of duplex sonography findings and portal pressure in 375 patients with portal hypertension. AJR Am J Roentgenol 1999;172(3):631–635.
25. Schneider AW, Kalk JF, Klein CP. Hepatic arterial pulsatility index in cirrhosis: correlation with portal pressure. J Hepatol 1999;30(5):876–881.
26. Piscaglia F, Donati G, Cecilioni L, et al. Influence of the spleen on portal haemodynamics: a non-invasive study with Doppler ultrasound in chronic liver disease and haematological disorders. Scand J Gastroenterol 2002;37(10):1220–1227.
27. Berzigotti A, Casadei A, Magalotti D, et al. Renovascular impedance correlates with portal pressure in patients with liver cirrhosis. Radiology 2006;240(2): 581–586.
28. Nunez D, Russell E, Yrizarry J, et al. Portosystemic communications studied by transhepatic portography; Radiology 1978;127(1):75–79.
29. Subramanyam BR, Balthazar EJ, Madamba MR, et al. Sonography of portosystemic venous collaterals in portal hypertension. Radiology 1983;146(1):161–166.
30. Henseler KP, Pozniak MA, Lee FT Jr, Winter TC 3rd. Three-dimensional CT angiography of spontaneous portosystemic shunts. Radiographics 2001;21(3): 691–704.
31. Bosch J, Bordas JM, Rigau J, et al. Noninvasive measurement of the pressure of esophageal varices using an endoscopic gauge: comparison with measurements by variceal puncture in patients undergoing endoscopic sclerotherapy. Hepatology 1986;6(4):667–672.
32. Lane MJ, Jeffrey RB Jr, Katz DS. Spontaneous intrahepatic vascular shunts. AJR Am J Roentgenol 2000;174(1):125–131.
33. Park JH, Cha SH, Han JK, Han MC. Intrahepatic portosystemic venous shunt. AJR Am J Roentgenol 1990;155(3):527–528.
34. Okuda K, Benhamou J. Portal hypertension: Clinical and physiological aspects. Tokyo, Springer-Verlag, 1991, p 569.
35. De Gaetano AM, Lafortune M, Patriquin H, et al. Cavernous transformation of the portal vein: patterns of intrahepatic and splanchnic collateral circulation detected with Doppler sonography. AJR Am J Roentgenol 1995;165:1151–1155.
36. Gallego C, Velasco M, Marcuello P, et al. Congenital and acquired anomalies of the portal venous system. Radiographics 2002;22(1):141–159.
37. Lopez-Machado E, Mallorquin-Jimenez F, Medina-Benitez A, et al. Aneurysms of the portal venous system: ultrasonography and CT findings. Eur J Radiol 1998; 26:210–214.
38. Lee J, Kim KW, Lee H, et al. Semiautomated spleen volumetry with diffusion-weighted MR imaging. Magn Reson Med 2012;68(1):305–310.
39. Bezerra AS, D'Ippolito G, Faintuch S, et al. Determination of splenomegaly by CT: is there a place for a single measurement? AJR Am J Roentgenol 2005;184(5): 1510–1513.

40. Bolognesi M, Merkel C, Sacerdoti D, et al. Role of spleen enlargement in cirrhosis with portal hypertension. Dig Liver Dis 2002;34(2):144–150.

41. Kamel IR, Kruskal JB, Warmbrand G, et al. Accuracy of volumetric measurements after virtual right hepatectomy in potential donors undergoing living adult liver transplantation. AJR Am J Roentgenol 2001;176(2):483–487.

42. Williams DM, Cho KJ, Aisen AM, Eckhauser FE. Portal hypertension evaluated by MR imaging. Radiology 1985;157(3):703–706.

43. Shah TU, Semelka RC, Voultsinos V, et al. Accuracy of magnetic resonance imaging for preoperative detection of portal vein thrombosis in liver transplant candidates. Liver Transpl 2006;12(11):1682–1688.

44. Stankovic Z, Csatari Z, Deibert P, et al. Normal and altered three-dimensional portal venous hemodynamics in patients with liver cirrhosis. Radiology 2012;262(3):862–873.

45. Applegate GR, Thaete FL, Meyers SP, et al. Blood flow in the portal vein: velocity quantitation with phase-contrast MR angiography. Radiology 1993;187(1):253–256.

46. Kashitani N, Kimoto S, Tsunoda M, et al. Portal blood flow in the presence or absence of diffuse liver disease: measurement by phase contrast MR imaging. Abdom Imaging 1995;20(3):197–200.

47. Annet L, Materne R, Danse E, et al. Hepatic flow parameters measured with MR imaging and Doppler US: correlations with degree of cirrhosis and portal hypertension. Radiology 2003;229(2):409–414.

48. Gouya H, Vignaux O, Sogni P, et al. Chronic liver disease: systemic and splanchnic venous flow mapping with optimized cine phase-contrast MR imaging validated in a phantom model and prospectively evaluated in patients. Radiology 2011;261(1):144–155.

49. Thomsen C, Christoffersen P, Henriksen O, Juhl E. Prolonged T1 in patients with liver cirrhosis: an in vivo MRI study. Magn Reson Imaging 1990;8(5):599–604.

50. Katsube T, Okada M, Kumano S, et al. Estimation of liver function using T1 mapping on Gd-EOB-DTPA-enhanced magnetic resonance imaging. Invest Radiol 2011;46(4):277–283.

51. Friedrich-Rust M, Muller C, Winckler A, et al. Assessment of liver fibrosis and steatosis in PBC with FibroScan, MRI, MR-spectroscopy, and serum markers. J Clin Gastroenterol 2010;44(1):58–65.

52. Lemoine M, Katsahian S, Ziol M, et al. Liver stiffness measurement as a predictive tool of clinically significant portal hypertension in patients with compensated hepatitis C virus or alcohol-related cirrhosis. Aliment Pharmacol Ther 2008;28(9):1102–1110.

53. Vizzutti F, Arena U, Romanelli RG, et al. Liver stiffness measurement predicts severe portal hypertension in patients with HCV-related cirrhosis. Hepatology 2007;45(5):1290–1297.

54. Nedredal GI, Yin M, McKenzie T, et al. Portal hypertension correlates with splenic stiffness as measured with MR elastography. J Magn Reson Imaging 2011;34(1):79–87.

55. Talwalkar JA, Yin M, Venkatesh S, et al. Feasibility of in vivo MR elastographic splenic stiffness measurements in the assessment of portal hypertension. AJR Am J Roentgenol 2009;193(1):122–127.

Chapter 4: Indirect Portal Pressure Measurement and Carbon Dioxide Wedged Hepatic Portography

Bill S. Majdalany and Minhaj S. Khaja

Introduction

The development of portal hypertension and cirrhosis is the final common pathway for chronic liver diseases, resulting in ascites, hepatic encephalopathy, and massive variceal hemorrhage among many other clinical manifestations. Noninvasive imaging advances in ultrasound, magnetic resonance imaging (MRI), and computed tomography (CT) have markedly improved the assessment of these patients. In many cases, these imaging tools are routinely used for screening and morphological assessment of the hepatic parenchyma and vasculature. However, portal pressure measurement remains a vital tool in the management of patients with chronic liver disease and is typically performed in conjunction with a transjugular liver biopsy in the form of the hepatic venous pressure gradient (HVPG). Similarly, while wedged CO_2 portography is rarely used for diagnostic imaging of the portal veins, it maintains a crucial procedural role during TIPS placement. The rationale and technical aspects of indirect portal pressure measurement and wedged CO_2 portography will be discussed.

Indirect Portal Pressure Measurement

Historically, portal pressures were directly measured through surgical, percutaneous transhepatic, or transjugular catheterization of the portal vein. Given the invasive nature and associated procedural risks, direct portal pressure measurement was rarely performed. Publications in 1951 by Myers and Taylor and separately by Friedman and Weiner described occlusive hepatic venous catheterization in humans, cats, and dogs.[1-3] Advancing the catheter to the terminus of the hepatic venule transduces the sinusoidal pressure, which is termed the wedged hepatic venous pressure (WHVP), and is an indirect reflection of the portal venous pressure. However, because the WHVP can be spuriously elevated due to increased intraabdominal pressure, for example from ascites, the free hepatic venous pressure (FHVP) is also measured by retracting the catheter into a nonocclusive position within the vein. Subtracting the FHVP from the WHVP results in the hepatic venous pressure gradient (HVPG), which is not subject to intraabdominal pressure changes. In the forthcoming sections, technical considerations and prognostic implications are discussed.

Comparison of End-Hole and Balloon Catheters for HVPG Measurement

Indirect portal pressure can be measured by advancing any variety of end-hole catheters into a wedged position within a hepatic vein (▶ Fig. 4.1; ▶ Fig. 4.2). Functionally, the pressure measurements represent only a small area in the liver with smaller veins representing smaller areas of liver, and increased potential for discrepancy. Repeating measurements requires the end-hole catheter to be removed and then repositioned into the same vein. Moreover, an end-hole catheter may be subject to kinking or partial obstruction resulting in spurious values. In 1979,

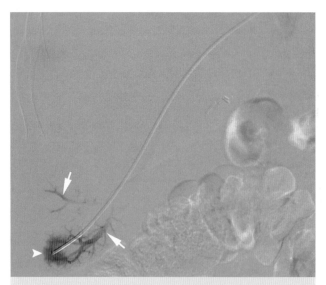

Fig. 4.1 Wedged end-hole catheter: Fluoroscopic image with an end-hole catheter in a wedged position. Iodinated contrast was hand injected to blush the hepatic parenchyma (*arrowhead*) with reflux across the hepatic sinusoids, opacifying portal radicals (*arrows*).

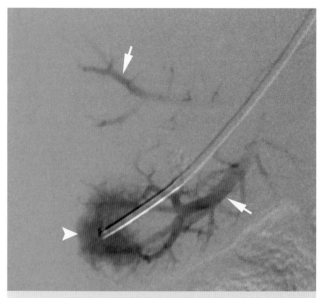

Fig. 4.2 Magnification wedged end-hole catheter. Magnification fluoroscopic image with an end-hole catheter in a wedged position. Iodinated contrast was hand injected to blush the hepatic parenchyma (*arrowhead*) with reflux across the hepatic sinusoids, opacifying portal radicals (*arrows*).

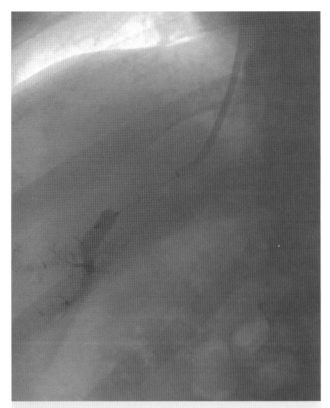

Fig. 4.3 Confirmation of balloon occlusion. Fluoroscopic image with the balloon inflated. After the wedged hepatic measurement was recorded and before deflating the balloon, contrast is injected to confirm that the balloon was occluding the hepatic vein.

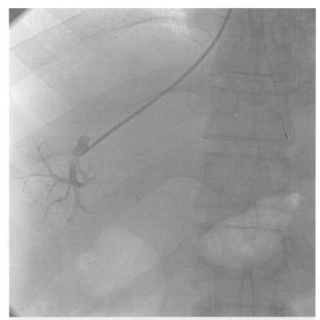

Fig. 4.4 Confirmation of balloon occlusion, a second example: Fluoroscopic image with a balloon occlusion catheter in a wedged position. Iodinated contrast was hand injected to confirm stasis in the hepatic vein. Care is taken not to reflux across the hepatic sinusoids.

Barth and Udoff reported on the use of balloon catheters for indirect portal pressure measurement.[4] Balloon catheters can occlude larger hepatic venous branches, allowing measurement of pressures across more sinusoids (▸ Fig. 4.3; ▸ Fig. 4.4). Repeat measurements are performed by deflating and inflating the balloon, providing reproducible measurements from the same area more easily.

Several studies have compared the reliability and reproducibility of indirect portal pressure measurements between end-hole and balloon catheters spanning over 40 years. Thalheimer and associates performed a meta-analysis of 11 studies on 320 patients over 44 years and ultimately found that wedged hepatic venous pressure did indeed reflect the portal venous pressure.[5] It is notable that 7 of the 11 studies used an end-hole catheter and that the 3 most recent studies were with the balloon technique.

The most recent studies comparing balloon with end-hole catheters for the measurement of HVPG were performed by Zipprich et al in 2010, Maleux et al in 2011, and Smith et al in 2011.[6-8] Zipprich et al compared the two methods head to head and noted that the assessment of the WHVP was the most striking weakness of the end-hole catheter. Moreover, they note the heterogeneity of liver disease and the possibility of sampling variability covering smaller areas of the liver and inherent peripheral positioning of the end-hole catheter to measure a WHVP as weaknesses of the technique. The balloon catheter produced more consistent results that were more closely correlated with the portal pressure.[6] Maleux et al compared end-hole catheter measurements with balloon catheter measurements and noted

that both corresponded well with a direct portal measurement. However, in this publication the agreement with direct portal pressure was "clearly much better" with the balloon catheter and there was more variability with the end-hole catheter measurements.[7] Smith et al noted significant overall differences between the two techniques, particularly in patients with fibrosis.[8] Overall differences in the HVPG were small. Collectively, these studies comprise nearly 300 patients and generally found improved accuracy, reproducibility, and reliability with occlusion balloon catheters versus end-hole catheters for the measurement of WHVP.

Technique

Performing the procedure in a reproducible manner in similar conditions is of paramount importance, particularly if a patient requires repeated measurements to monitor disease progression. Herein is a summary of the technique as published by Groszmann and Wongcharatrawee and reiterated in a separate publication by Groszmann, Vorobioff, and Gao.[9,10] Groszmann et al recommend a quartz pressure transducer, which has been calibrated against a known external pressure, and a recorder which can trace the pressure values at a slow recording speed of approximately 1-2 mm/s (▸ Fig. 4.5).

Using an occlusion balloon catheter and a scale measurement up to 30-40 mm Hg, the transducer should be positioned at the level of the right atrium in the mid-axillary line. The IVC pressure should be recorded; then the catheter can be advanced into the liver for measurement of the FHVP, WHVP, and mean pressure. Of note, the FHVP should be no more than 1 mm Hg greater than the IVC pressure (▸ Fig. 4.6). Moreover, when performing occlusion measurements, a check for total occlusion is performed at the end of the measurement by injecting contrast. The authors recommend pressure tracings to continue for 45 to 60 seconds,

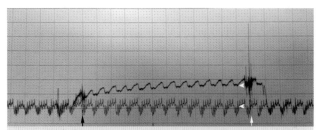

Fig. 4.5 Pressure tracing with free and wedged hepatic venous pressure. Pressure tracing strip shows a baseline pressure of the free hepatic vein. The balloon is inflated (*black arrow*) revealing a divergence between a wedged hepatic venous pressure (*top line*) and free hepatic venous pressure (*baseline*). The difference between the lines (*arrowheads*) is the hepatic venous pressure gradient. After deflating the balloon (*white arrow*) the two lines converge.

and measurements should be repeated at least three times to ensure reproducibility.

Generally, benzodiazepine sedatives will not significantly affect the accuracy of hepatic venous pressure measurements, though the patient should be similarly medicated each time if undergoing serial measurements.[11] In contradistinction, Reverter et al found that if patients were not awake and under deeper levels of sedation, as would be achieved with propofol and remifentanil, there would be increased variability and uncertainty of the

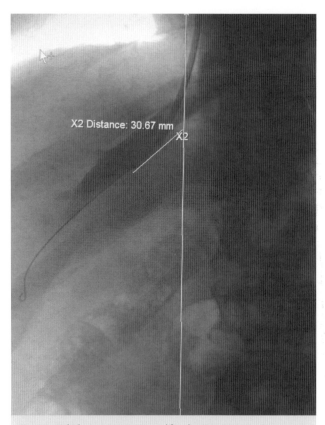

Fig. 4.6 Right hepatic venogram and free hepatic venous pressure. Fluoroscopic image of the sheath in the right hepatic vein, which is filled with iodinated contrast. The sheath tip is approximately 3 cm from a vertical white line, which demarcates the hepatic venous confluence with the inferior vena cava. Free hepatic venous measurements should be within 1 mm Hg of the IVC pressure.

measurements attributable both to a change in the respiratory pattern and the hemodynamic effects of the sedatives.[12]

The Use and Prognostic Implications of Indirect Portal Pressure Measurement

Indirect portal pressure measurement has added tremendously to the body of knowledge regarding the pathophysiology, treatment, and research regarding portal hypertension. Indirectly measuring the portal pressure not only is diagnostic of portal hypertension, but can help differentiate the underlying etiology. Normal portal pressure ranges between 1 and 5 mm Hg with values above 5 mm Hg reflecting increased resistance through the portal circuit, portal hypertension. The pattern of the acquired pressure measurements (FHVP, WHVP, and HVPG) in conjunction with biopsy can help differentiate portal hypertension into pre-hepatic, intra-hepatic, and post-hepatic etiologies with the large majority, viral hepatides, causing intra-hepatic portal hypertension. For instance, post-hepatic causes typically have elevation of the FHVP and WHVP, but a normal HVPG, while pre-hepatic etiologies will have a normal WHVP despite clinical signs of portal hypertension.[13,14]

However, the clinical utility of this value transcends strict diagnosis as it can provide important prognostic information in cirrhotics, predict the development of complications of portal hypertension, and monitor therapeutic response in portal hypertensives to support clinical decisions. D'Amico et al systematically reviewed 118 studies to evaluate the natural history and prognostic indicators of survival in cirrhotics, finding that measurement of the portal pressure was predictive of death in 67% of the studies.[15] For the manifestations of portal hypertension such as ascites and varices to develop, the threshold portal pressure of 10 mm Hg must be reached. Above a portal pressure of 12 mm Hg, the risk for variceal hemorrhage exists.[16,17] When diagnosed with portal hypertension, patients are treated with beta-blockers and nitrates to help decrease the portal pressure, thereby decreasing the risk of variceal hemorrhage.[18] Generally, a decrease of the HVPG by 20% is the goal of therapy, and monitoring the response with repeated HVPG measurements will delineate which patients may be nonresponders and warrant more aggressive therapy.[19,20]

Wedged CO_2 Portography

Historically, portography was performed either through visceral arteriography, a direct percutaneous transhepatic approach, or through wedged hepatic portography, which forces a contrast medium across the hepatic sinusoids in a retrograde manner (from hepatic venules through the sinusoids and refluxing back into the portal venules). Presently, neither arteriography nor direct percutaneous access is commonly performed for the sole purpose of imaging the portal vein. Refinements in ultrasound technology, MRI, and CT coupled with the wide availability of these exams allow rapid, accurate, and noninvasive assessments of the liver, portal veins, and flow dynamics. However, while wedged CO_2 portography is not considered an essential prerequisite for TIPS placement, it is routinely performed intraprocedurally prior to TIPS placement to evaluate and localize potential portal venous radicals thereby decreasing needle passes and procedure time.

Characteristics of Carbon Dioxide

Carbon dioxide is colorless, odorless, widely available, inexpensive, and safe. One of the important features of CO_2 as a gas contrast is that it is highly soluble and does not readily create long-lasting "air-locks," or rather, "gas-locks" in the studied area. Initially, CO_2 use as a venous contrast agent was described in the 1950s for the evaluation of pericardial effusion and since then it has been applied to many various interventional procedures including peripheral arterial disease, intra-abdominal hemorrhage, venous disease, abdominal aortic aneurysm repair, and TIPS placement among other procedures.[21,22] Cho studied the effects of various intravenous CO_2 volumes on cardiopulmonary parameters and confirmed that a single dose up to 1.6 cc/kg resulted in no adverse consequence, though caution should be exercised in patients with pulmonary hypertension. Because CO_2 is continuously produced and exhaled, the small volumes needed for imaging can be repeatedly injected every 30 seconds to 60 seconds. Moreover, as an endogenously produced substance, CO_2 poses no risk of allergy, hepatotoxicity, or nephrotoxicity. This is of particular importance when considering that many patients with vascular or liver disease may be susceptible to contrast induced nephrotoxicity either from impaired renal function or depletion of their intravascular volume.[23]

Key characteristics of CO_2 gas compared with other contrast agents include its buoyancy, low viscosity, and high solubility. Although CO_2 rapidly dissolves in blood and is quickly cleared, it does not mix with blood in the same manner as iodinated contrast would. Instead, because CO_2 is buoyant, it remains in the anti-dependent position, floating anterior to blood in a supine patient. With digital subtraction techniques, this displacement of blood decreases the intravascular density and results in a negative contrast image. Taken together with low viscosity and high solubility, these properties allow rapid reflux of large volumes across the hepatic sinusoids. Any extravasation of CO_2 is cleared quickly, and because it is a negative contrast agent, any residual CO_2 does not create a parenchymal stain which may obscure wires or catheters.[24] However, because CO_2 is buoyant and is of low viscosity and thus can reflux readily, CO_2 portography is not reflective of portal hemodynamics (for example, whether the portal flow is petal or fugal).

Preparation and Use of CO_2

Several delivery systems exist for CO_2 injection ranging from simple syringe hand injection, automatic and mechanical injectors, to prepackaged carbon dioxide kits from multiple vendors. Two technical challenges in the handling and delivery of this gas are present: air contamination and "explosive delivery" during hand injection.[22,25,26] In serial publications, Hawkins and Caridi described the essential components of a modified plastic bag system with an O-ring, syringe, stopcocks and connectors, and medical grade CO_2 cylinder.[27,28] This system allows controlled delivery and decreases potential contamination with room air. The plastic bag is purged three times through the O-ring filter with medical grade CO_2 and will subsequently serve as the CO_2 reservoir. The reservoir is connected with a three-way stopcock and connectors to a 50-mL syringe and connector tubing. CO_2 from the reservoir is used to fill the syringe and purge the air out of the tubing, which is attached to a second three-way stopcock and then connected to the angiographic catheter. At the second

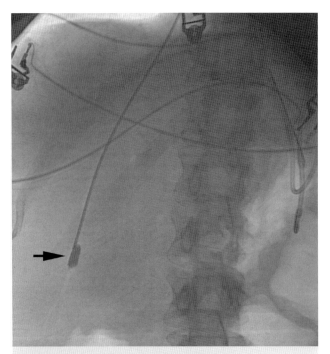

Fig. 4.7 Wedging of balloon occlusion catheter prior to CO_2 portography. Fluoroscopic image of a balloon occlusion catheter (*black arrow*) with the balloon inflated in the distal right hepatic vein. Balloon occlusion is performed in preparation of CO_2 injection.

three-way stopcock, it is crucial to elicit a small amount of back bleeding from the catheter and then to purge the blood from the catheter with CO_2. This step functions to minimize the "explosive delivery" or "sudden give" that is noted when CO_2 hand injection is performed. If the catheter is full of fluid, a forceful injection of CO_2 is required to clear the fluid because CO_2 is compressible. Upon clearing the catheter, the "sudden give" is felt as there is a rapid expansion of the CO_2 and "explosive delivery" is realized. Priming the catheter as described allows for controlled, direct, and gentle injections of CO_2.[22,25] Digital subtraction angiography is performed at three to four frames per second. Stacking of images and inversion imaging is also used to increase the sensitivity and specificity of CO_2 imaging[24] (▶ Fig. 4.7; ▶ Fig. 4.8).

Comparison of Iodinated Contrast with CO_2

To image the portal veins angiographically, one of three techniques can be employed: indirect portography through superior mesenteric and splenic arteriography with delayed imaging, percutaneous transhepatic access and direct injection of the portal veins, or reflux of contrast across the sinusoids from the hepatic to the portal veins during wedged hepatic venography (WHV) (▶ Fig. 4.9).

Martinez-Cuesta et al compared WHV with indirect arterial portography and concluded that CO_2 WHV was safe and effective, demonstrating the main portal vein in 90%, the right portal vein in 95%, and the left portal vein in 90% of patients. The superior mesenteric vein, splenic vein, gastroesophageal varices, and splenorenal shunts were visualized in less than 65% of patients.[29] However, it is important to note that arteriography is rarely if ever performed at the time of TIPS placement and would add both the

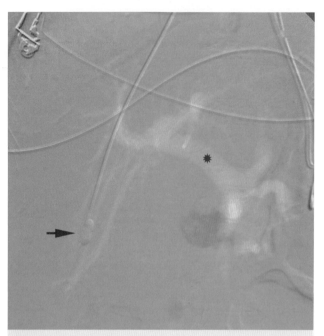

Fig. 4.8 Digital subtraction CO_2 portogram: balloon occlusion catheter (*black arrow*) with balloon inflated. Approximately 50 cc of CO_2 was hand injected and refluxed across the sinusoids to fill the main portal vein (*star*) and beyond.

risk and delay associated with an additional procedure. Similarly, percutaneous transhepatic portography is not performed during TIPS placement routinely and would pose additional risk with little if any benefit to the patient.

During WHV, a contrast medium can be gently hand injected to opacify the sinusoids and portal venous structures. Various

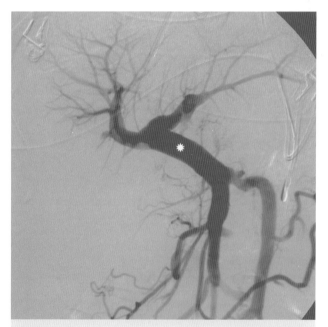

Fig. 4.9 Transjugular intrahepatic portogram. A transjugular intrahepatic access was gained from the right hepatic vein to the right portal vein. Iodinated contrast was injected to fill to portal system. The main portal vein (*star*) is well visualized and correlates to the CO_2 portogram.

contrasts have been injected, the most common being iodinated contrasts and CO_2, and subsequently studies comparing the media have emerged. Rees et al reported successful visualization of the portal system in 10 of 12 patients prior to TIPS.[30] Sheppard and associates compared CO_2 and iodinated contrast WHV during the placement of TIPS and concluded that in all three cases CO_2 was quick, effective, and should be used more frequently during TIPS.[31] Yang et al retrospectively evaluated 43 TIPS patients for the identification of the portal vein between CO_2 and iodinated contrast WHV and concluded that CO_2 was more likely to correctly and completely identify the portal vein.[32] Debernardi-Venon et al compared iodinated contrast with CO_2 WHV in 100 patients undergoing an evaluation of portal hypertension.[33] They noted that CO_2 WHV yielded markedly superior visualization of the portal venous system noting that the portal system was better visualized by CO_2. Krajina et al confirmed the superiority of CO_2 over iodinated contrast during TIPS placement, retrospectively comparing 36 patients who underwent iodinated contrast WHV and 45 patients who underwent CO_2 WHV prior to TIPS.[34] In the iodinated contrast cohort, the portal vein bifurcation was visualized in 25% of patients, while in the CO_2 cohort, the portal vein bifurcation was visualized in 87% of patients. Most recently, Maleux and associates compared pre-TIPS CO_2 WHV with direct catheter portography after TIPS creation in 163 patients.[35] While they concluded that CO_2 was safe, efficient, and reliable in identifying the right and left portal veins, it could not opacify the entire portal trunk as well as direct catheter portography.

Complications of Wedged CO_2 Portography

With respect to venography, no report of gas embolism is present. As discussed earlier, caution should be taken in patients who have respiratory disease as they may not be able to clear CO_2 readily. When in doubt, arterial blood gas should be checked between injections, which may also be separated by greater intervals of time.[23,36] Small case series have described severe liver injury during the performance of wedged CO_2 venography at the time of TIPS placement. During the placement of TIPS, Rees et al reported on inconsequential small subcapsular hematomas from the extravasation of CO_2 gas. Semba et al, Kantermann et al, and Theuerkauf et al each published cases of patients who suffered hepatic lacerations during wedged CO_2 portography prior to TIPS placement, and collectively the increased risk of laceration was attributed to patient coagulopathy, the presence of ascites, and the over-injection of CO_2 distally in the hepatic vein within 2 cm of the hepatic capsule.[37–39] Anecdotally, these hepatic capsular lacerations are not uncommonly fatal or near fatal especially in the setting of coagulopathy. Hepatic vein embolization and quick TIPS-creation (to divert blood away from the hepatic parenchyma) is recommended without delay.

References

1. Taylor WJ, Myers JD. Studies on pressures in an occluded hepatic venule and their possible relationship to portal venous pressure. Am J Med 1951;11:251.
2. Myers JD, Taylor WJ. An estimation of portal venous pressure by occlusive catheterization of an hepatic venule. J Clin Invest 1951;30:662.
3. Friedman EW, Weiner RS. Estimation of hepatic sinusoid pressure by means of venous catheter and estimation of portal pressure by hepatic vein catheterization. Am J Phys 1951;166:527.

4. Barth KH, Udoff EJ. Transfemoral balloon catheterization for hepatic wedge pressure measurements. Radiology 1980;135:779–780.

5. Thalheimer U, Leandro G, Samonakis DN, Triantos CK, Patch D, Burroughs AK. Assessment of the agreement between wedge hepatic vein pressure and portal vein pressure in cirrhotic patients. Dig Liver Dis 2005;37:601–608.

6. Zipprich A, Winkler M, Seufferlein T, Donllinger MM. Comparison of balloon vs. straight catheter for the measurement of portal hypertension. Ailment Pharmacol Ther 2010;32:1351–1356.

7. Maleux G, Willems E, Fieuws S, et al. Prospective study comparing different indirect methods to measure portal pressure. J Vasc Interv Radiol 2011;22: 1553–1558.

8. Smith TP, Kim CY, Smith AD, et al. Hepatic venous pressure measurements: comparison of end-hole and balloon catheter methods. *J Vasc Interv Radiol* 2012;23(2):219–226, e6.

9. Groszmann RJ, Wongcharatrawee S. The hepatic venous pressure: anything worth doing should be done right. Hepatology 2004;39:280–282.

10. Groszmann R, Vorobioff JD, Gao H. Measurement of portal pressure: when, how, and why to do it. Clin Liver Dis 2006;10:499–512.

11. Steinlauf AF, Guadalupe G, Zakko MF, et al. Low-dose Midazolam sedation: An option for patients undergoing serial hepatic venous pressure measurements. Hepatology 1999;29:1070–1073.

12. Reverter E, Blasi A, Abraldes JG, et al. Impact of deep sedation on the accuracy of hepatic and portal venous pressure measurements in patients with cirrhosis. Liver Int 2014;34:16–25.

13. Groszmann RJ, Atterbury CE. The pathophysiology of portal hypertension: a basis for classification. Semin Liver Dis 1982;2:177–186.

14. Vorobioff J, Groszmann RJ, Picabea E, et al. Prognostic value of hepatic venous pressure measurement in alcoholic cirrhosis: a ten year prospective study. Gastro 1996;111:701–9.

15. D'Amico G, Garcia-Tsao G, Pagliaro L. Natural history and prognostic indicators of survival in cirrhosis: a systematic review of 118 studies. J Hepatol 2006; Jan;44(1):217–231.

16. Viallet A, Marleau D, Huet M, et al. Hemodynamic evaluation of patients with intrahepatic portal hypertension. Relationship between bleeding varices and the portohepatic gradient. Gastroenterology 1975;69:1297–1300.

17. Garcia-Tsao G, Groszmann RJ, Fisher RL, et al. Portal pressure, presence of gastroesophageal varices and variceal bleeding. Hepatology 1985;5:419–424.

18. Albraldes JG, Tarantino I, Turnes J, et al. Hemodynamic response to pharmacological treatment of portal hypertension and long-term prognosis of cirrhosis. Hepatology 2004;37:902–8.

19. Villanueva C, Aracil C, Colomo A, et al. Acute hemodynamic response to beta-blockers and prediction of long-term outcome in primary prophylaxis of variceal bleeding. Gastroenterology 2009 Jul;137(1):119–28.

20. D'Amico G, Pagliaro L, Bosch J. Pharmacological treatment of portal hypertension: an evidence-based approach. Semin Liver Dis 1999;19:475–505.

21. Paul RE, Durant TM, Oppenheimer MJ, Stauffer HM. Intravenous carbon dioxide intracardiac gas contrast in the roentgen diagnosis of pericardial effusion and thickening. *Am J Roentgenol RadiumTher Nucl Med* 1957;78(2):24–225.

22. Hawkins IF Jr, Caridi JG. Carbon dioxide (CO_2) digital subtraction angiography: 26-year experience at the University of Florida. Euro Radiol 1998;3:391–402.

23. Cho KJ. CO_2 as a venous contrast agent: safety and tolerance. In: KJ Cho, IF Hawkins, eds. *Carbon Dioxide Angiography: Principles, Techniques and Practices*. New York: Informa Healthcare; 2007:37–44.

24. Cho KJ. CO_2 for wedged hepatic venography. In: KJ Cho, IF Hawkins, eds. *Carbon Dioxide Angiography: Principles, Techniques and Practices*. New York: Informa Healthcare; 2007:171–80.

25. Kerns SR, Hawkins IF Jr. Carbon dioxide digital subtraction angiography: Expanding applications and technical evolution. AJR 1995;164:735–41.

26. Cho KJ, Cho DR, Hawkins IF Jr. Potential air contamination during CO_2 angiography using a hand-held syringe. Theoretical considerations and gas chromatography. Cardiovasc Interv Radiol 2006;29:637–41.

27. Hawkins IF Jr, Caridi JG, Kerns SR. Plastic bag delivery system for hand injection of carbon dioxide. AJR 1995;165:1487–9.

28. Hawkins IF Jr, Caridi JG, Klioze SD, et al. Modified plastic bag system with O-ring fitting connection for carbon dioxide angiography. AJR 2001;176:229–32.

29. Martinez-Cuesta A, Elduayen B, Vivas I, et al. CO_2 wedged hepatic venography: technical considerations and comparison with direct and indirect portography with iodinated contrast. Abdom Imaging 2000;25:576–582.

30. Rees CR, Niblitt RL, Lee SP, Diamond NG, Crippin JS. Use of carbon dioxide as a contrast medium for transjugular approach for intrahepatic portosystemic shunt placement. J Vasc Interv Radiol 1994;5:383–386.

31. Sheppard DG, Moss J, Miller M. Imaging of the portal vein during transjugular intrahepatic portosystemic shunt procedures: A comparison of carbon dioxide and iodinated contrast. Clin Radiol 1998;53:448–50.

32. Yang L, Bettmann MA. Identification of the portal vein: Wedge hepatic venography with CO_2 or iodinated contrast medium. Acad Radiol 1999;6:89–93.

33. Debernardi-Venon W, Bandi JC, Garcia-Pagan JC, et al. CO_2 wedged hepatic venography in the evaluation of portal hypertension. Gut 2000;46:856–860.

34. Krajina A, Lojik M, Chovanec V, et al. Wedged hepatic venography for targeting the portal vein during TIPS: Comparison of carbon dioxide and iodinated contrast agents. Cardiovasc Interv Radiol 2002;25:171–175.

35. Maleux G, Nevens F, Heye S, et al. The use of carbon dioxide wedged hepatic venography to identify the portal vein: Comparison with direct catheter portography with iodinated contrast medium and analysis of predictive factors influencing level of opacification. J Vasc Interv Radiol 2006;17:1771–1779.

36. Caridi JG, Hawkins IF Jr. CO_2 digital subtraction angiography: Potential complications and their prevention. J Vasc Interv Radiol 1997;8:383–91.

37. Semba CP, Saperstein L, Nymann U, Dake MD. Hepatic laceration from wedged venography performed before transjugular intrahepatic portosystemic shunt placement. J Vasc Interv Radiol 7:143–146.

38. Kantermann RY. Hepatic laceration from wedged venography transjugular intrahepatic protosystemic shunt placement: One survivor. J Vasc Interv Radiol 7:776–777.

39. Theuerkauf I, Strunk H, Brensing KA, Schild HH, Pfeifer U. Infarction and laceration of liver parenchyma caused by wedged CO_2 venography before TIPS insertion. Cardiovasc Intervent Radiol 2001;Jan-Feb;24(1):64–7.

Chapter 5: Hemodynamic Evaluation of the Liver and Transjugular Liver Biopsy

George Behrens and Hector Ferral

Introduction

Because portal hypertension (PHT) is the earliest and most important consequence of cirrhosis and underlies most of the clinical complications of the disease, hemodynamic evaluation of the liver carries the most useful and critical information to diagnose, stratify their risks, and monitor of the efficacy of medical treatment of these patients.[1] Recent studies have shown that measurement of hepatic venous pressure gradient (HVPG) has a greater diagnostic accuracy than liver biopsy in the diagnosis of cirrhosis even though liver biopsy remains the "gold standard" in the diagnosis of cirrhosis.[2]

Transjugular catheterization of a hepatic vein with measurement of the HVPG is considered the gold standard method to determine the portal pressure in clinical practice.[3,4] It is calculated as the difference between the wedged hepatic venous pressure (WHVP) optimally obtained by an inflated catheter balloon in the mid or distal hepatic vein and the free hepatic venous pressure (FHVP) with the balloon deflated.[1-3] This method, in the absence of presinusoidal obstruction, indirectly reflects the portal pressure.

Several longitudinal studies have shown that WHVP provides an accurate estimation of the portal pressure in alcoholic and viral related cirrhosis.[1,5,7,13] Thus, the HVPG has a greater diagnostic accuracy than liver biopsy in the diagnosis of cirrhosis. In addition to the degree of PHT, the HVPG provides an excellent tool to evaluate response to the pharmacologic and nonpharmacologic interventions as well to reliably predict the outcomes in patients with cirrhosis-related PHT.[10-12]

In addition to the hemodynamic pressure measurements, other procedures can be performed during hepatic vein catheterization. These procedures include transjugular liver biopsy (which is discussed at the end of this chapter), CO_2 portography, and right heart catheterization in suspected congestive hepatopathy or investigation of cardiopulmonary complications caused by cirrhosis.

The most frequent procedure performed in conjunction with pressure measurement is transjugular liver biopsy (TJLB).[14,15] In the past, aspiration specimens obtained by a transjugular approach were considered to be inferior or less satisfactory compared with the percutaneous approach because they were smaller and more fragmented.[16] However, with the improvement and widespread use of new Tru-Cut type needles and technique improvement, the samples are now considered equal for the diagnosis and almost comparable for staging and grading chronic liver disease.[14,17]

Hemodynamic Evaluation of the Liver

Material Required for the Procedure

- Ultrasound machine with linear array probe
- State-of-the-art angiography suite
- Micropuncture set (Cook Medical, Bloomington, IN) or 18-gauge access needle
- 9-French × 35-cm bright tip or 10-Fr × 45-cm flexor vascular sheath
- 180-cm × 135-cm Bentson guidewire (Cook Medical)
- 6.5-Fr flow-directed balloon catheter made by Cook Medical
- 8.5- to 11.5-mm, 6-Fr Berenstein occlusion balloon catheter (Boston Scientific, Natick, MA)
- Pressure transducer system

Preprocedure Preparation

- Obtain informed consent.
- Ensure no contrast allergy; otherwise, CO_2 can be used as contrast media; ensure a platelet count greater than 50,000/µL.
- The patient should have nothing by mouth for 4 to 6 hours before the procedure.
- Coagulation profile: platelets: should be greater than 5000 to 10,000; international normalized ratio should be less than 3.0 to 3.5.

Technique

1. **Sedation:** Almost all cases can be done with conscious sedation, providing comfort during the procedure. General anesthesia could be used in claustrophobic or pediatric patients. Conscious sedation is obtained with midazolam, up to 0.02 mg/kg at 0.5- to 1-mg increments, and fentanyl, 0.05 to 2 g/kg at 25 to 50 mcg per increment, and is generally well tolerated. Higher doses of midazolam or deep sedation significantly alter pressure measurements.

2. **Monitoring:** As recommended by the American Society of Anesthesia, all patients should be monitored for blood pressure, heart rate, oxygen saturation, end-tidal CO_2, and electrocardiography. Cardiac ectopies and arrhythmias have been reported during catheterization of the hepatic veins, particularly in patients with electrolyte abnormalities.

3. **Venous access:** Venous access is obtained under real-time ultrasound guidance using a micropuncture access needle set (Cook Medical) or an 18-gauge needle. At our institution, all access is obtained using a micropuncture access set. The right jugular vein (RJV) has been the main vessel access. The theory behind supported by straighter anatomy for the access of the hepatic veins in comparison with the left IJ. However, our unpublished experience shows no significant difference. Right internal jugular vein obstruction may become a problem in patients with end-stage renal disease or previous history of RJV catheterization; in these cases, alternative access such as the external jugular, left internal jugular, or subclavian approach should be used. In these circumstances, the patients usually just are slightly more uncomfortable requiring more sedation. After venous access is obtained, a 9-Fr, 45-cm bright tip or 10-Fr flexor vascular sheath (Cook Medical) is advanced over a 0.035-inch

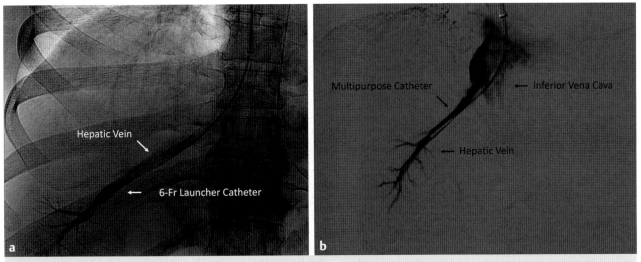

Fig. 5.1 (a) Hepatic vein catheterization. Frontal spot view venogram demonstrates the use of a reverse curve catheter (Launcher) to gain access in a middle hepatic vein. Catheterization of this vein had been attempted with a multipurpose catheter but had failed. (**b**) Hepatic venogram. Posterior-anterior projection (PA) digital subtraction venogram demonstrates a patent middle hepatic vein. Note the more central and caudal course of this vein.

guidewire into the inferior vena cava (IVC). It is always recommended to exclude the presence of an IVC filter before advancing the guidewire. There are some reports in the literature of IVC filter migration and guidewire entrapment within a filter.

4. **Hepatic vein catheterization:** A 5-Fr multipurpose catheter is then used to perform selective catheterization of the right or middle hepatic vein. When the access into the hepatic veins is difficult given the patient anatomy or in overweight or transplanted patients, reverse-curve catheters such as AL-1.5 6-Fr Guiding Launcher, 5-Fr Simmons-1 Cobra, or even, a Shetty catheter is recommended. Our personal experience shows that the 6-Fr Launcher catheter is the best catheter to obtain access into the hepatic vein after failure of a multipurpose catheter (▸ Fig. 5.1A).

5. **Hepatic venogram:** A hepatic venogram is suggested to confirm the position and the patency of the selected hepatic vein (▸ Fig. 5.1B). The multipurpose catheter is then exchanged for an occlusion balloon catheter, and wedge hepatic and free hepatic venous pressures are then obtained. The balloon catheter is positioned at the mid hepatic vein level, estimated by the hepatic vein venogram (▸ Fig. 5.2). If the hepatic vein is extremely large in diameter, then the catheter is positioned more distally.

6. **Transducer calibration:** Most transducers come precalibrated. The transducer is placed at the level of the heart, preferably at an approximate level of the mid right atrium. With transducer open to air (zero pressure), adjust the transducer to read zero.

7. **Pressure tracings and scale:** Permanent records should be captured either on paper or electronically. Use an appropriate scale for venous pressure measurements (full range up to 50 mm Hg) with appropriate visualization of the baseline because the normal right atrial pressure could be from –5 mm Hg.

8. **FHVP:** The FHVP is measured by maintaining the tip of the catheter "free" in the mid hepatic vein. The FHVP should be close to IVC pressure; if the difference between these

pressure values is more than 2 mm Hg, it is likely that the catheter is inadequately placed. In these cases, IVC pressure should be used for calculating HVPG.

9. **WHVP:** The WHVP is measured by occluding the hepatic vein, either by "wedging" the catheter into a small branch of a hepatic vein or by inflating a balloon-catheter. Occlusion of the hepatic vein by inflating a balloon is preferred because the volume of the liver circulation transmitting portal pressure is much larger than that attained by wedging the catheter. This reduces the variability of the measurements. Adequate occlusion of the hepatic vein is confirmed by slowly injecting 5 mL of contrast into the vein with the balloon

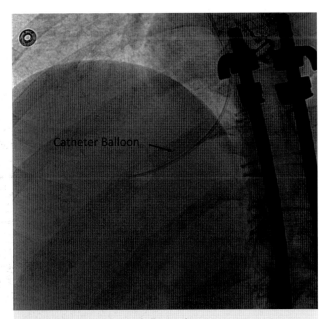

Fig. 5.2 Wedge position on a balloon catheter. Posterior-anterior projection (PA) spot film demonstrates the occlusion-balloon catheter inflated with air. The catheter is positioned in a central location within the right hepatic vein.

45

inflated. No reflux of the contrast or washout through communications with other hepatic veins should be observed. Otherwise, WHVP might underestimate portal pressure.

10. **Number of pressure measurements:** All measurements should be taken at least in three times. The final value is calculated as the mean of these measurements.

Complications

Overall, the hemodynamic evaluation of the liver is a really safe procedure with almost no major complications.[15] Minor complications reported are infrequent and include bleeding and/or hematoma at the puncture site. Most reported major complications are caused by the transjugular liver biopsy part rather than hemodynamic evaluation.[17]

Interpretation of the Hepatic Venous Pressure Gradient

Hepatic venous pressure gradient measurement has evolved from diagnostic purposes to be considered the most reliable tool to assess the severity, prognosis, and response to treatment of chronic liver disease and liver cirrhosis, including the risk of the complications such as ascites, variceal bleeding, encephalopathy, and hepatorenal syndrome.[9] Because the HVPG is a strong and independent predictor of outcomes in both compensated and decompensated cirrhosis, a new clinical classification system of cirrhosis that incorporates histologic, clinical, hemodynamic, and biologic features has been developed (▶ Table 5.1). This new classification is necessary for overcoming the limitation of prematurely concluding cirrhosis as an end stage of chronic liver disease. This system classified the distinction of compensation and decompensation, which is mainly defined by clinical outcome.[4] This classification uses the METAVIR scoring system to stage the degree of fibrosis found on the liver specimens, from no fibrosis as F0 to cirrhosis as F4. F1 to F3 are considered different degrees of fibrosis in the periportal regions to bridging fibrosis between the portal tracts.

Multiple studies have been shown that an HVPG greater than 10 mm Hg correlates with the presence of gastroesophageal varices.[1,2,4] Ripoll et al found that HVPG of 10 mm Hg or greater predicts the likelihood of developing hepatic decompensation in 40%

at 4 years and development of hepatocellular carcinoma (HCC).[18,19] For this reason, the term "clinically significant PHT" has been recognized when the HVPG is greater than 10 mm Hg. Patients with compensated cirrhosis gain 10% risk of decompensation at 5 years for each 1-mm Hg increase of the HVPG.[18,20]

The HVPG is also important in patients with decompensated cirrhosis, providing the mortality risk during the following years. In the patient with an acute variceal hemorrhage, a gradient of more than 20 mm Hg is an independent predictor of rebleeding and death.[12,21] For this reason, 16 mm Hg is considered the optimum cutoff value in decompensated cirrhosis.[6,22]

In patients with compensated cirrhosis, a gradient of 10 mm Hg or more is an independent predictor for developing HCC with a sixfold increased risk compared with patients with a gradient less than 10 mm Hg.[19] The gradient also has an important role in the treatment of HCC. In patients with compensated cirrhosis with a resectable HCC, the presence of a gradient greater than 10 mm Hg markedly increases the risk of hepatic decompensation 3 months after surgery. For this reason, surgical resection for HCC is reserved only in patients without clinically significant PHT (HVPG <10 mm Hg).[23]

Variceal bleeding occurs when HVPG is greater than 12 mm Hg. Longitudinal studies have demonstrated that if the gradient decreases to less than 12 mm Hg or at least 20% from the baseline by medical treatment (drug therapy), spontaneously, or by a transjugular intrahepatic portosystemic shunt (TIPS) procedure, the variceal bleeding is prevented, and varices decrease in size.[24,25] In patients who survive a variceal bleeding episode, the reduction of the gradient less than 12 mm Hg or more than 20% from the baseline is the strongest independent predictor of protection from subsequent bleeding episode, as well as other PHT-related complications such as ascites, spontaneous bacterial peritonitis, or hepatorenal syndrome. Two studies have shown that evaluation of the acute HVPG response to intravenous administration of propranolol is a practical tool in predicting the efficacy of nonselective beta-blockers in preventing variceal bleeding.[26,27] The acute HVPG response to propranolol was independently associated with survival in these patients.

Transjugular Liver Biopsy

Despite rapidly improving serologic, biomolecular testing, and noninvasive methods to assess the degree of cirrhosis, liver

Table 5.1 Clinical Stages of Cirrhosis and Portal Hypertension

Classification			Stages		
METAVIR	F1–F3	F4	F4	F4	F4
HVPG (mm Hg)		> 6	> 10	> 12	> 16
Clinical class		Stage 1	Stage 2	Stage 3	Stage 4
	No cirrhosis	Compensated	Compensated	Decompensated	Decompensated
			Varices	Variceal bleeding Ascites Encephalopathy	Variceal bleeding Ascites Encephalopathy Bacterial infection Hepatorenal syndrome
1-yr mortality rate (%)		1	3	10–30	60–100

HVPG: hepatic venous pressure gradient.

Box 5.1 Indications for Transjugular Liver Biopsy

Hemodynamic evaluation
Coagulopathy
Ascites
Massive adipose patients
Follow-up after liver transplant

Box 5.2 Contraindications for Transjugular Liver Biopsy

No clear contraindications
Lack of patent central veins (jugular veins or subclavian)
Assessing focal liver lesions

biopsy still considered the "gold standard" for the evaluation of acute and chronic liver diseases. Histologic assessment provides critical prognostic information and is frequently pivotal in therapeutic decisions not only for diagnosis but also to assess progression and response to therapy of chronic liver diseases.

Since Paul Elrich in 1883 described the first liver biopsy aspirate, several approaches have been developed to obtain liver tissue, including open surgical biopsy, percutaneous with or without image guidance (ultrasonography or computed tomography), laparoscopic, or transjugular. A transjugular approach was proposed by Dotter in 1964 in an experimental model,[28] and it was not until 1967 when the first case was performed by Hanafee et al.[29]

For most of the individuals, liver biopsy is safely and efficiently performed by the standard percutaneous approach. However, in patients with advanced liver disease with or without coagulopathy, for whom liver biopsy findings may be most critical and the associated risk of percutaneous approach carries an unacceptable bleeding risk, the transjugular approach becomes an excellent method to obtain tissue diagnosis.

Transjugular liver biopsy consists of obtaining liver tissue through a rigid cannula introduced into one of the hepatic veins via the jugular approach, which reduces the risk of intraabdominal hemorrhage after biopsy because the liver capsule is not violated and any bleeding resulting from the biopsy needle will drain into the hepatic veins.

This procedure was originally indicated in patients who had a contraindication to percutaneous biopsy such as those with a coagulopathy, including ascites,[17,30] acute liver failure,[31] large amount of adipose tissue, congenital clotting disorders,[32,33] and after liver transplantation. Currently, the main indication for TJLB is the possibility of being performed during the hemodynamic evaluation of the liver,[33] diminishing the added risk of a percutaneous liver biopsy (▶ Box 5.1).

There are no clear contraindications for a transjugular approach; however, it is not recommended during evaluation of focal liver masses or if there is a known history of central venous occlusion (▶ Box 5.2).

Materials

- Transjugular liver biopsy kit system. The LABS-100 or LABS-200 set with its either 18- or 19-gauge Quick-Core needle made by Cook Medical or the TLAB system also with its 18- or 19-gauge Flexcore needle recently acquired by Argon Medical Devices (Athens, TX). These two sets are Food and Drug Administration approved for this purpose. Both systems contain the following materials:
  - 7-Fr × 49-cm plastic sheath over angled metal sheath stiffener
  - 5-Fr multipurpose catheter for hepatic vein catheterization
  - 8-Fr dilator

Transjugular Liver Biopsy Technique

After completing the hemodynamic evaluation and in cases when liver tissue is required for a complete assessment of the liver or portal disease, a transjugular liver biopsy can be performed. This procedure can be safely performed in no more than 10 minutes.

1. **Cannula placement for biopsy:** The occlusion balloon placed for the estimation of the HVPG is removed over a wire, and the TJLB guiding cannula is advanced distally into the selected hepatic vein. In some instances, a guidewire with more support is required to advance the rigid cannula into the hepatic vein. A 0.035-in × 135-cm Rosen or even a super-stiff Amplatz guidewire is suggested (▶ Fig. 5.3).

2. **Needle biopsy:** Next, the liver samples are obtained using the selected TJLB needle system. It is important to remember the orientation of the needle in relation of the cannula. The Cook LABS 100 or 200 set recommend the needle spring-fire system should be facing upward toward the angulation of the cannula. If the set selected is the TLAB, the spring-fire red portion of the needle should be pointing toward the red mark in the cannula.

3. **Orientation of the cannula during biopsy:** If the catheterized vein is the right hepatic vein, an anterior orientation of the stiff cannula is recommended. This anatomic guideline is based in cross-sectional imaging where almost the entire right lobe of the liver is in an anterior location. However, careful attention must be present during the catheterization of the middle hepatic vein because the amount of liver parenchyma is less. This may increase the risk of capsular perforation or gallbladder perforation. In our experience, in three of five hemobilia cases with middle hepatic vein access with the cannula pointing anterior, lateral or even posterior

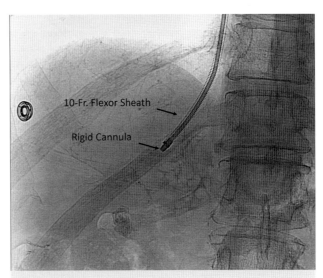

Fig. 5.3 Placement of the guiding cannula. Posterior-anterior (PA) spot film demonstrates the rigid cannula within the 10-Fr sheath, placed into the hepatic vein. The cannula is in a good position to obtain a liver sample.

orientation of the cannula is suggested. Similar findings are seen in previous reports. Our standardized protocol includes at least two peripheral samples of the liver and two central specimens. We found this as a critical aspect in the procedure, particularly in cases of chronic and diffuse liver disease, such as viral hepatitis.

4. **Evaluation of the specimen:** From a technical standpoint, we considered an optimal sample if the specimen is at least 75% of the needle throws. We follow the idea of at least 20 mm of peripheral and 20 mm of central specimens. Of course, at the end, the number of samples obtained per procedure is determined by the operator's judgment.

5. The rigid cannula and the vascular sheath are removed, and pressure is applied at the puncture site.

Complications

Transjugular liver biopsy is considered a safe procedure with few minor and major complications. Minor complications reported are small subcapsular hematoma, hemorrhage, and abdominal pain. Major complications occur in around 0.6% of the cases; hemobilia occurs most frequently. The overall mortality rate has been estimated in 0.1%.[15]

Specimens

The liver tissue obtained during the TJLB procedure should be immediately placed in a sterile cup containing formalin to be sent immediately to pathology for histologic evaluation.

An adequate biopsy specimen is critical for accurate histologic interpretation. Current recommendations are that an adequate liver biopsy specimen must be at least 15 mm long and contain at least six complete portal tracts (CPTs) to be considered optimal for diagnosis of diffuse liver disease.[30] However, recently, it has been demonstrated that reliable grading and staging of liver disease require a biopsy of at least 20 mm in length and at least 11 CPT.[34,35] The number of CPTs is considered to be the most important parameter in determining both the grade and stage of diffuse liver disease. The quality of TJLB specimens has been questioned because in theory, the specimens obtained with the transjugular biopsy needles are small and prone to fragmentation.[30] Recent advances in the design of transjugular spring-fire needle systems should yield liver samples useful for histologic evaluation.

Multiple reports have criticized the transjugular method, arguing that the specimens obtained are suboptimal for the evaluation of chronic liver diseases, particularly in chronic hepatitis, both for grading and staging purposes.[36] In this regard, it is very important to distinguish between the value of individual specimens and the total amount of tissue submitted for evaluation. Standish et al have emphasized the importance of submitting multiple liver specimens to improve the diagnostic and prognostic yield of liver biopsies.[36] Previous studies support the concept that a transjugular liver biopsy procedure can yield sufficient information if at least three individual nonfragmented specimens are submitted for evaluation.[36,37] Our group showed that the information obtained from a single liver sample is insufficient for diagnosis as well as for grading and staging. An average of four individual liver cores samples are required to achieve a specific histologic diagnosis in 96% of the cases. In addition, a retrospective study by Behrens et al demonstrated that the Flexcore needle

(TLAB) was superior to the Quick-Core needle (Cook Medical), obtaining a significantly higher mean number of CPT and therefore is significantly more useful for both staging and grading the liver disease.

References

1. Bosch J, Abraldes JG, Berzigotti A, et al. The clinical use of HVPG measurements in chronic liver disease. Nat Rev Gastroenterol Hepatol 2009;6:576–582.
2. Garcia-Tsao G, Friedman S, Iredale J, Pinzani M. Now there are many (stages) where before there was one: In search of a pathophysiological classification of cirrhosis. Hepatology 2010;51:1445–1449.
3. Krook H. Estimation of portal venous pressure by occlusive hepatic vein catheterization. Scand J Clin Lab Invest 1953;5:285–229.
4. D'Amico G, Garcia-Tsao G, Pagliaro L. Natural history and prognostic indicators of survival in cirrhosis: a systematic review of 118 studies. J Hepatol 2006;44:217–231.
5. Suk KT, Kim HC, Namkung S, et al. Diagnostic accuracy of hepatic venous pressure gradient measurement in the prediction of stage 1 compensated liver cirrhosis in patients with chronic hepatitis B. Eur J Gastroenterol Hepatol 2013;25:1170–1176.
6. Patch D, Armonis A, Sabin C, et al. Single portal pressure measurement predicts survival in cirrhotic patients with recent bleeding. Gut 1999;44:264–269.
7. Vinel JP, Cassigneul J, Levade M, et al. Assessment of short-term prognosis after variceal bleeding in patients with alcoholic cirrhosis by early measurement of portohepatic gradient. Hepatology 1986;6:116–117.
8. Merkel C, Montagnese S. Hepatic venous pressure gradient measurement in clinical hepatology. Dig Liver Dis 2011;43:762–767.
9. Albillos A, Garcia-Tsao G. Classification of cirrhosis: the clinical use of HVPG measurements. Dis Markers 2011;31:121–128.
10. Groszmann RJ, Garcia-Tsao G, Bosch J, et al. Beta-blockers to prevent gastroesophageal varices in patients with cirrhosis. N Engl J Med 2005;353:2254–2261.
11. Vlachogiannakos J, Kougioumtzian A, Triantos C, et al. Clinical trial: The effect of somatostatin vs. octreotide in preventing post-endoscopic increase in hepatic venous pressure gradient in cirrhotics with bleeding varices. Aliment Pharmacol Ther 2007;26:1479–1487.
12. Monescillo A, Martinez-Lagares F, Ruiz-del-Arbol L, et al. Influence of portal hypertension and its early decompression by TIPS placement on the outcome of variceal bleeding. Hepatology 2004;40:793–801.
13. Rincon D, Lo Iacono O, Tejedor M, et al. Prognostic value of hepatic venous pressure gradient in patients with compensated chronic hepatitis C-related cirrhosis. Scand J Gastroenterol 2013;48:487–495.
14. Behrens G, Ferral H, Giusto D, et al. Van Thiel transjugular liver biopsy: comparison of sample adequacy with the use of two automated needle systems. J Vasc Interv Radiol 22;(2011):341–345.
15. Behrens G, Ferral H. Transjugular liver biopsy. Semin Intervent Radiol 2012;29(2):111–117.
16. Lebrec D. Various approaches to obtaining liver tissue—choosing the biopsy technique. J Hepatol 1996;25(Suppl 1):20–24.
17. Kalambokis G, Manousou P, Vibhakorn S, et al. Transjugular liver biopsy—indications, adequacy, quality of specimens, and complications—a systematic review. J Hepatol 2007;47:284–294.
18. Ripoll C, Groszmann R, Garcia-Tsao G, et al. Hepatic venous pressure gradient predicts clinical decompensation in patients with compensated cirrhosis. Gastroenterology 2007;133:481–488.
19. Ripoll C, Groszmann RJ, Garcia-Tsao G, et al. Hepatic venous pressure gradient predicts development of hepatocellular carcinoma independently of severity of cirrhosis. J Hepatol 2009;50:923–928.
20. Suk KT. Hepatic venous pressure gradient: clinical use in chronic liver disease. Clin Mol Hepatol 2014;20(1):6–14.
21. Garcia-Pagan JC, Escorsell A, Feu F, et al. Propranolol plus molsidomine vs propranolol alone in the treatment of portal hypertension in patients with cirrhosis. J Hepatol 1996;24(4):430.
22. Berzigotti A, Rossi V, Tiani C, et al. Prognostic value of a single HVPG measurement and Doppler-ultrasound evaluation in patients with cirrhosis and portal hypertension. J Gastroenterol 2011;46(5):687–695.
23. Bruix J, Sherman M. Management of hepatocellular carcinoma. Hepatology 2005;42(5):1208–1236.
24. Groszmann RJ, Bosch J, Grace ND, et al. Hemodynamic events in a prospective randomized trial of propranolol versus placebo in the prevention of a first variceal hemorrhage [see comments]. Gastroenterology 1990;99(5):1401–1407.

25. Feu F, Garcia-Pagan JC, Bosch J, et al. Relation between portal pressure response to pharmacotherapy and risk of recurrent variceal haemorrhage in patients with cirrhosis. Lancet 1995;346(8982):1056–1059.

26. La Mura V, Abraldes JG, Raffa S, et al. Prognostic value of acute hemodynamic response to i.v. propranolol in patients with cirrhosis and portal hypertension. J Hepatol 2009;51(2):279–287.

27. Villanueva C, Aracil C, Colomo A, et al. Acute hemodynamic response to beta-blockers and prediction of long-term outcome in primary prophylaxis of variceal bleeding. Gastroenterology 2009;137(1):119–128

28. Dotter CT. Catheter biopsy. Experimental technique for transvenous liver biopsy. Radiology 1964;82:312–314.

29. Hanafee W, Weiner M. Transjugular percutaneous cholangiography. Radiology 1967;88:35–39.

30. Bravo AA, Sheth SG, Chopra S. Liver biopsy. N Engl J Med. 2001;344:495–500.

31. Miraglia R, Luca A, Gruttadauria S, et al. Contribution of transjugular liver biopsy in patients with the clinical presentation of acute liver failure. Cardiovasc Intervent Radiol 2006;29:1008–1010.

32. Dawson MA, McCarthy PH, Walsh ME, et al. Transjugular liver biopsy is a safe and effective intervention to guide management for patients with a congenital bleeding disorder infected with hepatitis C. Intern Med J 2005;35:556–559.

33. Azoulay D, Raccuia JS, Roche B, et al. The value of early transjugular liver biopsy after liver transplantation. Transplantation 1996;6:406–409.

34. Guido M, Rugge M. Liver fibrosis: natural history may be affected by the biopsy sample. Gut 2004;53:1878; author reply 1878.

35. Colloredo G, Guido M, Sonzogni A, et al. Impact of liver biopsy size on histological evaluation of chronic viral hepatitis: the smaller the sample, the milder the disease. J Hepatol 2003;39:239–244.

36. Standish RA, Cholongitas E, Dhillon A, et al. An appraisal of the histopathological assessment of liver fibrosis. Gut 2006;55:569–578.

37. Cholongitas E, Quaglia A, Samonakis D, et al. Transjugular liver biopsy in patients with diffuse liver disease: comparison of three cores with one or two cores for accurate histological interpretation. Liver Int 2007;27:646–653.

Section II

Medical, Endoscopic, Percutaneous, and Surgical Management

Chapter 6: Medical Management of Portal Hypertension Complications

Wissam Bleibel and Abdullah M.S. Al-Osaimi

Introduction

Portal hypertension (PHT) is caused by increased resistance to portal outflow and increased portal inflow resulting in portal venous pressure greater than 5 mm Hg. These hemodynamic changes result in increased blood volume in the splanchnic venous system and reduced circulating volume in the arterial and systemic venous systems. This abnormal distribution of blood volume leads to pathologic changes in most of the body's systems, including the cardiovascular, renal, immune, central nervous, and pulmonary systems[1,2] This chapter focuses on the medical managements of cirrhosis and PHT; endoscopic and interventional management will be discussed in a separate chapter.

Anatomy and Physiology

The vast majority of the blood draining from the gastrointestinal (GI) tract and spleen flows through the liver via the portal venous system. This allows the liver to manifest its significant metabolic, detoxifying, synthetic, and immunologic functions. The liver receives less than 25% of its blood supply via the hepatic artery, and in the hepatic sinusoids, arterial and portal venous blood mix together and drain into the hepatic vein. Branches of the portal venous system communicate with the vena cava system via watershed areas in the distal esophagus, superior and middle hemorrhoidal veins, paraumbilical veins, splenic venous bed and left renal vein, and retroperitoneum. In normal hemodynamic conditions, blood flow through these communications is minimal, but in cases of PHT and increased resistance in the portal venous routes, these communicating vessels significantly enlarge, thereby shunting major volumes of blood into the vena cava system (▶ Fig. 6.1).[2]

Clinical Pathophysiology

Portal hypertension can be classified based on the site of vascular resistance leading to increased venous pressure. Most cases of PHT are caused by cirrhosis, which is the most common cause of intrahepatic PHT. Other causes leading to intrahepatic (also known as sinusoidal) PHT include primary biliary cirrhosis, primary sclerosing cholangitis, alcoholic hepatitis, acute hepatitis, nodular regenerative hyperplasia, and infiltrative liver diseases. Prehepatic (presinusoidal) PHT is most commonly seen in cases of schistosomiasis (▶ Table 6.1). Other causes of prehepatic PHT include portal vein thrombosis, splenic vein thrombosis, and extrinsic compression on the portal vein. The third form of PHT is postsinusoidal, which is caused by increased pressure in the hepatic venous system in cases of right-sided congestive heart failure, tricuspid valve disease, constrictive pericarditis, Budd-Chiari syndrome, and veno-occlusive disease (▶ Table 6.1).[3]

In cases of increased portal venous pressure, blood flow is diverted toward collateral of lower resistance. These collaterals are in the watershed areas that communicate with the systemic venous system. The communicating vessels enlarge over time and develop large vascular structures known as varices. Although these collaterals shunt large amounts of blood, they are not able to effectively decompress the portal venous system and reduce the pressure back to normal.[3]

The portosystemic shunts associated with PHT reduce the pressure in the portal venous system, yet they are associated with pathologic manifestations. The massive dilatation of these vascular structures predisposes them to bleeding, clinically known as variceal hemorrhage. In addition, the immunologic and detoxifying roles of the liver can be significantly reduced by the portosystemic shunting of blood, thereby leading to increased systemic inflammatory response and hepatic encephalopathy (HE). Increased pressure in the portal venous system leads to development of ascites and hepatic hydrothorax (HH). This pathologic accumulation of fluid predisposes it to microbial infection known as spontaneous bacterial peritonitis (SBP). The hemodynamic disturbances associated with pooled blood in the portal venous system and away from the systemic veins lead to disturbances in the renal and pulmonary vascular systems, which clinically manifest as hepatorenal, hepatopulmonary, and portopulmonary syndromes.[4]

Gastrointestinal Varices

Progression of PHT necessitates further decompression of the congested portal venous system via further dilatation of portosystemic collateral or varices (▶ Fig. 6.1). At a certain point, these vascular structures become overwhelmed by their increased intraluminal pressure and blood flow. The clinically most significant forms of GI varices include esophageal, gastric, rectal, and less commonly ectopic varices of the GI tract. Esophageal varices are of the highest clinical significance because their rupture is the number one cause of death related to complications of cirrhosis.

Esophageal Varices

In the cirrhosis population, 8% of patients develop esophageal varices de novo annually, and preexisting small varices become large at the same annual rate.[5] Varices are less commonly seen in well-compensated cirrhosis (40% of patients with Child-A cirrhosis), yet with progression of liver failure, the risk of varices (up to 85% of patients with Child-C cirrhosis) and variceal hemorrhage increases. Around 60% of the cases of variceal hemorrhage do not spontaneously stop, and each episode of bleeding continues to carry a mortality rate of 20% despite the currently available treatment. Survivors carry a 60% risk of rebleeding within 1 to 2 years.[6–8]

Medical management of esophageal varices is directed at three levels: primary prophylaxis, treatment of active or recent hemorrhage, and secondary prophylaxis of variceal bleeding. ▶ Fig. 6.2 and ▶ Fig. 6.3 show our proposed algorithms for the management of esophageal varices and upper GI bleeding in patients with known or suspected PHT. Given the high risk of developing varices

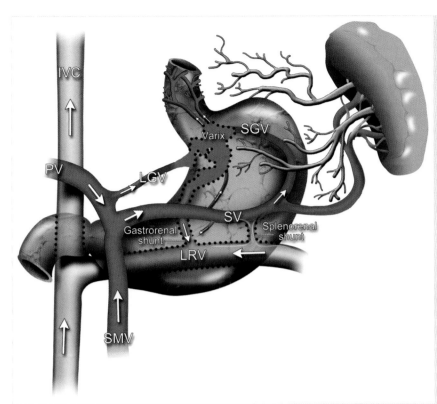

Fig. 6.1 Anatomy of the portal circulation. Gastric varices caused by splenic vein thrombosis (SVT) tend to arise from the short gastric veins running from the hilum of the spleen to the greater curvature aspect of the stomach rather than through splenorenal or gastrorenal shunts common with portal hypertensive fundal varices. IVC: inferior vena cava; LGV: left gastric vein; LRV: left renal vein; PV: portal vein; SGV: short gastric vein; SMV: superior mesenteric vein; SV: splenic vein.

and their associated bleeding complication, screening guidelines have been set by various hepatology societies. The predicted risk for esophageal variceal bleeding is determined by endoscopic evaluation and is based on the location of the varices (a higher risk is at the gastroesophageal junction and the palisade zone), size of the varices (larger varices are associated with higher risk to rupture), endoscopic finding of high-risk signs (red wale marks, cherry red spots, hematocystic spots, and diffuse erythema), and clinical manifestations of decompensated liver function. The 1-year risk of bleeding can be determined based on cumulative effect of these factors. This risk can be as low as 6% in a Child-A patient with small esophageal varices (grade F1) without high-risk stigmata and as

high as 76% in a Child-C patient with large (grade F3) esophageal varices with significant high-risk stigmata (▶ Fig. 6.4).[8,9]

Pharmacologic therapy of high-risk varices is targeted at reducing portal resistance and portal pressure by using vasoconstrictors or venodilators. Splanchnic vasoconstriction can be achieved by using nonselective beta-blockers, vasopressin and its analogues, or somatostatin and its analogues. Splanchnic vasoconstriction results in reduction of portal venous inflow. Nitrates lead to reduction in systemic arterial pressure with resultant reduction in arterial hepatic blood flow and subsequent reduction in sinusoidal and portal pressures. The combination of a vasoconstrictor and a vasodilator has a synergistic effect on reducing portal pressure.[7,8,10]

Table 6.1 Causes of Noncirrhotic Portal Hypertension

Intrahepatic Presinusoidal PHN	Sinusoidal PHN	Extrahepatic Postsinusoidal PHN
Hepatic schistosomiasis	Cirrhosis	Budd-Chiari syndrome
Congenital hepatic fibrosis	Noncirrhotic alcoholic liver disease	Right heart failure
Noncirrhotic portal fibrosis	Infiltrative disorders:	Constrictive pericarditis
Nodular regenerative hyperplasia	• Amyloidosis • Systemic mastocytosis	Suprahepatic IVC thrombosis
Primary biliary cirrhosis or primary sclerosing cholangitis	• Malignancy • Myeloproliferative disorder	Pulmonary hypertension
		Tricuspid valve regurgitation
Extrahepatic Presinusoidal PHN		**Intrahepatic Postsinusoidal PHN**
Portal vein thrombosis		Veno-occlusive disease
Superior mesenteric vein thrombosis	Peliosis hepatis	
Splenic vein thrombosis	Hypervitaminosis A	

IVC: inferior vena cava; PHN: portal hypertension.
(Adapted with modifications from Molina E, Reddy KR. Noncirrhotic portal hypertension. Clin Liver Dis 2001;5:769–787.[72])

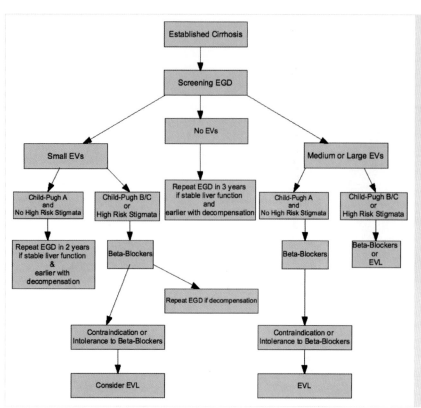

Fig. 6.2 Algorithm for the screening and management of varices. Decompensation is defined as worsening of liver function by laboratory or clinical findings or decreasing platelet count to less than 100,000/mL. EGD: esophagogastroduodenoscopy; EVs: esophageal varices; EVL: endoscopic variceal band ligation.

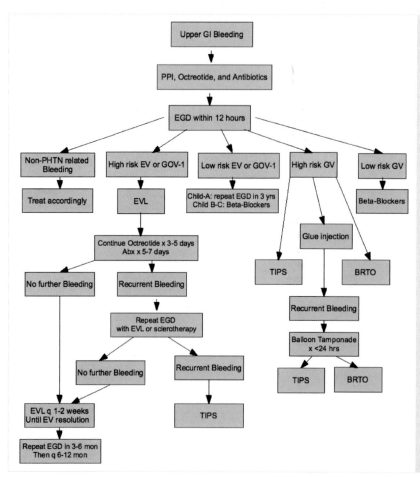

Fig. 6.3 Algorithm for management of variceal bleeding. Abx: antibiotics; BRTO: balloon-retrograde transvenous obliteration; EGD: esophagogastroduodenoscopy; EV: esophageal varices; EVL: endoscopic band ligation; GI: gastrointestinal; GOV: gastroesophageal varices; GV: gastric varices; PHTN: portal hypertension; PPI: proton pump inhibitor; TIPS: transjugular intrahepatic portosystemic shunt.

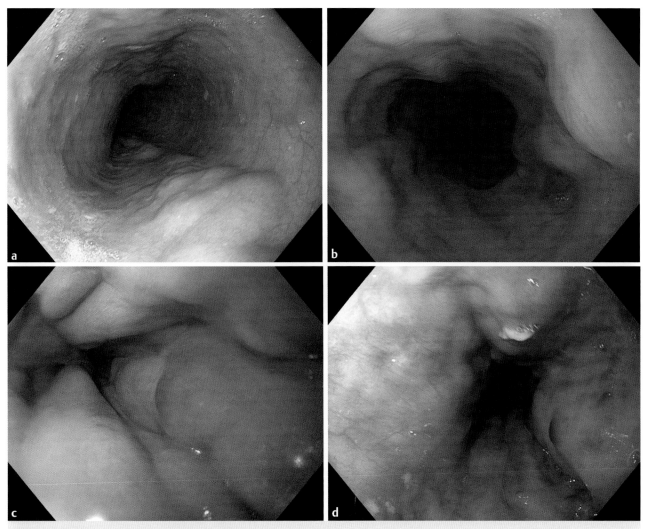

Fig. 6.4 Classification of esophageal varices. (**a**) Small, low-risk esophageal varices (or F1), almost flattened out with insufflation. (**b**) Medium-sized, low-risk esophageal varices (F2) that did not flatten with insufflation. (**c**) Large esophageal varices larger than one third of the esophageal lumen with some high-risk stigmata (red marks or wheals). (**d**) Esophageal varices with high-risk stigmata for recent bleeding and rebleeding with red marks and a nipple sign or fibrin plug.

Primary Prophylaxis

Nonselective beta-blockers (e.g., propranolol, nadolol, and carvedilol) have been shown to reduce the risk of first variceal bleeding (i.e., primary prophylaxis). The use of beta-blockers as primary prophylaxis is indicated for patients with small, medium, or large esophageal varices and decompensated liver disease (Child-A or -B cirrhosis). Although beta-blockers have been shown to reduce the risk of first bleeding from small esophageal varices in patients with Child-A cirrhosis, the risk of bleeding and the benefit of primary prophylaxis is small; therefore, the use of these medications is not currently recommended for this patient population (see ▶ Fig. 6.2).[7,8,11,12]

A meta-analysis of 11 trials that included 1189 patients showed that the risk of first variceal bleeding in patients with medium- or large-sized varices is significantly reduced by beta-blockers (30% in control participants vs. 14% in beta-blocker–treated patients) and indicated that treating 10 patients with beta-blockers results in preventing 1 variceal hemorrhage and reduces mortality in this patient group. The therapeutic target of beta-blockers is to reach a 25% reduction of heart rate from the baseline heart or to reach the maximum tolerated dose. When beta-blocker therapy is stopped, the PHT increases back to pretreatment levels; therefore, these medications should be given indefinitely.[11,12,13]

Reducing the hepatic venous pressure gradient to less than 12 mm Hg significantly diminishes the risk of variceal bleeding. Achieving this goal is not possible in many cases because of side effects of beta-blockers. About 15% of patients have contraindications for the use of beta-blockers, and another 15% of patients have to stop the medication because of significant side effects. Studies have shown a 10% to 20% reduction in hepatic venous pressure gradient significantly decreases the risk of variceal bleeding.[14]

Treatment of Variceal Hemorrhage

Survival analyses have shown reduction in mortality rates associated with active variceal bleeding with the currently available treatment. The management options include general medical measures, medical treatment, endoscopic interventions, interventional radiologic procedures, and surgery (▶ Fig. 6.3).[15]

The initial management measures include admission to intensive care setting, fluid resuscitation, and airway management to prevent aspiration and respiratory complications. Variceal bleeding could be massive, thereby leading to hemorrhagic shock with multiorgan failure. Caution should be taken not to overtransfuse with blood products and fluids because doing so may increase the portal venous pressure and thereby may increase the risk or rebleeding. Thus, the current recommendations indicate a hemoglobin level of 8.0 g/dL as a target for transfusion. Using recombinant factor VIIa (rFVIIa) may be of benefit in cases of difficult-to-control variceal bleeding (see ▶ Fig. 6.3).[16–18]

In addition to resuscitative measures, the prophylactic use of intravenous (IV) or oral antibiotics has been shown to reduce the mortality rate of patients with variceal bleeding. This recommendation is based on studies showing a higher risk of bacterial infections in patients with cirrhosis who have upper GI bleeding.[19] The most commonly used antibiotic regimens include an IV quinolone or ceftriaxone or oral norfloxacin for 7 days.[20]

Pharmacologic therapy should be initiated in patients with suspected variceal bleeding even before diagnostic or therapeutic endoscopy. Studies have shown that treatment with vasopressin and nitroglycerin, terlipressin, somatostatin, or octreotide to reduce death associated with variceal hemorrhage (see ▶ Fig. 6.3). Pharmacologic treatment should be continued for at least 2 days after endoscopic intervention because studies have showed that the hepatic venous pressure gradient increases for 48 hours after band ligation and for more than 5 days after sclerotherapy of esophageal varices.[7,21]

Vasopressin is the most potent splanchnic vasoconstrictor, yet it is associated with a number of systemic side effects that limit its use in variceal hemorrhage. Coadministration of nitrates attenuates these side effects to some degree, but it does not render it as safe as the other available medications.[22,23]

Terlipressin is a synthetic analogue of vasopressin with a longer biologic activity and significantly fewer side effects. It has been widely used in Europe with studies showing its efficacy at controlling variceal bleeding and lowering its associated mortality rate, but currently it is not approved by the U.S. Food and Drug Administration.[23]

Somatostatin and analogues such as octreotide and vapreotide reduce portal pressure via a local vasodilatory effect. Recent meta-analysis has shown a limited value of octreotide as a single agent without endoscopic intervention. This could possibly be due to tachyphylaxis associated with its use.[24]

Secondary Prophylaxis

After an episode of variceal hemorrhage, close monitoring of hemodynamics for at least 24 hours is recommended. Shortly, after hemodynamic stability and with no further evidence of rebleeding, secondary prophylaxis should be initiated (see ▶ Fig. 6.3). If secondary prophylaxis is not undertaken, the risk of rebleeding could be as high as 60% within 2 years. If nonselective beta-blockers are used, then this risk may be reduced to less than 43%. Beta-blockers do not have to be used in patients who had surgical or radiologic portosystemic shunts. A combination of nonselective beta-blocker and a nitrate may be more efficient at reducing the risk of variceal bleeding, yet this regimen carries a higher rate of side effects, thereby limiting the practicality of its use. The combination of pharmaceutical and

endoscopic treatment is most likely superior to either treatment alone in reducing the risk of variceal rebleeding with data showing that this risk may be reduced to 14% to 23% with the combined treatment.[11,25]

Gastric Varices

Gastric varices are less prevalent than esophageal varices and are present in 5% to 33% of patients with PHT with a reported incidence of bleeding of about 25% in 2 years, with a higher bleeding incidence for fundal varices (▶ Fig. 6.5; ▶ Fig. 6.6). The efficacy of pharmacologic treatment is not clear in cases of gastric variceal bleeding because of the limited number of studies. Vasoconstrictors and venodilators may be of little benefit in managing gastric variceal bleeding because of the difference in hemodynamics from esophageal variceal and the presence of large portosystemic shunts except for cases of gastroesophageal varices I (▶ Fig. 6.5a), which are typically treated as esophageal varices (see ▶ Fig. 6.3).[24,26] The endoscopic and radiologic treatments of gastric variceal hemorrhage are discussed in separate chapters of this book.

Hepatic Encephalopathy

Hepatic encephalopathy or portosystemic encephalopathy is a syndrome of largely reversible impairment of the central nervous system occurring in patients with acute or chronic liver failure or in patients with major portosystemic shunts. This condition

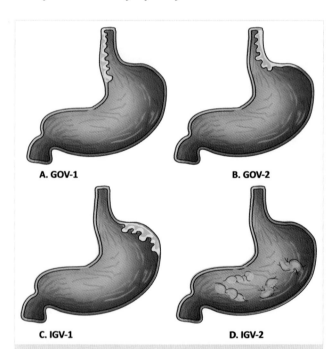

A. GOV-1   **B. GOV-2**

C. IGV-1   **D. IGV-2**

Fig. 6.5 Schematic diagram of Sarin's classification of gastric varices. Type 1 gastroesophageal varices (GOV-1) are typically a continuation of esophageal varices onto the lesser curvature. The fundal varices are included in two groups. Type 2 gastroesophageal varices (GOV-2) occur when the esophageal and fundal varices are present in continuity over the cardia; these might include type 1 isolated gastric varices (IGV-1), which are usually isolated gastric fundal varices. Type 2 isolated gastric varices (IGV-2) are gastric varices at ectopic sites in the stomach outside the cardiofundal region or the first part of the duodenum.

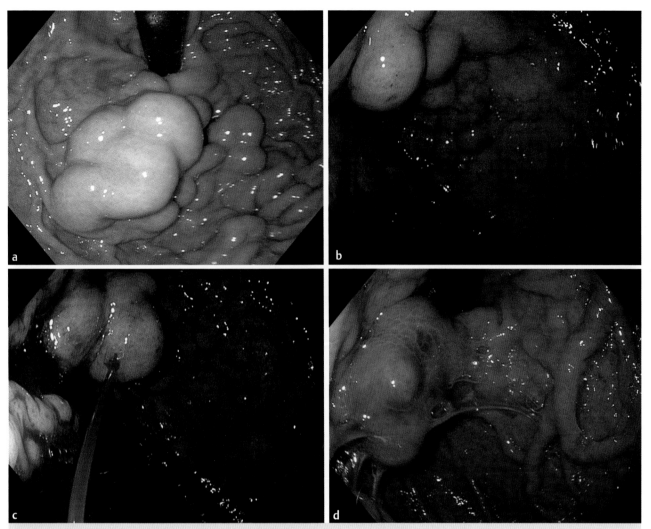

Fig. 6.6 Photographs of gastric varices. (**a**) Large (>3 cm) gastric varices (IGV-1) with no stigmata of bleeding. (**b**) A large IGV-1 with evidence of recent bleeding (blood in the stomach and a nipple or dimple sign). (**c**) The nipple sign area with active bleeding. (**d**) Mosaic (snake skin–like appearance) pattern of post–balloon retrograde transvenous obliteration (BRTO) findings of a GOV-2.

is associated with a wide spectrum of neurologic impairments ranging from subclinical disease to coma. The underlying cause of this disorder is a combination of impairment of liver function caused by hepatocellular disease and major portosystemic shunting, both of which result in large volumes of portal venous blood being poorly filtered through the liver or completely bypassing the detoxifying effect of the liver directly into the systemic venous system; then these toxins (ammonia and toxic fatty acids) attain a direct access to the brain.[27]

A precipitating cause of (rather than worsening of) hepatocellular function can be identified and successfully treated in more than 80% of cases of HE, and half of these cases are caused by an underlying infection such as urinary tract infection, pneumonia, or SBP. In addition to infectious causes, medication noncompliance, constipation, renal failure, electrolyte imbalance, use of sedative medications, and recent increased systemic stress caused by surgery or other illness may precipitate HE.[28–30] ▶ Fig. 6.7 proposes a pathway for management of a patient with HE.

In addition to targeting the precipitating factor, reducing systemic ammonia and other toxins load has been widely used to improve brain function and resolve manifestations of HE. This could be achieved via either reducing ammonia production in the GI tract or facilitating its elimination. Synthetic disaccharides (lactulose and lactitol) have shown to be more effective than placebo in resolving HE, but this may not significantly affect patients' mortality rate. Colonic bacteria digest these disaccharides with production of short chain fatty acids that lower the colonic pH and lead to conversion of NH_3 to nonabsorbable NH_4. Furthermore, the cathartic effect of these medications increases fecal nitrogen excretion by up to fourfold. The therapeutic target of these medications is to achieve two or three soft bowel movements per day (see ▶ Fig. 6.7).[31–33]

Lowering arterial ammonia levels can be achieved via altering the GI microflora, favoring less ammonia-producing bacteria. This has been achieved by the use of various oral antibiotics, including neomycin, rifaximin, metronidazole, paromomycin, and vancomycin. Nowadays, neomycin is less commonly used in practice because of its nephrotoxic and ototoxic side effects in addition to the availability of effective and less toxic alternatives. Rifaximin is increasingly being used and has a good safety profile with a very low rate of intestinal absorption. Studies have shown treatment with rifaximin to be

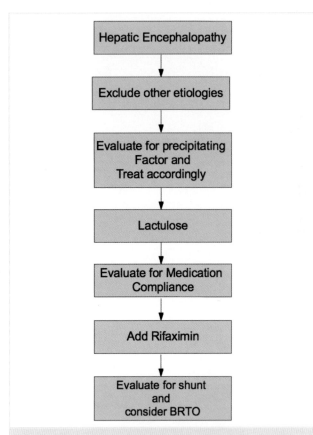

Fig. 6.7 Algorithm for management of hepatic encephalopathy. BRTO: balloon-retrograde transvenous obliteration.

associated with a higher response rate, faster effect, and fewer side effects than lactulose. It has also been shown to improve patients' quality of life, reduce the recurrence rate of overt HE, reduce the length of hospitalization and health care costs, and improve psychomotor abnormalities of minimal HE (see ▶ Fig. 6.7).[31,32]

Alteration of GI microflora via oral administration of probiotics, prebiotics, or synbiotics has been shown to improve the manifestations of HE. These supplementations may lead to predominance of nonproteolytic non–urease-producing bacteria, thereby reducing the ammonia load delivered into the systemic venous system.[31,32]

Major spontaneous portosystemic shunts should be suspected in cases of refractory HE. Several reports have shown that occluding these shunts by surgical or radiologic approaches may improve HE (see ▶ Fig. 6.7).[34] The details of balloon-occluded retrograde transvenous obliteration of portosystemic shunts are discussed in detail in separate chapters.

Protein restriction has been shown to aggravate HE via inducing proteolysis with resultant production of urea and ammonia in addition to increased muscle wasting. In addition, data have shown that muscles contribute to the ammonia metabolism by converting it into glutamine. Thus, a balanced protein diet should be recommended to patients with cirrhosis and HE.[35]

Liver transplantation is the ultimate treatment for HE. Studies have shown that cognitive function significantly improves after liver transplantation, yet some degree of irreversible brain damage can persist. After each episode of overt HE, residual brain damage could be detected by specialized neurocognitive tests and magnetic resonance imaging. The severity of this irreversible

neurocognitive impairment (or chronic HE) has been shown to correlate with the number of episodes of overt HE.[36,37]

Post-TIPS Hepatic Encephalopathy

Transjugular intrahepatic portosystemic shunts (TIPS) allows portal vein blood flow to pass the liver without detoxification, which can result in HE, termed post-TIPS HE. This form of HE has a higher incidence in the first 30-days after TIPS. The management of this type of HE is similar to other causes of HE, in addition the consideration of TIPS reduction or closure in refractory cases. The details of the pathogenesis and treatment options are further discussed in the section of complications of TIPS.

Ascites

Ascites is the third most common complication of cirrhosis after variceal bleeding and HE. The development of ascites is indicative of decompensated liver function and is associated with a poor prognosis (▶ Fig. 6.8).[38,39]

Treatment of ascites caused by PHT is mainly based on sodium restriction to less than 2000 mg/day and the use of oral diuretics. In ▶ Fig. 6.9, we propose a pathway for the management of ascites. Sodium restriction is of more importance than fluid restriction. Thorough nutritional education is required to ensure that the patient understands how to determine his or her daily sodium intake. The goal of using diuretics is to increase urinary excretion of sodium to more than 78 mmol/day. A random "spot" urine sodium concentration greater than the potassium concentration correlates with a 24-hour sodium excretion greater than 78 mmol/day with approximately 90% accuracy.[38,40–42]

The diuretic regimen recommended to treat ascites consists of a combination of furosemide and spironolactone. These medications are started at daily doses of 40 mg and 100 mg, respectively. The combination of both drugs is more efficacious and results in fewer side effects than either drug alone (see ▶ Fig. 6.9). The doses can be increased simultaneously every 3 to 5 days (maintaining the 40 mg:100 mg ratio) to reach a maximum daily dose of 160 mg of furosemide and 400 mg of spironolactone.[16,17] Amiloride or eplerenone can be substituted for spironolactone in patients with tender gynecomastia. Triamterene, metolazone, and hydrochlorothiazide have also been used to treat ascites.[39,41]

Chronic hyponatremia is not uncommon in patients with cirrhosis particularly with chronic diuretic use, and it may reflect worsening liver disease. In most cases, hyponatremia does not result in significant symptoms except when it develops or worsens acutely or when the sodium level drops below 110 mmol/L. Severe hyponatremia (with sodium level below 120 mmol/L) should be treated with fluid restriction and adjustment of diuretic doses. Aquaretic agents such as tolvaptan and conivaptan have been shown to improve hyponatremia in cirrhosis. Because of the high expense of these medications, they should be reserved for patients with severe and refractory hyponatremia.[43]

Dietary sodium restriction and a dual diuretic regimen with spironolactone and furosemide have been shown to be effective in more than 90% of patients in achieving a reduction in the volume of ascites to acceptable levels.[44]

With failure of these measures to control the fluid status or when the use of diuretics is restricted (e.g., patients with renal dysfunction or severe hyponatremia), more invasive treatment

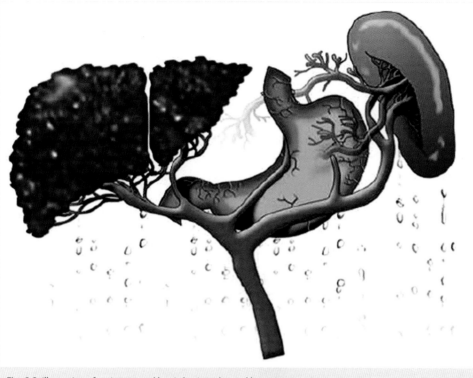

Fig. 6.8 Illustration of ascites caused by cirrhosis and portal hypertension.

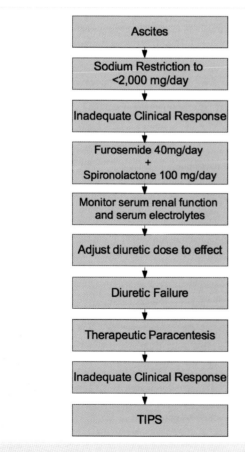

Fig. 6.9 Algorithm for management of ascites. TIPS: transjugular intrahepatic portosystemic shunt.

options should be considered. The second line of treatment is large-volume paracentesis followed by TIPS.[40,41]

Large-Volume Paracentesis

Large-volume paracentesis is a relatively safe outpatient procedure that results in rapid relief of tense ascites and its related symptoms. Because of the rapid volume shifts with draining more than 5 L of ascitic fluid, 6 to 10 g of IV albumin is recommended for each liter of drained fluid. Serial paracenteses deplete proteins and predispose to infection; thus, this procedure should be reserved for patients with diuretic-resistant ascites.[40,41,45]

Transjugular Intrahepatic Portosystemic Shunt

Transjugular intrahepatic portosystemic shunt is a side-to-side portosystemic shunt that is placed by interventional radiology. This procedure has been shown to reduce the hepatic venous pressure gradient, thereby reducing ascitic fluid accumulation. Studies have shown the efficacy of TIPS in controlling ascites, yet this procedure is invasive and carries a risk for various complications, including worsening or de novo development of HE, decompensation of heart failure, acute-on-chronic liver failure, and even death. The indications and possible complications of this procedure are explained in detail in other chapters.

Hepatic Hydrothorax

In patients with PHT, fluid accumulation in the pleural space with or without the presence of ascites is termed HH. This condition is seen in 5% to 12% of patients with cirrhosis, and it can be associated with significant respiratory distress.[46] In 59% of cases, the pleural effusion is right sided; in 17%, it is left sided; and it is bilateral in the remaining 24%, as determined by computed tomography.[47]

The pathogenesis of HH is related to PHT and ascites. Although the majority of these patients have concomitant ascites, a small percentage may have no detected ascites.[48] It is widely accepted that ascitic fluid leaks from the peritoneal cavity into the pleural space through diaphragmatic defects and is also driven by the negative thoracic pressure during inhalation.[48,49]

Hepatic hydrothorax can be associated with significant symptoms, including dyspnea, hypoxia, nonproductive cough, and chest pain.[48] Furthermore, similar to ascitic fluid, HH is at risk for spontaneous bacterial pleuritis or empyema, which may carry a mortality rate of up to 38%.[50]

Hepatic hydrothorax diagnosis is based on a high clinical suspicion with exclusion of intrathoracic malignancy and cardiopulmonary etiologies in addition to pleural fluid analysis, which is consistent with transudative process.[47,48] In a study by Gurung et al,[47] the authors reported that the serum albumin pleural fluid to albumin gradient was 1.5 (standard deviation, 0.41). Rarely, the diagnosis requires confirmation by injecting radiolabeled albumin into the peritoneal space to document its migration into the pleural cavity.[47,48]

Management of HH is mainly based on sodium restriction and the use of diuretics as recommended for treatment of ascites. When these measures fail, therapeutic thoracentesis can be performed on an as-needed basis. This treatment option provides rapid relief of symptoms, yet it carries a risk of infection, pulmonary edema, bleeding, nutritional and electrolyte disturbances, and a resultant decrease in quality of life. Thus, when thoracentesis is required frequently, other treatment options should be considered.[48] These options include TIPS, pleurodesis, and surgical repair of diaphragmatic defects. In appropriate settings, TIPS can result in improvement or resolution of symptoms in more than 75% of patients.[51]

Liver Transplantation

Development of ascites is a complication of end-stage liver disease that indicates poor survival outcome; hence, the severity of ascites is a component of Child-Pugh classification. Liver transplantation is the ultimate treatment of liver failure and thereby a significant therapeutic modality for ascites and HH.

Spontaneous Bacterial Peritonitis

Ascitic fluid is at risk for infection, or SBP, which is a major cause of morbidity and mortality in the cirrhotic population. The diagnosis is based on detecting the causative bacteria in the ascitic fluid or elevated ascitic fluid neutrophilic count above 250 cells/mL in the absence of a surgical cause of peritonitis. The most common bacterial pathogens detected in SBP are *Escherichia coli*, *Klebsiella pneumoniae*, and pneumococci. In recent years, the widespread use of quinolones in SBP prophylaxis has led to more SBP cases caused by gram-positive pathogens and quinolone-resistant bacteria.[52]

The diagnosis of SBP cannot be based on clinical suspicion without performing diagnostic paracentesis. After the diagnosis of SBP is established, the treatment should be started emergently given the high morbidity and mortality rates of untreated patients. A broad-spectrum antibiotic is recommended, and the drug of choice can be changed based on results of bacterial culture. In a small percentage of patients with SBP, early paracentesis may not show an elevated neutrophil count; thus, with a high clinical suspicion, empiric antibiotic treatment should be initiated pending bacterial cultures. A 5- to 10-day course of IV cefotaxime, or another third-generation cephalosporin may be used as first-line treatment. Ceftriaxone is widely used for the treatment of SBP, although it may have a lower bioavailability in the ascitic fluid than cefotaxime. In properly selected patients, an oral course of ofloxacin may be safe and effective in treating SBP. IV albumin has been shown to decrease the mortality rate of patients with SBP. The recommended dosage is 1.5 g/kg of body weight on day 1 followed by 1.0 g/kg of body weight on day 3.[41,53]

Spontaneous bacterial peritonitis should be distinguished from peritonitis caused by bowel perforation or intraabdominal infection such as an abscess (secondary bacterial peritonitis). The treatment of secondary bacterial peritonitis is different and frequently requires early surgical or radiologic intervention. In contrast to SBP, the ascitic fluid analysis in secondary bacterial peritonitis exhibits a very high neutrophilic count, low serum-ascites albumin gradient, elevated protein and lactate dehydrogenase, low glucose levels, and polymicrobial culture.[54]

Patients with a history of SBP are at risk for recurrent episodes of SBP. In addition, patients with ascitic fluid protein level of less than 1 g/dL and those with recent variceal bleeding are at risk of developing SBP. Studies have shown that antibiotic prophylaxis prevents the development of SBP in these patient groups. The recommended antibiotic regimens are 400 mg/day of norfloxacin, 400 mg/day of ofloxacin, 750 mg once a week of ciprofloxacin, or 5 doses of double-strength trimethoprim–sulfamethoxazole per week. It is important to mention that antibiotic prophylaxis has been shown to result in a shift in the microorganism, causing SBP from predominantly gram-negative bacteria to gram-positive bacteria.[53,55]

Hepatorenal Syndrome

The diagnosis of hepatorenal syndrome (HRS) is based on development of functional renal failure in the setting of cirrhosis and ascites. Other causes or renal failure, such as intravascular volume depletion, diuretic use, drug-induced renal dysfunction, shock, or intrinsic renal disease, should be excluded. Intravascular volume depletion is excluded after withholding diuretics, nephrotoxic drugs, and volume expansion with 1 g/kg up to a maximum of 100 g of IV albumin (▶ Table 6.2).[56]

Two types of HRS have been described, a rapidly progressive type I in which patients double their serum creatinine in less than 2 weeks and the less progressive type II in which the renal function slowly deteriorates over a prolonged period of time.[57]

Triple therapy with albumin, midodrine, and octreotide is the currently recommended treatment for HRS. This has been shown to reduce the mortality rate of patients with HRS. Other agents tried in treatment of HRS include dopamine, norepinephrine, and terlipressin. TIPS with and without terlipressin has been shown to improve renal function in patients with HRS type I.[41,58,59]

Renal replacement therapy is frequently used to control azotemia as a bridge to liver transplantation. With a prolonged course of renal failure because of HRS, the kidney may lose some of the potential to recover. Without liver transplantation, patients requiring renal replacement therapy caused by HRS have a low chance of survival.[56,57]

Table 6.2 Criteria for the Diagnosis of Hepatorenal Syndrome

Cirrhosis with ascites
Serum creatinine > 1.5 mg/dL
No improvement of serum creatinine (decrease to a level of ≤ 1.5 mg/dL) after at least 2 days with diuretic withdrawal and volume expansion with albumin
Absence of shock
No current or recent treatment with nephrotoxic drugs
Absence of parenchymal kidney disease
Adapted from Salerno F, Gerbes A, Ginès P, et al. Diagnosis, prevention and treatment of hepatorenal syndrome in cirrhosis. Gut 2007;56:1310–1318.[60]

Portopulmonary Hypertension

Portopulmonary hypertension (PoPH) refers to pulmonary arterial hypertension in the setting of PHT with the exclusion of other etiologies of pulmonary hypertension. This is an uncommon complication of PHT with or without cirrhosis.[61] It affects 2% to 5% of patients with cirrhosis and up to 12% of those being evaluated for liver transplantation,[62] and it carries a high mortality rate of around 60% in 5 years.[63,64]

The exact mechanism that leads to the development of PoPH has not yet been well elucidated. Several factors, including vasoactive mediators (endothelin-1, prostacyclin, and thromboxane), inflammatory processes, and shear stress, have been proposed in the pathogenesis of PoPH.[65,66] In the initial phase, these mechanisms lead to pulmonary arterial vasospasm with resultant increased resistance and pressure. Subsequently, this vasospasm leads to smooth muscle hyperplasia and hypertrophy, microthrombosis, necrotizing vasculitis, and concentric intimal fibrosis. The second phase of the disease carries a significant component of irreversibility.[67]

Most cases of PoPH are subclinical, and the symptomatic cases are associated with dyspnea, orthopnea, fatigue, syncope, chest pain, and heart failure. On physical examination, no specific physical findings are present. Patients may have hypoxia and findings of right heart strain or failure. Thus, the diagnosis requires a high index of suspicion in the correct clinical settings. In the liver transplant settings, patients are screened for pulmonary hypertension with echocardiography. If the right ventricular systolic pressure is greater than 50 mm Hg, a right heart catheterization is recommended.[66,67]

The criteria for the diagnosis include a mean pulmonary arterial pressure exceeding 25 mm Hg at right heart catheterization with increased pulmonary vascular resistance to above 240 dynes.s.cm⁻⁵, normal cardiac output and pulmonary artery opening pressure, and a pulmonary capillary wedge pressure less than 15 mm Hg. With pressure exceeding 35 mm Hg, the PoPH is considered to be of moderate severity, and when the pressure is over 45 mm Hg, the condition is classified as severe.[63,64]

Medical treatment of PoPH is based on reducing the pulmonary artery resistance. Various drug groups have been used for this purpose, including prostanoids, endothelin receptor antagonists, phosphodiesterase-5 inhibitors, and nitric oxide.[66]

Prostanoids (epoprostol, treprostinil, and iloprost) are potent inhibitors of vascular tone. Epoprostol is the most commonly used drug of this group. It is mainly given as a continuous IV infusion.[68]

Endothelin receptor inhibitors reduce vascular resistance via elevation of intracellular calcium levels. This group includes bosentan, ambrisentan, atrasentan, and sitaxsentan. Bosentan

has been rarely used in treatment of PoPH because of its associated risk of hepatotoxicity. In a small study, ambrisentan was shown to be effective and safe in the treatment of PoPH.[69]

Phosphodiesterase-5 inhibitors such as sildenafil, vardenafil, and tadalafil reduce pulmonary pressure by preventing the breakdown of cyclic guanosine monophosphate, the mediator of nitric oxide. Sildenafil is well tolerated and has been shown to be effective in the treatment of PoPH.[68]

Inhaled nitric oxide is a very effective yet very expensive pulmonary vasodilator that can be effective in treatment of intubated patients with PoPH.[68]

Medical treatment of PoPH has been shown to improve survival (up to 45% at 5 years compared with 14% in an untreated group) and is an effective bridge to liver transplantation, which may be a more effective treatment for this condition.[70] With severe PoPH, the surgical mortality rate of liver transplantation is extremely high; thus, a pulmonary arterial pressure of more than 50 mm Hg is a contraindication for liver transplantation.[71]

Conclusion

Complications of PHT with or without end-stage liver disease and cirrhosis are associated with significant morbidity and mortality. The management of these complications needs to be tailored to the individual patient and usually requires a multidisciplinary approach. The knowledge of these complications and their medical management and potential options is imperative for successful outcomes as discussed in this chapter.

Clinical Pearls

- Esophageal and gastric varices are common among patients with liver cirrhosis and PHT.
- The risk of variceal hemorrhage correlates with Child-Pugh classification and platelet counts below 100,000/mL.
- Management of patients with of PHT includes screening, primary prevention, acute intervention, and secondary prevention of complications.

References

1. Thalheimer U, Bellis L, Puoti C, Burroughs AK. Should we routinely measure portal pressure in patients with cirrhosis, using hepatic venous pressure gradient (HVPG) as a guide for prophylaxis and therapy of bleeding and rebleeding? Eur J Intern Med 2011;22:5–7.
2. Pinzani M, Rosselli M, Zuckermann M. Liver cirrhosis. Best Pract Res Clin Gastroenterol 2011;25:281–290.

3. Martell M, Coll M, Ezkurdia N, et al. Physiopathology of splanchnic vasodilation in portal hypertension. World J Hepatol 2010;2:208–220.

4. Rahimi RS, Rockey DC. Complications and outcomes in chronic liver disease. Curr Opin Gastroenterol 2011;27:204–209.

5. Groszmann RJ, Garcia-Tsao G, Bosch J, et al. Beta-blockers to prevent gastroesophageal varices in patients with cirrhosis. N Engl J Med 2005;353:2254–2261.

6. El-Serag HB, Everhart JE. Improved survival after variceal hemorrhage over an 11-year period in the Department of Veterans Affairs. Am J Gastroenterol 2000; 95:3566–3573.

7. Garcia-Tsao G, Bosch J. Management of varices and variceal hemorrhage in cirrhosis. N Engl J Med 2010;362:823–832.

8. Garcia-Tsao G, Sanyal AJ, Grace ND, et al. Prevention and management of gastroesophageal varices and variceal hemorrhage in cirrhosis. Hepatology 2007;46:922–938.

9. North Italian Endoscopic Club for the Study and Treatment of Esophageal Varices. Prediction of the first variceal hemorrhage in patients with cirrhosis of the liver and esophageal varices. A prospective multicenter study. N Engl J Med 1988;319:983–989.

10. Garcia-Pagan JC, Feu F, Bosch J, Rodés J. Propranolol compared with propranolol plus isosorbide-5-mononitrate for portal hypertension in cirrhosis. A randomized controlled study. Ann Intern Med 1991;114:869–873.

11. Villanueva C, Balanzo J. Variceal bleeding: pharmacological treatment and prophylactic strategies. Drugs 2008;68:2303–2324.

12. Minano C, Garcia-Tsao G. Clinical pharmacology of portal hypertension. Gastroenterol Clin North Am 2010;39:681–695.

13. Abraczinskas DR, Ookubo R, Grace ND, et al. Propranolol for the prevention of first esophageal variceal hemorrhage: a lifetime commitment? Hepatology 2001; 34:1096–1102.

14. Zhang C, Thabut D, Kamath PS, Shah VH. Oesophageal varices in cirrhotic patients: from variceal screening to primary prophylaxis of the first oesophageal variceal bleeding. Liver Int 2011;31:108–119.

15. Chalasani N, Kahi C, Francois F, et al. Improved patient survival after acute variceal bleeding: a multicenter, cohort study. Am J Gastroenterol 2003;98: 653–659.

16. Cardenas A. Management of acute variceal bleeding: emphasis on endoscopic therapy. Clin Liver Dis 2010;14:251–262.

17. Kravetz D, Sikuler E, Groszmann RJ. Splanchnic and systemic hemodynamics in portal hypertensive rats during hemorrhage and blood volume restitution. Gastroenterology 1986;90:1232–1240.

18. Sass DA, Chopra KB. Portal hypertension and variceal hemorrhage. Med Clin North Am 2009;93:837–853, vii–viii.

19. Pauwels A, Mostefa-Kara N, Debenes B, et al. Systemic antibiotic prophylaxis after gastrointestinal hemorrhage in cirrhotic patients with a high risk of infection. Hepatology 1996;24:802–806.

20. Fernandez J, Ruiz del Arbol L, Gómez C, et al. Norfloxacin vs ceftriaxone in the prophylaxis of infections in patients with advanced cirrhosis and hemorrhage. Gastroenterology 2006;131:1049–1056.

21. Avgerinos A, Armonis A, Stefanidis G, et al. Sustained rise of portal pressure after sclerotherapy, but not band ligation, in acute variceal bleeding in cirrhosis. Hepatology 2004;39:1623–1630.

22. Kalambokis G, Tsiouris S, Tsianos EV, et al. Effects of terlipressin and somatostatin on liver and thorax blood volumes in patients with cirrhosis. Liver Int 2010;30:1371–1378.

23. Dell'Era A, de Franchis R, Iannuzzi F. Acute variceal bleeding: pharmacological treatment and primary/secondary prophylaxis. Best Pract Res Clin Gastroenterol 2008;22:279–294.

24. Thabut D, Bernard-Chabert B. Management of acute bleeding from portal hypertension. Best Pract Res Clin Gastroenterol 2007;21:19–29.

25. Gonzalez R, Zamora J, Gomez-Camarero J, et al. Meta-analysis: combination endoscopic and drug therapy to prevent variceal rebleeding in cirrhosis. Ann Intern Med 2008;49:109–122.

26. Hashizume M, Akahoshi T, Tomikawa M. Management of gastric varices. J Gastroenterol Hepatol 2011;26Suppl 1:102–108.

27. Prakash R, Mullen KD. Mechanisms, diagnosis and management of hepatic encephalopathy. Nat Rev Gastroenterol Hepatol 2010;7:515–525.

28. Bass NM, Mullen KD, Sanyal A, et al. Rifaximin treatment in hepatic encephalopathy. N Engl J Med 2010;362:1071–1081.

29. Sharma P, Agrawal A, Sharma BC, Sarin SK. Prophylaxis of hepatic encephalopathy in acute variceal bleed: a randomized controlled trial of lactulose versus no lactulose. J Gastroenterol Hepatol 2011;26:996–1003.

30. Shawcross D, Jalan R. Dispelling myths in the treatment of hepatic encephalopathy. Lancet 2005;365:431–433.

31. Bismuth M, Funakoshi N, Cadranel JF, Blanc P. Hepatic encephalopathy: from pathophysiology to therapeutic management. Eur J Gastroenterol Hepatol 2011;23:8–22.

32. Mullen KD. The treatment of patients with hepatic encephalopathy: review of the latest data from EASL 2010. Gastroenterol Hepatol (NY) 2010;6:1–16.

33. Mortensen PB. The effect of oral-administered lactulose on colonic nitrogen metabolism and excretion. Hepatology 1992;16:1350–1356.

34. Kato T, Uematsu T, Nishigaki Y, et al. Therapeutic effect of balloon-occluded retrograde transvenous obliteration on portal-systemic encephalopathy in patients with liver cirrhosis. Intern Med 2001;40:688–691.

35. Córdoba J, López-Hellín J, Planas M, et al. Normal protein diet for episodic hepatic encephalopathy: results of a randomized study. J Hepatol 2004;41:38–43.

36. Riggio O, Ridola L, Pasquale C, et al. Evidence of persistent cognitive impairment after resolution of overt hepatic encephalopathy. Clin Gastroenterol Hepatol 2011;9:181–183.

37. Garcia-Martinez R, Rovira A, Alonso J, et al. Hepatic encephalopathy is associated with post-transplant cognitive function and brain volume. Liver Transpl 2011;17:38–46.

38. Sandhu BS, Sanyal AJ. Management of ascites in cirrhosis. Clin Liver Dis 2005; 9:715–732.

39. Salerno F, Guevara M, Bernardi M, et al. Refractory ascites: Pathogenesis, definition and therapy of a severe complication in patients with cirrhosis. Liver Int 2010;30:937–947.

40. Ginès P, Cárdenas A, Arroyo V, Rodés J. Management of cirrhosis and ascites. N Engl J Med 2004;350:1646–1654.

41. Runyon BA. AASLD Practice Guidelines Committee: management of adult patients with ascites due to cirrhosis: an update. Hepatology 2009;49:2087–2107.

42. El-Bokl MA, Senousy BE, El-Karmouty KZ, et al. Spot urinary sodium for assessing dietary sodium restriction in cirrhotic ascites. World J Gastroenterol 2009;15:3631–3635.

43. Arroyo V, Colmenero J. Ascites and hepatorenal syndrome in cirrhosis: pathophysiological basis of therapy and current management. J Hepatol 2003;38: S69–S89.

44. Stanley MM, Ochi S, Lee KK, et al. Peritoneovenous shunting as compared with medical treatment in patients with alcoholic cirrhosis and massive ascites. Veterans Administration Cooperative Study on Treatment of Alcoholic Cirrhosis with Ascites. N Engl J Med 1989;321:1632–1638.

45. Hou W, Sanyal AJ. Ascites: diagnosis and management. Med Clin North Am 2009;93:801–817.

46. Alberts WM, Salem AJ, Solomon DA, Boyce G. Hepatic hydrothorax: cause and management. Arch Intern Med 1991;151:2383–2388.

47. Gurung P, Goldblatt M, Huggins JT, et al. Pleural fluid analysis and radiographic, sonographic, and echocardiographic characteristics of hepatic hydrothorax. Chest 2011;140:448–453.

48. Roussos A, Philippou N, Mantzaris GJ, Gourgouliannis KI. Hepatic hydrothorax: pathophysiology diagnosis and management. J Gastroenterol Hepatol 2007;22: 1388–1393.

49. Emerson PA, Davies JH. Hydrothorax complicating ascites. Lancet 1955;268: 487–488.

50. Chen CH, Ho-Chang, Liu HC, et al. Outcome predictors of cirrhotic patients with spontaneous bacterial empyema. Liver Int 2011;31:417–424.

51. Dhanasekaran R, West JK, Gonzales PC, et al. Transjugular intrahepatic portosystemic shunt for symptomatic refractory hepatic hydrothorax in patients with cirrhosis. Am J Gastroenterol 2010;105:635–641.

52. Bernardi M. Spontaneous bacterial peritonitis: from pathophysiology to prevention. Intern Emerg Med 2010;5:S37–S44.

53. Koulaouzidis A, Bhat S, Saeed AA. Spontaneous bacterial peritonitis. World J Gastroenterol 2009;15:1042–1049.

54. Akriviadis EA, Runyon BA. Utility of an algorithm in differentiating spontaneous from secondary bacterial peritonitis. Gastroenterology 1990;98:127–133.

55. Saab S, Hernandez JC, Chi AC, Tong MJ. Oral antibiotic prophylaxis reduces spontaneous bacterial peritonitis occurrence and improves short-term survival in cirrhosis: a meta-analysis. Am J Gastroenterol 2009;104:993–1001.

56. Testino G, Ferro C. Hepatorenal syndrome: a review. Hepatogastroenterology 2010;57:1279–1284.

57. Munoz SJ. The hepatorenal syndrome. Med Clin North Am 2008;92:813–837.

58. Angeli P, Volpin R, Gerunda G, et al. Reversal of type 1 hepatorenal syndrome with the administration of midodrine and octreotide. Hepatology 1999;29: 1690–1697.

59. Esrailian E, Pantangco ER, Kyulo NL, et al. Octreotide/midodrine therapy significantly improves renal function and 30-day survival in patients with type 1 hepatorenal syndrome. Dig Dis Sci 2007;52:742–748.

60. Salerno F, Gerbes A, Ginès P, et al. Diagnosis, prevention and treatment of hepatorenal syndrome in cirrhosis. Gut 2007;56:1310–1318.

61. Hopps E, Valenti A, Caimi G. Portopulmonary hypertension. Clin Invest Med 2011;34: E111–E118.

62. Kochar R, Nevah Rubin MI, Fallon MB. Pulmonary complications of cirrhosis. Curr Gastroenterol Rep 2011;13:34–39.

63. Krowka MJ, Mandell MS, Ramsay MA, et al. Hepatopulmonary syndrome and portopulmonary hypertension: a report of the multicenter liver transplant database. Liver Transpl 2004;10:174–182.

64. Krowka MJ, Miller DP, Barst RJ, et al. Portopulmonary hypertension: a report from the US-based REVEAL registry. Chest, 2012;141:906–915.

65. Tsiakalos A, Hatzis G, Moyssakis I, et al. Portopulmonary hypertension and serum endothelin levels in hospitalized patients with cirrhosis. Hepatobiliary Pancreat Dis Int 2011;10:393–398.

66. Ramsay M. Portopulmonary hypertension and right heart failure in patients with cirrhosis. Curr Opin Anaesthesiol 2010;23:145–150.

67. Mukhtar NA, Fix OK. Portopulmonary hypertension. J Clin Gastroenterol 2011; 45:703–710.

68. Sussman NL, Kochar R, Fallon MB. Pulmonary complications in cirrhosis. Curr Opin Organ Transplant 2011;16:281–288.

69. Cartin-Ceba R, Swanson K, Iyer V, et al. Safety and efficacy of ambrisentan for the treatment of portopulmonary hypertension. Chest 2011;139:109–114.

70. Swanson KL, Wiesner RH, Nyberg SL, et al. Survival in portopulmonary hypertension: Mayo Clinic experience categorized by treatment subgroups. Am J Transplant 2008;8:2445–2453.

71. Umeda N, Kamath PS. Hepatopulmonary syndrome and portopulmonary hypertension. Hepatol Res 2009;39:1020–1022.

72. Molina E, Reddy KR. Noncirrhotic portal hypertension. Clin Liver Dis 2001;5: 769–787.

Chapter 7: Endoscopic Classification and Management of Varices

David M. Arner and Abdullah M.S. Al-Osaimi

Introduction

Gastrointestinal (GI) varices represent a serious complication of portal hypertension (PHT) and can lead to life-threatening hemorrhage. Although there are many possible causes of noncirrhotic PHT (► Table 7.1), the most common cause is cirrhosis. Liver remodeling with fibrosis and regenerative nodule formation in cirrhosis increases venous resistance and portal pressure. Intrahepatic vasoconstriction secondary to decreased nitric oxide, and increased endothelin-1 further increases portal pressure.[1] Portosystemic collaterals can form in several anatomic areas along the GI tract. PHT is defined as hepatic venous pressure gradient (HVPG) greater than 5 mm Hg. The HVPG is calculated as the wedged hepatic venous pressure minus the free hepatic vein pressure. Varices do not occur until the HVPG rises above 10 mm Hg, and variceal hemorrhage can occur if HVPG is greater than 12 mm Hg.[2,3]

Esophageal varices (EVs) and gastric varices (GVs) are the most common PHT-induced GI varices because they provide the largest portosystemic collateral flow via the short and left gastric veins; however, ectopic varices are becoming increasingly recognized on endoscopic and radiologic evaluation (► Fig. 7.1). A variety of treatment options are used for PHT-induced GI varices depending on their location, the acuity of the situation (i.e., bleeding vs. nonbleeding varices), and the patient's underlying vascular anatomy. Such options include pharmacologic therapy with vasoactive drugs; endoscopic management with band ligation; sclerotherapy; glue injection; stenting; balloon tamponade (BT); or interventional radiologic management with balloon-occluded retrograde transvenous obliteration (BRTO), transjugular intrahepatic portosystemic shunt (TIPS), or venous embolization. With the increased effectiveness and availability of endoscopic and interventional radiologic treatment methods, surgical portosystemic shunt operations are less commonly used but still may play a role in select situations. This chapter reviews endoscopic management of PHT-induced varices.

Esophageal Varices

Esophageal varices exist in approximately 45% of individuals with cirrhosis and correlate with the severity of liver disease (► Fig. 7.2). Child class A patients with cirrhosis have a nearly 40% likelihood of having EVs on routine screening upper endoscopy, whereas Child class C patients with cirrhosis have an approximately 80% probability.[4] Varices enlarge at a rate of 4% to 10% annually. Large varices are more likely to rupture, and the 2-year probability of first bleed ranges from 7% among small varices up to 30% with large varices.[5,6] Up to 50% of variceal bleeding episodes stop spontaneously. Variceal hemorrhage carries a 6-week mortality rate of 20%, and up to 70% of untreated individuals die within 1 year of their initial hemorrhage. Predictors of hemorrhage include large varices, red marks (red wale sign or cherry red spots) (► Fig. 7.2d), alcoholic cirrhosis, and decompensated Child class B or C cirrhosis.

Screening

Evaluation of EVs has traditionally been performed by esophagogastroduodenoscopy (EGD) (see ► Fig. 6.2). Alternative screening modalities have been evaluated, including computed tomography (CT), esophageal capsule endoscopy (ECE), and ultrathin endoscopy. In a prospective study comparing CT with endoscopy, CT had 90% sensitivity but only 50% specificity for identifying large EVs. The sensitivity of detecting GVs by CT was 87% compared with EGD.[7] A multicenter study of 120 patients with

Table 7.1 Causes of Noncirrhotic Portal Hypertension

Intrahepatic Presinusoidal PHT	Sinusoidal PHT	Extrahepatic Postsinusoidal PHT
Hepatic schistosomiasis	Cirrhosis	Budd-Chiari syndrome
Congenital hepatic fibrosis	Noncirrhotic alcoholic liver disease	Right heart failure
Noncirrhotic portal fibrosis	Infiltrative disorders:	Constrictive pericarditis
Nodular regenerative hyperplasia	• Amyloidosis • Systemic mastocytosis	Suprahepatic IVC thrombosis
Primary biliary cirrhosis, sclerosing cholangitis	• Malignancy • Myeloproliferative disorder	Pulmonary hypertension
		Tricuspid valve regurgitation
Extrahepatic Presinusoidal PHN		
Portal vein thrombosis		**Intrahepatic Postsinusoidal PHN**
Superior mesenteric vein thrombosis	Peliosis hepatis	Veno-occlusive disease
Splenic vein thrombosis	Hypervitaminosis A	

IVC: inferior vena cava; PHT: portal hypertension.
(Adapted with modifications from Molina E, Reddy KR. Noncirrhotic portal hypertension. Clin Liver Dis 2001;5:769–787.[70])

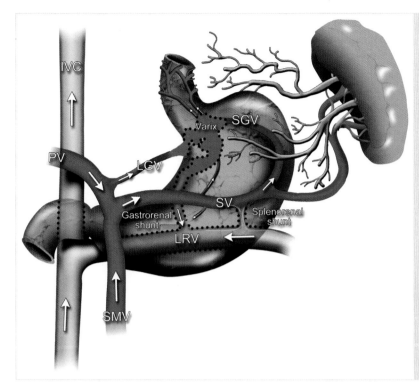

Fig. 7.1 Anatomy of the portal circulation. Gastric varices caused by splenic vein thrombosis (SVT) tend to arise from the short gastric veins and run from the hilum of the spleen to the greater curvature aspect of the stomach. PHT-induced gastric fundal varices arise from splenorenal or gastrorenal shunts. IVC: inferior vena cava; LGV: left gastric vein; LRV: left renal vein; PV: portal vein; SGV: short gastric vein; SMV: superior mesenteric vein; SV: splenic vein.

cirrhotic and noncirrhotic PHT compared ECE with EGD for EV screening and found a sensitivity of 77% and specificity of 86%.[8] A meta-analysis by Lu and colleagues showed similar rates of sensitivity and specificity.[9] The benefits of CT or ECE over EGD include little discomfort and sedation-less convenience with immediate return to normal activities. Disadvantages of CT include radiation exposure and the possibility of incidental findings of no clinical significance that could prompt further workup and incur additional costs. No serious complications have been reported with ECE, although a low rate of capsular retention has been reported (0.7%–2.2%), usually due to unknown esophageal strictures.[10] CT or ECE may be used as treatment modalities among patients who are unwilling to undergo EV screening evaluation with EGD. As opposed to CT and ECE, EGD also affords definitive endoscopic management of varices at the time of the procedure.

Another technique evaluated as a possible screening tool for EV is ultrathin endoscopy. Ultrathin endoscopy is a 3.1-mm battery-powered esophagoscope that can be comfortably used without sedation. One study of 28 patients who underwent both ultrathin endoscopy and routine EGD found ultrathin endoscopy to have a sensitivity of 100% and a specificity of 93% for detection of EV, and the ultrathin endoscope was well tolerated.[11] The ultrathin esophagoscope does not allow for treatment of varices if identified.

Classification

Several endoscopic classification schemes have been used to grade EVs. In the early 1980s, the Japanese Research Society for Portal Hypertension recommended that endoscopists describe the color, location, and form or size of varices in addition to any possible red marks.[12] In 1988, the North Italian Endoscopic Club grouped them into small (F1), medium (F2), and large varices (F3) with or without red marks (▶ Fig. 7.2). Small varices are minimally elevated above the esophageal mucosa and typically flatten with air insufflation (▶ Fig. 7.2a). Medium vessels occupy less than one third of the esophageal lumen but do not flatten with insufflation (▶ Fig. 7.2b). Large EVs occupy greater than one-third the diameter of the esophageal lumen (▶ Fig. 7.2c). In an effort to further simplify EV classification, recommendations were made at the Baveno I Consensus Conference to categorize varices as either small or large, with a suggested cutoff diameter of 5 mm.[13,14] Red marks or nipple signs should still be identified because they represent high-risk features of hemorrhage (▶ Fig. 7.2d). Most endoscopists use one of the last two classification schemes, and we recommend using the low- or high-risk classification method.

Management: Primary Prophylaxis

Current guidelines suggest a benefit to screening all patients with cirrhosis for EV, and EGD is the most widely used screening method.[14] EGD surveillance is recommended at a 1- to 3-year interval based on the patient's liver disease (compensated or decompensated cirrhosis) and prior findings (presence and grade of varices). Follow-up endoscopies are not required among patients with low-risk varices who are on appropriately dosed beta-blockade therapy (see ▶ Fig. 6.2).

After EGD has been performed, patients with nonbleeding EVs can be risk stratified based on their risk of hemorrhage. Small nonbleeding EVs without high-risk features can be conservatively monitored with surveillance EGD. Small EVs with high-risk features can be managed with medical pharmacologic therapy alone and/or with endoscopic variceal band ligation (EVL). Nonselective beta-blockers is to decrease cardiac output and cause splanchnic vasoconstriction. Patients with nonbleeding large EVs can

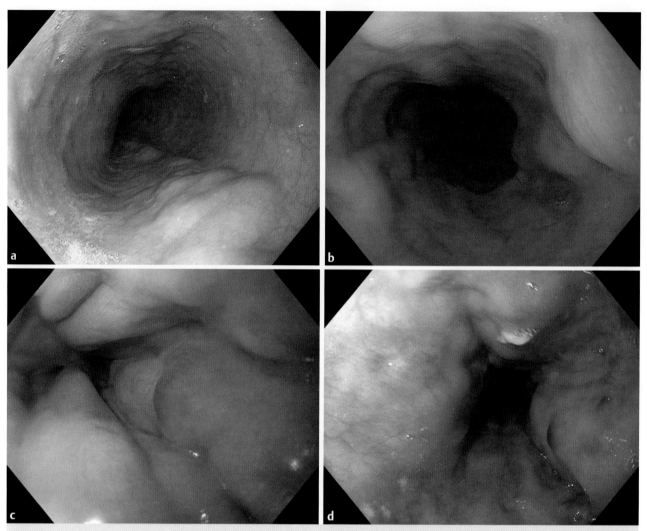

Fig. 7.2 Classification of esophageal varices. (**a**) Small, low-risk esophageal varices (or F1), almost flattened out with insufflation. (**b**) Medium-sized, low-risk esophageal varices (F2) that did not flatten with insufflation. (**c**) Large esophageal varices larger than one third of the esophageal lumen with some high-risk stigmata (red marks or wheals). (**d**) Esophageal varices with high-risk stigmata for recent bleeding and rebleeding with red marks and a nipple sign or fibrin plug.

be treated with beta-blockade therapy, which has been shown to lower rates of first variceal bleeding and mortality.[15] However, other treatment options are available for large EVs with high-risk features or among individuals who do not tolerate maximal beta-blockade therapy. Endoscopic treatment modalities primarily include endoscopic sclerotherapy (EST) or EVL.[14] TIPS and surgical shunt therapy has also been evaluated for primary prophylaxis.[14]

Endoscopic Sclerotherapy

Endoscopic sclerotherapy involves direct injection of a chemical sclerosant into the varices. EST has been used as primary prophylactic treatment of EV since the 1980s. Initial trials showed a significant survival benefit in addition to lower rates of first bleeding events.[16-18] However, further studies did not support these data and actually suggested that EST could provoke bleeding when used as primary prophylaxis.[19,20] One study comparing prophylactic sclerotherapy with sham therapy for EV treatment had to be terminated prematurely because the mortality rate

was significantly higher in the sclerotherapy group.[21] Complications of EST, such as ulcer or stricture formation, perforation, and chest pain, led to the development of alternative treatment options, primarily EVL. Therefore, EST is not recommended as primary prevention of variceal hemorrhage. The technique of EST is described elsewhere in this chapter.

Endoscopic Variceal Ligation

The first reported case of EVL was performed on dogs in 1986 with a 92% success rate. After its safety and efficacy had been assessed, it became available for endoscopic use in humans in 1988 (▶ Fig. 7.3). Since then, several randomized controlled trials and two meta-analyses have shown EVL to be at least equivalent and possibly superior to nonselective beta-blockers in primary prevention of an initial variceal bleeding episode and to have fewer complications.[22-26] Complication rates of EVL are low but include chest pain, ulceration, bleeding, stricture formation, and perforation.[27] EVL is a recommended treatment option for patients

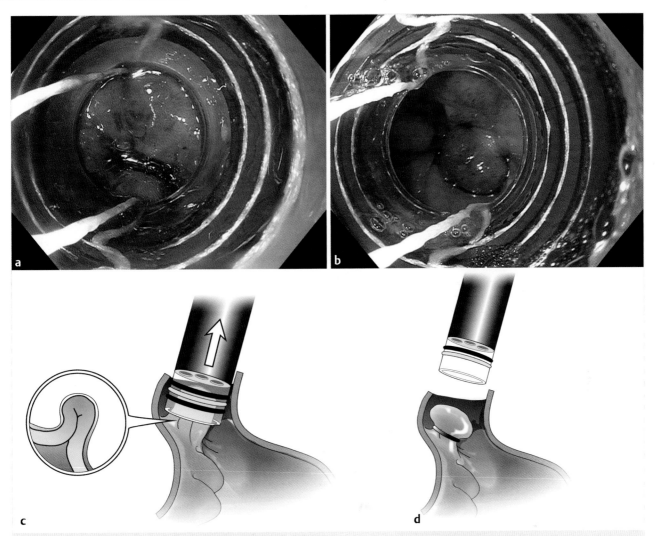

Fig. 7.3 (a,b) A transparent cap that is attached to the end of the endoscope with strings that acts as a tripwire and deploys the bands as seen on these images. (The bands are black, and the yellow band indicates the one before the last band; thus, repeated band placement is feasible.) **(c,d)** Illustrations of the transparent cap that is attached to the end of the endoscope with depiction of the suctioning maneuver of the varix inside the cap and then the deployment of the band.

with nonbleeding large varices who cannot tolerate beta-blocker therapy or large varices with high-risk features of hemorrhage. Compared with no active treatment, EVL is associated with a relative risk reduction of first bleeding episode of 64% with a number needed to treat of four to prevent a bleeding episode.[28,29]

Technique

Banding devices have evolved, and a variety of EVL devices are available for use. Each has a transparent cap that attaches onto the end of the endoscope and carries 1 to 10 stretched bands (▶ Fig. 7.3). A string that acts as a tripwire attaches the cap to the control handle via the accessory channel of the endoscope. The control handle contains a small wheel that can be rotated to draw the string back and deploy the band(s) when ready. After EVs have been identified, the scope is removed, the banding device is set up and attached to the endoscope, and then the endoscope is readvanced to the most distal varix. With the attached cap placed

directly onto the targeted varix, suction is then applied to the varix until it is brought up into the cap. The band is then deployed onto the suctioned varix by turning the trigger wheel. This process can be repeated with the remaining bands on residual varices (▶ Fig. 7.3b). Banding from the distal end and working proximally is the best method for decompressing varices, allows for complete visualization of the esophagus, and prevents possibly dislodging bands that have already been placed.

Shunt Surgery Operations and TIPS

Although portosystemic shunt surgery is effective at relieving PHT and decreasing EV formation and variceal hemorrhage, studies have shown more episodes of encephalopathy and higher mortality rates associated with this surgery.[30] This is likely due to decreasing portal blood flow to the liver.[31] TIPS has the same underlying physiologic mechanism as surgical shunt therapy, and because they both carry risks of encephalopathy, liver failure, and procedural complications, neither shunt surgery nor TIPS can be recommended as primary prevention of EV hemorrhage.

Management of Esophageal Varices Hemorrhage

Up to 90% of patients with cirrhosis will eventually develop EV, and nearly one third of them will have an episode of variceal hemorrhage (see ▶ Fig. 6.3). Advances in medical care over the past three decades has dramatically improved survival rates among EV bleeding with a mortality rate of 42% in the 1980s to current rates of 15% to 20%.[32,33] Medical therapy should be initiated as early as possible and involves volume resuscitation and hemodynamic support in an intensive care unit setting with goal hemoglobin of 7 to 8 g/dL except in patients with active ongoing bleeding or known ischemic cardiac disease. Care should be taken to not overtransfuse the patient to avoid elevated portal pressures and worsened bleeding. If the patient is having active hematemesis, intubation for airway protection should be strongly considered. Prophylactic antibiotics should be initiated to prevent spontaneous bacterial peritonitis, and octreotide or terlipressin (outside the United States) should be started. Beta-blockers should not be used in the setting of acute hemorrhage. Endoscopic therapy is considered the first-line definitive treatment option and should be performed as early as possible. If unsuccessful or the patient is not hemodynamically stable for upper endoscopy, TIPS or surgical shunting is pursued based on local expertise. As an emergent temporizing measure, balloon tamponade (BT) can be used to control active hemorrhage. BT is effective up to 80% of the time and should be considered if definitive management is not readily available as a temporizing modality.[34] Several BT devices are available with the most widely used being the Sangstaken-Blakemore and Minnesota tubes. Esophageal stents have also been evaluated as a tamponade device for uncontrollable EV hemorrhage.

Rebleeding can occur after initial hemostasis and is defined as recurrent variceal hemorrhage after a 24-hour bleed-free interval. Several factors have been associated with rebleeding or failure to control active bleeding and include active spurting varices, Child class C cirrhosis, bacterial infection, portal vein thrombosis, or HVPG greater than 20 mm Hg.[35,36]

Endoscopic Variceal Ligation

Endoscopic variceal ligation is the most common and recommended treatment method for actively bleeding EV. Approximately 80% to 90% of patients with an active EV bleed achieve hemostasis with EVL; the remaining 10% to 20% of individuals have either unsuccessful hemostasis with EVL or early rebleeding after band ligation.[30] The technique used with EVL has been described previously in this section (▶ Fig. 7.3). When treating an active EV bleed, the endoscopist may start banding at the GE (gastroesophageal) junction and work more proximally. Alternatively, a band may initially be placed on the bleeding or highest risk appearing varix and then additional bands placed from that point. The band causes thrombosis of the varix with necrosis of the mucosa, and the bands typically fall off within a few days with a residual superficial mucosal ulceration that heals and eventually scars. Repeat sessions should be performed at 2- to 4-week intervals until there is complete obliteration of varices.[14,32]

Endoscopic Sclerotherapy

Endoscopic sclerotherapy is generally used as second-line therapy in an actively bleeding EV or when bleeding precludes adequate visualization to perform band ligation. A variety of sclerosing agents are available, and all appear to be equally effective. The most commonly used sclerosants include sodium morrhuate (5%) and ethanolamine oleate (5%). EST involves initially drawing up the desired amount of sclerosant into a syringe and then attaching it to a needle injector and flushing the injector with sclerosant. The injector is then advanced through the scope channel, and under direct endoscopic visualization, the desired varix can then be injected with 1 to 2 cc of sclerosant and then briefly monitored for bleeding cessation. Varices can be reinjected if needed. Injection adjacent to the varices (paravariceal) is sometimes also performed to assist in thrombosis of the varix by causing inflammation of the surrounding mucosa. EST is typically started at the likely site of active bleeding. If unable to identify this, then it is recommended to inject distally near the GE junction and then advance proximally along the esophagus. A total of 10 to 15 cc of sclerosant is generally used, and both intravariceal and paravariceal injections are effective. EST is a good treatment option when there is significant blood within the esophagus precluding adequate visualization of the bleeding varix. It does come with potential complications as noted previously, primarily esophageal ulcers with possible bleeding, esophageal strictures, perforation, mediastinitis, pericarditis, chylothorax, and acute respiratory distress syndrome.[37,38]

Esophageal Stents

A few case series have been published on treatment of acute EV hemorrhage with endoscopic stent placement. These stents have been specially developed to not require fluoroscopic guidance. The stent is placed over a guidewire previously passed to the stomach by EGD. The stent has a distal balloon that is inflated with a syringe to ensure proper location in the cardia and lower esophagus.[39–41] When in location, the stent can be deployed to tamponade the bleeding EV. It can be left in place for up to 14 days and can then be retrieved endoscopically with a hook system.

Self-expandable metal stents (SEMS) have primarily been evaluated as salvage therapy after failure of hemostasis with traditional endoscopic approaches. In a case series of 10 patients who failed initial endoscopic management and had contraindications to TIPS or BT, SEMS was successfully placed in 9 patients. Bleeding was not controlled in three patients, although two of them had GVs.[40] A pilot study of 20 patients who failed pharmacologic and endoscopic therapy had SEMS placed with a reported 100% success rate and no significant complications.[41] Of the 20 patients, 8 were Child class B and 12 Child class C. The stents were left in place for 2 to 14 days, and bleeding was immediately controlled after placement of the stent in all cases. All of the stents were extracted without complication. Data on SEMS in acute variceal hemorrhage is limited, but it might offer an additional choice to salvage therapy in select patients.

Transjugular Intrahepatic Portosystemic Shunt

TIPS is an effective method of controlling EV bleeding because it significantly lowers the HVPG. TIPS results in a communication between the hepatic vein and one of the intrahepatic portal vein branches, which effectively decompresses the portal system and achieves immediate hemostasis in more than 90% of actively bleeding EV.[42] Compared with endoscopic therapy, TIPS reduces rebleeding (19% vs. 47%) but increases encephalopathy (34% vs. 19%) and liver failure without survival or cost benefit.[43–45] Because of this, TIPS has primarily been used as salvage therapy in cases of EV hemorrhage with inadequate control of bleeding after one or two endoscopic therapy sessions or rebleeding.

A recent randomized multicenter study demonstrated reductions in treatment failure and mortality with earlier use of TIPS among patients with cirrhosis hospitalized for acute variceal bleeding and at high risk for treatment failure. Patients were randomized to either early TIPS (performed within 72 hours) or pharmacotherapy, and EVL with TIPS used as rescue therapy as needed. Among the early TIPS group, there was significant improvement in control of bleeding, decreased rebleeding rates, and a 30% mortality absolute risk reduction. The author of this study concluded that in patients with Child class B or C cirrhosis and HVPG greater than 20 mm Hg, early TIPS may be a reasonable first-line therapy choice in the setting of acute variceal bleeding. Notably, patients with Child class C scores above 13 were excluded from the study.[46]

Absolute contraindications to TIPS include severe congestive heart failure, severe pulmonary hypertension, severe hepatic failure, multiple hepatic cysts, uncontrolled systemic infection, or unrelieved biliary obstruction. Hepatoma, severe coagulopathy (international normalized ratio >5), thrombocytopenia (<20,000), and portal vein thrombosis are all relative contraindications to TIPS. The MELD (Model of End Stage Liver Disease) score can accurately predict mortality after TIPS.

Surgical Decompression

With the development of additional endoscopic and interventional radiologic approaches to the treatment of actively bleeding varices, surgical decompression of EV bleeding has dramatically declined in the United States and is now only rarely used as rescue therapy. Because of this, many surgeons no longer receive training in shunt operations, and TIPS is generally considered the rescue treatment of choice in most centers.

Gastric Varices

Gastric varices have been reported in 20% to 25% of patients with PHT and have an approximate 25% risk of bleeding within 2 years, with fundal varices carrying the highest bleeding rates[14] (▶ Fig. 7.4). Although GV bleeding occurs less frequently than bleeding from EVs, it tends to be more severe and has higher rebleeding and mortality rates (▶ Fig. 7.5).[14,32]

GVs have been classified by Sarin et al as gastroesophageal varices (GOVs) and isolated gastric varices (IGVs) based on their location (▶ Fig. 7.4).[47] GOVs are an extension of EV. Whereas GOV type 1 lesions traverse the lesser curvature, GOV-2 varices extend along the fundus and tend to be more tortuous (▶ Fig. 7.4a,b; ▶ Fig. 7.5d). IGVs are categorized as IGV-1 lesions if located in the fundus or IGV-2 lesions if located in the body, antrum, or pylorus (▶ Fig. 7.4c,d; ▶ Fig. 7.5a,b,c).[48] IGV-1 are much less common than IGV-2 but have a higher risk of bleeding (▶ Fig. 7.5d). They

should also prompt evaluation of possible splenic vein thrombosis, and if found, splenectomy might be a potential therapeutic option.

As GOV-1 are extensions of EV, they should be treated the same as EV, primarily with EVL. Several therapeutic options have been evaluated for the treatment of high-risk and actively bleeding GVs, including EST, EVL, cyanoacrylate injection, BRTO, and TIPS. High-risk GVs are defined as GOV-2 IGV-1 with stigmata of recent bleeding (i.e., fibrin plug or clot), or any GV in the setting of a recent bleed with no definite stigmata but no identifiable source of bleeding (▶ Fig. 7.5b,c). Studies have shown glue injection to have higher initial hemostasis rates and lower rebleeding and mortality rates compared with EST and EVL.[49,50] Cyanoacrylate glue injection has been shown to have 36% and 46% lower 2- and 3-year rebleeding rates than gastric variceal band ligation.[51,52]

Cyanoacrylate Injection

Current practice guidelines recommend glue injection with tissue adhesives such as cyanoacrylate as the preferred treatment option for control of GV bleeding with TIPS being a consideration in patients in whom hemorrhage from fundal varices cannot be controlled or in cases of rebleeding[14] (see ▶ Fig. 6.3).

The most common cyanoacrylates used are Histoacryl or Glubran (-butyl-2-cyanoacrylate), Dermabond (2-octyl-cyanoacrylate), and Indermil (N-butyl-cyanoacrylate). Cyanoacrylates polymerize rapidly upon contact with weak bases, such as

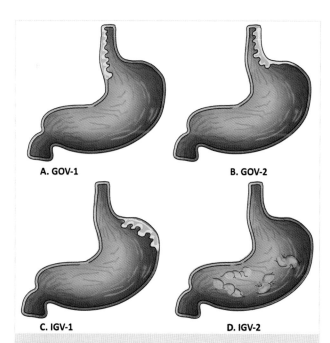

A. GOV-1 **B. GOV-2**

C. IGV-1 **D. IGV-2**

Fig. 7.4 Schematic diagram of Sarin's classification of gastric varices. Type 1 gastroesophageal varices (GOV-1) are typically a continuation of esophageal varices onto the lesser curvature. The fundal varices are included in two groups. Type 2 gastroesophageal varices (GOV-2) occur when the esophageal and fundal varices are present in continuity over the cardia; these might include type 1 isolated gastric varices (IGV-1), which are usually isolated gastric fundal varices. Type 2 isolated gastric varices (IGV-2) are gastric varices at ectopic sites in the stomach outside the cardiofundal region or the first part of the duodenum.

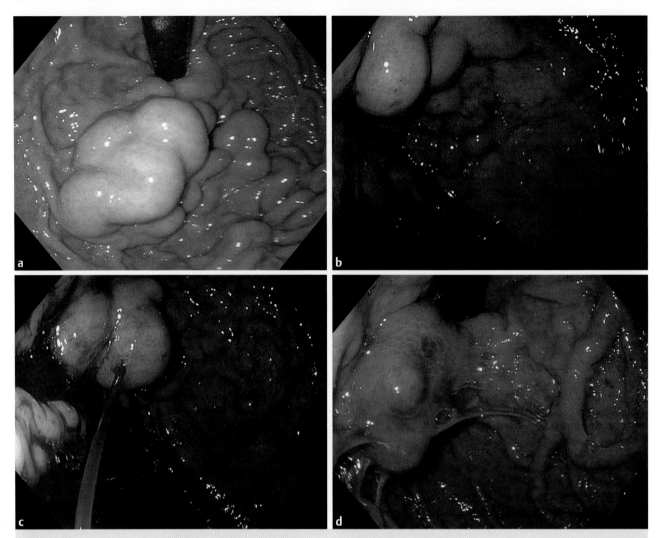

Fig. 7.5 Photographs of gastric varices. (**a**) Large (>3 cm) gastric varices (IGV-1) with no stigmata of bleeding. (**b**) A large IGV-1 with evidence of recent bleeding (blood in the stomach and a nipple or dimple sign). (**c**) The nipple sign area with active bleeding. (**d**) Mosaic (snake skin–like appearance) pattern of post–balloon-occluded retrograde transvenous obliteration (BRTO) findings of a GOV-2.

blood, but the polymerization time varies by compound. When injected intravascularly, they solidify and form a cast within the varix. Partial occlusion of the vein occurs immediately, and there is generally total occlusion within hours. The glue cast may remain for months to years. Initial hemostasis rates with glue injection of GV ranges from 90% to 100% with rebleeding rates ranging from 5% to 30%, approximately the same rates as TIPS. GV glue injection carries a 2% to 5% risk of serious complication, including fever, chest pain, embolism, infarction, needle impaction, sepsis, and death. Scope damage from the tissue adhesive can also occur. It should be noted that cyanoacrylates are not approved by the Food and Drug Administration for GV treatment.

Technique

We use Indermil for glue injection of GV, and it must remain refrigerated before use. Indermil is drawn up into two to three 10-cc syringes with varying quantity depending on the number and size of the GV. A 3-way stopcock is then attached to a 23-gauge needle injector and a 10-cc syringe of olive oil. The Indermil syringes are then attached to the stopcock. A flexible sigmoidoscope is used to perform the EGD given its greater viewing angles. After the GV is identified, the surrounding mucosa is cleaned with simethicone. The injector needle is then advanced through the channel and flushed with olive oil to prevent premature polymerization of the Indermil in the scope channel. The Indermil is then injected until a few drops exit the injector needle. The injector needle is advanced directly into the GV, and several milliliters of Indermil are injected into the varix immediately followed by a water flush and removal of the injector needle. This process is then repeated until all GVs are adequately treated. The scope can then be removed and cleaned with acetone and a cleaning brush. The patient should be treated with antibiotics for 1 week. We perform follow-up EGD with EUS (endoscopic ultrasonography) in 48 to 72 hours with Doppler assessment for residual varices (▶ Fig. 7.5d). Repeat glue injection can be performed until GV obliteration.

Balloon-Occluded Retrograde Transvenous Obliteration and Transjugular Intrahepatic Portosystemic Shunt

BRTO was first described by Kanagawa et al[53] in 1992 and is an interventional radiologic procedure used to treat gastric or ectopic varices with a spontaneous splenorenal or gastrorenal shunt and is described in greater detail in Chapter 29. The therapeutic efficacies of cyanoacrylate glue injection and BRTO appear to be similar based on one small prospective study with glue injection possibly having a higher rebleeding rate than BRTO. Additionally, BRTO may be a reasonable salvage therapy in failed or rebleeding glue cases.[54] Obliteration of splenorenal or gastrorenal shunts during BRTO likely increases portal pressure and the subsequent risk of EV hemorrhage in the long term, with one study showing no difference in EV bleeding rates at 1 and 3 year follow-up but a significant increase in bleeding rates at 5 and 7 years in the BRTO group.[55] TIPS is effective at controlling active bleeding from GV and was shown to be more effective than other forms of variceal obturation in preventing recurrent hemorrhage.[56] Each treatment option carries potential adverse effects, and each is reviewed in greater detail elsewhere in this book.

Our preference at our institution is to perform BRTO as the initial treatment for bleeding or high-risk GV if the patient has an accessible splenorenal or gastrorenal shunts. If the patient's anatomy precludes BRTO, we perform cyanoacrylate glue injection. We primarily use TIPS with embolization of the GV feeders as salvage therapy.

Ectopic Varices

Ectopic varices are any portosystemic shunt secondary to PHT that occur within the GI tract outside the gastroesophageal region. This includes varices in the duodenum, jejunum, ileum, colon, rectum, and ostomy sites. Ectopic varices account for up to 5% of all variceal bleeding episodes and typically present with sudden onset profuse hematochezia or melena and carry a mortality rate of up to 40%.[57-59] Urgent EGD should be performed followed by colonoscopy. If no bleeding lesion is identified, consideration should be made for angiography to identify the bleeding source.

Duodenal varices (DVs) originate from either the superior mesenteric vein (SMV) or the portal vein trunk via either the superior or inferior pancreaticoduodenal veins, which then drain into the inferior vena cava (IVC). Although they can occur anywhere in the duodenum, more than 80% of DVs are in the descending duodenum.[60] DVs are sometimes misidentified as other lesions and biopsied for further evaluation, and this can trigger massive bleeding requiring urgent treatment. Caution should be taken when evaluating duodenal lesions in patients with cirrhosis, and EUS can be used to better localize and differentiate suspected DVs from other lesions. Management options are outlined below.

Small bowel varices have become more recognized with our increased ability to visualize the entire small bowel either with balloon enteroscopy or capsule endoscopy. The prevalence of small bowel (other than DV) varices ranges from 1.9% to 8.7% among patients evaluated for obscure GI bleeding to nearly 70% of patients with known PHT who undergo capsule endoscopy.[61-63] They arise from collateral vessel formation between jejunal and ileal branches of the superior and inferior mesenteric veins (SMV and IMV, respectively) and the systemic venous circulation. They can also occur without PHT in the event of splenic or mesenteric vein thrombosis or congenital vascular malformations.[64]

Colonic varices occur in approximately 40% of patients with cirrhosis and arise from enlarged collaterals between ileocolic, right and middle colic vessels, and the systemic venous circulation.[65] Rectal varices must be distinguished from hemorrhoids and arise from communication between superior hemorrhoidal veins and the middle or inferior hemorrhoidal vein that eventually drains into the IVC. Rectal varices occur in up to 40% of patients with cirrhosis and extend more than 4 cm above the anal verge. Rectal varices collapse with digital pressure, but hemorrhoids do not. Stomal varices occur in up to 30% of patients with cirrhosis who have undergone colon surgery, and they develop at the mucocutaneous border of the stoma or just proximal to it.[66] Most commonly, this occurs in patients with inflammatory bowel disease and primary sclerosing cholangitis–induced cirrhosis who have undergone proctocolectomy with formation of ileostomy. These varices may not be obvious and may only be identified by a blue halo surrounding the stoma.

Management

Ectopic varices can be challenging to treat because they can be difficult to locate endoscopically. There are no substantiated data on primary prophylaxis of ectopic varices, but beta-blocker therapy is a reasonable option to decrease portal pressure and subsequent varix wall tension. The goal pulse rate should be 55 to 60 beats/min, similar to beta-blocker therapy when treating other varices. No further recommendations can be made on primary prophylaxis of ectopic varices.

Medical treatment of actively bleeding ectopic varices should be similar to other variceal hemorrhage medical management, with hemodynamic support, octreotide, and antibiotic therapy. Several studies have reported successful therapy of ectopic varices with EVL, EST, or glue injection. EVL has limited success when the ectopic varix measures larger than 15 mm, and other treatment options should be considered in these circumstances. EST has been used with the same sclerosants mentioned earlier for treatment of all ectopic varices, including peristomal varices; however, EST may result in stomal injury.[67] Glue injection can be performed on ectopic varices as in GV treatment. Another described method is initially clipping the bleeding vessel followed by intravariceal sclerotherapy or glue injection for definitive hemostasis. If there is failure to achieve initial hemostasis or rebleeding occurs, the next treatment option is venous embolization, which involves occluding the feeding vein on the portal venous side to the ectopic varices.[68,69] If bleeding persists, BRTO, TIPS, or surgical shunt should then be considered. In cases of bleeding stomal varices, surgical ligation or cautery can be effective. Because there are no substantiated controlled data to guide management of ectopic varices, endoscopic management of these lesions is left to the discretion and expertise of the endoscopist and treatment facility capabilities.

Conclusion

Variceal complications from cirrhosis and PHT are common and can have serious consequences. The treatment of variceal bleeding is complex and is best managed in a and is best managed in a multidisciplinary approach. Primary prophylaxis is indicated in certain cases, but available therapies for active or recent variceal bleeding are multifaceted, as discussed in this chapter.

Clinical Pearls

- Esophageal varices occur in approximately 45% of patients with cirrhosis.
- Esophageal varices severity correlates with Child-Pugh classification.
- Variceal hemorrhage carries a 6-week mortality rate of 20%, and up to 70% of untreated individuals die within 1 year of their initial hemorrhage.
- Primary prophylaxis of esophageal varices consists of beta-blockers or band ligation; variceal banding is the usual treatment of choice for variceal bleeding. TIPS is reserved for uncontrolled bleeding.
- Gastric varices occur in up to 20% to 25% of patients with PHT with or without cirrhosis.
- Gastric varices have an approximate 25% risk of bleeding within 2 years, with fundal varices carrying the highest bleeding rates.
- Gastric variceal bleeding is usually managed with cyanoacrylate therapy or BRTO, but is based on the expertise of the endoscopist and local medical institution.

References

1. Pinzani M, Milani S, De Franco R, et al. Endothelin 1 is overexpressed in human cirrhotic liver and exerts multiple effects on activated hepatic stellate cells. Gastroenterology 1996;110:534–548.
2. Garcia-Tsao G, Groszmann RJ, Fisher RL, at al. Portal pressure, presence of gastroesophageal varices and variceal bleeding. Hepatology 1985;5:419–424.
3. Lebrec D, De Fleury P, Rueff B, et al. Portal hypertension, size of esophageal varices, and risk of gastrointestinal bleeding in alcoholic cirrhosis. Gastroenterology 1980;79:1139–1144.
4. Pagliaro L, D'Amico G, Pasta L, et al. Portal hypertension in cirrhosis: natural history. In: Bosch J, Groszmann RJ. Portal Hypertension. Pathophysiology and Treatment. Oxford, UK, Blackwell Scientific, 1994, pp 72–92.
5. Merli M, Nicolini G, Angeloni, S, et al. Incidence and natural history of small esophageal varices in cirrhotic patients. Hepatology 2003;38:266–272.
6. Conn HO, Grace ND, Bosch J, et al. Propranolol in the prevention of the first variceal hemorrhage from esophagogastric varices: a multicenter randomized clinical trial. the Boston-New Haven-Barcelona Portal Hypertension Study Group. Hepatology 1991;13:902–912.
7. Perri RE, Chiorean MV, Fidler JL, et al. A prospective evaluation of computerized tomography (CT) scanning as a screening modality for esophageal varices. Hepatology 2008;47:1587–1594.
8. Lapalus MG, Ben Soussan E, Gaudric M, et al. Esophageal capsule endoscopy vs. EGD for the evaluation of portal hypertension: a French prospective multicenter comparative study. Am J Gastroenterol 2009;104:1112–1118.
9. Lu Y, Gao R, Liao Z, et al. Meta-analysis of capsule endoscopy in patients diagnosed or suspected with esophageal varices. World J Gastroenterol 2009;15:1254–1258.
10. Waterman M, Grainek IM. Capsule endoscopy of the esophagus. J Clin Gastroenterol 2009;7:605–612.
11. Madhotra R, Mokhashi M, Willner I, et al. Prospective evaluation of a 3.1mm battery-powered esophagoscope in screening for esophageal varices in cirrhotic patients. Am J Gastroenterol 2003;98:807.
12. Beppu K, Inokuchi K, Koyanagi N, et al. Prediction of variceal hemorrhage by esophageal endoscopy. Gastrointest Endosc 1981;27:213–218.
13. de Franchis R, Pascal JP, Burroughs AK, et al. Definitions, methodology and therapeutic strategies in portal hypertension. A consensus development workshop. J Hepatol 1992;15:256–261.
14. Garcia-Tsao G, Sanyal AJ, Grace ND, et al. Prevention and management of gastroesophageal varices and variceal hemorrhage in cirrhosis. Hepatology 2007; 46:922–938.
15. D'Amico G, Pagliaro L, Bosch J. Pharmacological treatment of portal hypertension: an evidence-based approach. Semin Liver Dis 1999;19:475–505.
16. Paquet KJ. Prophylactic endoscopic sclerosing treatment of the esophageal wall in varices: a prospective controlled randomized trial. Endoscopy 1982; 14:4–5.
17. Piai G, Cipolletta L, Claar M, et al. Prophylactic sclerotherapy of high-risk esophageal varices: results of a multicentric prospective controlled trial. Hepatology 1988;8:1495–1500.
18. Witzel L, Wolbergs E, Merki H. Prophylactic endoscopic sclerotherapy of oesophageal varices: a prospective controlled study. Lancet 1985;1:773–775.
19. The Veterans Affairs Cooperative Variceal Sclerotherapy Group. Prophylactic sclerotherapy for esophageal varices in men with alcoholic liver disease: a randomized, single-blind, multicenter clinical trial. N Engl J Med 1991;324:1779–1784.
20. Santangelo WC, Dueno MI, Estes BL, et al. Prophylactic sclerotherapy of large esophageal varices. N Engl J Med 1988;13:814–818.
21. The Veterans Affairs Cooperative Variceal Sclerotherapy Group. Sclerotherapy for esophageal varices in men with alcoholic liver disease. A randomized, single-blind, multicenter clinical trial. Hepatology 1994;20:618–625.
22. Khuroo MS, Khuroo NS, Farahat KL, et al. Meta-analysis: endoscopic variceal ligation for primary prophylaxis of oesophageal variceal bleeding. Aliment Pharmacol Ther 2005;21:347–361.
23. Garcia-Pagan JC, Bosch J. Endoscopic band ligation in the treatment of portal hypertension. Nat Clin Pract Gastroenterol Hepatol 2005;2:526–535.
24. Lo GH, Chen WC, Chen MH, et al. Endoscopic ligation vs. nadolol in the prevention of first variceal bleeding in patients with cirrhosis. Gastrointest Endosc 2004;59:333–338.
25. Schepke M, Kleber G, Nurnberg D, et al. Ligation versus propranolol for the primary prophylaxis of variceal bleeding in cirrhosis. Hepatology 2004;40:65–72.
26. Lay CS, Tsai YT, Lee FY, et al. Endoscopic variceal ligation versus propranolol in prophylaxis of first variceal bleeding in patients with cirrhosis. J Gastroenterol Hepatol 2006;21:413–419.
27. Wehrmann T, Riphaus A, Feinstein J, et al. Hemorrhoidal elastic band ligation with flexible videoendoscopes: a prospective, randomized comparison with the conventional technique that uses rigid proctoscopes. Gastrointest Endosc 2004;60:191–195.
28. Imperiale TF, Chalasani N. A meta-analysis of endoscopic variceal ligation for primary prophylaxis of esophageal variceal bleeding. Hepatology 2001;33: 802–807.
29. Triantos C, Vlachogiannakos J, Armonis A, et al. Primary prophylaxis of variceal bleeding in cirrhotics unable to take B-blockers: a randomized trial of ligation. Aliment Pharmacol Ther 2005;21:1435–1443.
30. D'Amico G, Pagliaro L, Bosch J. The treatment of portal hypertension: a meta-analytic review. Hepatology 1995;22:332–354.
31. Boyer TD, Haskal ZJ. The role of transjugular intrahepatic portosystemic shunt in the management of portal hypertension. Hepatology 2005;41:386–400.
32. Grace ND. Diagnosis and treatment of gastrointestinal bleeding secondary to portal hypertension. American College of Gastroenterology Practice Parameters Committee. Am J Gastroenterol 1997;92:1081–1091.
33. The North Italian Endoscopic Club for the Study and Treatment of Esophageal Varices: prediction of the first variceal hemorrhage in patients with cirrhosis of the liver and esophageal varices. A prospective multicenter study. N Engl J Med 1988;319:983–989.
34. Avgerinos A, Armonis A. Balloon tamponade technique and efficacy in variceal haemorrhage. Scand J Gastroenterol Suppl 1994;207:11–16.
35. Moitinho E, Escorsell A, Bandi JC, et al. Prognostic value of early measurements of portal pressure in acute variceal bleeding. Gastroenterol 1999;117:626–631.
36. D'Amico G, de Franchis R. Upper digestive bleeding in cirrhosis. Post-therapeutic outcome and prognostic indicators. Hepatology 2003;38:599–612.
37. Villanueva C, Colomo A, Aracil C, et al. Current endoscopic therapy for variceal bleeding. Best Pract Res Clin Gastroenterol 2008;22:261–278.
38. Baillie J, Yudelman P. Complications of endoscopic sclerotherapy of esophageal varices. Endoscopy 1992;24:284–291.
39. Kumbhari V, Saxena P, Khashab MA. Self-expandable metallic stents for bleeding esophageal varices. Saudi J Gastroenterol 2013;19:141–143.
40. Wright G, Lewis H, Hogan B, et al. A self-expanding metal stent for complicated variceal hemorrhage: experience at a single center. Gastrointest Endosc 2010;71:71–78.
41. Hubmann R, Bodlaj G, Czompo M, et al. The use of self-expanding metal stents to treat acute esophageal variceal bleeding. Endoscopy 2006;38:896–901.
42. Azoulay D, Castaing D, Majno P, et al. Salvage transjugular intrahepatic portosystemic shunt for uncontrolled variceal bleeding in patients with decompensated cirrhosis. J Hepatol 2001;35:590–597.
43. Sanyal AJ, Freedman AM, Luketic VA, et al. Transjugular intrahepatic portosystemic shunts for patients with active variceal hemorrhage unresponsive to sclerotherapy. Gastroenterology 1996;111:138–146.

44. Meddi P, Merli M, Lionetti R, et al. Cost analysis for the prevention of variceal rebleeding: a comparison between transjugular intrahepatic portosystemic shunt and endoscopic sclerotherapy in a selected group of Italian cirrhotic patients. Hepatology 1999;29:1074–1077.

45. Luca A, D'Amico G, La Galla R, et al. TIPS for prevention of recurrent bleeding in patients with cirrhosis: meta-analysis of randomized clinical trials. Radiology 1999;212:411–421.

46. García-Pagán JC, Caca K, Bureau C, et al. Early use of TIPS in patients with cirrhosis and variceal bleeding. N Engl J Med 2010;362:2370–2379.

47. Sarin S, Kumar A. Gastric varices: profile, classification and management. Am J Gastroenterol 1989;84:1244–1249.

48. Sarin SK, Lahoti D, Saxena SP, et al. Prevalence, classification and natural history of gastric varices: a long-term follow-up study in 568 portal hypertension patients. Hepatology 1992;16:1343–1349.

49. Ryan BM, Stockbrugger RW, Ryan JM. A pathophysiologic, gastroenterologic, and radiologic approach to the management of gastric varices. Gastroenterology 2004;126:1175–1189.

50. Sarin SK, Jain AK, Jain M, Gupta R. A randomized controlled trial of cyanoacrylate versus alcohol injection in patients with isolated fundic varices. Am J Gastroenterol 2002;97:1010–1015.

51. Tan PC, Hou MC, Lin HC, et al. A randomized trial of endoscopic treatment of acute gastric variceal hemorrhage: N-butyl-2-cyanoacrylate injection versus band ligation. Hepatology 2006;43:690–697.

52. Lo GH, Lai KH, Cheng JS, et al. A prospective, randomized trial of Butyl cyanoacrylate injection versus band ligation in the management of bleeding gastric varices. Hepatology 2001;33:1060–1064.

53. Kanagawa H, Mima S, Kouyama H, et al. A successfully treated case of fundic varices by retrograde transvenous obliteration with balloon. Jpn J Gastroenterol 1991;88:1459–1462.

54. Hong CH, Kim HJ, Park JH, et al. Treatment of patients with gastric variceal hemorrhage: endoscopic N-butyl-2-cyanoacrylate injection versus balloon-occluded retrograde transvenous obliteration. J Gastroenterol Hepatol 2009;24:372–378.

55. Choi YS, Lee JH, Sinn DH, et al. Effect of balloon-occluded retrograde transvenous obliteration on the natural history of coexisting esophageal varices. J Clin Gastroenterol 2008;42:974–979.

56. Lo GH, Liang HL, Chen WC, et al. A prospective, randomized controlled trial of transjugular intrahepatic portosystemic shunt versus cyanoacrylate injection in the prevention of gastric variceal rebleeding. Endoscopy 2007;39:679–685.

57. Hosking SW, Smart HL, Johnson AG, et al. Anorectal varices, haemorrhoids, and portal hypertension. Lancet 1989;1:349–352.

58. Weisner RH, LaRusso NF, Dozois RR. Peristomal varices after proctocolectomy in patients with primary sclerosing cholangitis. Gastroenterol 1986;90:316–322.

59. Khouqeer F, Morrow C, Jordan P. Duodenal varices as a cause of massive upper gastrointestinal bleeding. Surgery 1987;102:548–552.

60. Watanabe N, Toyonaga A, Kojima S, et al. Current status of ectopic varices in Japan: results of a survey by the Japan Society for Portal Hypertension. Hepatol Res 2010;40:763–776.

61. Arakawa D, Ohmiya N, Nakamura M, et al. Outcome after enteroscopy for patients with obscure GI bleeding: diagnostic comparison between double-balloon endoscopy and videocapsule endoscopy. Gastrointest Endosc 2009;69:866–874.

62. Tang SJ, Zanati S, Dubcenco E, et al. Diagnosis of small-bowel varices by capsule endoscopy. Gastrointest Endosc 2004;60:129–135.

63. Figueiredo P, Almeida N, Lerias C, et al. Effect of portal hypertension in the small bowel: an endoscopic approach. Dig Dis Sci 2008;53:2144–2150.

64. Sugiyama S, Yashiro K, Nagasako K, et al. Extensive varices of ileo-cecum report of a case. Dis Colon Rectum 1992;35:1089–1091.

65. Chen LS, Lin HC, Lee FY, et al. Portal hypertensive colopathy in patients with cirrhosis. Scand J Gastroenterol 1996;31:490–494.

66. Fucini C, Wolff BG, Dozois RR. Bleeding from peristomal varices—perspectives on prevention and treatment. Dis Colon Rectum 1991;34:1073–1078.

67. Spier BJ, Fayyad AA, Lucey MR, et al. Bleeding stomal varices: case series and systematic review of the literature. Clin Gastroenterol Hepatol 2008;6:346–352.

68. Barbish AW, Ehrinpreis MN. Successful endoscopic injection sclerotherapy of a bleeding duodenal varix. Am J Gastroenterol 1993;88:90–92.

69. Bhasin DK, Sharma BC, Sriram PV, et al. Endoscopic management of bleeding ectopic varices with histoacryl. HPB Surg 1999;11:171–173.

70. Molina E, Reddy KR. Noncirrhotic portal hypertension. Clin Liver Dis 2001;5:769–787.

Chapter 8: Paracentesis and the LeVeen and Denver Shunts

Louis G. Martin

Introduction

Large-volume paracentesis (LVP) and peritoneovenous shunts (PVS) are two of four commonly used methods of treating ascites that is refractory to optimal medical management (the other two, transjugular intrahepatic portosystemic shunt [TIPS] and liver transplant [LT], are discussed in other chapters of this book). All four methods compete for the same patient population, that is, patients with end-stage portal hypertension (PHT). It is not a fair competition. LT is the only one of the four that will significantly extend patient survival. Active alcohol or substance abuse, HIV or other systemic infections, life-limiting medical conditions (advanced cardiac, pulmonary, neurologic, or neoplastic conditions), uncontrolled psychiatric disorders, inability to comply with pre- and posttransplant regimens, and advanced age may eliminate a patient from consideration for LT. Patients with refractory ascites who are not candidates for LT or are waiting for a liver to become available are candidates for LVP and PVS placement.

One of the most serious signs of decompensated liver disease is refractory ascites, which has a prevalence of 5% to 10% in patients with advanced PHT and a survival rate as low as 50% at 12 to 24 months after diagnosis.[1] Ascites is considered refractory when it cannot be relieved by dietary sodium restriction and diuretic treatment. Sodium restriction to 2 g/day (88 mmol/day) and diuretics are the mainstay of therapy for cirrhotic ascites. Together these measures achieve successful diuresis in more than 90% of patients. About 10% to 15% of patients have sufficient spontaneous natriuresis to be managed by sodium restriction without the need for diuretics. The remainder requires oral diuretics; those recommended by the American Association for the Study of Liver Diseases (AASLD) are a combination of 100 mg of spironolactone and 40 mg of furosemide administered as a single morning dose.[2] If necessary, these doses can be raised until a maximum of 400 mg and 160 mg, respectively, are reached. One or more additional diuretics may be added in low doses to treat inadequate diuresis. Potassium disturbances or painful gynecomastia may necessitate a reduction in the dose of spironolactone and the substitution of amiloride. Failure to control ascites by these measures may be due to an insufficient response to sodium restriction and diuretic therapy, termed *diuretic-resistant ascites*, or the occurrence of diuretic-induced complications such as hyperkalemia, hyponatremia, renal insufficiency, or hepatic encephalopathy, termed *diuretic-intractable ascites*. Contraindications to diuretic use include hepatic encephalopathy, a serum sodium level lower than 120 mmol/L, and renal insufficiency with a serum creatinine level above 2 mg/dL. Diuretics should be discontinued and other therapeutic options considered if any of these adverse events occurs.[3]

The main factor contributing to the development of ascites in a patient with cirrhosis is PHT, which results from increased intrahepatic resistance to blood flow and is exacerbated by splanchnic vasodilatation as a result of local production of vasodilators. A commonly accepted theory of ascites formation in PHT is that it develops secondary to the continuous retention of sodium. Splanchnic vasodilation caused by PHT causes arterial system underfilling (hypovolemia); as a result, vasopressin activity increases and causes fluid retention. The body is eventually unable to maintain homeostasis, and fluid starts leaking into the peritoneal cavity. Sodium and water retention develop as the sympathetic nervous system and renin–angiotensin–aldosterone system are activated to compensate for the arterial hypovolemia. This theory is believed to explain the development of hepatorenal syndrome (HRS) and dilutional hyponatremia seen in patients with refractory ascites. The splanchnic circulation remains patent in PHT as a result of its own production of vasodilators such as prostaglandin E, prostacyclin, and nitric oxide, causing low vascular resistance, increased cardiac output, and decreased blood pressure. As a result of elevated hepatic sinusoidal pressure, there is an increase in venous blood flow and therefore increased lymph formation, which exceeds the flow rate that can be transported by the thoracic duct into the central venous system, resulting in fluid leaks into the peritoneal cavity (i.e., ascites).

Large-Volume Paracentesis

Paracentesis was the only treatment available for ascites from the time of Hippocrates until the advent of dietary sodium restriction and oral diuretics in the 20th century. For the past 2000 years, a rather large, hollow-bore metallic cannula was used access the ascitic collection; this has been replaced over the past 60 years by much smaller needles and catheters and a more stringent attention to aseptic technique.[1] Despite our progress during the past century, LVP is not a benign procedure; complications, including hyponatremia, renal failure, severe infection, gastrointestinal and abdominal wall bleeding, and paracentesis-induced circulatory dysfunction (PICD), occur in 20% to 50% of patients. In an era when moderate obesity is the norm and morbid obesity is not unusual, it is not always easy to diagnose even a large peritoneal fluid collection on physical examination. The classic signs of bulging flank and distended abdomen, shifting dullness to percussion, a fluid wave, auscultatory percussion, and the "puddle sign" (periumbilical dullness to percussion after the patient has been on his or her hands and knees for several minutes) can be masked by the patient's girth. Thankfully, ultrasonography, which can detect as little as 100 mL of fluid, has become the "gold standard" and is readily available to any radiologist.

Having determined that the patient has ascites, does he or she need paracentesis for relief of symptoms? Paracentesis can often give temporary relief of chest pain, dyspnea, abdominal pain, and anorexia. The AASLD practice guideline suggests a single LVP of 4 to 6 L followed by dietary sodium restriction and diuretic therapy for tense ascites; for patients with refractory ascites, the AASLD practice guideline recommends serial LVP sessions as needed. These guidelines consider albumin infusion as optional for LVP of more than 5 L but do not recommend it for paracentesis of lesser volume.[2] Patients with tense ascites are frequently treated by the removal of 7 to 10 L of ascitic fluid. Removal of such large volumes has been determined to cause PICD, a disorder characterized by marked activation of the renin–angiotensin axis secondary to the further increase of an already established arteriolar vasodilatation, which is a frequent and potentially harmful complication of paracentesis of greater than 6 L. Although PICD is clinically silent, it has been associated with a rapid recurrence of tense ascites and shorter survival times. The rate of fluid extraction, mechanical modifications (caused by abdominal decompression), and release of vasodilator molecules (e.g., nitric oxide) from the vascular endothelium are postulated to play a major role in development of PICD. The main feature of PICD is a marked activation of the renin–angiotensin and sympathetic nervous system without changes in plasma volume, heart rate, or hematocrit. Therefore, the rationale for using plasma expanders such as albumin after paracentesis is to maintain the circulatory status and to prevent the subsequent activation of vasoconstrictor systems. In a prospectively randomized study by Sola-Vera et al,[4] the incidence of PICD was significantly higher ($P = 0.03$) in the saline group versus the albumin group receiving total paracentesis; however, no significant differences were found when less than 6 L of ascitic fluid was evacuated (6.7% vs. 5.6% in the saline and albumin groups, respectively). Complications other than PCID were almost twice as frequent in the saline group in this study. Albumin was better than saline in the prevention of PICD. The incidence of PICD in patients receiving saline in Sola-Vera et al's study is similar to that reported in patients treated with dextran 70 (34%) or polygeline (38%); therefore, these are inferior substitutes for albumin.[4]

Disseminated intravascular coagulation (DIC) and an acute abdomen requiring surgery are the only absolute contraindications to paracentesis. Significant bleeding was below 0.3% in 5337 patients with coagulopathy or thrombocytopenia in two retrospective studies. In both studies, an increased bleeding rate was associated with significant renal failure.[5,6] Prophylactic

transfusion with fresh frozen plasma did not reduce the rate of bleeding in one of the studies.[5] Ultrasound guidance is mandatory if the patient in question has had an LT or abdominal surgery, which increase the likelihood of bowel adhesions and a lead to high probability of collateral veins on the abdominal wall that must be avoided. The patient should be asked to empty his or her bladder before the procedure. Prophylactic antibiotics should be given to cover the most common organisms (*Escherichia coli*, *Klebsiella pneumoniae*, and pneumococci) pending culture of the causative agent if the polymorphonuclear count is above 250 per cubic millimeter. Overviews of the indications, contraindications, preprocedure testing, and patient management related to LVP are summarized in ▸ Table 8.1.

Procedure

As is frequently the case in interventional radiology (IR) procedures, the materials used are not as important as how they are used. Paracentesis and thoracentesis kits are sold by many companies; some interventionalists prefer to use the centesis trocar supplied in these kits; others prefer a multi-sidehole catheter introduced by the Seldinger technique for LVP. The procedure can be performed with little or no sedation. Informed consent and aseptic technique are mandatory. Examination of the abdomen by ultrasonography immediately before paracentesis is recommended but not mandatory for all cases. The standard of care demands that preventive measures be followed in determining the needle-entry site for paracentesis.

1. When the midline approach is taken, the needle should not be entered cephalad to the umbilicus because the recanalized

Table 8.1 Large-Volume Paracentesis

Diagnostic indications	Fluid evaluation to determine the etiology of new-onset ascites, suspected spontaneous or secondary bacterial peritonitis, detection of cancer cells
Therapeutic indications	Chest pain, respiratory compromise, anorexia, abdominal pain or pressure (including abdominal compartment syndrome) secondary to ascites
Absolute contraindications	Hyperfibrinolysis, disseminated intravascular coagulopathy, acute abdomen that requires surgery
Relative contraindications	Abdominal wall cellulitis, intraabdominal adhesions, distended bowel or bladder, pregnancy
Procedural complications	Hyponatremia, hyperkalemia, renal failure, severe infection, GI bleeding, intraperitoneal bleeding, SBP, PCID, shortened survival time
Preprocedure Laboratory Tests[16]	
INR	Routinely recommended for patients with liver disease
aPTT	Routinely recommended for patients receiving IV UFH
Platelet count	Not routinely recommended
Hematocrit	Not routinely recommended
Preprocedure Patient Management[16]	
INR > 2.0	Threshold for treatment (i.e., FFP, vitamin K)
PTT and Hct	No consensus
Platelet count < 50,000/μL	Transfusion recommended
Clopidogrel	Withhold for 5 days before procedure
Aspirin	Do not withhold
LMWH	Withhold one dose before procedure

aPTT: activated partial thromboplastin time; FFP: fresh-frozen plasma; GI: gastrointestinal; Hct: hematocrit; INR: international normalized ratio; IV: intravenous; LMWH: low-molecular-weight heparin; PICD: paracentesis-induced circulatory dysfunction; SBP: spontaneous bacterial peritonitis; UFH: unfractionated heparin.

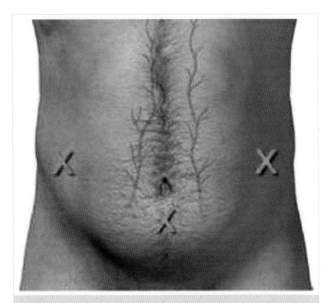

Fig. 8.1 Puncture sites for paracentesis should be through the linea alba below the umbilicus to avoid puncture of recanalized umbilical veins through the abdominal wall lateral to the linea alba to avoid puncture of the inferior superficial epigastric artery and vein, which are marked on the abdominal wall of this figure.

umbilical vein commonly underlies the abdominal wall in this location.

2. The needle must be inserted under ultrasound guidance several centimeters from surgical scars to avoid perforating loops of bowel adherent to the peritoneal surface of the abdomen.

3. Needle puncture should be performed under ultrasound guidance and below the umbilicus in patients who have had LT to avoid adhesions between the abdominal wall and the intestines.

4. Whether performed above or below the umbilicus, needle puncture should be through the linea alba or lateral to the rectus muscle sheath to avoid trauma to the deep and superficial branches of the inferior epigastric arteries that lies under this muscle (▶ Fig. 8.1).

5. Tunneling the needle for several centimeters in a zig-zag course through the subcutaneous tissue before entering the peritoneal space is recommended to prevent leakage of residual or reaccumulated ascitic fluid through the paracentesis puncture site.

Analysis of the ascitic fluid is only needed on the initial paracentesis and includes a cell count, culture, albumin level, and total protein level on the ascitic fluid and the serum albumin level. The serum-ascites albumin gradient or gap (SAAG) is a calculation used to determine the cause of ascites. A value over 1.1 mg/dL indicates a greater than 97% probability of PHT, and below 1.1 mg/dL indicates that PHT is very unlikely.

Peritoneovenous Shunts

Development of refractory ascites is associated with a 1-year mortality rate of up to 50%. Patients with cirrhosis who develop ascites should therefore be evaluated for LT. A treatment algorithm must be developed for patients with refractory ascites who are not candidates for LT. Some consider PVS as a third line of treatment

behind LT and LVP; others contend that there is "no role for PVS" in the present care of the patient with PHT.[7] PVS may be the only remaining option for treatment with expectations of a reasonably acceptable quality of life in a patient with refractory ascites and HRS or encephalopathy. The major criticism of the Denver Shunt is that it requires high maintenance and has a high complication rate that includes an increased risk of spontaneous bacterial peritonitis (SBP), which may jeopardize successful LT. First, not all patients with refractory ascites who have failed LVP are candidates for LT. Second, not all transplant surgeons believe that PVS has no place in the care of LT candidates; some endorse peritoneovenous shunting of ascites as a bridge to LT.[8] A recent review of 1491 consecutive adult patients undergoing LT at the University of Pittsburgh identified 80 patients (5.4%) who had at least one episode of SBP before LT. There was no difference in the long-term mortality rate between the two groups during a mean 4-year follow-up.[9] The issue of Denver Shunt use in a patient who is a candidate for LT may still be considered "open." Each practice will depend on the feelings of local transplant hepatologists and surgeons.

The Denver Shunt has proven useful for treatment of abdominal and pleural cirrhotic ascites but of course has no place in control of variceal bleeding. Better results can be expected in patients with lower Child-Pugh and model for end-stage liver disease (MELD) scores. Timing may be a critical factor; evidence shows that physiologic and quality of life improvement is enhanced by early placement of the shunt before the patient has deteriorated to the point that short-term survival is threatened.[10] End-stage renal failure requiring dialysis, sepsis, uncorrectable coagulopathy, morbid obesity, and septation of the peritoneal cavity caused by previous infection or surgery are contraindications to the procedure. To maintain Denver Shunt patency, the valve must be compressible against a firm, stable structure (i.e., a rib or the sternum), so the patient's body habitus is an important factor that must be evaluated individually. HRS and liver function have been reported to improve after shunt placement; therefore, low levels of functional impairment are not contraindications. Early and advanced age are not contraindications to Denver Shunt use nor does age significantly affect expected benefit.[10,11] TIPS offers relief to those with cirrhotic ascites but at the cost of accelerated hepatic failure and hepatic encephalopathy. Placement of a pleurovenous or PVS, which before the introduction of TIPS and LT was the only recourse available to this patient population, is generating renewed interest among hepatologists, transplant surgeons, and interventional radiologists. There are not many options for the patients with cirrhosis with diuretic refractory ascites who are not candidates for LT.

In the days before the TIPS procedure, Harry H. LeVeen designed a permanently implantable PVS to transmit ascitic fluid from the peritoneal cavity back into the central venous system, where it could be eliminated by the kidneys. A one-way valve in the LeVeen Shunt controlled antegrade flow of ascitic fluid through the shunt, allowing flow to occur when the peritoneal pressure was 3 to 5 cm H_2O higher than the intrathoracic venous pressure.[12] In 1979, Lund and Newkirk introduced the Denver Shunt, which was a modification of a ventriculoperitoneal shunt they had originally developed for the treatment of hydrocephalus.[13] This shunt has one or two silicone miter (duckbill) valves located in the pump chamber that permit flow in only one direction. The valves are designed so that their inner surfaces coapt when the pressure gradient between the peritoneal or pleural cavity and the central venous system falls below 3 to 5 cm H_2O, slide against each other when manually pumped to reduce buildup on the valves, and open to allow continuous flow when the peritoneovenous pressure gradient exceeds 5 cm H_2O. The Denver Shunt is currently marketed by the CareFusion Corporation (3750 Torrey View Court, San Diego, CA 92130); the LeVeen Shunt is no longer in production. The Denver Shunt it is offered in two French sizes and with either a single or a double valve. These one-way (unidirectional) valves prevent the reflux of blood into the venous limb of the shunt. The second valve acts as a "check valve" to prevent reflux of ascitic fluid or blood from the venous limb of the shunt into the valve chamber while it is refilling following compression "pumping." Therefore, the two-valve model is more effective at preventing reflux and is the shunt most commonly placed; however, the one-valve shunt should be chosen when the ascitic fluid is very viscous or when the daily production of ascites is unusually large. The venous limb of the shunt can be obtained with either 11.5-or 15.5-Fr tubing (catheter). The smaller tubing may be chosen when the shunt is placed via the subclavian vein, where the larger tubing may occlude the vein as it passes between the first rib and the clavicle, or via the saphenous vein, where larger tubing may cause venous obstruction or patient discomfort. Overviews of the indications, contraindications, preprocedure testing, and patient management related to the PVS are summarized in ▶ Table 8.2.

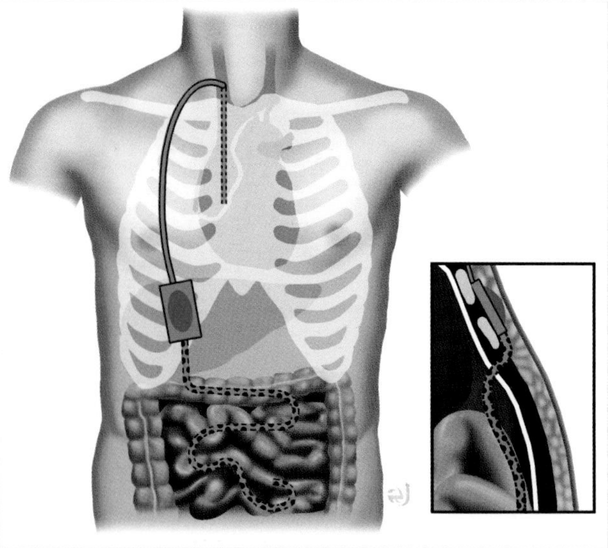

Fig. 8.2 Denver Shunt valve placed over the costochondral margin of the right lower rib cage so that the valve can be compressed over an immovable structure.

Procedure

We currently prefer to admit the patient for overnight observation after Denver Shunt placement. The shunt is routinely placed under moderate sedation. Broad-spectrum prophylactic antibiotics are given before the procedure and for 7 to 10 days after the procedure. The compressible valve must be placed over a firm, immobile area of the rib cage or sternum (▶ Fig. 8.1). The venous access can be jugular, subclavian, or saphenous; it is preferable to use the small-caliber catheter (11.5 Fr) when opting for a subclavian or saphenous access because the larger caliber catheter (15.5 Fr) can become occlusive in these veins. Operative patient preparation and nuances of the shunt placement are presented in ▶ Fig. 8.2, ▶ Fig. 8.3, ▶ Fig. 8.4, and ▶ Fig. 8.5.

Patients are discharged with prescriptions for oral analgesics and antibiotics; a contact phone number; and most important

Table 8.2 Peritoneovenous Shunt

Diagnostic indications	None
Therapeutic indications	Chest pain, respiratory compromise, anorexia, abdominal pain or pressure (including abdominal compartment syndrome) secondary to ascites, HRS
Absolute contraindications	Hyperfibrinolysis, disseminated intravascular coagulopathy, acute abdomen that requires surgery, sepsis, morbid obesity, end-stage renal disease requiring dialysis, septation of the peritoneal cavity caused by previous infection or surgery, abdominal wall cellulitis, SBP
Relative contraindications	Lack of access to health-care provider to oversee daily maintenance of shunt, likelihood of receiving a liver transplant
Preprocedure Laboratory Testing[16]	
INR	Routinely recommended
aPTT	Routinely recommended for patients receiving IV UFH
Platelet count	Not routinely recommended
Hematocrit	Not routinely recommended
Preprocedure Patient Management[16]	
INR > 2.0	Threshold for treatment (i.e., FFP, vitamin K)
PTT and Hct	No consensus
Platelet count < 50,000/μL	Transfusion recommended
Clopidogrel	Withhold for 5 days before procedure
Aspirin	Do not withhold
LMWH	Withhold one dose before procedure

aPTT: activated partial thromboplastin time; FFP: fresh-frozen plasma; Hct: hematocrit; HRS: hepatorenal syndrome; INR: international normalized ratio; IV: intravenous; LMWH: low-molecular-weight heparin; SBP: spontaneous bacterial peritonitis; UFH: unfractionated heparin.

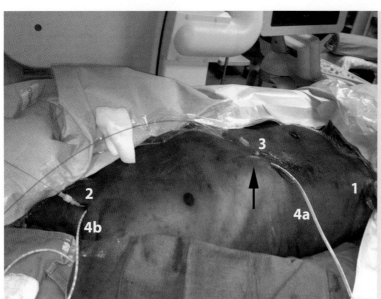

Fig. 8.3 Paracentesis in right lower quadrant (1); right internal jugular vein access (2); puncture from the right lower rib margin to the right lower quadrant peritoneal cavity (3); Denver Shunt catheter drawn through a subcutaneous tract between the peritoneal cavity access (4a) and the right internal jugular vein dermatotomy (4b); arrow points to the Denver Shunt valve that has been drawn into a pocket created over the right costochondral margin.

of all, instructions on how and when to compress the shunt pump. We recommend a return visit in 2 to 3 weeks to make sure everything is proceeding properly. It is vitally important that the venous limb of the shunt is compressed while pressure on the single-valve chamber is released (not while it is being compressed). If this is not done, blood will be drawn by negative pressure into the venous limb and eventually the shunt chamber. This point is stressed in the instruction manual that the company supplies for the patient. It is a good idea to highlight this paragraph and read it to the patient and caregiver. Moreover, flow through the shunt is affected by patient position. Maximal flow will occur in the supine

position, significantly less if the head and shoulders are elevated 45 degrees, and little or no flow if the patient is upright or sitting in a chair. Therefore, manual pumping of the chamber should only be performed while the patient is in the supine position. The most frequently encountered problem is that the patient or caregiver is not pumping the valve properly or frequently enough. It is imperative that the interventional radiologist invests sufficient time to make sure they understand how to pump the shunt properly before the patient is discharged. A recommended practice is to have the patient, caregiver, or both describe their maintenance methods at the time of discharge and on each return visit.

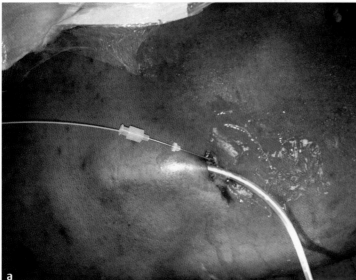

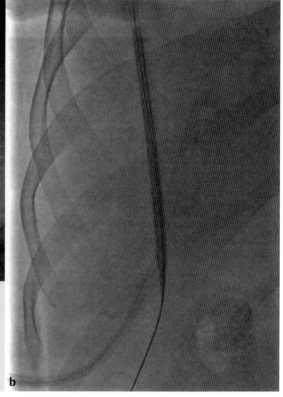

Fig. 8.4 (a) Denver Shunt valve has been pulled into a subcutaneous pocket. The peritoneal limb of the shunt is ready to be introduced into the peritoneal cavity into which a stiff guidewire has been introduced via the Seldinger technique using the zig-zag technique to lessen the chance of fluid leak along the catheter track. (b) Fluorocapture of the peritoneal track being dilated before introduction of the peritoneal limb of the shunt. Note the position of the shunt valve.

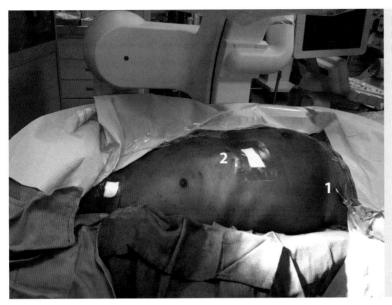

Fig. 8.5 Note abdominal swelling as normal saline is being introduced into peritoneal drain (1); marks on the skin to help identify location of pump valve for compression (2).

Shunt Evaluation and Repair

It is important to be able evaluate the Denver Shunt and its components.[14] A shunt chamber that is firm and difficult to compress indicates an obstruction of the venous limb or coagulated blood in the chamber. A shunt chamber that is slow to refill after compression indicates an obstruction of the peritoneal limb. Flow within the limbs of the shunt can be evaluated by Doppler ultrasonography. When it is necessary to access the shunt for diagnostic or therapeutic purposes, it is best to use a noncoring needle such as a Huber needle or an 18-guage Chiba needle with the stylet in place. These can be placed into the shunt chamber and either limb without causing significant damage. Contrast can be injected to identify and dislodge any accumulated material blocking the valve or limbs. To rule out reflux caused by valvular damage, the venous limb of the shunt should be compressed cephalad to the needle while contrast is injected. Contrast reflux into the valve or from the valve into the peritoneal limb will identify a defective valve that requires replacement. Injection of contrast into the shunt limb below the valve should reflux into the peritoneal cavity when the limb is compressed between the needle and the valve or flow through the valve if compressed caudad to the needle puncture site. These infusions should flush out debris that was blocking the shunt system. Shunt function should be restored after repriming the system by pumping the valve. A guidewire placed into the shunt limb through the Chiba needle will most often dislodge debris that is blocking the lumen. If the peritoneal limb of the shunt becomes lodged between bowel loops or inflammatory adhesions, the shunt catheter should be repositioned using means similar to those used to reposition peritoneal dialysis catheters. Furthermore, the peritoneal and venous limbs can be replaced and repositioned if the attempts to recanalize them are unsuccessful. It may be possible to fibrinolyze the clotted blood in the pump chamber that cannot be removed otherwise by directly injecting tissue plasminogen activator into the clot. Replacement pumps are not sold separately, but it should be possible to replace the defective pump while retaining the functioning venous and peritoneal limbs by splicing a new pump to the existing limbs using nylon tubing connectors available from the manufacturer.

Care after Denver Shunt placement should include observation for consumptive coagulopathy or disseminated intravascular coagulopathy (DIC) and fluid overload. A hematocrit; DIC profile (DIC Screen), which includes prothrombin time (PT), active partial thromboplastin time (aPTT), fibrinogen, D-dimer, and ATIII activity; serum creatinine; and measurement of 24-hour urine volume should be performed. The author sees the patient in 7 to 10 days for a postoperative evaluation and counseling. More information about Denver Shunt design, care, and management is available at the manufacturer's website.[15]

Clinical Pearls: Ascites

- Ascites is a sign of very serious cirrhotic liver failure.
- It is associated with an up to 50% mortality in 12 to 24 months after diagnosis.
- Elevated hepatic sinusoidal pressure results in an increase in venous blood flow and therefore increased lymph formation that exceeds the flow rate that can be transported by the thoracic duct into the central venous system, resulting in fluid leaks into the peritoneal cavity (i.e., ascites).
- Salt restriction and diuretics are the first-line therapy.
  - Salt restriction alone may be sufficient for 10% to 15% of patients.
  - An insufficient response to sodium restriction and diuretic therapy is termed *diuretic-resistant ascites.*
  - The occurrence of diuretic-induced complications such as hyperkalemia, hyponatremia, renal insufficiency, and hepatic encephalopathy is termed *diuretic intractable ascites.*

Clinical Pearls: Large-Volume Paracentesis

- Paracentesis was the only treatment available for ascites from the time of Hippocrates until the advent of dietary sodium restriction and oral diuretics in the 20th century.

- Complications, including hyponatremia, renal failure, severe infection, GI and abdominal wall bleeding, and paracentesis-induced circulatory dysfunction, occur in 20% to 50% of patients.
- The AASLD practice guideline suggests a single LVP of 4 to 6 L followed by dietary sodium restriction and diuretic therapy for tense ascites.
- The AASLD practice guidelines consider albumin infusion as optional for LVP of more than 5 L but do not recommend it for paracentesis of lesser volume.

Clinical Pearls: Paracentesis-Induced Circulatory Dysfunction

- The main feature of PICD is a marked activation of the renin–angiotensin and sympathetic nervous system without changes in plasma volume, heart rate, or hematocrit.
- PCID is predominantly caused by an accentuation of the arteriolar vasodilation already present in untreated patients with cirrhosis who have ascites.
- PICD is associated with increased levels of renin and norepinephrine and is associated with a significant reduction in systemic vascular resistance and an increase in the HVPG.
- The role of plasma expanders such as albumin after paracentesis is to maintain the circulatory status and to prevent the subsequent activation of the renin–angiotensin and other vasoconstrictor systems.

Clinical Pearls: Peritoneovenous Shunt

- PVS is associated with a higher incidence of SBP, which may jeopardize future LT.
- Some LT surgeons endorse PVS as a bridge to LT.
- High Childs-Pugh and MELD scores predict a reduced benefit from PVS.
- End-stage renal failure requiring dialysis, sepsis, uncorrectable coagulopathy, morbid obesity, and septation of the peritoneal cavity caused by previous infection or surgery are contraindications to PVS.
- HRS and liver function have been reported to improve after PVS placement.

Clinical Pearls: Spontaneous Bacterial Peritonitis

- SPB is the infection of previously sterile ascitic fluid.
- SBP has no intraabdominal source.
- SBP is thought to result from intestinal bacteria crossing the bowel wall into the peritoneal cavity.
- The incidence of SBP is as high as 30% in patients with cirrhosis admitted to the hospital.
- SBP must be distinguished from secondary bacterial peritonitis which may require surgery or additional IR drainage procedures to control.

Clinical Pearls: Disseminated Intravascular Coagulopathy (Consumptive Coagulopathy)

- DIC, which is characterized by widespread activation of coagulation resulting in thrombotic occlusion of small- and medium-sized blood vessels, may present as severe bleeding.
- DIC may occur in 30% to 50% of patients with gram-negative or -positive sepsis.
- Cell-specific membrane components of the microorganism may activate the cytokine network because of sepsis, trauma, cancer, vascular and immunologic disorders, and toxins.
- There is no single laboratory test that can diagnose or rule out the diagnosis of DIC.
  - Severe liver disease and DIC have the same laboratory characteristics.
  - Clinical studies have shown that hypofibrinogenemia and schistocytes on blood smear are diagnostically useful in very severe cases.
- A continuous infusion of low-dose heparin (300–500 U/hr) is probably useful in severe cases.
- High doses of antithrombin III have resulted in a significant reduction of mortality in a meta-analysis of nonrandomized trials.

References

1. Runyon BA. Management of adult patients with ascites due to cirrhosis. Hepatology 2004;39(3):841–856.
2. Runyon BA. AASLD practice guidelines. Management of adult patients with ascites due to cirrhosis: an update. 2009. http://www.aasld.org/practiceguidelines/Documents/Bookmarked%20Practice%20Guidelines/ascites%20Update6-2009.pdf.
3. Wong F. Management of ascites in cirrhosis. J Gastroenterol Hepatol 2012;27(1):11–20.
4. Sola-Vera J, Minana J, Ricart E, et al. Randomized trial comparing albumin and saline in the prevention of paracentesis-induced circulatory dysfunction in cirrhotic patients with ascites. Hepatology 2003;37(5):1147–1153.
5. McVay PA, Toy PT. Lack of increased bleeding after paracentesis and thoracentesis in patients with mild coagulation abnormalities. Transfusion 1991;31(2):164–171.
6. Pache I, Bilodeau M. Severe haemorrhage following abdominal paracentesis for ascites in patients with liver disease. Aliment Pharmacol Ther 2005;21(5):525–529.
7. Wongcharatrawee S, Garcia-Tsao G. Clinical management of ascites and its complications. Clin Liver Dis 2001;5(3):833–850.
8. Dumortier J, Pianta E, Le Derf Y, et al. Peritoneovenous shunt as a bridge to liver transplantation. Am J Transplant 2005;5(8):1886–1892.
9. Mounzer R, Malik SM, Nasr J, et al. Spontaneous bacterial peritonitis before liver transplantation does not affect patient survival. Clin Gastroenterol Hepatol 2010;8(7):623–628.
10. Oida T, Mimatsu K, Kawasaki A, et al. Early implantation of Denver shunt. Hepatogastroenterology 2011;58(112):2026–2028.
11. Abbas M, El Damarawy M, Seyam M, et al. Denver peritoneovenous shunt in the management of refractory ascites due to chronic liver diseases: impact of patients selection on its outcome. J Egypt Soc Parasitol 2007;37(3 suppl):1159–1174.
12. LeVeen HH, Christoudias G, Ip M, et al. Peritoneo-venous shunting for ascites. Ann Surg 1974;180(4):580–591.
13. Kirsch WM, Newkirk JB, Predecki PK. Clinical experience with the Denver shunt: a new silicone-rubber shunting device for the treatment of hydrocephalus. Technical note. J Neurosurg 1970;32(2):258–264.
14. Martin LG. Percutaneous placement and management of peritoneovenous shunts. Semin Intervent Radiol 2012;29(2):129–134.
15. CareFusion. Denver Shunts. For patients with refractory ascites. 2011. http://www.carefusion.com/pdf/Interventional_Specialties/Denver_shunt_brochure.pdf.
16. Patel IJ, Davidson JC, Nikolic B, et al. Consensus guidelines for periprocedural management of coagulation status and hemostasis risk in percutaneous image-guided interventions. J Vasc Interv Radiol 2012;23(6):727–736.

Chapter 9: Surgical Management of Portal Hypertension

Kaj H. Johansen

Introduction

In the 15 years since publication of the second edition of this book, the once preeminent role of the general surgeon in the management of portal hypertension (PHT) has virtually vanished. The ever-wider application of percutaneous catheter–based portal decompressive methodologies, more aggressive pharmacologic and endoscopic approaches, and the maturation of liver transplantation into a technically feasible and predictably successful treatment for end-stage liver disease have supplanted the role of the general surgeon in the contemporary management of patients with bleeding varices. Randomized trial evidence that percutaneous transjugular intrahepatic portacaval shunt (TIPS) construction results in survival and variceal rebleeding outcomes equivalent to those after surgical shunt underscored this progression.[1] Portosystemic shunt and esophagogastric devascularization procedures, for a half century the mainstay of the management of patients with cirrhosis and PHT, are now so rarely performed that few currently active general surgeons have carried any of them out in the past quarter century. Such operations are no longer even part of the training curriculum for general surgery residents.

This chapter is, therefore, to a substantial degree a reflection on general surgeons' historical involvement with the management of PHT and a testimonial to the inexorable advance of medical technologies. Others have offered similar valedictories.[2] Herein are archived general principles about the various types of portal decompressive shunts and devascularization procedures, perhaps of occasional contemporary use when the interventional radiology team is out of town and the airport is closed by bad weather or perhaps in the developing world where well-stocked angiography suites are rare but technically skilled surgeons are not.

General Considerations

The major complications associated with hepatic cirrhosis and PHT include gastrointestinal (GI) tract hemorrhage, ascites, hypersplenism, hepatic encephalopathy, and liver failure. The last two complications are commonly progressive and irreversible and, as markers for advanced liver disease, are indications for consideration of transplantation—a topic discussed elsewhere in this text.

Studies of the natural history of cirrhosis and PHT suggest that esophagogastric varices will develop in approximately 30% of patients with compensated cirrhosis and in 60% of patients with decompensated disease.[3] The risk of bleeding from large varices is 20% to 30% per year. After an initial bleed, the risk of rebleeding is 75% to 80%, with the highest risk being within the first 6 months to 1 year. Acute variceal bleeding carries a mortality rate of approximately 30% (range, 15%–50%), with most deaths occurring in poor-risk Child class C patients as the consequence of progressive liver failure.

Pathophysiologic studies of portal venous pressure have yielded several important observations: (1) normal portal venous pressure is 5 to 7 mm Hg; (2) variceal bleeding does not occur until the portal venous pressure exceeds 12 mm Hg; and (3) reduction of the portosystemic pressure gradient by 50%, or to an absolute pressure of ≤12 mm Hg, generally prevents variceal bleeding. PHT is defined as a portal pressure of greater than 10 mm Hg.

A majority of patients with PHT present with upper (or lower) GI tract hemorrhage from esophageal, gastric, hemorrhoidal, or stomal varices or from portal hypertensive gastropathy. In Western countries, the leading cause of portal hypertensive bleeding remains alcoholic liver disease; in developing countries, such hemorrhage arises most commonly as a consequence of various infectious disorders (viral hepatitis, schistosomiasis).

After the source of GI tract hemorrhage has been identified as portal hypertensive in origin, proper initial management includes blood and volume restitution, pharmacologic modification of portal venous pressure, and (for upper GI bleeding) endoscopic therapy by variceal sclerotherapy or banding. Because variceal rebleeding in this setting is commonplace, one or another form of percutaneous transjugular or direct TIPS construction is warranted. Transfer to a center where such procedures are frequently performed may be necessary.

Because anesthesia, major surgery, blood loss, and diversion of hepatic portal blood flow are tolerated poorly by decompensated Child class C cirrhotics, whenever possible, patients with persistent jaundice, intractable ascites, spontaneous encephalopathy, and advanced muscle wasting are better managed by endoscopic variceal therapy or banding or TIPS (or, when appropriate, orthotopic liver transplantation). Not all such patients are irreversibly ill; temporary control of bleeding followed by vigorous nutritional and metabolic resuscitation frequently can improve Child class and prognosis in patients with cirrhosis and therefore improve their likelihood of long-term survival. Similarly, documented abstinence from alcohol for 6 to 12 months in a previously recalcitrant alcoholic with cirrhosis makes consideration of liver transplantation ethically reasonable.[4]

Another important prognostic feature is the presence of a significant coagulopathy, defined as an international normalized ratio greater than 1.8 despite correction with blood products. Such patients have an excessive risk of intra- and postoperative hemorrhage, and surgery should be withheld. Thrombocytopenia from hypersplenism is commonplace in patients with variceal bleeding, with platelet counts commonly around 60,000/mL. Successful portal decompression generally reverses hypersplenism and restores platelet counts to normal levels.[5]

Special concerns accompany the anesthetic management of the patient with cirrhosis, especially those undergoing shunts or liver transplantation.[6,7] Generalized arteriovenous shunting in these patients may involve the pulmonary circulation, resulting in significant hypoxemia. Hepatocellular dysfunction may result in slowed clearance of anesthetic agents and sedatives that are normally metabolized by the liver. Cirrhosis is associated with an upregulation of benzodiazepine receptors in the brain, thus making the use of such sedative agents relatively contraindicated. Fluid and electrolyte disorders, such as extracellular volume excess, respiratory alkalosis, and total body potassium deficiency, can be anticipated. Repletion of blood volume in an actively bleeding patient may result in numerous problems with volume shifts and dilutional coagulopathy. Endotracheal intubation of a patient who has recently bled is fraught with the risk of aspiration of gastric contents—a problem that may be exacerbated when concurrent ascites results in significantly raised intraabdominal pressure.

Intravenous vasopressin or octreotide predictably diminishes portal pressure and may be administered, especially for the acute control of bleeding. However, coronary vasoconstriction leading to myocardial ischemia (perhaps worsened by alcoholic cardiomyopathy) can result from administration of vasopressin. Concurrent administration of nitroglycerin with vasopressin may significantly reduce the latter agent's coronary vasoconstrictive side effects. The plasma volume of a patient with hypoalbuminemia and sodium excess should be restituted using a noncrystalloid volume replacement, such as plasma, albumin, or hetastarch.

Patients with variceal hemorrhage often are both acutely and chronically ill, with multiple medical comorbidities complicating their hospital course and the conduct of any procedure performed. Their appropriate treatment(s) will depend on many factors, such as the cause of PHT, the urgency with which variceal hemorrhage must be treated, and the patient's clinical status. The patient's clinical status may change significantly for better or for worse, so therapeutic options may develop or be eliminated by the passage of time and new clinical findings. Care in a center where all such options are available is optimal.

Acute Management of Recalcitrant Variceal Bleeding

A certain percentage of patients may experience early recurrence of bleeding or will have continued hemorrhage despite vasopressin or octreotide administration and endoscopic variceal sclerotherapy or banding. Virtually all such early recurrent or persistent bleeding can be controlled with esophagogastric balloon tamponade. In fact, persistent bleeding in the face of these maneuvers raises the likelihood of a nonvariceal bleeding source such a peptic ulcer diathesis, postsclerotherapy ulceration, or a Mallory-Weiss tear. In a patient whose bleeding is temporarily controlled by balloon tamponade, definitive portal decompressive management must be planned within the next 48 to 72 hours, by which time balloon tamponade must be discontinued.

Emergent Management of Active Variceal Bleeding

Although general anesthesia and major surgery in a hypovolemic, malnourished, coagulopathic, chronically ill patient with cirrhosis might seem to result in an overwhelmingly elevated morbidity and mortality, Orloff and Bell successfully performed emergency side-to-side portacaval shunts (PCSs) in more than 450 patients.[8] Although the early post-shunt mortality rate was 16%, further variceal bleeding was eliminated, and the 5-year survival rate exceeded 70%. However, others have reported mortality rates of 30% to 50% after emergency PCS surgery.

Today almost all such patients would optimally be treated initially with endoscopic therapy and then by TIPS, with immediate control of bleeding in virtually all such patients. However, when TIPS is performed on an emergency basis in actively bleeding patients who are inadequately resuscitated, the mortality rate remains excessive.

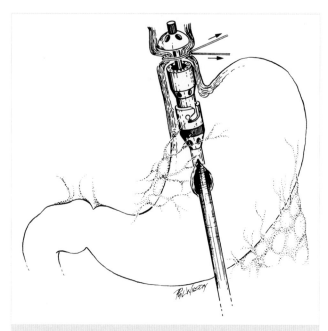

Fig. 9.1 Esophageal transection using the end-to-end anastomosis stapling device. The stapler is introduced into the distal esophagus via a high gastrostomy. The distal esophagus has been carefully dissected, with careful attention to the identification and preservation of the vagus nerves. A heavy monofilament suture is then tied around the "open" central rod of the stapler, after which the stapler is fired and removed. The tissue "donut" from the stapler, which is the area of the esophageal transection and reanastomosis, is checked for completeness, and the gastrostomy is closed.

Devascularization Procedures

Laparotomy and transgastric staple transection of the esophagus may be the optimal approach for emergency control of esophageal variceal bleeding in which endoscopic treatment has failed and for some reason TIPS is not feasible. Such a procedure is rapid, relatively straightforward, and effective (at least in the short term), and it does not significantly interfere with consideration of a shunt or liver transplantation if the patient survives to be a candidate for either (► Fig. 9.1).

Direct operative attack on bleeding esophageal and gastric varices has been a well-established therapeutic concept for more than a century. The aim is to reduce inflow to the bleeding gastroesophageal varices and is dependent on the extent of devascularization, with better bleeding control being achieved with more extensive procedures.

Certain approaches, such as direct oversewing of variceal columns after thoracotomy and longitudinal esophagotomy, are obsolete. Other variations on the devascularization theme combine splenectomy; gastroesophageal variceal plexus ligation; and occlusion of the coronary, gastroepiploic, and short gastric veins.[9] It is important that a sufficient length of esophagus (at least 7 cm) is mobilized to be devascularized from below the diaphragm. Moreover, gastric devascularization should totally devascularize the entire greater curvature and lesser curvature of the stomach in a manner similar in extent to a highly selective vagotomy. An extremely aggressive devascularization procedure, originally promoted by Sugiura and Futagawa, entails a staged thoracotomy and laparotomy to perform splenectomy, esophageal mucosal transection, and a painstaking ligation of esophagogastric venous collaterals.[10] The incidence of encephalopathy is 10% or less after devascularization but depends on the underlying liver disease and its severity.

Staple transection of the esophagus obviously does not treat gastric varices or portal hypertensive gastropathy. It may be rendered more difficult or impossible to perform if the esophagus is edematous, inflamed, or scarred because previous endoscopic variceal therapy. Because the vagus nerves may be divided during esophageal transection, pyloroplasty may be required to prevent postoperative gastric outlet obstruction.

Devascularization procedures can be used for patients who have extensive portal venous thrombosis and who continue to have significant gastric or esophageal variceal bleeding despite pharmacologic and endoscopic therapy. Extensive devascularization for these patients can reduce the risk of major bleeding for several years and may be the only reasonable therapeutic solution in bleeding patients who have no shuntable splanchnic vessels.

Portal Decompressive Shunt Surgery

Because variceal hemorrhage results from underlying PHT, reduction of portal pressure to normal physiologic levels invariably halts such bleeding. Bypassing splanchnic venous outflow obstruction by connecting the hypertensive portal system to the systemic venous circulation, either directly or by means of various autogenous or synthetic conduits, once proved to be a highly effective means of halting variceal hemorrhage.

In 1877, Eck performed the first PCS in dogs. Pavlov et al performed the first substantive investigations of the metabolic effects of portosystemic shunts in 1893. Vidal, in 1903, performed the first PCS in a patient with ascites. The patient died 4 months later, probably from sepsis, liver failure, and encephalopathy. A resurgence of interest in total portosystemic shunts paralleled the beginning of arterial reconstructive surgery in the 1940s and 1950s, and such procedures, usually end-to-end or side-to-side PCS, became commonplace therapy for patients with variceal hemorrhage in the two decades after the Second World War.[11]

Several complicating factors became evident. A characteristic neuropsychiatric disorder of memory loss; altered levels of consciousness; behavioral changes; and (in its advanced stages) stupor, coma, and death was noted to be a frequent and unpredictable result in patients who had undergone portosystemic shunt.[12] This syndrome, hepatic or portosystemic encephalopathy ("hepatic coma"), remains incompletely understood and, in varying degrees, has continued to plague all forms of portal decompression. Pavlov had shown that dogs undergoing PCS become listless and anorectic, suffer premature death, and have hepatic atrophy at autopsy. Extensive investigations in the 1950s and 1960s, summarized most elegantly by Starzl et al, suggested that an equivalent phenomenon in humans undergoing PCS, accelerated hepatic atrophy and progressive loss of hepatocellular function occur because diversion of portal flow deprives the liver of a splanchnic venous trophic factor (insulin seemed a likely candidate) necessary for normal hepatocellular function and regeneration.[13]

General acceptance of the "hepatotrophic theory," combined with the demonstration that PCS improved survival only minimally in prospective randomized trials, led to a significant decline in the performance of PCS after the 1980s. Recognizing, on the

one hand, the ability of PCS to control bleeding but, on the other hand, the evident advantage of maintaining portal perfusion following devascularization procedures, Warren et al introduced the concept of selective shunts for variceal decompression in the 1960s.[14] Even later, in the 1980s, the concept of partial PCSs, designed to lower portal pressures to nonbleeding but not "subnormal" levels, was advanced.

Three types of surgical decompression have been used to treat gastroesophageal varices. All aim to reduce variceal pressure and provide durably effective control of variceal bleeding. *Total* shunts divert *all* portal venous blood flow from the liver, *selective* shunts divert only the gastric and splenic components of portal flow, and *partial* shunts reduce the portal pressure but may maintain some portal flow. The more central the shunt, the greater the continuing patency rate—because of the high flow—but the more certain is loss of first-pass portal perfusion of the liver. Use of prosthetic materials increases the risk of thrombosis. Factors that determine the choice of shunt are technical feasibility based on preoperative evaluation of the splanchnic vessels, the surgeon's preference and experience, and the subsequent possibility of liver transplantation.

Operative approaches to each of these procedures will not be described in great detail but will be diagrammed; specifics can be found in reference texts. The key steps are adequate operative exposure of the vessels to be connected and careful operative technique in fashioning the veno-venous anastomoses. The overall perioperative management of the condition of patients with underlying cirrhosis and impaired liver function is the other key factor in a successful outcome.

Total Portosystemic Shunts

The goal of a total portosystemic shunt is *complete* portal decompression. Theoretically, such shunts have the highest likelihood of protecting against further variceal rebleeding. Total shunts include PCSs, mesocaval shunts, and proximal or central splenorenal shunts. The shunts are usually 15 to 25 mm in diameter (▶ Fig. 9.1; ▶ Fig. 9.2; ▶ Fig. 9.3; ▶ Fig. 9.4; ▶ Fig. 9.5).

In experienced hands, the patency rate of PCSs is more than 90%, with excellent control of variceal bleeding. In some 1700 PCSs performed by Orloff, fewer than 10 (<0.1%) have been associated with proven variceal rebleeding (Orloff MJ, personal communication). However, others have reported higher rebleeding rates, ranging from 3% to 17%. Shunt failure, when it occurs, almost always results from an attempt to anastomose a partially or completely thrombosed portal vein to the inferior vena cava (IVC) rather than performing an alternative portal decompressive procedure.

Unfortunately, total PCS is associated with a substantial risk of encephalopathy (30%–50%) and acceleration of liver failure. Notwithstanding the fact that a number of such patients with postoperative neuropsychological deterioration can be treated medically (protein-restricted diet, oral antibiotics, and/or lactulose) with mitigation of symptoms, most authorities discouraged and discarded this particular shunt construction.

Drapanas et al theorized that a conduit from a tributary of the portal vein (such as the superior mesenteric vein [SMV]) to the systemic venous circulation might preserve prograde portal flow (and continued hepatic portal perfusion) and still afford adequate portal decompression and protect against further variceal

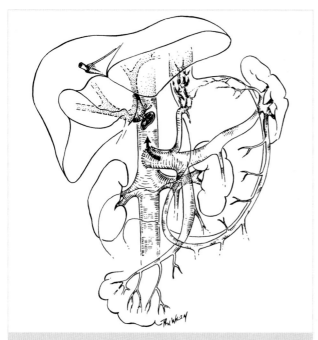

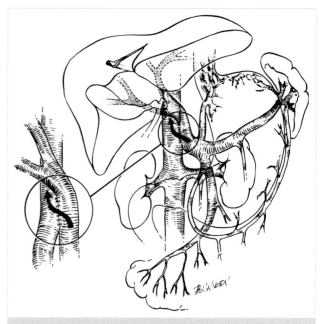

Fig. 9.2 Classic end-to-side total portacaval shunt. An extensive Kocher maneuver is needed to expose the infrahepatic inferior vena cava (IVC). Then the portal vein is exposed, generally by incising the peritoneum over the lateral hepatoduodenal ligament. Mobilization of the portal vein may require suture ligation of any large side branches, such as the coronary vein(s) and the large posterolateral portal vein tributary from the head of the pancreas. Then the main portal vein is divided. The hepatic limb of the portal vein near the hilum is suture ligated. The splanchnic end of the main portal vein is directly anastomosed to the IVC. Note that the coronary vein is not ligated.

Fig. 9.3 Classic side-to-side total portacaval shunt (PCS). The inferior vena cava (IVC) and portal vein are exposed in the same manner as for the end-to-side PCS. If necessary, part of the often-hypertrophied caudate lobe is resected. A parallel cavotomy and portal venotomy are performed. The anastomosis is accomplished by apposition of the anterior and posterior walls of the IVC to the portal vein using 4-0 or 5-0 monofilament sutures.

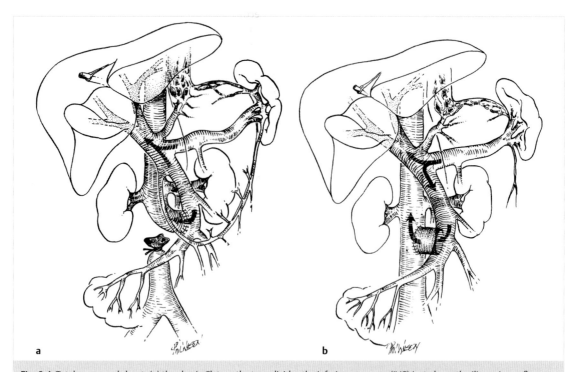

Fig. 9.4 Total mesocaval shunt: (a) the classic Clatworthy type divides the inferior vena cava (IVC) just above the iliac vein confluence. The distal end is suture ligated, and the proximal end is rotated medially and anastomosed to the superior mesenteric vein in an end-to-side fashion. (b) Alternatively, an interposition prosthetic graft is interposed between the superior mesenteric vein and the IVC.

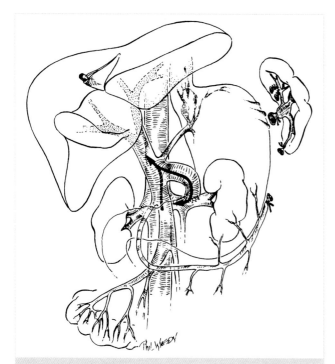

Fig. 9.5 The central splenorenal shunt. After splenectomy, the mesenteric end of the splenic vein is anastomosed to the anterosuperior aspect of the left renal vein in an end-to-side fashion.

hemorrhage.[15] Development of the prosthetic interposition mesocaval shunt quickly followed. Although mesocaval shunts continue to be performed, their long-term efficacy is questionable. Initially constructed using large-caliber Dacron grafts, mesocaval shunts resulted in slow flow through a thrombogenic synthetic conduit, with predictable shunt thrombosis and variceal rebleeding. Interposition of autologous tissue (most commonly internal jugular vein) as mesocaval graft was shown to produce the highest likelihood of long-term patency.[16] Importantly, the underlying premise that hepatic portal venous perfusion can be preserved by a mesocaval shunt has not been borne out; such patients have a likelihood of postoperative complications equivalent to that of patients undergoing standard PCS.

Portacaval Shunt

The relative anatomic proximity of the portal vein and the IVC makes direct anastomosis between the two relatively technically straightforward. Extensive venous collaterals may be found in the subcutaneous tissue of the abdominal wall while performing the initial incision. Abdominal exploration generally will reveal ascites, a substantially enlarged spleen, fragile portosystemic venous collaterals in the retroperitoneum, and a cirrhotic liver. The liver should be examined carefully for concurrent hepatocellular carcinoma, especially in patients with a history of hepatitis. Extreme caution must be adopted in dissecting medially beneath the common bile duct because one to four large, fragile, high-pressure coronary veins reside there and are extremely difficult to control if inadvertently avulsed.

End-to-side PCS (▶ Fig. 9.2) is performed by dividing the portal vein as close to the hepatic hilum as possible, preferably even by dividing the right and left portal veins just cephalad to the portal vein bifurcation. This usually permits a relatively tension-free anastomosis to the side of the infrahepatic IVC. The portacaval anastomosis is constructed between the end of the portal vein and the IVC. If total decompression is intended, the target portacaval pressure gradient (portal vein pressure minus IVC pressure) should not exceed 5 mm Hg.

The side-to-side PCS (▶ Fig. 9.3) is believed by some to be technically more difficult than end-to-side shunt because increased tension between the two vessels to be anastomosed may result from the distance between them or by the intervening hypertrophied caudate lobe of the liver. This, in fact, should rarely be a problem. Complete dissection of an adequate length of portal vein and IVC and resection (if necessary) of some of the caudate lobe should permit a tension-free side-to-side portacaval anastomosis. The shunt is constructed by performing a longitudinal anteromedial cavotomy and a posterolateral portal venotomy as close to the liver as possible. Each venotomy should be 2.5 to 3.0 cm in length. The venotomies are then anastomosed with fine monofilament vascular suture, "parachuting" down the posterior wall after initial suture placement.

Circumstances in which a standard total PCS may be warranted have classically included the need for emergency portal decompression, the treatment of acute Budd-Chiari syndrome uncomplicated by retrohepatic caval obstruction, and in rare cases of refractory ascites.

Mesocaval Shunt

Connecting the SMV and the IVC was initially thought to offer the possibility of variceal decompression while simultaneously preserving portal perfusion of the liver. This is now known to be untrue; the mesocaval shunt (▶ Fig. 9.4) is hemodynamically equivalent to a total PCS. The procedure is carried out by dissecting out the SMV at the base of the great mesentery and the anterior surface of the infrarenal IVC after a generous Kocher maneuver of the duodenum. An autogenous or, more commonly, a prosthetic graft is passed between the two vessels through a plane traversing the C-loop of the duodenum followed by end-to-side anastomoses of the graft to the SMV and the vena cava. Relief of ascites and hypersplenism and acceleration of encephalopathy and liver decompensation are equivalent for mesocaval shunts as for other total portal decompressive procedures. The lower incidence of encephalopathy observed in some series probably relates to the higher likelihood of thrombosis of mesocaval shunts.

An alternative, rarely performed autogenous mesocaval shunt designed by Clatworthy uses the divided and medially rotated IVC as the decompressive shunt (▶ Fig. 9.4). This has uncommonly been constructed except in children.

Central Splenorenal Shunt

The central splenorenal shunt is hemodynamically equivalent to a standard PCS or mesocaval shunt (▶ Fig. 9.5). The central splenorenal shunt is generally performed through a midline laparotomy or a transverse left upper quadrant incision. Splenectomy is performed, and the splenic vein is dissected centrally from its intimate attachment to the back of the pancreas. The left renal vein is exposed from beneath the pancreas and the transverse mesocolon. Gonadal or adrenal tributaries of the renal vein may be ligated and divided to free up this vessel. An end-to-side anastomosis of the splenic vein to the upper surface of the left renal vein is then accomplished, making sure that the splenic vein is not kinked acutely around the lower border of the pancreas. Similar to the mesocaval shunt, the central splenorenal shunt has the advantage of effective portal decompression without involving the hilum of the liver. Notwithstanding early hopes to the contrary, this is a totally decompressing shunt, with the same risk of encephalopathy and accelerated liver failure as a PCS.

Selective Shunts

Despite their excellent and virtually permanent protection against variceal rebleeding, total portosystemic shunts may result in accelerated liver failure as well as an increased risk of portosystemic encephalopathy. Warren et al designed the distal splenorenal shunt to provide isolated or "selective" decompression of the gastroesophageal variceal plexus, with preservation of portal venous perfusion to the liver.[14]

The distal splenorenal shunt (▶ Fig. 9.6) has two parts: anastomosis of the splenic end of the divided splenic vein to the left renal vein and meticulous ligation and division of all potential venous collaterals between the portomesenteric and gastrosplenic venous beds. The splenic vein is dissected away from the pancreas from above and behind (through the lesser sac) or from below the lower border of the pancreas, after which it is anastomosed end to side to the upper aspect of the left renal vein. Initial reports suggested dissection of just enough of the splenic vein to permit its anastomosis to the left renal vein. However,

subsequent finding that the low-pressure shunt attracts collaterals from the high-pressure portomesenteric circulation through the pancreatic "siphon" led to the modification of splenopancreatic dissociation, in which meticulous dissection, ligation, and division of all connections between the pancreas and the splenic vein are performed throughout its entire length. Because the Warren shunt avoids the hepatic hilum, it is considered by many to be the optimal shunt in patients who may be liver transplant candidates in the future.

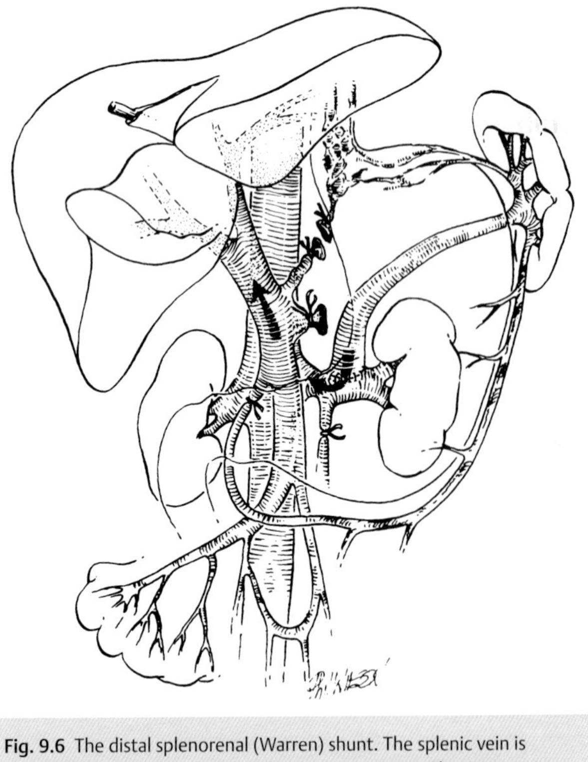

Distal splenorenal shunt became the portal decompressive approach of choice in many medical centers during the 1970s and 1980s. Variceal bleeding is controlled in more than 90% of patients, and the encephalopathy rate is 10% to 15%. The rate of encephalopathy appears to correlate primarily with the underlying disease and its progression. Prospective randomized comparisons of selective and total shunts have not demonstrated a survival advantage in patients undergoing selective shunt.

Distal splenorenal shunt cannot be performed in patients who have previously undergone splenectomy. It is also believed to be contraindicated in patients with ascites; with poor hepatocellular function (Child class C); or in circumstances in which preoperative angiography demonstrates abnormalities of the splenic or left renal veins, such as unfavorable anatomic displacement, diminutive vessel caliber, or areas of thrombosis. Because the procedure (especially with the addition of splenopancreatic dissociation) is lengthy, it is generally not indicated as an emergency decompressive operation.

Partial Portosystemic Shunts

Partial portosystemic shunts are created as either a side-to-side PCS or mesocaval shunt with an interposed small diameter (8 to 10 mm) graft (venous or synthetic) or as a small-stomal side-to-side PCS.

The possibility that prograde flow could be maintained by forming a smaller, higher resistance portosystemic shunt was investigated initially by Marion et al and Bismuth et al. In the 1980s, Sarfeh et al introduced the concept of the small-caliber polytetrafluoroethylene (PTFE) interposition H portacaval graft (▶ Fig. 9.7).[17] By systematic studies, they showed that grafts of 8 mm diameter reduced the portacaval pressure gradient to 12 mm Hg while maintaining prograde portal flow in the portal vein in 83% of patients. Variceal bleeding was controlled in approximately 90% of the cases, and the rate of encephalopathy was approximately 15%. However, shunt stenosis or occlusion has been a documented problem in 10% to 20% of cases. These can be treated with interventional radiologic techniques.

The portal interposition H graft of Sarfeh et al has the virtue of relative technical ease and the disadvantage of the placement of a thrombogenic prosthetic graft in the venous system. In this procedure, a 6- or 8-mm PTFE graft is interposed between the portal vein and the anterior surface of the infrahepatic IVC. A direct small-caliber PCS avoids use of a potentially thrombogenic graft but may be slightly more technically difficult. The shunt is performed in the same manner as a total PCS but, instead of a 2.5- to 3.0-cm anastomosis, a much smaller cavotomy and portal venotomy are performed. A 12- to 15-mm venotomy generally results in a portacaval pressure gradient of 7 to 12 mm Hg.[18,19] Collateral ligation is not considered important; persistent filling of varices post-shunt can be readily embolized using interventional radiologic techniques.

Fig. 9.6 The distal splenorenal (Warren) shunt. The splenic vein is divided near its confluence with the mesenteric vein. The mesenteric end of the splenic vein is suture ligated, as are the coronary vein, right gastroepiploic vein, and left gonadal vein. In addition, all small, fragile venous tributaries to the pancreas must be exposed and ligated. The other end of the splenic vein is rotated inferiorly and anastomosed to the anterosuperior aspect of the left renal vein in an end-to-side fashion.

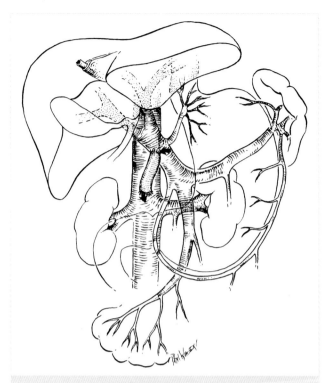

Fig. 9.7 The small-caliber prosthetic H portacaval graft. The exposure of the vena cava and the portal vein are as for total end-to-side or side-to-side portacaval shunts. The interposed polytetrafluoroethylene (PTFE) graft is constructed as short as possible.

In 50 consecutive patients undergoing direct side-to-side small-stomal PCS and postoperative duplex ultrasonography, Johansen showed consistent loss of portal perfusion of the liver despite the relatively high resistance of the shunt (10 mm Hg portacaval pressure gradient).[18,19] However, an incidence of encephalopathy of only 6% in these patients suggested that maintenance of first-pass portal perfusion of the liver might not be relevant to the development of post-shunt encephalopathy. In a prospective comparison, patients undergoing partial portal decompression had a late mortality rate of 13% and an encephalopathy rate of 8% compared with total shunt patients' late mortality risk of 39% ($P < 0.05$) and an encephalopathy risk of 56% ($P < 0.0001$).[18] All patients in both groups had lost portal perfusion of the liver at the time of postoperative duplex ultrasonography.

More recently, the need to avoid operating in the right upper quadrant in patients who might undergo a liver transplant in the future spurred a significant rebirth of interest in mesocaval interposition grafts. The current practice is to use an 8- to 10-mm ringed PTFE interposition conduit. Paquet et al have reported effective portal decompression with good durability and only a modest risk of postoperative PSE with this approach.[20]

Whether partially decompressing PCSs protect against encephalopathy and liver failure by preserving prograde portal flow or by maintaining "physiologic" splanchnic venous pressures remains unclear. The unacceptably high incidence of post-shunt complications after total portal decompression and the ever-increasing technical complexity of the distal splenorenal shunt have resulted in increased interest in the concept of partial portal decompression when operative portal decompression is required. Interestingly, selection of a 10-mm caliber for the standard TIPS stent was derived from prior studies of partial portal decompressive shunts (Ernest Ring MD, personal communication).

Special Circumstances

Budd-Chiari Syndrome

In patients with Budd-Chiari syndrome, congenital or acquired thrombotic occlusion of the hepatic veins or the suprahepatic vena cava leads to acute hepatic congestion, with severe right upper quadrant pain, massive ascites, and progressive hepatic dysfunction. It may be managed by interventional radiologic techniques. When such measures are unsuccessful, operative therapy is warranted because the condition is otherwise often lethal. Bismuth and Sherlock demonstrated that relatively acute-onset Budd-Chiari syndrome, without massive centrilobular necrosis or scarring present on liver biopsy, can effectively be treated by operative portal decompression.[21] When advanced hepatocellular destruction is present, optimal management of chronic Budd-Chiari syndrome is orthotopic liver transplantation.

Careful imaging of the IVC is crucial in patients with Budd-Chiari syndrome. If the IVC is patent, a side-to-side PCS may be performed. Others prefer a mesocaval shunt to avoid the subhepatic scarring that might complicate later liver transplantation. In patients in whom there is caval obstruction at or above the level of the liver, PCSs will not work. However, a mesoatrial shunt, connecting the SMV to the right atrium or the right atrial appendage, may satisfactorily decompress the portal system.[22] Patients whose Budd-Chiari syndrome arises as a result of a hypercoagulable state may be at higher risk for treatment failure because of a heightened risk of shunt or graft hepatic artery thrombosis.

Extrahepatic Thrombosis of the Portal Vein

Creating a TIPS in a patient with variceal bleeding caused by extrahepatic portal vein thrombosis may be very difficult, although advanced transcatheter techniques to disobliterate and recanalize the portal vein are increasingly successful. If such efforts fail and surgical portal decompression is required, it most commonly has been accomplished by central splenorenal or mesocaval shunt construction. Because hepatic function in patients with portal vein thrombosis frequently is either normal or only minimally diminished, these individuals may have excellent long-term prognoses.[23]

Almost all such patients requiring therapy for PHT are infants and children. Endoscopic therapy of bleeding esophageal varices in such patients is initially indicated and may be highly effective. But "breakthrough" hemorrhage, especially from gastric varices or portal hypertensive gastropathy, can be torrential; furthermore, hypersplenism can render these patients both severely leukopenic and thrombocytopenic. Pediatric patients are usually not candidates for percutaneous transhepatic efforts at portal vein recanalization or other similar approaches, and standard portal decompressive shunts must be based on smaller portal tributaries such as the splenic or SMVs.

The Rex shunt (or bypass), originally developed as a solution to portal vein thrombosis in liver transplant patients, is an elegant solution to this problem. As demonstrated (▶ Fig. 9.8), a bypass graft is constructed from the SMV to the intrahepatic left portal vein in the Rex recess, thus simultaneously decompressing the

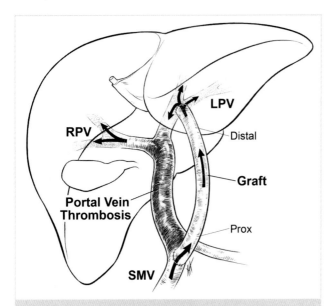

Fig. 9.8 The Rex bypass for the treatment of portal hypertension caused by extrahepatic portal vein thrombosis. A conduit (preferably autogenous internal jugular or great saphenous vein) is anastomosed to the upper superior mesenteric vein (SMV), with the outflow anastomosis to the left portal vein (LPV) in the Rex recess.

hypertensive splenomesenteric venous circulation and restoring prograde portal perfusion to the liver. Particularly when autogenous vein is used, the Rex bypass has efficacy and long-term patency rates approaching 100%.[24,25] The Rex bypass has not commonly been performed in adults with extrahepatic portal vein obstruction.

Patients with extrahepatic portal vein thrombosis in the presence of postnecrotic cirrhosis must be carefully screened by serum alpha-fetoprotein levels and hepatic imaging for presence of an underlying hepatocellular carcinoma. PHT resulting from diffuse splanchnic venous thrombosis, commonly arising as a result of a hematologic disorder, may be difficult to treat. In some circumstances in which the portal, splenic, and SMVs are diffusely thrombosed, the inferior mesenteric vein may be patent and can be anastomosed to the left renal vein.[26] If this option is unavailable, devascularization by esophagogastrectomy or a variant of the Sugiura procedure may be the best option.[27,28]

In patients with cavernomatous transformation of the portal vein or diffuse mesenteric venous thrombosis, intraabdominal variceal collaterals may be huge. But the temptation to anastomose one of these collaterals to the systemic venous circulation must be resisted because such "makeshift" shunts rarely remain patent.

Isolated Splenic Vein Thrombosis

The splenic vein may thrombose as a result of chronic pancreatic inflammation, usually secondary to alcoholic pancreatitis. In such a setting, an isolated left upper quadrant venous hypertension, manifested by massive splenomegaly and gastric varices, may occur. Bleeding can be torrential, and pancytopenia caused by hypersplenism may be significant. Splenectomy is curative. Polyvalent vaccine directed against encapsulated bacterial species (pneumococcus, *Haemophilus influenzae*, and *Neisseria meningitidis*) must

be administered to diminish the risk of subsequent postsplenectomy sepsis.

Surgical Management of Intractable Ascites

Ascites as a complication of PHT actually confers an even greater negative prognostic significance than does variceal bleeding. Ascites is usually a sign of decompensation of the underlying hepatic cirrhosis. Spontaneous bacterial peritonitis and hepatorenal syndrome are known complications.

The pathogenesis of ascites includes a combination of PHT, altered renal sodium and water handling, and hypoalbuminemia. Initial management of ascites is primarily medical. Dietary sodium restriction to 1 to 2 g/day is implemented, along with the use of appropriate diuretics. Spironolactone (Aldactone) is the first-line treatment to counteract the secondary hyperaldosteronism. When ascites is refractory to medical management, the next line of treatment is serial large-volume paracentesis. This is, however, useful only for symptomatic relief. A total side-to-side portacaval or large-caliber mesocaval shunt (*not* a selective or partial shunt) would be expected to resolve intractable ascites but at an excessive mortality and morbidity risk. TIPS commonly results in resolution of intractable ascites[29] and, not uncommonly, reversal of hepatorenal failure.[30] Because, as noted, such patients' liver function has deteriorated significantly, the risk of post-total shunt or post-TIPS hepatic encephalopathy is substantial, and orthotopic liver transplantation may be these patients' best chance for long-term survival.

The use of surgically inserted peritoneovenous shunts for the management of intractable ascites has been abandoned over the past 25 years.

References

1. Henderson JM, Boyer TD, Kutner MH, et al. Distal splenorenal shunt versus transjugular intrahepatic portal systemic shunt for variceal bleeding: a randomized trial. Arch Surg 2007;142:219–221.
2. Orozco H, Mercado MA. Rise and downfall of the empire of portal hypertension surgery. Gastroenterology 2006;130:1643–1651.
3. Graham DY, Smith JL. The course of patients after variceal hemorrhage. Gastroenterology 1981;80:800–809.
4. Moss AH, Siegler M. Should alcoholics compete equally for liver transplantation? JAMA 1991;265:1295–1298.
5. Soper NJ, Rikkers LF. Effect of operations for variceal hemorrhage on hypersplenism. Am J Surg 1982;144:700–703.
6. Agarwal S. Anesthetic management during liver transplantation. Transplantation Proc 1994;26:321–324.
7. Canton EG, Rettke SR, Plevak D, et al. Perioperative care of the liver transplant patient. Anesth Analg 1994;28:120–133.
8. Orloff MJ, Bell RH Jr. Long-term survival after emergency portacaval shunting for bleeding varices in patients with alcoholic cirrhosis. Am J Surg 1986;151:176–183.
9. Hassab MA. Gastroesophageal decongestion and splenectomy in the treatment of esophageal varices in bilharzial cirrhosis: further studies with the report of 355 operations. Surgery 1967;61:169–176.
10. Sugiura M, Futagawa S. Results of six hundred thirty-six esophageal transections with paraesophagogastric devascularization in the treatment of esophageal varices. J Vasc Surg 1984;1:254–260.
11. Whipple AO. The problem of portal hypertension in relation to the hepatosplenopathies. Ann Surg 1945;122:449–456.
12. Sherlock S, Summerskill WHJ, White LP, et al. Portosystemic encephalopathy: neurological complications of liver disease. Lancet 1954;2:453–456.
13. Starzl TE, Porter KA, Francavilla JA. *One Hundred Years of the Hepatotrophic Controversy:* Hepatotrophic Factors CIBA Symposium. Amsterdam, The Netherlands: Elsevier Excerpta Medica;1978.

14. Warren WD, Zeppa R, Foman JS. Selective transsplenic decompression of gastro-esophageal varices by distal splenorenal shunt. Ann Surg 1967;166:437–455.

15. Drapanas T, LoCicero J, Dowling JB. Hemodynamics of the interposition meso-caval shunt. Ann Surg 1975;181:523–533.

16. Stipa S, Ziparo V, Anza M, et al. A randomized controlled trial of mesentericocaval shunt with autologous jugular vein. Surg Gynecol Obstet 1981;153:353–356.

17. Sarfeh IJ, Rypins E, Conroy RM, el al. Portacaval H-graft: relationship of shunt diameter, portal flow patterns and encephalopathy. Ann Surg 1983;197:422–426.

18. Johansen KH. Partial portal decompression for variceal hemorrhage. Am J Surg 1989;157:479–482.

19. Johansen KH. Prospective comparison of partial versus total portal decompression for bleeding esophageal varices. Surg Gynecol Obstet 1992;175:528–534.

20. Paquet KJ, Mercado MA, Gad HA. Surgical procedures for bleeding esophagogastric varices when sclerotherapy fails: a prospective study. Am J Surg 1990;160:43–47.

21. Bismuth H, Sherlock DJ. Portasystemic shunting versus liver transplantation for the Budd-Chiari syndrome. Ann Surg 1991;214:581–589.

22. Tilamus HW. Budd-Chiari syndrome. Br J Surg 1995;82:1023–1030.

23. Webb LJ, Sherlock S. The etiology, presentation and natural history of extrahepatic portal venous obstruction. Q J Med 1979;48:627–639.

24. Emre S, Dugan C, Frankenburg T, et al. Surgical portasystemic shunts and the Rex bypass in children: a single-centre experience. HPB J 2009;11:252–257.

25. Lautz TB, Keys LA, Melvin JC, et al. Advantages of the meso-Rex bypass compared with portasystemic shunts in the management of extrahepatic portal vein obstruction in children. J Am Coll Surg 2013;216:83–89.

26. Gorini P, Johansen K. Use of the inferior mesenteric vein for portal decompression. HPB Surg 1998;10:365–370.

27. Orloff MJ, Orloff MS, Daily PO, et al. Long-term results of radical esophagogastrectomy for bleeding varices due to unshuntable extra-hepatic portal hypertension. Am J Surg 1994;167:96–103.

28. Caps MT, Helton WS, Johansen K. Left upper quadrant devascularization for "unshuntable" portal hypertension. Arch J Surg 1996;131:834–839.

29. Albillos A, Banares R, Gonzalez M, et al. A meta-analysis of transjugular portasystemic shunt versus paracentesis for refractory ascites. J Hepatol 2005;43:990–996.

30. Rossle M. TIPS for the treatment of refractory ascites, hepatorenal syndrome and hepatic hydrothorax: a critical review. Gut 2010;59:988–1000.

Chapter 10: Percutaneous Management of Surgically Placed Portosystemic Shunts

Wael E.A. Saad

Introduction

The first line of treatment for acute recurrent gastroesophageal variceal bleeding is medical management with endoscopic banding or sclerosis of varices. Where available, percutaneous transjugular intrahepatic portosystemic shunts (TIPS) have largely replaced surgical shunting. Elective surgery is still preferred by some authorities for portal decompression in patients with relatively good liver function (Child's A) and who fail endoscopic treatment.[1,2] These clinicians believe that surgical shunts are associated with longer periods of patency and a lower incidence of encephalopathy. They reserve the use of TIPS for Child's B patients as a bridge to liver transplantation.

The most popular types of portal decompressive surgery include the placement of small-diameter interposition portocaval or mesocaval shunts and the splenorenal shunt.[3]

Shunt malfunction is usually the result of kinking, build-up of a thick mural thrombus, or complete thrombotic occlusion. The incidence of shunt occlusion is estimated to be 7% to 10%, based on rebleeding episodes, angiography, surgery, and autopsy.[4] However, the true incidence of shunt stenosis is probably in the range of 30% or more, because shunts can become stenotic or occluded without recurrent variceal bleeding (hemodynamic stenosis without clinical dysfunction). Percutaneous recanalization of dysfunctional shunts is often such a simple operation that it should be considered a first–intention procedure for treating patients with active esophageal variceal bleeding.[5] Moreover, adhesion and fibrosis around the surgical shunt may hinder surgical revisions of these surgically established portosystemic shunts.[4]

Diagnosis of Shunt Dysfunction

The evaluation of shunt patency is most commonly performed by Doppler ultrasound, which is reasonably accurate when shunt flow is visualized and when the cephalad segment of the superior mesenteric vein is noted to be wider than its caudal segment.[6] However, moderate shunt stenosis can be missed. Shunts may not be visible in the presence of intestinal gas and in large abdomens. Although magnetic resonance angiography and cross-sectional imaging are probably more accurate in defining shunt patency, these studies are not commonly used, especially if the patient is actively bleeding. In stable patients the author (WS) prefers portal venous phase CT. Adjunct Doppler ultrasound to evaluate for patency and dysfunction of flow within the portal vein is also used.

When a patient with a history of having a surgical shunt is admitted with variceal hemorrhage and has failed endoscopic therapy, he or she should be considered for emergency percutaneous shunt catheterization.[7–11] If the shunt is found to have a residual lumen, then it usually can be easily and safely reopened to lower the portocaval pressure gradient to a safe level. Recanalization of a malfunctioning portosystemic shunt via the inferior vena cava (IVC) is safe, quick, and requires only standard catheter and angioplasty balloon technology. Stent placement is usually reserved for lesions that are recalcitrant to balloon angioplasty or have frequent recurrences after balloon angioplasty.

Indirect Portography

Celiac and superior mesenteric arteriography can be performed to assess the patency and hemodynamics of the shunt and portal circulation. At least 50 to 70 mL higher-concentration radiopaque media must be injected in each vessel to obtain good opacification of the portal system. For more precise visualization of H-shunts it is suggested that the mesenteric arteriogram be performed after an intraarterial vasodilator is instilled into the artery and imaging performed in a left posterior oblique position. Opacification of the shunt and the IVC indicates some degree of patency, which can allow subsequent transcaval dilatation. The reverse is not true, because some hemodynamically occluded shunts can still be recanalized (see ▶ Fig. 6.3). Opacification of the IVC alone can occur through large natural splenorenal shunts and cannot therefore be of use as a sign of surgical shunt patency.

Shunt Catheterization Through the Inferior Vena Cava

It is important to obtain from the operative notes information on the type and location of shunts that were placed. Without such information it is difficult to assess from surgical clip patterns the site of shunt anastomosis into the IVC or renal vein (RV). Surgeons should be encouraged to place metal markers at the caval entrance of the graft into the IVC for later angiographic guidance, as recommended by Scudamore et al.[2] If preliminary attempts at indirect shunt imaging have been successful in identifying the course of the shunt, then it is quite simple to catheterize it selectively in a retrograde direction from the IVC or RV. Noninvasive imaging (such as contrast enhanced CT) is very important to plan for the shunt catheterization. The standard access site is the right femoral vein; it may at times be easier to catheterize splenorenal shunts from the right internal jugular vein approach. Cobra-shaped catheters are adequate for catheterizing H-shunts; hockey-stock or Simmons catheters are more useful for probing the cephalad wall of the left RV for splenorenal or adrenal shunts. The normal mean portosystemic venous pressure gradient should be less than 8 to 10 mm Hg. One should be alert to the fact that portal hypertension with variceal bleed can be caused in part by caval hypertension resulting from circumferential compression of the IVC by cirrhotic nodules.

If no shunt flow is demonstrable by imaging, then it is still possible to catheterize the shunt through either a residual pinpoint opening of the proximal anastomosis or through a soft occlusive thrombus by careful methodical probing of the caval or RV wall around the expected location of the thrombus.[7] If the shunt body is open but its distal anastomosis is severely narrowed or occluded by hyperplasia or kinking, this can also be quite easily catheterized.

It is also possible to quickly assess the presence of a residually patent mesocaval shunt by a balloon occlusion technique. A 3-cm occlusion-balloon catheter (Meditech, Boston Scientific Corp., Natick, Massachusetts) is inserted into the IVC through a 9-French sheath next to a 5-French cobra catheter. After the balloon has been expanded to occlude the IVC just below the renal veins, a cavagram is performed through the other catheter. Any residual shunt channel should fill in a retrograde manner and allow immediate catheterization with the cobra catheter.

Treatment of Dysfunctional Shunts

Balloon Dilatation of the Malfunctioning Shunt

Most plastic interposition portocaval or mesocaval H-shunts are 8 to 20 mm in diameter and can easily tolerate appropriately sized balloon dilatation on the caval side. For venous H-shunts, 8- to 10-mm balloon dilatation is appropriate. On the distal mesenteric side of the shunt, the venous anastomosis can tolerate dilatation to 8 to 10 mm, depending on vessel size. Because of elastic recoil, careful overdilation is mandatory. One should not be too aggressive in dilating recent shunt strictures because of potential anastomotic dehiscence from suture breakage.[9] Dilatation of stenotic veno-venous splenorenal shunt can be performed safely with 6- to 8-mm balloons.

Stenting of Strictured Shunts

The use of metallic stents has been described in only two case reports: one (11 mm) in a splenorenal and the other (12 mm) in a mesocaval shunt. Each had only a 4-month follow-up.[12,13]

Stents should be reserved for shunts that are recalcitrant to balloon angioplasty or have a high frequency of recurrence (symptomatic restenosis within 3 months for angioplasty).

Emergency Variceal Embolization and Sclerosis

One of the most useful aspects of successful trans-shunt catheterization is the ability to immediately access the gastroesophageal varices for embolization/sclerosis. This procedure, in concert with shunt dilatation, will help bring about cessation of bleeding. Occlusion of varices is performed most quickly by inserting coils alternately with sclerosants and/or gelfoam.[7]

Embolization techniques are also performed to control severe encephalopathy. Ruff et al used transhepatic or trans-shunt embolization of varices to isolate the portal from the splenic venous systems in patients with distal splenorenal shunts.[9] Uflacker et al used a balloon catheter to occlude a mesocaval shunt from a femoral vein access.[14] Koito et al showed that it is possible to sclerose bleeding gastric varices through surgical or spontaneous splenorenal or gastrorenal shunts.[15] This effective technique requires balloon occlusion of the dilated suprarenal vein or surgical shunt to allow retrograde injection of ethanol or ethanolamine. Embolization and/or sclerosis of varicies associated with dysfunctional surgically placed portosystemic shunts should be no different from embolization and/or sclerosis associated with TIPS dysfunction.

Thrombolysis of Clotted Shunts

Acute shunt thrombosis occurring within 1 to 2 weeks postoperatively is probably the result of surgical error, external shunt compression, or kinking.[2,3,11] Balloon angioplasty is ineffective because soft clot re-forms immediately after balloon dilatation. Reports have been published on thrombolytic therapy of the occluded shunt followed by angioplasty of portocaval (n = 1), and mesocaval (n = 1) shunts.[7,8] Streptokinase (Astra-Merck, Wayne, Pennsylvania; 4000 U/hour for 2 days) was used in one case. In the other, urokinase (Abbott Lab, North Chicago, Illinois) was infused at 50,000 U/hour for 1 to 3 days after an initial bolus of 100,000 U. The thrombolytic drug was infused directly into the shunt by embedding a multi-side-hole catheter into the thrombus. There was a no retroperitoneal hemorrhage, despite the recent surgery.

Follow-Up and Treatment of Shunt Dysfunction

Most chronic shunt strictures, whether they occur at anastomoses or within the body of the interposition graft, show significant elastic recoil after overdilation. Most will need to be redilated on an outpatient basis on a routine 3- to 6-month cycle to maintain an acceptable portosystemic pressure gradient. Alternatively, the patient can be treated when renewed structuring has developed on ultrasound imaging or when symptoms of bleeding or ascites are recurrent. In the author's experience of 16 patients, trans-shunt catheterization was possible in 14 and bleeding was controlled with the need for additional surgery in 12.[7]

Results and Discussion

Among the relatively few reports on the interventional management of symptomatic dysfunctional portosystemic shunts the published results show that percutaneous treatment is safe and efficacious and can be used to postpone or replace TIPS or a reshunting surgical procedure. Shunt patency has been observed to last from 15 to 30 months.[7,8,10] Many patients succumb from liver failure and rebleeding. The need for surgical portosystemic shunts has markedly decreased with the development of endoscopic transesophageal variceal sclerosis in the 1980s, followed in the 1990s by the use of TIPS and more effective liver transplantation techniques. However, surgical shunts are still being inserted, especially in patients with relatively good remaining liver function. It is important to remember that the quickest and simplest way to manage the 10% to 20% of patients who develop subsequent symptomatic shunt stenosis or occlusion, irrespective of whether they fail endoscopic sclerosis, is by percutaneous trans-shunt recanalization and variceal embolization.

References

1. Knechtle SJ, et al. Surgical portosystemic shunts for treatment of portal hypertensive bleeding: outcome and effect on liver function. Surgery 1999;126(4): 708–713.
2. Scudamore CH, et al. Medium aperture meso-caval shunts reliably prevent recurrent variceal hemorrhages. Am J Surg 1996;171(5):490–494.
3. Mercado MA, et al. Distal splenorenal shunt versus 10-mm low-diameter mesocaval shunt for variceal hemorrhage. Am J Surg 1996;171(6):591–595.

4. Mehigan DG, Zuidema GD, Cameron JL. The incidence of shunt occlusion following portosystemic decompression. Surg Gynecol Obstet 1980;150(5):661–663.

5. Soyer P, Roche A, Breittmayer F. [Percutaneous transluminal angioplasty of portosystemic shunts.] Gastroenterol Clin Biol 1991;15(4):280–284.

6. Grant EG, et al. Color Doppler imaging of portosystemic shunts. AJR Am J Roentgenol 1990;154(2):393–397.

7. Cope C. Dilatation of mesocaval shunts. Ann Radiol (Paris) 1986;29(2):178–180.

8. Grosso M, et al. [Percutaneous unblocking of porto-systemic shunts. Personal experience with 11 cases]. Radiol Med 1990;80(3):334–338.

9. Ruff RJ, et al. Percutaneous vascular intervention after surgical shunting for portal hypertension. Radiology 1987;164(2):469–474.

10. Henderson JM, El Khishen MA, Milikan WJ, et al. Management of stenosis of distal splenorenal shunt by balloon dilatation. Surg Gynecol Obstetr 1983;157:43–48.

11. Isaksson B, et al. Mesocaval interposition shunting in the treatment of bleeding oesophageal varices. Eur J Surg 1997;163(8):569–576.

12. Hausegger KA, et al. Stenosis of a surgical portosystemic shunt–treatment with angioplasty and placement of a Wallstent. Cardiovasc Intervent Radiol 1993;16(4):243–244.

13. Soyer P, Levesque M, Zeitoun G. Treatment of mesocaval shunt stenosis with a metallic stent. AJR Am J Roentgenol 1992;158(6):1251–1253.

14. Uflacker R, et al. Chronic portosystemic encephalopathy: embolization of portosystemic shunts. Radiology 1987;165(3):721–725.

15. Koito K, et al. Balloon-occluded retrograde transvenous obliteration for gastric varices with gastrorenal or gastrocaval collaterals. AJR Am J Roentgenoll 1996;167(5):1317–1320.

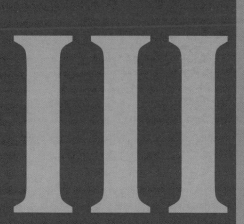

Section III

Endovascular Management: Shunts and Splenic Embolization

Chapter 11: Patient Selection and the Effect of Transjugular Intrahepatic Portosystemic Shunt on Liver and Kidney Function

Hector Ferral and George Behrens

Introduction

The management of portal hypertension (PHT) and its complications has changed drastically in the past 20 years.[1,2] Changes in the recommendations for the management PHT are a result of expert consensus conferences that have taken place between 1986 and 2010.[1,3] The role of the transjugular intrahepatic portosystemic shunt (TIPS) procedure in the management of patients with complications of PHT has changed as a result of these expert panel discussions.[4,5] The most common indications to perform a TIPS procedure have been control of esophageal variceal bleeding and management of refractory ascites.[4,6] The procedure is performed either in an emergency situation (active variceal bleeding) or in an elective fashion (recurrent bleed after failed medical and endoscopic therapy or for the management of ascites).

The purposes of this chapter are to convey an updated perspective of the role of TIPS in the management of patients with complicated PHT, emphasize the importance of careful patient selection before the procedure, and describe the hemodynamic effects of the shunt and its impact on liver and renal function.

The Role of Transjugular Intrahepatic Portosystemic Shunt in Patients with Variceal Bleeding

The first expert consensus conference was held in Baveno, Italy, in 1995.[1] The first Baveno conference in 1995 established that the first line of treatment for acute variceal hemorrhage should be based on endoscopic techniques; TIPS was recommended only in case of failure of endoscopic and pharmacologic therapy.[1] The concept of clinically significant PHT (hepatic venous pressure gradient [HVPG] >10 mm Hg) was introduced in the conference held in April 2000. There were no changes in recommendations regarding the role of TIPS in the management of variceal bleeding.[1] Endoscopic band ligation emerged as an alternative therapy for the management of bleeding esophageal varices during the conference held in 2005. Early TIPS was presented as an option in patients at high risk of rebleeding for the first time during the conference held in 2007,[1] and the recommendations for early TIPS in acute variceal bleeding were reinforced in the conference held in 2010.[1]

Current recommendations in the management of hemorrhagic PHT depend on the clinical stage of the disease. The clinical stages include: (i) patients with PHT who have not developed esophageal varices; (ii) patients with PHT with esophageal varices who have never bled; (iii) patients with acute variceal hemorrhage; and (iv) patients who have survived a bleeding episode and require treatment to prevent rebleeding.

Patients with Portal Hypertension Who Have Not Developed Esophageal Varices

These patients require no therapy, and management is focused on treating the cause of cirrhosis.

Patients with Portal Hypertension with Esophageal Varices Who Have Never Bled

In this stage, patients are further classified into high risk and low risk. High-risk patients are those with advanced cirrhosis (Child-Pugh class C) and large varices. Low-risk patients are those who have less severe cirrhosis (Child-Pugh class A or B) and small varices. Treatment options for patients at high risk of bleeding include nonselective beta-blockers and endoscopic variceal ligation (EVL). Studies have shown that EVL and nonselective beta-blockers are equally effective in preventing first variceal bleed; therefore, management decisions depend on local expertise and resources.[3] The downside of beta-blockers is that they are associated with side effects, and their use has to be discontinued in 15% to 20% of patients because of poor tolerance to the drug.[3] The problem with EVL is that it requires technical expertise, and it may be associated with postprocedural complications, the worst of which is the development of ulcers that may be associated with severe bleeding.[3] The focus in this stage is prophylaxis and the risks of beta-blocker side effects or EVL procedural complications need to be weighed against their potential clinical benefits.[3] In patients with advanced liver failure and small, low-risk varices, the recommendation is to treat them with nonselective beta-blockers instead of using endoscopic options.[3] Finally, in low-risk patients, the use of beta-blockers is optional. According to current recommendations, TIPS has no role in this prophylactic stage.

Patients with Acute Variceal Hemorrhage

This stage is a medical emergency. Patients are treated in intensive care units (ICUs) and require aggressive medical management, including airway control, transfusion of blood products, prophylactic antibiotics, and vasoactive drugs. A diagnostic endoscopy is mandatory and should be performed within 12 hours of admission.[1] EVL is the treatment of choice if varices are confirmed as the source of bleeding.[1] Sclerotherapy may be used if EVL proves to be technically difficult. TIPS procedure is indicated in patients who fail endoscopic and vasoactive treatment.[1] Recent reports have determined that approximately 10% to 20% of patients with acute variceal bleeding fail standard therapy,[3,7] and those are the patients who need to be evaluated for an emergency TIPS procedure. Clinical studies have reported the effectiveness of emergency TIPS procedure to treat acute esophageal and gastric variceal bleeding in patients who have failed medical and endoscopic therapy.[8]

Patients with a Child-Pugh class C, HPVG greater than 20 mm Hg and bleeding varices during diagnostic endoscopy are considered to be at high risk of failing standard therapy,[1] and this is the subgroup of patients that may benefit from an early TIPS procedure.[1,3,9] A recent prospective, randomized, multicenter trial conducted by Garcia-Pagan and coworkers[9] demonstrated that the application of early TIPS (within 72 hours of admission) resulted in a significant improvement in patient survival and a significant decrease in rebleeding rates in a group of patients with cirrhosis at high risk of conventional treatment failure. Careful patient evaluation before the procedure is crucial in selecting patients who may benefit from early TIPS. The clinical history, laboratory data, and diagnostic imaging studies must be reviewed.[6,9] The role of the interventional radiologist as a true clinical consultant is to determine if a patient is a suitable candidate to undergo a TIPS procedure after the patient's evaluation has been completed. The operator must also be able and willing to recommend alternative forms of endovascular therapy (i.e., balloon-occluded retrograde transvenous obliteration [BRTO] or direct embolization of varices) for patients who are not suitable candidates to undergo a TIPS procedure.[10,11]

It is important to point out that in this recent study by Garcia-Pagan, early TIPS was not performed in patients who had a Child-Pugh score greater than 13 points, who had isolated bleeding gastric varices, who were older than 75 years of age, who had hepatocellular carcinoma, who had portal vein thrombosis, and who had renal failure. Furthermore, a total of 22 patients in this study were excluded for nonspecified reasons. Therapeutic options offered to the patients who were excluded were not specified.[9]

Clinical studies have shown that patients who are Child-Pugh class C and have an APACHE II (Acute Physiology and Chronic Health Evaluation II) score greater than 18 have a very poor prognosis if they undergo an emergency TIPS procedure to control variceal bleed. The 30-day mortality rate for such patients is 98% to 100%.[12,13] Multiple variables have been associated with a poor prognosis in patients undergoing an emergency TIPS, including delayed admission to the ICU; presence of ascites; emergent requirement for mechanical ventilation; elevation of serum creatinine; elevated international normalized ratio (INR)[14]; and elevated serum bilirubin, especially if it reaches levels higher than 6 mg/dL.[12]

Chalasani and coworkers[15] studied 129 patients who underwent a TIPS procedure in a single center in the United States to evaluate the variables associated with early death. Only 16% of the patients in this series underwent an emergency TIPS; however, these authors identified four factors associated with 30-day mortality after TIPS: active variceal bleeding, emergency TIPS, prolonged prothrombin time (>17 sec), and bilirubin level greater than 3 mg/dL.[15]

Patch and coworkers[16] developed the prognostic index, a model specifically designed to predict mortality for patients undergoing an emergency TIPS. This predictive model was developed after the evaluation of 54 patients undergoing emergency TIPS for variceal bleeding.[16] In this study, five factors were associated with a poor prognosis: ascites (moderate or severe), need for emergent mechanical ventilation, white blood cell count, serum creatinine, and activated partial thromboplastin time (aPTT). Based on statistical methods, these authors developed a formula to calculate the prognostic score:

$$PI = 1.54 \text{ (ascites)} + 1.27 \text{ (ventilation)} + 1.38 \log e \text{ (white blood cell count)} + 2.48 \log e \text{ (aPTT)} + 1.55 \log e \text{ (creatinine)} - 1.05 \log e \text{ (platelet count)}.$$

The patients with a higher score had higher mortality rates. Overall, the 6-week mortality rate in this series was 48%.[16] Using this model, these investigators found that the 6-week mortality rate was 100% in patients with a prognostic index greater than

18.52.[16] The model was prospectively tested in an additional group of 31 patients undergoing emergency TIPS. From this group, there were 11 deaths (35%) within the 6-week period. All patients who had an early death had a prognostic index greater than 17.1.[6,16] In essence, these authors demonstrated that the 6-week mortality rate was 100% for any patient with a prognostic score greater than 18.52.

Scores to predict early mortality have been applied and tested clinically in patients with acute variceal bleeding; however, most of these scores have not been validated with further studies.[6] The scores are useful guides and allow the consulting interventional radiologist to give referring physicians, patients, and family members a realistic opinion on what to expect after the procedure if it is at all performed.[6] In our practice, we apply the APACHE II score to patients who are being considered for an emergency TIPS. If the APACHE II score is greater than 18 or the patient has more than one of the previously mentioned high-risk factors, we recommend against the TIPS and offer alternative options, including BRTO or even direct variceal embolization.

Patients Who Have Survived a Bleeding Episode and Require Treatment to Prevent Rebleeding

The risk of rebleeding in a patient who has survived an episode of acute variceal bleed is high, ranging between 50% to 60%.[1,17] Two groups of patients are identified within this clinical category: (i) patients who underwent a TIPS procedure and (ii) patients who responded to medical and endoscopic therapy. Patients who underwent a TIPS procedure require surveillance of the shunt but do not require drugs to prevent rebleeding.[1,18] Patients who responded to medical therapy require continued prophylactic therapy with nonselective beta-blockers.[1] In this latter group, either TIPS or surgical shunts are indicated for those who rebleed despite medical and endoscopic treatment.[1,3] TIPS procedures performed in this setting are considered to be either emergent or even elective; thus, these patients in general have a better prognosis. Evaluation of the clinical history, laboratory examinations, and imaging studies is still very important.

At least five prognostic scores have been described to try to determine the survival prognosis of patients undergoing a TIPS procedure.[6,19] The scores that have been more commonly used in clinical practice for this purpose include the Child-Pugh score and the model for end-stage liver disease (MELD) score.[6]

The Child-Pugh score (▶ Table 11.1) has been used to predict outcomes in patients undergoing portal hypertensive surgery since 1973 and was adopted to predict outcomes in patients undergoing TIPS since 1989.[20] The application of the Child-Pugh score divides the patients in three groups: A (score, 5–6), B (score, 7–9), and C (score, 10–15). The higher the score, the worse the liver function.[21] Patients with high scores (10–15) are considered to be poor operative risks.[22] The Child-Pugh score has some disadvantages; the calculation includes two subjective variables: ascites and degree of encephalopathy.[23] In addition, it is subject to the so-called ceiling effect.[6] This is considered to be a major disadvantage of the Child-Pugh score.[24] Despite these theoretical disadvantages, the Child-Pugh scoring system has withstood the test of time and is still very effective in predicting outcomes in patients with end-stage liver disease undergoing TIPS procedures[25–28]; it

Table 11.1 The Child-Pugh Classification

Variable	Points*		
	1	2	3
Ascites	None	Easily controlled	Poorly controlled
Albumin	> 3.5 g/dL	2.8–3.5 g /dL	< 2.8 g/dL
Bilirubin	< 2 mg/dL	2–3 mg/dL	> 3 mg/dL
Encephalopathy	Absent	Grades 1–2 (minimal)	Grades 3–4 (advanced)
Prothrombin (sec > control)	< 4.0	4–6	> 6

*Point modification for bilirubin values in patients with primary biliary cirrhosis: Bilirubin (mg/dL): 1–4: 1 point; > 4–10: 2 points; > 10: 3 points.
Child-Pugh score:
  A: 5–6, good prognosis
  B: 7–9, moderate
  C: 10–15, poor prognosis

has been compared with other recently described predictive scoring systems and has performed very well in patients undergoing both emergency[25] and elective TIPS.[26] In general, most authors coincide in the opinion that a Child-Pugh class C patient with a score of 12 or higher is at a very high risk of having an early death after a TIPS procedure.[13,29,30]

Malinchoc and coworkers[23] developed a model specifically designed to predict mortality in patients undergoing elective TIPS procedures. The model was developed based on a group of 231 consecutive patients with cirrhosis who underwent an elective TIPS procedure.[23] Four variables were identified as predictors of survival using the Cox proportional-hazards regression: serum creatinine, serum bilirubin, INR, and cause of cirrhosis.[23] These investigators developed a formula to calculate a risk score by using these four prognostic variables. The authors found this model to be quite effective in the prediction of patient survival after elective TIPS, with a sensitivity of 77%, specificity of 79%, positive predictive value of 63%, and negative predictive value of 88%.[23] The original model developed by Malinchoc was tested, and its formula was slightly modified; minor changes in the formula included deletion of the cause of cirrhosis as an adverse factor and multiplying the score by 10 to make it easier to apply.[28,31] The new model was called the model for end-stage liver disease score, better known as the MELD score. The MELD score has been validated in clinical studies and is now extensively used for patients undergoing TIPS and in patients with end-stage liver disease awaiting a liver transplant.[31–34] Most reports have confirmed that a MELD score greater than 18 is associated with an unfavorable prognosis with significantly lower 3-month survival rates.[27] Angermayr and colleagues[26] evaluated a total of 475 patients who underwent elective TIPS placement in 5 different hospitals in Austria in a 10-year period. These authors confirmed that patients with a MELD scores greater than 18 have significantly lower survival rates. The 3-month survival rate was 40% for patients with MELD scores of 18 or greater compared with 90% for patients with MELD scores of 18 or less; the difference was statistically significant ($P = 0.002$).[26] Other reports have demonstrated even more significant differences in survival if lower MELD score thresholds are selected to evaluate the patients.[27,34] Ferral and coworkers[27] tested the MELD score in a group of 166 patients who underwent elective TIPS in 2 different institutions in the United States. These authors found that the 30-day mortality rate was 0% in patients with MELD scores of 10 or less as opposed to an early mortality rate of 42% in patients with MELD scores of 25 or greater.[27] Furthermore, the 3- and 6-month mortality rates were 65.5% and 74.2%, respectively, for patients with MELD scores of 25 or greater.[27] In a recent retrospective study comparing multiple scoring systems, Gaba and coworkers[19] documented that the MELD and MELD-Na scores were the most accurate in predicting patient prognosis after a TIPS procedure.

The use of prognostic scores in this set of patients is useful in the sense that again, it allows the interventional radiologist to give a reasonable perspective of the expectations after the procedure to patients, referring physicians, and patient family members. The consensus is that TIPS should probably be withheld in patients with MELD scores greater than 25, and alternative options should be investigated to take care of the patient's clinical problem.

The Role of Transjugular Intrahepatic Portosystemic Shunt in Patients with Ascites

Ascites is a common complication seen in patients with cirrhosis. The development of ascites in a patient with cirrhosis indicates a poor prognosis.[2] The standard treatment for a patient with cirrhosis who develops ascites is medical management, including fluid and sodium restriction and the administration of diuretics.[2] Medical therapy fails in 5% to 10% of patients with ascites.[35] These patients are classified as having either refractory ascites or diuretic-intractable ascites.[2] Refractory ascites is the condition in which the fluid cannot be eliminated despite daily doses of 400 mg of spironolactone or 30 mg of amiloride plus 160 mg of furosemide. The patient must have been compliant with dietary sodium restriction. The group classified as diuretic intractable ascites is a specific group of patients who develop complications with diuretic therapy.[2] TIPS and large-volume paracentesis (LVP) have been used as therapeutic options for patients who cannot tolerate or do not respond to medical therapy.[2] Prospective clinical studies comparing LVP and TIPS have shown that TIPS is better to control the accumulation of fluid; however, it does not improve the patient's survival and requirement for hospital admissions. In addition, patients undergoing TIPS have a significantly higher incidence of encephalopathy after treatment.[36] For this reason, there is current controversy on which therapeutic option to use in these patients.[2,37]

Two factors separate the patients being treated for ascites from patients treated for bleeding: (i) patients with ascites have a poorer prognosis,[34,37] and (ii) TIPS procedures performed to treat ascites are always elective and aimed to improve patient's quality of life. For this reason, careful patient evaluation is even more important when deciding to perform a TIPS procedure in a patient with ascites difficult to control.[6] Another factor to consider is the development of encephalopathy after TIPS. The development of this complication ranges between 20% and 50% depending on the series reviewed.[38]

Taking all of these factors into consideration, careful clinical patient evaluation and the application of the MELD score and Child-Pugh score are useful to decide the therapeutic approach for these patients. The performance of a TIPS procedure for the management of ascites should probably be withheld in patients with MELD scores greater than 18 unless the patient is a liver transplant candidate.[2,28,39] Along the same lines, TIPS should not be performed to manage ascites in patients with MELD scores higher than 24 because the 30-day mortality rate in this group of patients ranges between 40% and 60%, and in our opinion, this is prohibitively high for an elective procedure.[39]

Kim and coworkers developed the MELD-Na score, which includes serum sodium as a variable in the formula.[37,40] The MELD-Na score appears to be more precise than the standard MELD score for the prediction of outcomes in patients undergoing elective TIPS procedures.[37] In a retrospective review of the outcomes of 148 patients who underwent an elective TIPS procedure, Guy and coworkers found that a MELD-Na score of 15 was the optimal cutoff point for prognostic prediction in their group of patients. This concept is probably even more important in patients who undergo TIPS for the management of ascites because these patients have a well-known derangement in the handling of serum sodium.[2,41] The lower the serum sodium, the higher the mortality rate as predicted by the MELD-Na score.[37] These patients should continue with LVP, creation of a Denver Shunt, or placement of a tunneled peritoneal drain (abdominal Pleur-x), especially if they are not suitable liver transplant candidates.[42]

Effect of Transjugular Intrahepatic Portosystemic Shunt on Liver and Kidney Function

TIPS is a nonselective portosystemic shunt, and if properly created, it causes profound hemodynamic changes. First, there is a well-documented and significant decrease in the portosystemic gradient.[43–45] Given its nature as a nonselective shunt, the immediate effect of a properly created TIPS is often a complete portal venous flow diversion in which the entire flow to the portal vein is shunted directly into the right atrium; even the intrahepatic portal vein branches may show flow reversal into the shunt.[46,47] This shunting of blood flow causes increases in central venous pressure, cardiac index, end-diastolic volume index, and a decrease in the systemic vascular resistance index.[43] These hemodynamic changes have effects both on kidney and liver function. Persistent improvement of the kidney function has been documented after successful TIPS procedures, with significant decreases in the serum creatinine levels as soon as 1 week after the procedure.[43,48] This improvement in renal function is most probably

related to the increased cardiac preload, which subsequently increases organ perfusion.[43] In addition, the increase in central venous pressure distends the right atrium and triggers the release of atrial natriuretic factor (ANF). This change in the ANF is followed by an increase in urinary sodium, and this mechanism is thought to participate in the improvement of the sodium balance after TIPS and explains the improvement of ascites.[2] By the same token, a deterioration of the liver function has been documented[43] after successful TIPS, and this is probably related to the portal flow diversion. After the portal flow is diverted, proper maintenance of liver function depends on the appropriate increase in flow from the hepatic artery, the so-called hepatic arterial buffer response.[46,47,49–53] If the hepatic artery flow does not increase in proportion to the percentage of portal flow loss, the relative lack of adequate flow to the liver places the patient at a high risk for a potential decompensation of liver function.[43]

Anderson and coworkers found that TIPS in general increases the MELD score, which is a reflection of worsening hepatic function. However, patients with renal dysfunction (not on dialysis) had improved renal function reflected by a reduction in the serum creatinine.[48] Moreover, in patients with normal renal function, the MELD score became worse after TIPS. However, in patients with renal dysfunction (not on dialysis), the MELD score decreased or remained stable after TIPS.[48]

Regarding the performance of TIPS in patients with renal failure, on hemodialysis, the literature on this topic is scarce.[54] In a small series of six patients, Haskal et al pointed out that in patients who are dialysis dependent and who undergo a TIPS procedure, the performance of hemodialysis shortly after the procedure is essential to improve the patient's short-term survival. In this report, Haskal et al also pointed out that the incidence of encephalopathy seems to be higher in this group of patients. In general, our interpretation of these results is that the performance of a TIPS procedure is not indicated in patients who are on hemodialysis unless the clinical situation of the patient is such that TIPS is the best possible option to manage the patient's clinical problem.

Conclusion

The role of TIPS has changed drastically in the past 10 years. The use of early TIPS for patients with acute variceal bleeding and at high risk needs to be evaluated further before it is established as an accepted option. The most useful prognostic scores are still the MELD, MELD-Na, and Child-Pugh scores. These scores are helpful as guides to understand the risks and prognosis of patients undergoing both emergency and elective TIPS procedures. In general, it is not our policy to refuse to perform a TIPS based on scores indicating a poor prognosis. There will always be certain variants and individual conditions pertaining each patient considered or evaluated that are not included in the scores (i.e., patient age, presence of renal failure, portal vein thrombosis, associated cancers) that may completely change a final clinical decision.

Clinical Pearls

- A total of 10% to 20% of patients with cirrhosis who have acute variceal bleeding fail standard therapy (beta-blockers or endoscopic management), and those are the patients who need to be evaluated for emergent TIPS.

- The 30-day mortality rate of patients undergoing emergent TIPS is 98% to 100% in patients with a Child-Pugh class C and an APACHE II score greater than 18.
- Other prognostic factors of poor survival for emergent TIPS include moderate to severe ascites, need for emergent mechanical ventilation, increased white blood cell count, increased serum creatinine, and increased aPTT.
- The components of the Child-Pugh score are ascites, albumin, bilirubin, encephalopathy, and prothrombin time or INR. Both ascites and encephalopathy are subjective components.
- A Child-Pugh class of C (score of 10–15) carries a poor prognosis after TIPS.
- The components of the MELD score are bilirubin, creatinine, and INR with a demarcation for dialysis.
- The MELD score has no subjective components and, as a result, is used primarily in the United States for defining transplant waiting lists and organ procurement.
- A MELD score of 18 or greater carries a poor prognosis after TIPS.
- The 3-month survival rates after TIPS are approximately 0% for MELD scores less than 10, 40% for MELD scores of 10 to 17, and 90% for MELD scores of 18 or greater.
- Refractory ascites is the condition in which ascetic fluid cannot be eliminated despite a daily dose of one of the following:
  - 400 mg of spironolactone
  - 30 mg of amiloride + 160 mg of furosemide
- Patients with the primary indication of ascites for TIPS have a poorer prognosis than those patients with a primary indication of variceal bleeding.
- Hepatic encephalopathy occurs in 20% to 50% of patients after TIPS.
- The MELD-Na score is probably more important in patients who undergo TIPS for management of refractory ascites because patients with ascites have a well-known derangement in handling of serum sodium.
- In general, TIPS causes worse hepatic function (an increase in the MELD score) and improved renal function. The worsening MELD score is thought to be transient. As a result, patients with normal renal function have an increase in MELD after TIPS, and patients with renal dysfunction (not on dialysis) have an improvement (reduction) in the MELD score.

References

1. Bari K, Garcia-Tsao G. Treatment of portal hypertension. World J Gastroenterol 2012;18(11):1166–1175.
2. Wong F. Management of ascites in cirrhosis. J Gastroenterol Hepatol 2012; 27(1):11–20.
3. Garcia-Tsao G, Bosch J. Management of varices and variceal hemorrhage in cirrhosis. N Engl J Med 2010;362(9):823–832.
4. Boyer TD, Haskal ZJ. The Role of Transjugular intrahepatic portosystemic shunt (TIPS) in the management of portal hypertension: update 2009. Hepatology 2010;51(1):306.
5. Riggio O, Ridola L, Lucidi C, Angeloni S. Emerging issues in the use of transjugular intrahepatic portosystemic shunt (TIPS) for management of portal hypertension: time to update the guidelines? Dig Liver Dis 2010;42(7):462–467.
6. Ferral H, Patel NH. Selection criteria for patients undergoing transjugular intrahepatic portosystemic shunt procedures: current status. J Vasc Interv Radiol 2005;16(4):449–455.
7. Boyer TD, Haskal ZJ. The role of transjugular intrahepatic portosystemic shunt in the management of portal hypertension. Hepatology 2005;41(2):386–400.
8. Chau TN, Patch D, Chan YW, et al. "Salvage" transjugular intrahepatic portosystemic shunts: gastric fundal compared with esophageal variceal bleeding. Gastroenterology 1998;114(5):981–987.
9. Garcia-Pagan JC, Caca K, Bureau C, et al. Early use of TIPS in patients with cirrhosis and variceal bleeding. N Engl J Med 2010;362(25):2370–2379.
10. Saad WE, Darcy MD. Transjugular intrahepatic portosystemic shunt (TIPS) versus Balloon-occluded retrograde transvenous obliteration (BRTO) for the management of gastric varices. Semin Intervent Radiol 2011;28(3):339–349.
11. Saad WE, Sabri SS. Balloon-occluded retrograde transvenous obliteration (BRTO): technical results and outcomes. Semin Intervent Radiol 2011;28(3): 333–338.
12. Brensing KA, Raab P, Textor J, et al. Prospective evaluation of a clinical score for 60-day mortality after transjugular intrahepatic portosystemic stent-shunt: Bonn TIPSS early mortality analysis. Eur J Gastroenterol Hepatol 2002;14(7):723–731.
13. Rubin RA, Haskal ZJ, O'Brien CB, et al. Transjugular intrahepatic portosystemic shunting: decreased survival for patients with high APACHE II scores. Am J Gastroenterol 1995;90(4):556–563.
14. Azoulay D, Castaing D, Majno P, et al. Salvage transjugular intrahepatic portosystemic shunt for uncontrolled variceal bleeding in patients with decompensated cirrhosis. J Hepatol 2001;35(5):590–597.
15. Chalasani N, Clark WS, Martin LG, et al. Determinants of mortality in patients with advanced cirrhosis after transjugular intrahepatic portosystemic shunting. Gastroenterology 2000;118(1):138–144.
16. Patch D, Nikolopoulou V, McCormick A, et al. Factors related to early mortality after transjugular intrahepatic portosystemic shunt for failed endoscopic therapy in acute variceal bleeding. J Hepatol 1998;28(3):454–460.
17. Boyer TD, Haskal ZJ. American Association for the Study of Liver Diseases practice guidelines: the role of transjugular intrahepatic portosystemic shunt creation in the management of portal hypertension. J Vasc Interv Radiol 2005;16(5):615–629.
18. Huang Q, Wu X, Fan X, et al. Comparison study of Doppler ultrasound surveillance of expanded polytetrafluoroethylene-covered stent versus bare stent in transjugular intrahepatic portosystemic shunt. J Clin Ultrasound 2010;38(7):353–360.
19. Gaba RC, Couture PM, Bui JT, et al. Prognostic capability of different liver disease scoring systems for prediction of early mortality after transjugular intrahepatic portosystemic shunt creation. J Vasc Interv Radiol 2013;24(3):411–420.
20. Richter GM, Noeldge G, Palmaz JC, Roessle M. The transjugular intrahepatic portosystemic stent-shunt (TIPSS): results of a pilot study. Cardiovasc Intervent Radiol 1990;13(3):200–207.
21. Haskal ZJ, Rees CR, Ring EJ, et al. Reporting standards for transjugular intrahepatic portosystemic shunts. Technology Assessment Committee of the SCVIR. J Vasc Interv Radiol 1997;8(2):289–297.
22. Pugh RN, Murray-Lyon IM, Dawson JL, et al. Transection of the oesophagus for bleeding oesophageal varices. Br J Surg 1973;60(8):646–649.
23. Malinchoc M, Kamath PS, Gordon FD, et al. A model to predict poor survival in patients undergoing transjugular intrahepatic portosystemic shunts. Hepatology 2000;31(4):864–871.
24. Forman LM, Lucey MR. Predicting the Prognosis of chronic liver disease: an evolution from Child to MELD. Hepatology 2001;33:473–475.
25. Schepke M, Roth F, Fimmers R, et al. Comparison of MELD, Child-Pugh, and Emory model for the prediction of survival in patients undergoing transjugular intrahepatic portosystemic shunting. Am J Gastroenterol 2003;98(5):1167–1174.
26. Angermayr B, Cejna M, Karnel F, et al. Child-Pugh versus MELD score in predicting survival in patients undergoing transjugular intrahepatic portosystemic shunt. Gut 2003;52(6):879–885.
27. Ferral H, Gamboa P, Postoak DW, et al. Survival after elective transjugular intrahepatic portosystemic shunt creation: prediction with model for end-stage liver disease score. Radiology 2004;231(1):231–236.
28. Kamath PS, Kim WR. The model for end-stage liver disease (MELD). Hepatology 2007;45(3):797–805.
29. Encarnacion CE, Palmaz JC, Rivera FJ, et al. Transjugular intrahepatic portosystemic shunt placement for variceal bleeding: predictors of mortality. J Vasc Interv Radiol 1995;6(5):687–694.
30. Banares R, Casado M, Rodriguez-Laiz JM, et al. Urgent transjugular intrahepatic portosystemic shunt for control of acute variceal bleeding. Am J Gastroenterol 1998;93(1):75–79.
31. Kamath PS, Wiesner RH, Malinchoc M, et al. A model to predict survival in patients with end-stage liver disease [see comments]. Hepatology 2001;33(2):464–470.
32. Wiesner RH, McDiarmid SV, Kamath PS, et al. MELD and PELD: application of survival models to liver allocation. Liver Transpl 2001;7(7):567–580.
33. Said A, Williams J, Holden J, et al. Model for end stage liver disease score predicts mortality across a broad spectrum of liver disease. J Hepatol 2004;40(6): 897–903.
34. Heinzow HS, Lenz P, Kohler M, et al. Clinical outcome and predictors of survival after TIPS insertion in patients with liver cirrhosis. World J Gastroenterol 2012;18(37):5211–5218.
35. Ferral H, Bjarnason H, Wegryn SA, et al. Refractory ascites: early experience in treatment with transjugular intrahepatic portosystemic shunt. Radiology 1993;189(3):795–801.

36. Sanyal AJ, Genning C, Reddy KR, et al. The North American Study for the Treatment of Refractory Ascites. Gastroenterology 2003;124(3):634–641.

37. Guy J, Somsouk M, Shiboski S, et al. New model for end stage liver disease improves prognostic capability after transjugular intrahepatic portosystemic shunt. Clin Gastroenterol Hepatol 2009;7(11):1236–1240.

38. Riggio O, Nardelli S, Moscucci F, et al. Hepatic encephalopathy after transjugular intrahepatic portosystemic shunt. Clin Liver Dis 2012;16(1):133–146.

39. Montgomery A, Ferral H, Vasan R, Postoak DW. MELD score as a predictor of early death in patients undergoing elective transjugular intrahepatic portosystemic shunt (TIPS) procedures. Cardiovasc Intervent Radiol 2005;28(3):307–312.

40. Kim WR, Biggins SW, Kremers WK, et al. Hyponatremia and mortality among patients on the liver-transplant waiting list. N Engl J Med 2008;359(10):1018–1026.

41. Salerno F, Guevara M, Bernardi M, et al. Refractory ascites: pathogenesis, definition and therapy of a severe complication in patients with cirrhosis. Liver Int 2010;30(7):937–947.

42. Martin LG. Percutaneous placement and management of the Denver Shunt for portal hypertensive ascites. AJR Am J Roentgenol 2012;199(4):W449–W453.

43. Saugel B, Phillip V, Gaa J, et al. Advanced hemodynamic monitoring before and after transjugular intrahepatic portosystemic shunt: implications for selection of patients—a prospective study. Radiology 2012;262(1):343–352.

44. Angermayr B. Transjugular intrahepatic portosystemic shunt—current status in 2011. Acta Gastroenterol Belg 2011;74(4):553–559.

45. Albillos A, Garcia-Tsao G. Classification of cirrhosis: the clinical use of HVPG measurements. Dis Markers. 2011;31(3):121–128.

46. Foshager MC, Ferral H, Finlay DE, et al. Color Doppler sonography of transjugular intrahepatic portosystemic shunts (TIPS). AJR Am J Roentgenol 1994;163(1):105–111.

47. Ferral H, Foshager MC, Bjarnason H, et al. Early sonographic evaluation of the transjugular intrahepatic portosystemic shunt (TIPS). Cardiovasc Intervent Radiol 1993;16(5):275–279.

48. Anderson CL, Saad WE, Kalagher SD, et al. Effect of transjugular intrahepatic portosystemic shunt placement on renal function: a 7-year, single-center experience. J Vasc Interv Radiol 2010;21(9):1370–1376.

49. Walser E, Ozkan OS, Raza S, et al. Hepatic perfusion as a predictor of mortality after transjugular intrahepatic portosystemic shunt creation in patients with refractory ascites. J Vasc Interv Radiol 2003;14(10):1251–1257.

50. Kelly DM, Zhu X, Shiba H, et al. Adenosine restores the hepatic artery buffer response and improves survival in a porcine model of small-for-size syndrome. Liver Transpl 2009;15(11):1448–1457.

51. Mathie RT, Alexander B. The role of adenosine in the hyperaemic response of the hepatic artery to portal vein occlusion (the "buffer response"). Br J Pharmacol 1990;100(3):626–630.

52. Rocheleau B, Ethier C, Houle R, et al. Hepatic artery buffer response following left portal vein ligation: its role in liver tissue homeostasis. Am J Physiol 1999;277(5 Pt 1):G1000–G1007.

53. Siebert N, Cantre D, Eipel C, Vollmar B. H2S contributes to the hepatic arterial buffer response and mediates vasorelaxation of the hepatic artery via activation of K(ATP) channels. Am J Physiol Gastrointest Liver Physiol 2008;295(6):G1266–G1273.

54. Haskal ZJ, Radhakrishnan J. Transjugular intrahepatic portosystemic shunts in hemodialysis-dependent patients and patients with advanced renal insufficiency: safety, caution, and encephalopathy. J Vasc Interv Radiol 2008;19(4):516–520.

Chapter 12: Hepatic and Portal Venous Anatomy Relative to the Transjugular Intrahepatic Portosystemic Shunt Procedure

Nael E. Saad and Kathryn J. Fowler

Introduction

Portal hypertension (PHT) is a condition that results from portal venous flow obstruction. Transjugular intrahepatic portosystemic shunt (TIPS) is an artificial channel created between the portal venous inflow and the hepatic vein outflow of the liver. This channel acts as a conduit through which the venous flow of the splanchnic circulation can bypass the liver parenchyma in a way that obviates the risk of life-threatening hemorrhage that can result from variceal rupture. TIPS has become the mainstay of management of PHT complications and has supplanted surgical shunt creation.

Many factors affect the success of TIPS. Anatomy plays an essential role in preprocedural planning and ultimate success. The size of the shunt is important for ensuring adequate reduction of portal pressures. Hence, the hepatic vein selected for TIPS must be of a suitable size to allow sufficient functional diameter of the TIPS. In addition to size, distance and angulation of the shunt tract are vital to successful decompression and long-term patency. An appropriate trajectory from hepatic vein to portal vein must be planned for creating a smoothly curved TIPS.[1] A thorough understanding of the standard liver, hepatic vein, and portal vein anatomy as well as common anatomic variants is paramount.

Liver Morphology and Anatomy

The liver is the largest solid organ in the body, weighing between 1400 and 1600 g in men and between 1200 and 1400 g in women.[2] The liver is located in the right upper quadrant; the upper margin is at the approximate T9 level, and the inferior border extends to the 11th rib (▶ Fig. 12.1). The size of the liver is subject to great variation, especially in patients with end-stage liver disease. Even in the healthy subjects, there are common variants of Riedel's lobe (right lobe extends into the right lower quadrant) and high variability of left lobe size (the left border of the liver may be to the right of the spine or extend several centimeters to the left). Common morphologic changes associated with cirrhosis include right lobe atrophy with left lobe or caudate hypertrophy, widening of the preportal space, a small shrunken liver, and displacement of the liver from the right abdominal wall caused by large-volume ascites (▶ Fig. 12.2).

Adjacent organs are at risk for inadvertent needlestick and injury. The liver is bordered inferiorly by the right kidney and hepatic flexure of the colon. The kidney is located within the retroperitoneum separated from the peritoneal cavity and liver surface by an investment of peritoneal fascia. The hepatic flexure may extend anterior and superior to the liver margin, creating the potential for inadvertent injury from needlestick. The

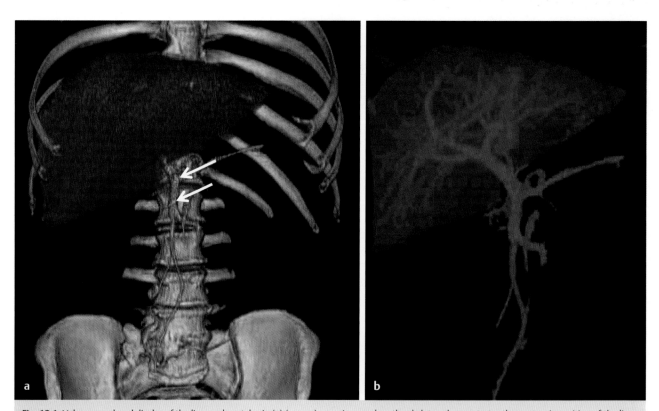

Fig. 12.1 Volume-rendered display of the liver and portal vein (**a**) (*arrows*) superimposed on the skeleton demonstrates the anatomic position of the liver in the right upper quadrant. Maximum intensity projection image of the liver and portal vein (**b**).

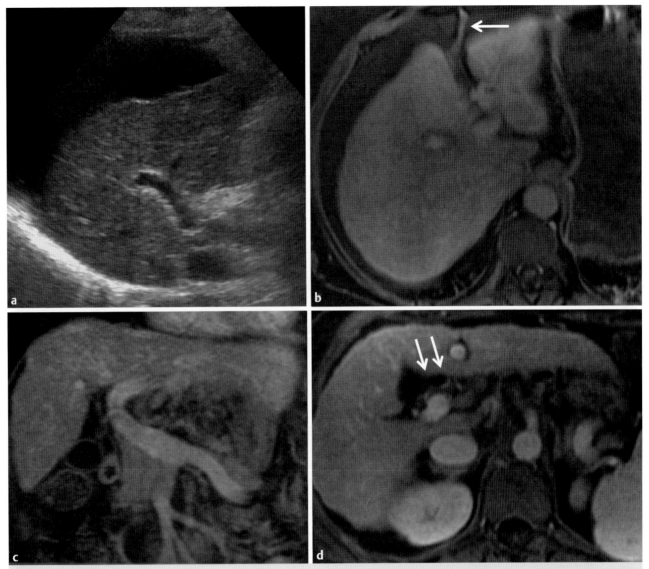

Fig. 12.2 Imaging features of cirrhosis. (a) Ultrasound image shows a coarse, nodular, shrunken liver with surrounding ascites. (b) Axial contrast-enhanced (CE) magnetic resonance image (MRI) shows recanalized paraumbilical vein. (c) Coronal CE MRI shows dilation of the portal and mesenteric vessels. (d) Axial CE MRI shows widening of the preportal space and a nodular small liver (*arrows*).

gallbladder is located within a fossa along the anterior inferior visceral surface of the liver between the medial left and anterior right hepatic sections. The duodenum and stomach together border the anterior-inferior margin of the left hemiliver.

Liver segmental and sectional anatomy is dictated by portal venous territories for surgical and radiological purposes. On the largest scale, the liver can be divided into right and left hemiliver along a boundary between the gallbladder fossa (interlobar fissure) and right margin of the middle hepatic vein–inferior vena cava (IVC) junction (Cantlie line).[3] The right hepatic artery and portal vein supply the right hemiliver, and the left hepatic artery and portal vein supply the left hemiliver. Each hemiliver can be further divided into two sections: right anterior, right posterior, left medial, and left lateral. The right sections are divided by the right hepatic vein and the left section by the falciform ligament/left hepatic vein. Each section is supplied by a corresponding major

portal venous branch. The caudate lobe is considered separately from the right and left hemilivers because it is invested by its own fascial covering and has independent portal and hepatic venous flow as well as variable arterial supply from either the right or left hepatic arteries. Furthermore, the liver may be divided into eight separate segments, first described in 1957 by Couinaud[4,5] (► Fig. 12.3).

Finally, a closer look at the hepatic parenchyma shows that the portal veins are located within the portal triads accompanied by arterial branches, bile ducts, and lymphatics. The close proximity of the hepatic arteries and bile ducts to the portal veins makes inadvertent sticks common during a TIPS procedure. The portal veins become progressively diminutive within the peripheral parenchyma supplying the inflow to the sinusoidal channels, the capillary network of the liver parenchyma (► Figs. 12.4 and ► 12.5).[6] On the other side of the sinusoidal channel or network,

SEGMENTATION OF THE LIVER

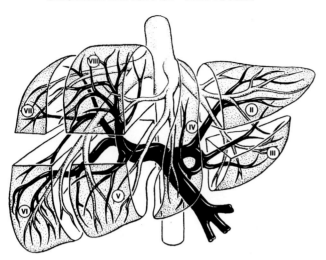

I	Caudate Lobe (not shown) Located Posterior, Behind IV
II	Posterior Aspect, Lateral Segment Left Lobe
III	Anterior Aspect, Lateral Segment Left Lobe
IV	Medial Segment, Left Lobe
V	Inferior Aspect, Anterior Segment Right Lobe
VI	Inferior Aspect, Posterior Segment Right Lobe
VII	Superior Aspect, Posterior Segment Right Lobe
VIII	Superior Aspect, Anterior Segment Right Lobe

Fig. 12.3 Schematic drawing of the Couinaud segments of the liver. The hepatic veins are in white, and the portal veins are in black.

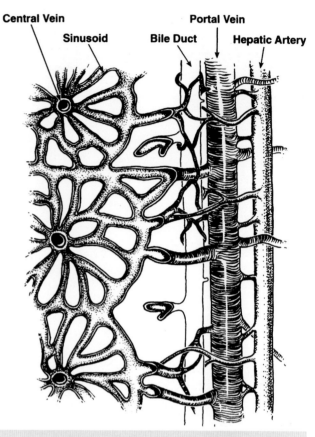

Fig. 12.4 Schematic diagram showing the microvascular bed of the liver parenchyma. The liver is histologically divided into lobules (see ► Fig. 12.5). The sinusoidal inflow is an admixture of "nutritive" blood from both the hepatic artery and the portal vein.

the blood drains into the terminal hepatic venules. The hepatic veins course independently from other vasculature with these small peripheral tributaries joining to form larger trunks more centrally that eventually drain into the IVC.

Hepatic Venous Anatomy

The hepatic veins constitute the only venous drainage of the liver. The right, middle, and left hepatic veins are the three largest hepatic veins and drain into the anterior surface of the IVC 1 cm below the diaphragm and 2 cm below the inferior border of the right atrium[7] (► Fig. 12.6).

Right Hepatic Vein

The right hepatic vein is the largest of the three main veins and drains the entire right hemiliver (segments V, VI, VII, and VIII). The diameter of the right hepatic vein is largest at the confluence with the IVC, measuring approximately 1 cm.[8] It can be challenging to differentiate the right from the middle hepatic vein during venography. The insertion of the right hepatic vein on the IVC is lateral and slightly superior to that of the middle hepatic vein. The marginal tributary characteristically helps identify the right hepatic vein as it arcs through the superior aspect of the right hemiliver to join the right hepatic vein centrally (► Fig. 12.7).

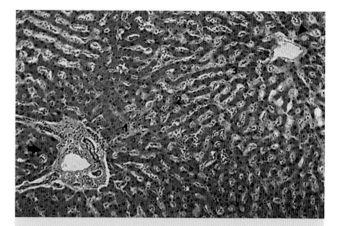

Fig. 12.5 The liver is divided histologically into lobules. The hepatic arteries, portal veins, and bile ducts, commonly referred to as the portal triad (*arrow*), are located in the periphery of the lobule, whereas the central vein (*arrowhead*) is at the center of the lobule. Functionally, the liver can be divided into three zones, based upon oxygen supply. Zone 1 encircles the portal tracts, where the oxygenated blood from hepatic arteries enters. Zone 3 is located around central veins, where oxygenation is poor. Zone 2 is located between zones 1 and 3.

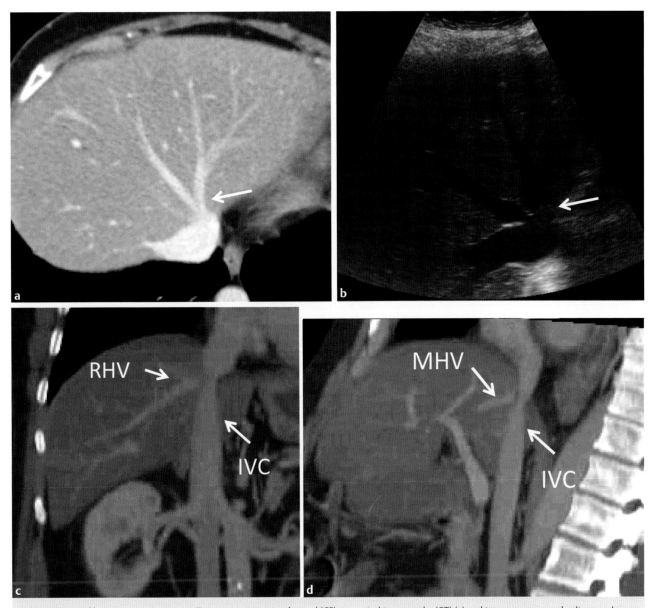

Fig. 12.6 Normal hepatic venous anatomy. Transverse contrast-enhanced (CE) computed tomography (CT) (**a**) and transverse gray-scale ultrasound (**b**) images show the normal right (RHV), middle (MHV), and left hepatic veins. Note the common trunk of the left and middle veins (*arrow*). Coronal (**c**) and sagittal (**d**) CE CT images show the normal relationship of the hepatic veins to the right atrium and inferior vena cava (IVC).

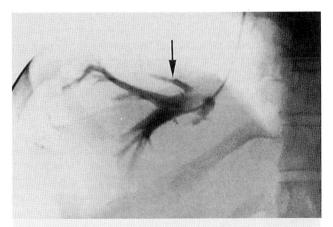

Fig. 12.7 Right hepatic venogram showing the marginal branch (*arrow*).

Middle Hepatic Vein

The middle hepatic vein commonly drains segment IV (left medial section) and often receives blood supply from the anterior right hepatic section (segments V and VIII). The middle hepatic vein ostium on the IVC is caudal to the right hepatic vein and located along the left anterior aspect of the IVC. The common trunk formed by the middle and left hepatic vein measures approximately 1 cm in length.[8] The middle hepatic vein may be a suitable alternative to the right hepatic vein for TIPS.

Left Hepatic Vein

The left hepatic vein is a short trunk formed by the union of drainage veins from segments II and III (left lateral section). The left hepatic vein often forms a common trunk with the middle hepatic

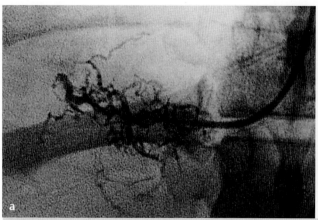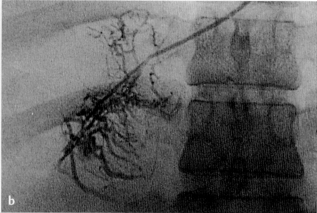

Fig. 12.8 Patient with acute Budd-Chiari syndrome undergoing placement of transjugular intrahepatic portosystemic shunt. Selective hepatic venogram of the (**a**) right and (**b**) middle hepatic veins shows the classic "spider web" appearance of the hepatic veins seen in this condition.

vein before draining to the IVC.[8] The size of the left hepatic vein is variable because of the variability in size of the left hemiliver. It is least commonly used for TIPS.

Variant Anatomy

In addition to the three main veins, numerous other smaller veins drain the inferior portion of the right lobe and the caudate. Variations are encountered in up to 30% of patients.[7,9–11] Supranumerary left hepatic veins are frequently present. An accessory inferior right hepatic vein is also frequently seen and is the largest accessory vein, potentially providing the dominant drainage of the right hemiliver. An accessory right inferior hepatic vein usually drains the inferior portion of the posterior right hepatic section via a sizable trunk connecting to the midportion of the retrohepatic IVC.[4] Additional common variants include multiple accessory right hepatic veins, absent right hepatic vein, a separate umbilical segment vein, and the accessory segment VIII branch draining into the middle hepatic vein. Helpful tips for differentiating the right from the middle hepatic vein during venography include the following:

- The right hepatic vein ostium is lateral and slightly superior.
- The marginal tributary arcs superior to join the right hepatic vein.
- The right hepatic vein is more horizontal in course (lateral projection may help).
- There may be an inflow artifact along the left lateral aspect of the middle hepatic vein from left vein drainage.
- A wedged hepatic venogram through the right hepatic vein will opacify the right portal vein first, but through the middle hepatic vein, the left and right portal veins opacify simultaneously.

In the setting of parenchymal fibrosis, there may be attenuation or "pruning" of the hepatic veins. In addition, hepatic vein-to-hepatic vein collaterals may become prominent. As fibrosis progresses, the size of the central hepatic veins may decrease, and the shrunken liver morphology and presence of ascites may alter the relationship of the hepatic veins with the IVC. An acute angle between the IVC and hepatic veins may make catheterization from a transjugular approach very difficult. Paracentesis and removal of large-volume ascites can improve this angle and facilitate cannulation for TIPS.

In Budd-Chiari syndrome, impedance of venous outflow may occur at the level of the small hepatic venules, the larger hepatic veins, or the IVC.[9,12–15] Thrombosis and obliteration at the level of the main hepatic veins is most common. Long-standing obstruction results in collateral pathways and development of the so-called spider-web appearance[16] (▶ Fig. 12.8). The caudate venous drainage is often spared, and venous collateralization and drainage of the entire liver may occur through the caudate lobe veins. As a result of venous outflow obstruction, the liver becomes enlarged, and compression of the intrahepatic IVC is typically present (▶ Fig. 12.9). When Budd-Chiari syndrome is caused by suprahepatic IVC obstruction, the hepatic veins are engorged and enlarged with many veno-venous collaterals present (▶ Fig. 12.10). Further discussion of TIPS creation in the difficult setting of Budd-Chiari syndrome is provided in Chapter 17.

Portal Venous Anatomy

The main blood supply to the normal liver is the portal vein. The portal venous inflow is formed by four major contributors: the splenic vein, superior mesenteric vein (SMV), inferior mesenteric vein (IMV), and coronary vein.[7,9] ▶ Figures 12.11 and ▶ 12.12 demonstrate normal portal venous anatomy. The splenic vein drains the spleen and greater curvature of the stomach, the SMV drains the small bowel and right and transverse colon, the IMV drains the left and rectosigmoid colon, and the coronary vein drains the distal esophagus and lesser curvature of the stomach. The portal vein is formed posterior to the neck of the pancreas, passing behind the duodenum and along the free edge of the lesser omentum to the porta hepatis. The main portal vein is located at the approximate T11 to L1 vertebral level in healthy patients.[17,18] The main portal vein is approximately 7 to 8 cm in length and just more than 1 cm in diameter in normal patients.[17,19]

The main portal vein bifurcates into a left and right branch, denoted as the portal bifurcation. The portal bifurcation may be extrahepatic in about half, intrahepatic in about a quarter, and located right at the entrance to the liver in a quarter of patients.[2,20] The hepatic artery and common hepatic duct travel alongside the main portal vein in the hepatic hilum. The typical spatial relationship at the porta hepatis is that the portal vein lies posterior to both the bile duct and artery.[8,21] This spatial relationship is often

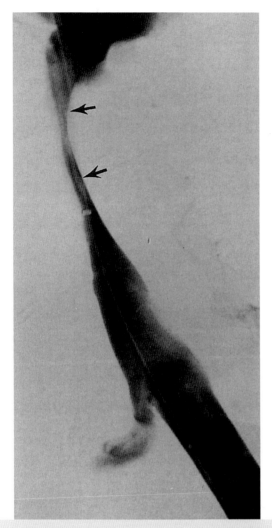

Fig. 12.9 Nonselective inferior venocavogram in the same patient in shows marked narrowing of the intrahepatic portion of the inferior vena cava (*arrows*) secondary to swelling of the liver caused by the venous engorgement.

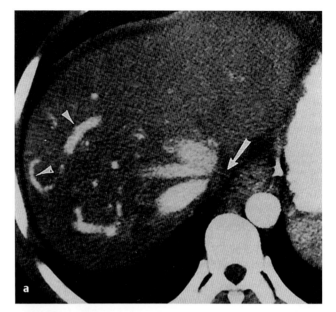

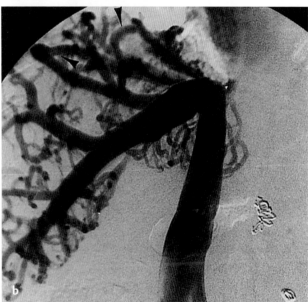

Fig. 12.10 A patient presents after orthotopic liver transplant with lower truncal and extremity edema. (**a**) Contrast-enhanced computed tomograph of the liver and (**b**) nonselective inferior venacavogram shows lack of contrast opacification (*arrow*) as a result of occlusion of the suprahepatic inferior vena cava at the surgical anastomosis and antegrade flow of contrast into the right atrium. Note the retrograde filling of the engorged hepatic veins. Prominent intrahepatic venous collaterals are present (*arrowheads*).

maintained within the hepatic parenchyma with the bile duct and artery located anterior to the portal vein within the portal triads.

Right Portal Vein

The right portal vein receives flow from the cystic vein, draining the gallbladder, and then enters the right hemiliver. The common right portal trunk is present in 90% of patients and is usually located between the 10th and 12th ribs and within 0.5 to 1.5 vertebral widths to the right of the lateral margin of the vertebral body.[19] The right portal vein trunk usually courses for several centimeters before bifurcating into anterior and posterior sectional branches. These supply the anterior and posterior right hepatic sections. The anterior branch then bifurcates into a superior segmental branch to segment VIII and an inferior segmental branch to segment V. The posterior sectional portal vein bifurcates into a superior segmental branch to segment VII and an inferior segmental branch to segment VI.

Left Portal Vein

The left portal vein is longer than the right but generally smaller in caliber. The intrahepatic left portal vein has two distinct segments: 1) proximal or transverse segment giving off branches to the caudate and 2) distal or umbilical segment giving off branches to segments II, III, and IV. In healthy patients, the umbilical segment of the left portal vein terminates in the ligamentum teres, which is the obliterated umbilical vein.[9,20]

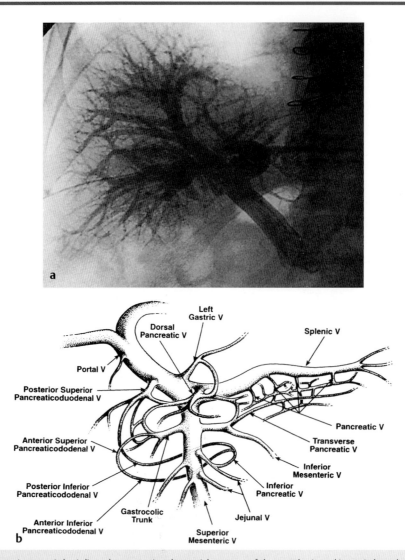

Fig. 12.11 (a) Portovenogram in a noncirrhotic liver, demonstrating the spatial anatomy of the portal vein and its main branches relative to the osseous structure. (b) Schematic drawing of the portal vein and its branches. V: Vein

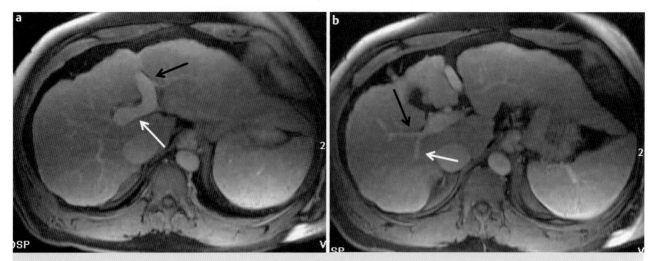

Fig. 12.12 Portal vein anatomy. Two transverse postcontrast magnetic resonance images show the transverse (**a**, *white arrow*) and umbilical segments (**a**, *black arrow*) of the left portal vein. Note the presence of cirrhosis with enlargement of the left hemiliver and portal vein caused by a recanalized periumbilical vein. The anterior (**b**, *black arrow*) and posterior (**b**, *white arrow*) branches of the right portal vein are small, reflecting the atrophy of the right hemiliver in the setting of cirrhosis.

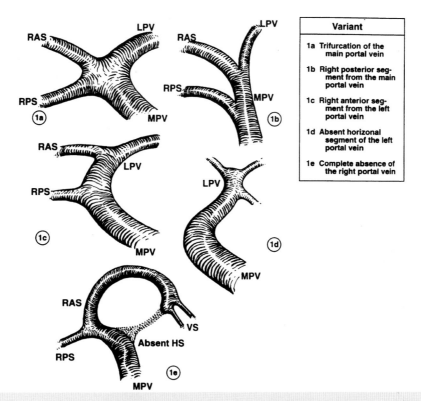

Fig. 12.13 Schematic diagram showing the variant anatomy of the portal vein. MPV: main portal vein; LPV: left portal vein; RAS: right anterior segment; RPS: right posterior segment; HS: horizontal segment; VS: vertical segment.

Anatomic Variants

Normal variations in anatomy occur in 10% to 15% of patients.[7,9,11,19,22,23] In 11% of patients, there is no right portal vein trunk, and the main portal vein trifurcates into right anterior, right posterior, and left portal branches.[9,23] Other common variants are the right posterior segment branch arising from the main portal vein (5% of patients) and the right anterior segment branch arising from the left portal vein (4% of patients). Other less common variants include an accessory left portal vein arising from the main portal vein, absence of the right portal vein, and absence of the horizontal segment of the left portal vein.[22] ► Figure 12.13 shows variant portal venous anatomy.

Pathophysiologic Variants

In the setting of PHT, flow within the portal vein may be reversed (hepatofugal or retrograde). In this setting, the portal venous flow contributes substantially less nutritive support to the liver, so hence hepatic arterial supply accounts for a greater contribution. In response to PHT, the portal vein initially becomes dilated, and portal vein velocities may be decreased. As PHT progresses, flow within the portal system may become stagnant or "to and fro" (► Fig. 12.14). This stagnation of portal flow predisposes patients to portal venous thrombosis.

Portal venous thrombosis may be nonocclusive and often laminar along the walls of the portal vein or occlusive with complete

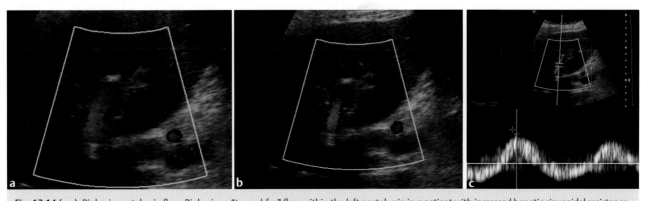

Fig. 12.14 (a-c) Biphasic portal vein flow. Biphasic or "to-and-fro" flow within the left portal vein in a patient with increased hepatic sinusoidal resistance caused by acute hepatitis. This pattern of flow can also be seen in portal hypertension. Normal portal vein phasicity should not dip below baseline (as is seen in the spectral analysis waveform (c)).

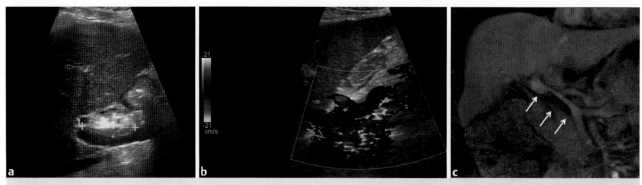

Fig. 12.15 Nonocclusive portal vein thrombosis. Gray scale (**a**) and color Doppler ultrasound (**b**) images show a nonocclusive thrombus in the main portal vein. Note the sluggish flow (indicated by the excessive background noise and low scale of the Doppler image). Coronal magnetic resonance imaging postcontrast image (**c**) from the same patient also shows the thrombus, which appears nearly black in signal intensity next to the enhancing lumen (*arrows*).

obstruction to flow (▶ Fig. 12.15). When occlusive thrombosis occurs and is long standing, cavernous transformation may occur (▶ Fig. 12.16). In the setting of cavernous transformation, many periportal venous collaterals become enlarged (▶ Fig. 12.17). These collaterals often course along the common bile duct, duodenum, and gallbladder. Large collaterals may be present, mimicking a patent main portal vein.

In addition to bland thrombus-related to altered flow dynamics, patients with cirrhosis are at risk for development of hepatocellular carcinoma, which can present with vascular invasion and tumor thrombus.[24,25]

Spatial Relationship of Hepatic and Portal Veins

The performance of successful TIPS requires an understanding of the spatial relationship of the portal vein to the hepatic vein. In most instances, the hepatic veins are superior or cephalad to the portal veins, requiring the transhepatic needle to be directed inferiorly. In general, the anteroposterior and medial-lateral relationship of the hepatic to portal veins can be anticipated. The main right portal vein is located anterior and inferior or inferomedial to the right hepatic vein and posterior and lateral to the middle hepatic vein.[8] The main left portal vein is located directly inferior to the middle hepatic vein and inferior and medial to the left hepatic vein.[8] It can be challenging to determine if the middle or right hepatic vein has been cannulated because both course in the same apparent direction when viewed in the anteroposterior projection. The list above describes useful tips to help differentiate. In general, the middle hepatic vein has a more vertical orientation compared with the more horizontal orientation of the right hepatic vein. As previously stated, the presence of a marginal vein arcing and joining the right hepatic vein can also be a useful indicator. Finally, the right hepatic vein confluence is located along the right lateral aspect of the IVC, and the middle hepatic vein confluence is located along the anterior aspect. Performing steep oblique or lateral projections (or both) may help in difficult cases as the right hepatic vein is more posterior than the middle hepatic vein. One additional clue is that there may be an inflow artifact along the left lateral aspect of the middle hepatic vein caused by inflow from the left hepatic vein in instances with a shared trunk.

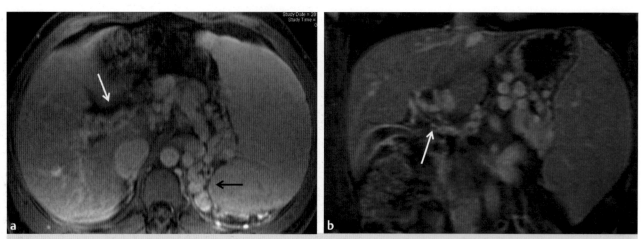

Fig. 12.16 (**a,b**) Cavernous transformation of the portal vein. Chronic occlusion results in extensive collaterals, which are shown by *arrows* in the transverse and coronal magnetic resonance images with contrast. Also note the extensive short gastric varices (*black arrow*).

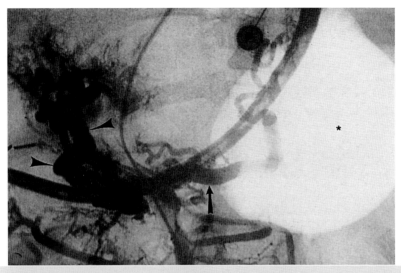

Fig. 12.17 Portomesogram shows occlusive thrombus in the main portal vein and opacification of multiple collateral veins (*arrowheads*) in the porta hepatis. The coronary vein is filling (*arrow*), and the gastric balloon of a Sengstaken-Blakemore tube is inflated (*asterisk*).

Pathophysiologic Variants

In small cirrhotic livers, the relationship of the hepatic veins to the portal veins is altered. The portal veins may be horizontal or cephalad to the hepatic veins, requiring an altered trajectory of the transhepatic needle. The presence of ascites may alter the angle of the hepatic veins relative to the IVC. In severe cirrhosis, the overall liver size may be diminutive, especially the right hemiliver, which may increase the technical difficulty of TIPS procedure and the risk for capsular perforation during the transhepatic portion of the procedure. Budd-Chiari syndrome presents many challenges to TIPS placement. Access to an accessory hepatic vein, direct intrahepatic portacaval shunt (DIPS), or direct shunting to the IVC may be options to consider.[26]

Imaging Options

Cross-sectional imaging with computed tomography, magnetic resonance imaging/magnetic resonance angiography, or ultrasonography with Doppler is essential to understand the anatomy before performing TIPS, especially in patients with end-stage liver cirrhosis.[27] Each modality has advantages and disadvantages (▶ Table 12.1). When noninvasive imaging fails to give confident depiction, angiography can be performed but with the attendant risks and excess cost of an invasive procedure.

Although portal venous puncture can be made using anatomic landmarks, wedged hepatic venography is recommended to provide safe targeting for portal vein access. The order in which the portal vein branches opacify can also help confirm the identity of the catheterized hepatic vein (right vs. middle). From a right hepatic vein approach, the right portal vein should opacify first. But from a middle hepatic vein approach, the left and right portal veins often opacify simultaneously. When performed correctly, wedged hepatic venography is generally safe and relatively quick and can provide information on appropriate hepatic vein choice and patency of the portal venous system and insight into the spatial relationship between the portal and hepatic vein.

New technologies exist that can help guide interventions. Electromagnetic navigation systems use sensors in the tips of needles to provide real-time three-dimensional visualization, tracking, and navigation toward a predefined target. Additionally, cone-beam systems can generate low-resolution reconstructed cross-sectional images using rotational digital fluoroscopy to provide better anatomic depiction during a procedure. These advanced imaging options may be useful for defining anatomy during challenging cases.

Table 12.1 Relative Advantages and Disadvantages of Noninvasive Cross-Sectional Imaging for Assessing Pre-TIPS Anatomy

Modality	Advantages	Disadvantages
Ultrasonography	Relatively inexpensive Doppler analysis can determine direction of flow and velocities No contrast is required	Operator dependent Limited by hepatic steatosis and overlying bowel gas
Computed tomography with contrast	Relatively accessible Provides thin slices than can be multiplanar reformatted Fast and not as affected by respiratory motion and ascites	Radiation exposure Timing of postcontrast phase may result in flow artifacts mimicking thrombus (non-opacified blood inflow) Iodinated contrast nephrotoxic
Magnetic resonance imaging	High soft tissue contrast depicts vessels well Multiple phases of contrast routinely obtained Gadolinium contrast not nephrotoxic	Limited by motion and ascites Flow artifacts may limit visualization of hepatic veins

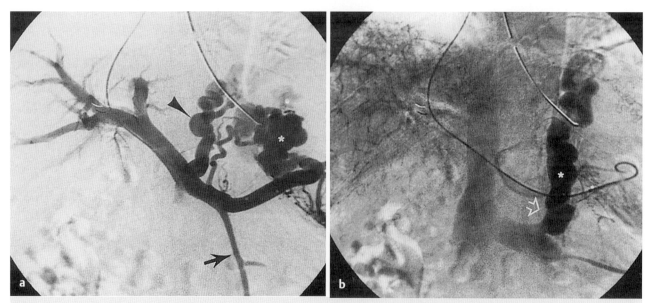

Fig. 12.18 (a) Early and (b) late phases of a splenoportogram shows reversal of flow in the inferior mesenteric vein (*arrow*), dilated left gastric (*arrowhead*), and short gastic (***) veins (*varices*), as well as a spontaneous splenorenal shunt (*open arrow*).

Portal Hypertension and Portosystemic Collaterals

Pressures in the normal liver range from 5 to 10 mm Hg,[28,29] constituting a high-flow, low-resistance parenchymal vascular bed. The pressure difference between the portal vein and the right atrium, denoted the portosystemic gradient, is normally between 3 and 6 mm Hg.[28,29] When increased resistance to flow occurs in the portal circulation, the portosystemic gradient increases, and PHT is defined as an absolute portal pressure greater than 10 mm Hg or a portosystemic gradient greater than 6 mm Hg.[28,29] Portal veins, hepatic veins, and sinusoidal channels lack valves or the ability to dictate directionality of flow. Impairment of venous return at any level between the bowel and the heart can elevate pressures and lead to retrograde transmission of pressure. This concept of increased portal pressure caused by increased portal resistance is termed the "backward-flow theory."[30] However, this concept may not capture the entire picture. After the development and progression of PHT, venous collaterals spontaneously occur and decompress portal circulation, allowing for reduced resistance within the portal venous system. However, portal pressures often remain elevated despite extensive collateralization. Some believe that splanchnic inflow is as much to blame for sustained PHT as is increased resistance within the portal circulation. An explanation for the amplified mesenteric and portal flow can be found in two separate theories: 1) a blunted response of mesenteric vessels to circulating vasoconstrictors; and 2) elevated levels of circulating vasodilators. Whichever the case may be, the development and maintenance of PHT is probably the result of a combination of increased portal resistance and increased splanchnic inflow ("forward-flow theory").[30]

The first morphologic changes associated with PHT are the increase in size of the portal, splenic, and mesenteric vessels and via "backward flow" the enlargement of the normal tributaries.[28,29]

The normal communications between the portal and systemic venous systems (hemorrhoidals, periumbilical, coronary vein) become enlarged. The coronary vein collateralizes with the azygous–hemiazygos system and when enlarged forms esophageal and gastric varices (▶ Fig. 12.18). Variceal bleeding may occur when the portosystemic gradient is greater than 12 mm Hg.[28,29,31,32] Gastric varices may also arise in the fundus from short gastric collaterals, which originate directly from the splenic vein along most of its course. Communication between small veins near the splenic hilum and the renal vein may also occur, causing a spontaneous "splenorenal shunt" (▶ Fig. 12.18). The normally obliterated umbilical vein can become recanalized coursing along the free margin of the falciform ligament to the surface of the liver, where it traverses to the umbilicus, providing a collateral pathway that results in the "caput medusa" appearance. A recanalized umbilical vein can create difficulty in TIPS if the left portal vein is punctured. The catheter and guidewire may be easily advanced in to one of these venous structures and be mistaken for a main portal vein in the anteroposterior projection.

Additional sites for varices include perisplenic, retrogastric, omental, splenolumbar, retroperitoneal, mesenteric, gastrorenal, peripancreatic, and pelvic. Ectopic varices (those arising outside the typical pathological variceal locations) have a higher rate of bleeding and are highly complex and variable in their anatomy.[33]

Conclusion

A thorough understanding of liver anatomy and vasculature is essential to successful TIPS placement. Anatomic variants, both congenital and acquired as a result of cirrhosis, may alter the spatial relationship between the portal veins and hepatic veins, making TIPS more challenging in some instances. Preprocedural imaging and intraprocedural guidance should be used to evaluate the anatomy and anticipate difficult scenarios.

Clinical Pearls

- Anatomy plays an essential role in preprocedural planning and ultimate success of TIPS.
- The performance of successful TIPS requires an understanding of the spatial relationship of the portal vein to the hepatic vein.
- Ideal curvature of TIPS is a smoothly curved TIPS.
- In the hepatic hilum, the portal vein lies posterior to the bile duct and hepatic artery.
- The right portal vein trunk is the most common target for portal venous access for TIPS.
- The common right portal trunk is present in 90% of patients and is usually located between the 10th and 12th ribs and within 0.5 to 1.5 vertebral widths to the right of the lateral margin of the vertebral body.

References

1. Saad N, Darcy M, Saad W. Portal anatomic variants relevant to transjugular intrahepatic portosystemic shunt. Tech Vasc Interv Radiol 2008;11(4):203–207.
2. Schultz SR, LaBerge JM, Gordon RL, Warren RS. Anatomy of the portal vein bifurcation: intra- versus extrahepatic location—implications for transjugular intrahepatic portosystemic shunts. J Vasc Interv Radiol 1994;5(3):457–459.
3. Myers M. Normal Anatomic Relationships and Variants. New York, Springer-Verlag, 1992.
4. Germain T, Favelier S, Cercueil JP, et al. Liver segmentation: practical tips. Diagn Interv Imaging 2014;95(11):1003–1016.
5. Bismuth H. Surgical anatomy and anatomical surgery of the liver. World J Surg 1982;6(1):3–9.
6. Healey J.Vascular anatomy of the liver. Ann NY Acad Sci 1970;170:8–17.
7. Saxon RR, Keller FS. Technical aspects of accessing the portal vein during the TIPS procedure. J Vasc Interv Radiol 1997;8(5):733–744.
8. Uflacker R, Reichert P, D'Albuquerque LC, de Oliveira e Silva A. Liver anatomy applied to the placement of transjugular intrahepatic portosystemic shunts. Radiology 1994;191(3):705–712.
9. Laberge J. Anatomy relevant to the transjugular intrahepatic portosystemic shunt procedure. Semin Intervent Radiol 1995;12:337–346.
10. Baird RA, Britton RC. The surgical anatomy of the hepatic veins: variations and their implications for auxiliary lobar transplantation. J Surg Res, 1973;15(5):345–7.
11. Kadir S. Atlas of Normal and variant Angiographic Anatomy. Philadelphia, WB Saunders, 1991.
12. Becker CD, Scheidegger J, Marincek B. Hepatic vein occlusion: morphologic features on computed tomography and ultrasonography. Gastrointest Radiol 1986;11(4):305–311.
13. Takayasu K, Moriyama N, Muramatsu Y, et al. Intrahepatic venous collaterals forming via the inferior right hepatic vein in 3 patients with obstruction of the inferior vena cava. Radiology 1985;154(2):323–328.
14. Park JH, Han JK, Choi BI, Han MC. Membranous obstruction of the inferior vena cava with Budd-Chiari syndrome: MR imaging findings. J Vasc Interv Radiol 1991;2(4):463–469.
15. Menu Y, Alison D, Lorphelin JM, et al. Budd-Chiari syndrome: US evaluation. Radiology 1985;157(3):761–764.
16. Harter LP, Gross BH, St Hilaire J, et al. CT and sonographic appearance of hepatic vein obstruction. AJR Am J Roentgenol 1982;139(1):176–178.
17. Doehner GA, Ruzicka FF, Hoffman G, Rousselot LM. The portal venous system: its roentgen anatomy. Radiology 1955;64(5):675–689.
18. Nakamura S, Tsuzuki T. Surgical anatomy of the hepatic veins and the inferior vena cava. Surg Gynecol Obstet 1981;152(1):43–50.
19. Darcy MD, Sterling KM. Comparison of portal vein anatomy and bony anatomic landmarks. Radiology 1996;200(3):707–710.
20. Yamane T, Mori K, Sakamoto K, Ikei S, Akagi M. Intrahepatic ramification of the portal vein in the right and caudate lobes of the liver. Acta Anat (Basel) 1988;133(2):162–172.
21. Bret PM, de Stempel JV, Atri M, et al. Intrahepatic bile duct and portal vein anatomy revisited. Radiology 1988;169(2):405–407.
22. Fraser-Hill MA, Atri M, Bret PM, et al. Intrahepatic portal venous system: variations demonstrated with duplex and color Doppler US. Radiology 1990;177(2):523–526.
23. Atri M, Bret PM, Fraser-Hill MA. Intrahepatic portal venous variations: prevalence with US. Radiology 1992;184(1):157–158.
24. Okuda K, Ohnishi K, Kimura K, et al. Incidence of portal vein thrombosis in liver cirrhosis. An angiographic study in 708 patients. Gastroenterology 1985;89(2):279–286.
25. Harbin WP, Robert NJ, Ferrucci JT Jr. Diagnosis of cirrhosis based on regional changes in hepatic morphology: a radiological and pathological analysis. Radiology 1980;135(2):273–283.
26. Gaba RC, Khiatani VL, Knuttinen MG, et al. Comprehensive review of TIPS technical complications and how to avoid them. AJR Am J Roentgenol 2011;196(3):675–685.
27. Scanlon T, Ryu RK. Portal vein imaging and access for transjugular intrahepatic portosystemic shunts. Tech Vasc Interv Radiol 2008;11(4):217–224.
28. Sherlock S. Portal circulation and portal hypertension. Gut 1978;19(1):70–83.
29. Galambos JT. Portal hypertension. Semin Liver Dis 1985;5(3):277–290.
30. Benoit JN, Womack WA, Hernandez L, Granger DN. "Forward" and "backward" flow mechanisms of portal hypertension. Relative contributions in the rat model of portal vein stenosis. Gastroenterology 1985;89(5):1092–1096.
31. Viallet A, Marleau D, Huet M, et al. Hemodynamic evaluation of patients with intrahepatic portal hypertension. Relationship between bleeding varices and the portohepatic gradient. Gastroenterology 1975;69(6):1297–1300.
32. Bosch J, Navasa M, Kravetz D, et al. Diagnosis and evaluation of portal hypertension. Z Gastroenterol 1988;26(suppl 2):8–14.
33. Saad WE, Lippert A, Saad NE, Caldwell S. Ectopic varices: anatomical classification, hemodynamic classification, and hemodynamic-based management. Tech Vasc Interv Radiol 2013;16(2):158–175.

Chapter 13: Technique for the Transjugular Intrahepatic Portosystemic Shunt Procedure

John A. Kaufman, Frederick S. Keller, and Josef Rösch

Historical Note

The origin of transjugular intrahepatic portosystemic shunt (TIPS) can be traced to inadvertent entries into intrahepatic portal branches during transjugular cholangiography done in the late 1960s to define biliary obstructions. This ability to access the portal vein from the transjugular approach led to the development of this technique in animal experiments for visualization of the portal venous system. Enlarging the tract in the liver between the hepatic and portal venous systems using dilatation catheters and maintaining patency by inserting Teflon tubing was the next step (▶ Fig. 13.1). These experimental shunts in canines, however, stayed patent for only 2 weeks and then thrombosed because of their small (4 to 6 mm) diameters and slow portal flow caused by a lack of portal hypertension (PHT). In a final report in 1971, the conclusion was that TIPS was a feasible technique. Even though one of the authors was able to demonstrate TIPS in human liver specimens and cadavers, technology at that time was not sufficiently advanced for TIPS to be clinically applicable.[1] Progress in technology has helped to advance TIPS from an experimental to a clinical procedure. Introduction of dilatation balloon catheters allowed Ronald Colapinto to perform the first clinical TIPS in the early 1980s.[2] However, even continuous 12-hour dilatation of the liver puncture tract offered only temporary results. Introduction of expandable metallic stents in the mid 1980s finally made TIPS a clinical reality. Palmaz explored using his balloon-expandable stents to create TIPS in dogs and achieved long-term primary patency.[3] The first clinical TIPS procedure using stents was performed in January 1988 in Freiburg, Germany, by Goetz Richter and associates using Palmaz stents.[4] Their success inspired many interventionalists to introduce TIPS procedures at their hospitals and contributed to a rapid expansion of this new technique. Introduction of a stent graft for TIPS in the late 1990s then brought further progress and significantly improved the long-term results of TIPS.

Present Status

Presently, 24 years after its clinical introduction, TIPS has become widely disseminated throughout the world and has been accepted as a minimally invasive treatment of the complications of PHT. More than 2300 citations on PubMed for "transjugular intrahepatic portosystemic shunt" speak for popularity and scientific interest in TIPS.

TIPS is a challenging procedure. Clinically, it requires detailed knowledge of patient's general condition and anatomy of his or her hepatic and portal venous systems. Technically, it calls for a skillful interventionalist experienced with jugular vein access, catheterization of hepatic veins, intrahepatic access to main portal branches, dilatation of the intrahepatic tract, and placement of the expandable stent or stent graft. Procedural success and freedom from complications were reported to be closely related to the experience of the operator. The average technical success rate of TIPS was reported at 97.3% with failure rate higher in those institutions having performed fewer than 100 procedures.[5] Similarly, the rate of fatal procedural complication was reported at 1.4% at institutions with more than 150 procedures and at 3% with fewer than 150 TIPS.[5]

In current practice, the majority (80%–90%) of TIPS procedures are performed on an elective basis.[6–9] The main indications for TIPS are prevention of recurrent bleeding from gastroesophageal or ectopic varices and management of refractory ascites or recurrent hepatic hydrothorax. An emergency "rescue" TIPS for acute uncontrollable variceal bleeding, which used to be a common indication for TIPS in earlier years, should be done only in patients with a reasonable chance of survival (see Chapter 21).

Procedure Planning

To facilitate the TIPS procedure, the interventionalist needs to become familiar with the anatomy of the liver and its venous and portal vasculature, which are often distorted by processes leading to PHT.[10,11] Abdominal ultrasonography, including duplex

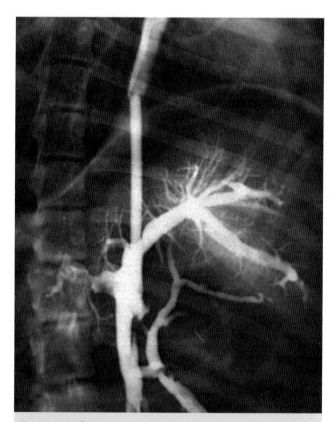

Fig. 13.1 The first successful experimental transjugular intrahepatic portosystemic shunt created in a canine in November 1968 with use of Teflon tubing. *Reprinted from Rösch J, Hanafee WN, Snow H. Transjugular portal venography and radiologic portacaval shunt: an experimental study. Radiology 1969;92:1112–1114; with permission from RSNA.*

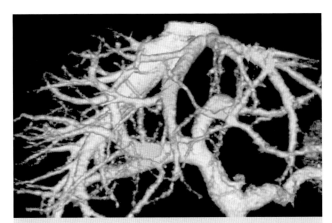

Fig. 13.2 Reformatted liver computed tomography scan demonstrating anatomic relation of hepatic veins and portal vein bifurcation.

evaluation of the portal and hepatic veins, has been often used for pre-TIPS evaluation. We prefer the cross-sectional liver imaging by computed tomography because it provides a detailed view of the liver anatomy and pathology (▶ Fig. 13.2).

In particular, the anatomic relationship between the hepatic and portal veins can be determined and the optimal site for intrahepatic portal vein entry selected.

Before the procedure, ascites is often drained. This lowers the position of the liver and thus facilitates catheterization of hepatic veins and introduction of the portal vein access set. Hepatic hydrothorax is not evacuated. All patients receive antibiotics before the procedure (1 g of cefazolin). In patients with significant penicillin allergy, vancomycin is used as an alternative.[12]

The Procedure

Some interventionalists perform TIPS with conscious sedation using a combination of fentanyl and midazolam. In patients with alcohol dependence, they augment sedation with droperidol.[12] Presently, we now perform TIPS with our patients under general anesthesia. General anesthesia is easier and safer in uncooperative patients and in all cases permits the interventionalist to concentrate completely on the procedure. The anesthesiologist can provide apnea during parts of the procedure such as intrahepatic puncture and filming. Electrocardiographic monitoring is required, especially during passing catheters across the right atrium.

Portal Vein Access Set

Presently, there are four commercially available transjugular access sets for TIPS in the United States. The Ring set, the Rösch-Uchida set (RUPS), and the Haskal set are all from Cook Medical (Bloomington, IN), and the fine-needle access set is from Angio-Dynamics (Lantham, NY). There are only minor differences among these sets, and the choice is mostly based on personal preference. We use the RUPS (▶ Fig. 13.3). With this equipment, the hepatic vein and portal vein puncture is done with a sharp 0.038 trocar stylet inside a well-tapered 5-Fr catheter. A curved 14-gauge stiffening cannula inside a curved 10-Fr catheter and a 10-Fr Flexor introducer sheath ensures stable position for the trocar puncture.

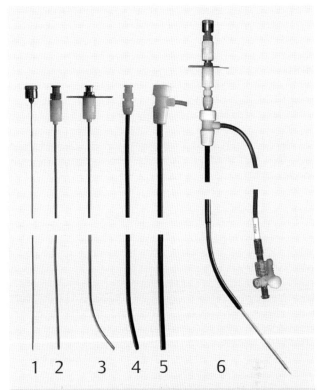

Fig. 13.3 The portal vein access set (Rösch-Uchida set [RUPS], Cook Medical). (1) 0.038-in trocar stylet; (2) Tapered 5-Fr catheter; (3) 14-gauge cannula; (4) 10-Fr catheter ; (5) 10-Fr flexor sheath; (6) Assembled RUPS.

The curved tip of the cannula can be manually adjusted depending on the anatomy of the hepatic veins.

Hepatic Vein Catheterization

The right internal jugular venous approach is most commonly used for TIPS because of its straight course to the inferior vena cava (IVC). The left internal jugular vein is used when the right vein is occluded and often in patients with high position of the liver. The left-sided approach gives the portal vein access set a more oblique orientation that favors catheterization of horizontally directed hepatic veins.

Jugular vein access is performed with a micropuncture (21-gauge) needle under ultrasonic guidance. The midportion of the neck is usually selected for access. After sterile skin preparation, a small skin incision with a scalpel that is dilated with a hemostat, the jugular vein is accessed. The access site is then dilated with the micropuncture catheter, and a 0.038-J guidewire is introduced and advanced through the right atrium into the IVC. The skin and subcutaneous tissue of the neck are then dilated with an 11-Fr dilator, and the RUPS access set without the trocar stylet is introduced. The hepatic vein is catheterized. This is accomplished using the curve of the metal cannula with the leading guidewire. If the guidewire will not exit the right atrium, it is withdrawn into the superior vena cava, and the curve of the metal cannula is used to orient the guidewire through the right atrium into the IVC and hepatic vein.

Selection of the correct hepatic vein for access to the portal vein is critical for successful TIPS because it determines the anterior or posterior orientation of the metal cannula for portal vein access. The right hepatic vein, when of sufficient size, is best suited for TIPS because of its location and relation to the portal vein. It lies superiorly, posteriorly, and slightly laterally to the right portal vein. If the right hepatic vein in a cirrhotic liver is small or cannot be safely be catheterized, then either the middle hepatic or left hepatic vein can be used to create TIPS. The middle hepatic vein lies superiorly and anteriorly and sometimes slightly medially to the right portal vein. The left hepatic vein is anterior, superior, and lateral to the left portal vein.[10,11]

Wedged Hepatic Venogram

Wedged hepatic venography gives useful information about the portal venous anatomy, particularly the position of the portal vein. We perform it using an occlusion balloon catheter and CO_2 as contrast material (► Fig. 13.4). When the 10-Fr sheath of the RUPS set is securely located in the preselected hepatic vein, the inner 5-Fr catheter, metal stiffening cannula, and 10-Fr Teflon catheter are removed. A 5-Fr occlusion balloon catheter is introduced into the sheath, and the balloon inflated with dilute contrast material sufficiently to wedge the catheter in the midportion of the catheterized hepatic vein. Thirty to 50 mL of sterile CO_2 is rapidly injected while digital subtraction images are obtained. We prefer the "balloon occlusion" technique to wedging an end-hole catheter peripherally in a small hepatic vein because it is more effective and safer.

Portal Vein Access

Portal vein access is initiated in the proximal 2 to 3 cm of the hepatic vein cephalad to the expected location of the target portal vein main branch. Visualization of the portal vein during hepatic wedged venography serves as guidance for orientation of the puncture.[13] The locked access set is rotated anteriorly in the right hepatic vein or posteriorly in the middle or left hepatic veins. The tip of the 10-Fr catheter is then wedged inferiorly against the hepatic vein wall. This step of wedging is essential for successful

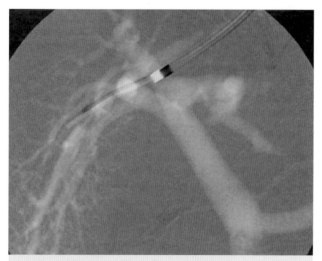

Fig. 13.4 Wedged hepatic venogram with CO_2.

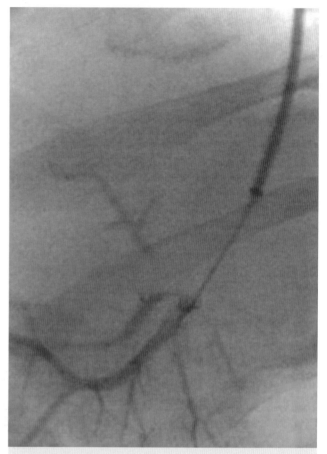

Fig. 13.5 Portal vein access under fluoroscopy with contrast material test injection confirming position of 5-Fr catheter in portal circulation.

liver puncture because if the tip of the 10-Fr catheter is free in hepatic vein, the needle slides along the vein wall rather than piercing it. Portal vein access should be about 2 cm lateral to the portal bifurcation. In this position, the liver parenchymal tract and the TIPS are almost a continuation of the portal vein, thus having optimal flow. Also, the superior portal vein wall is intra-parenchymal with no risk of extraparenchymal portal access. The puncture is performed with a sharp thrust of the locked trocar and 5-Fr catheter into the hepatic parenchyma for a distance of 3 to 5 cm. The trocar stylet is removed, and a 10-mL syringe containing contrast material is attached to the 5-Fr catheter. During its slow withdrawal, suction is applied. When blood is aspirated, contrast material is injected to confirm catheter position in the portal system (► Fig. 13.5).

When the portal system is not entered, the trocar stylet is reintroduced into the 5-Fr catheter, and the puncture is repeated in slightly medial or lateral projection. It can take several attempts to access the portal vein in proper location, particularly in patients with cirrhosis who have distorted portal anatomy. In difficult cases, we use a Siemens Acuson AcuNav 8- or 10-Fr ultrasound intravenous catheter introduced by the femoral approach. With its capability of side-view imaging up to 15 cm in depth, it provides visualization of the selected portion of the portal vein, facilitating access[14] (► Fig. 13.6). During all of these and subsequent maneuvers, rotation of the metal cannula should be maintained, but the operator should allow the portal vein access set to

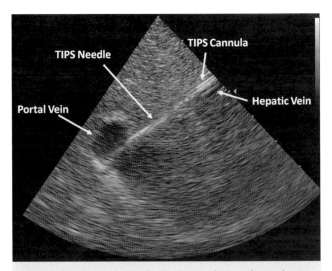

Fig. 13.6 Portal vein access under intravenous ultrasound control. TIPS: transjugular intrahepatic portosystemic shunt.

move slightly with inspiration and expiration.[6] When the portal vein is accessed, a 0.038-inch Bentson or an angled hydrophilic guidewire is introduced (▶ Fig. 13.7). It often advances laterally initially but then prolapses down into the main portal vein. If the guidewire does not go in the desired direction, a catheter with small radius curves such as the RIM or Binkert catheter is used to direct it into the portal vein.

With the 5-Fr catheter safely in the portal vein and while keeping the cannula wedged, the 10-Fr catheter is unlocked and advanced over the guidewire into the portal vein, dilating the liver parenchymal tract. At that point, often the sheath is also advanced into the portal vein. With a hard liver, the cannula can be advanced with the 10-Fr catheter to stiffen it and overcome the resistance of liver parenchyma and the portal vein wall. Exchange for an Amplatz stiff guidewire may help with this step. The 10-Fr catheter and metal cannula are removed, and the 10-Fr sheath is withdrawn to the right atrium. A calibrated sizing pigtail catheter is then introduced into the portal system for pressure measurement and portal venography.

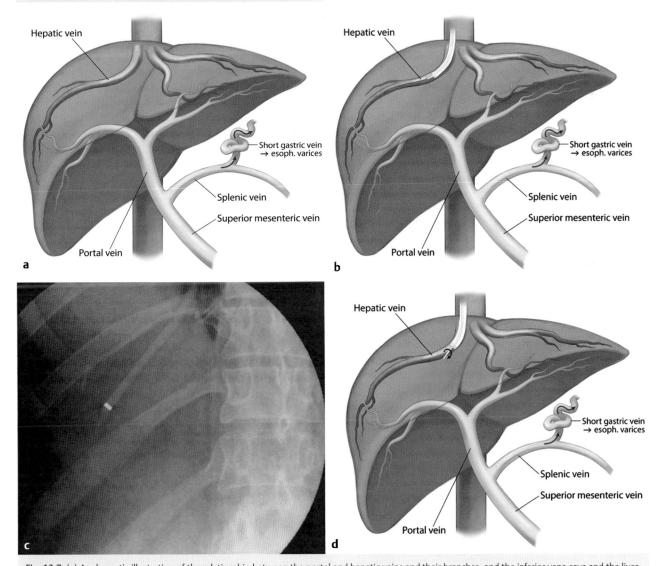

Fig. 13.7 (a) A schematic illustration of the relationship between the portal and hepatic veins and their branches, and the inferior vena cava and the liver. The *red arrows* depict the direction of blood flow with portal hypertension and varices. (b) A schematic illustration and (c) radiograph demonstrate the introduction of the TIPS set into the right hepatic vein over a guidewire. (d-f) A schematic illustration and radiographs show that the TIPs set is rotated anteriorly (counterclockwise). (*continued*)

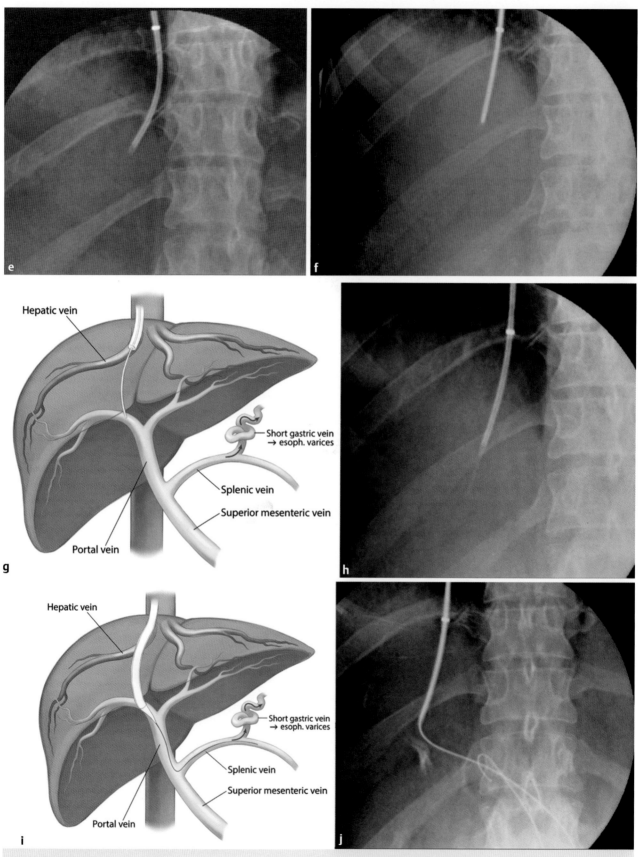

Fig. 13.7 (*Continued*) The radiographs depict the TIPs set (**e**) before and (**f**) after rotation. (**g,h**) A schematic illustration and radiograph show the needle puncturing from the hepatic to the portal vein. (**h**) The 5-French catheter is protruding distally from the TIPS set. Its tip is in the right portal vein. (**i,j**) A schematic illustration and radiograph show the completed puncture from the hepatic to the portal vein with a guidewire in the splenic vein (**i**) and the superior mesenteric vein (**j**). (*continued*)

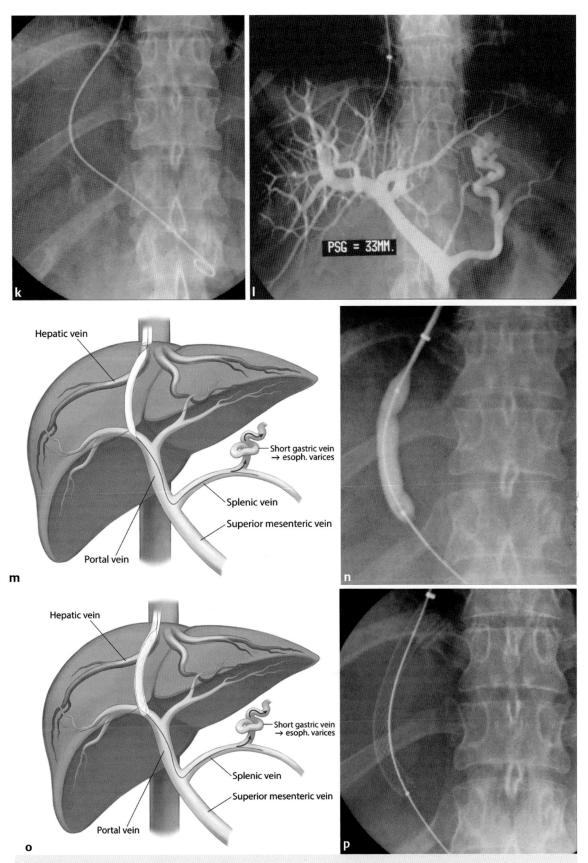

Fig. 13.7 (*Continued*) (**k**) Pigtail angiographic catheter in main portal vein before venogram. (**l**) Initial portal venogram, with a portosystemic gradient (PSG) of 33 mm Hg. (**m,n**) A schematic illustration and radiograph show dilation of the parenchymal track with an angioplasty balloon. The indentations on the balloon in (**n**) indicate the locations of the hepatic and portal vein walls at the site of their punctures. (**o,p**) Placement and deployment of the TIPS stent graft. (**o**) A schematic illustration shows the proper location to deploy the TIPS stent graft. (**p**) A radiograph shows the stent graft deployed. (*continued*)

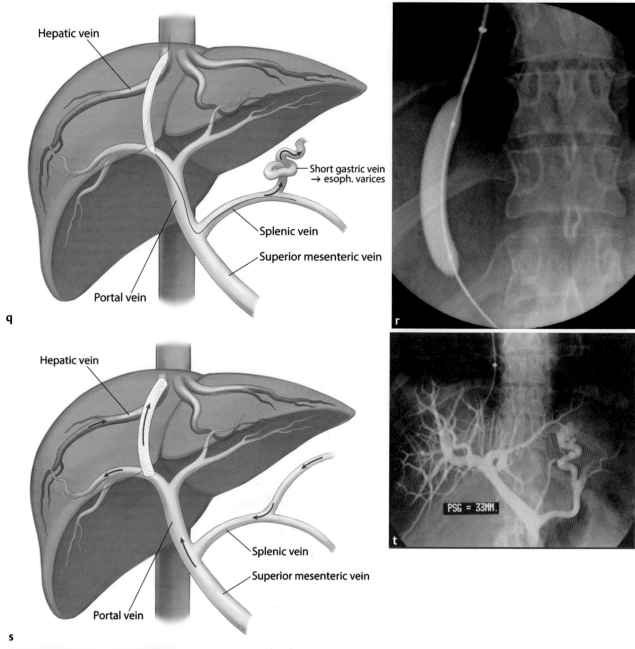

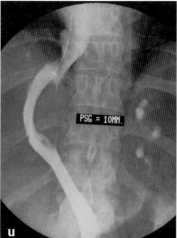

Fig. 13.7 (*Continued*) (**q,r**) A schematic illustration and radiograph show the dilation of the TIPS stent graft with an angioplasty balloon. (**s**) After TIPS all the portal system blood flow is up to the liver (*red arrows*) and no longer up to the esophageal varices. (**t,u**) Portal venograms before and after TIPS: (**t**) Prior to TIPS, the portosystemic gradient (PSG) is 33 mm Hg and there is flow up to the esophageal varices. (**u**) After TIPS, the portosystemic gradient is reduced to 10 mm Hg and portal blood flow is directed through the TIPS with no more flowing through the embolized varices.

Pressure Measurements and Portal Venography

Measurements of pressures in the portal system and the right atrium and portal venography are important parts of the TIPS procedure.[15] The difference between the pressure in the portal vein and the right atrial pressure is the portal systemic pressure gradient (PSPG). This provides information on the severity of PHT and is useful in determining the appropriate diameter of the stent graft. Portal pressure is measured with the pigtail catheter in the main portal vein. The venous systemic pressure is measured with the 10-Fr sheath retracted into the right atrium. In the normal liver, the PSPG does not exceed 5 mm Hg. PHT is defined with gradient exceeding 6 mm Hg. Clinical complications usually occur only when the PSPG exceeds 10 mm Hg.

Portal venography is important for evaluation of portal system anatomy and the location and extent of varices and to determine the length of the planned stent graft. Before portal venography, the 10-Fr sheath is first advanced to the origin of the hepatic vein, and its position is confirmed with a contrast injection. The sizing pigtail catheter is then advanced into the splenic vein. If evaluation of mesenteric or rectal collaterals is necessary, that catheter tip is placed into the superior or inferior mesenteric vein. Depending on the size and flow in portal circulation, 25 to 45 mL of contrast material is injected in 3 to 4 seconds. The distance between the accessed portal vein wall and the junction of the hepatic vein with the IVC, plus 1 cm, is the required length of the stent graft to be used (▶ Fig. 13.8). With a very curved tract, a 2-cm longer prosthesis is used.

Dilatation of the transhepatic tract is the next step. A stiff Amplatz-type exchange guidewire is introduced, and the pigtail catheter is removed. A high-pressure balloon catheter, 8 mm in diameter and 4 cm in length is then positioned across the transhepatic tract to cover both access sites in the hepatic and portal veins. The balloon is inflated with dilute contrast under fluoroscopic visualization. Although the liver parenchyma tract dilates easily, the wall of the portal vein offers considerable resistance, and a persistent waist is seen on the balloon until increased balloon inflation pressure is applied. Without general anesthesia, the patient feels considerable discomfort, and additional analgesia is required. After balloon deflation, the 10-Fr sheath is advanced into the portal vein for stent graft deployment, and the balloon catheter is removed. The guidewire remains.

Endograft Deployment

After long experience with various bare stents and repeated interventions to keep TIPS patent and functional, we now exclusively use ePTFE-coated stent grafts (Gore Viatorr) for all our TIPS (▶ Fig. 13.9). With proper placement of this device, TIPS stay

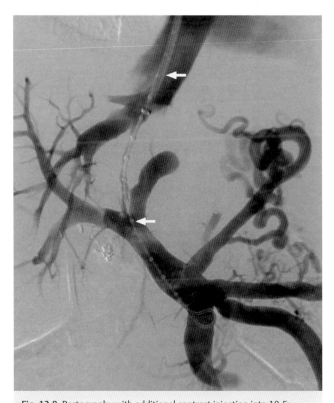

Fig. 13.8 Portography with additional contrast injection into 10-Fr sheath for measurement of the needed endograft length (8 cm in this case). The *arrows* indicate the top and bottom ends of the TIPS stent graft.

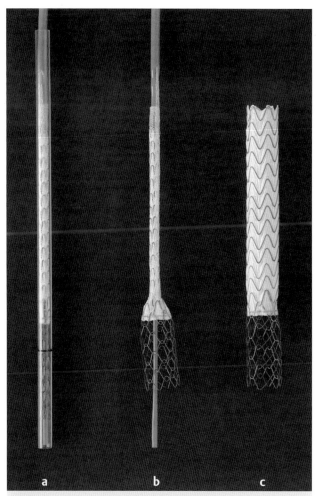

Fig. 13.9 Viatorr endoprosthesis (WL Gore). (a) Endoprosthesis contained by plastic access sleeve. (b) Expansion of the distal uncovered; the portal portion of the endoprosthesis after removal of the introducing sheath. (c) Fully expanded endoprosthesis.

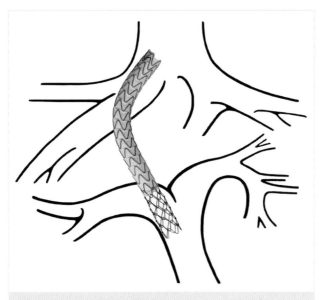

Fig. 13.10 Schematic drawing of ideal Viatorr endoprostesis position.

patent and function well (▶ Fig. 13.10). Although the Viatorr is more expensive than bare stents, its increased cost is well justified by the markedly decreased need for reintervention.

The final diameter of the endoprosthesis is influenced by the indication and the pressure gradients, but we generally use a 10-mm-diameter endograft.[16] For patients with bleeding, a lower final gradient is preferred, and thus the TIPS is often dilated to 10 mm. Patients with ascites are at higher risk of encephalopathy, and although we place a 10-mm-diameter graft, we often leave it at 8 mm diameter or less. Sometimes we place a constricting balloon-expandable stent in the parenchymal tract before endograft deployment for control of TIPS diameter (▶ Fig. 13.11).

Exact placement of the endograft is essential for long-term TIPS patency and function.[17] The endoprosthesis delivery catheter flushed with heparinized saline is introduced into the 10-Fr sheath over the 0.035-inch stiff guidewire and advanced to its tip that is deep in the portal vein. The 10-Fr sheath is then retracted about 3 cm, allowing the uncovered 2-cm-long portion of endoprosthesis to expand. The 10-Fr sheath with the delivering catheter is then slowly retracted to the accessed portal vein wall. The radiopaque marker at the beginning of the covered endoprosthesis should be at the portal vein wall. Slight compression of the junction of the bare and covered endoprosthesis (marked with a radiopaque ring) during withdrawal indicates that it is entering the portal vein wall. The endoprosthesis may then be advanced for 3 to 4 mm to ensure that its bare part is not in the parenchymal tract or deployed as is. The 10-Fr sheath is then retracted back into the IVC, and the covered part of the endoprosthesis is released by pulling the constraining cord. The delivery catheter is removed. A radiopaque marker at the upper end of endoprosthesis indicates its relation to the IVC. The deployed endoprosthesis is usually dilated with a 10-mm-diameter balloon catheter. A 5-Fr pigtail catheter is reintroduced for follow-up PSPG measurements and portal venography (▶ Fig. 13.12).

Generally, decrease of the PSPG to 12 mm Hg or less is an optimal result in bleeding patients. In patients with ascites, reducing the portosystemic gradient by half should be satisfactory.[16,18]

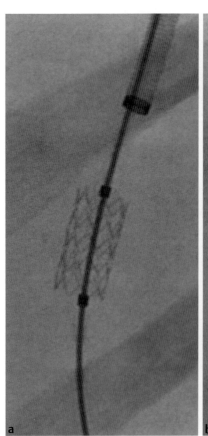
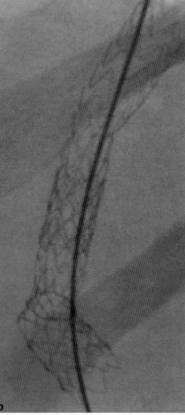

Fig. 13.11 Transjugular intrahepatic portosystemic shunt constricting stent placement for ascites. (**a**) A dilated Palmaz stent in the distal portion of the created intrahepatic tract. (**b**) Viatorr endoprosthesis after dilatation with an 8-mm balloon.

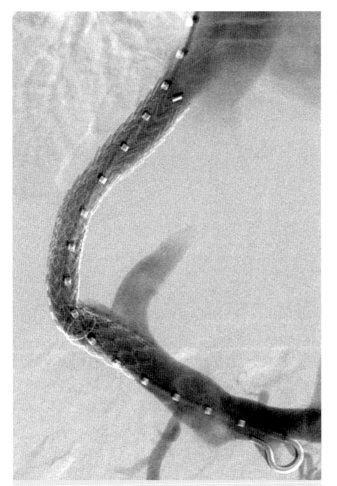

Fig. 13.12 Follow-up portogram after endoprosthesis deployment and its dilatation with a 10-mm balloon.

endoprosthesis wall. When indicated, a 5-Fr curved catheter is introduced for variceal embolization.

Variceal Embolization

There has been no consensus on the use and timing of variceal embolization during TIPS creation. After our extensive experience, we now perform variceal embolization in patients who are active by bleeding or with recent (7 to 10 days) history of variceal bleeding. It has been documented that embolization of varices in these patients prevents or decreases recurrent variceal bleeding.[19] As for the timing of embolization during the TIPS procedure, there is not consensus even among interventionalists in our institute. Some interventionalists embolize varices before endograft placement when the variceal flow is oriented in hepatofugal direction. Others perform embolization after creation of TIPS. They first concentrate on creation of TIPS, performing embolization secondarily even when follow-up venography shows decreased variceal filling. Selective catheterization and venography, however, gives good variceal visualization. Occlusion of varices prevents further hepatofugal flow and increases hepatopetal flow to both the liver and through the TIPS. Therefore, it theoretically may reduce the risk of hepatic encephalopathy.[19,20]

Mechanical occlusive devices such as stainless steel coils or Amplatzer occluders are used first to decrease flow. They have to be significantly oversized relative to varices or their feeding veins. After creating a large mechanical block, small coils are added as needed to further decrease flow, finally followed by a larger coil to prevent their dislocation into the portal system (▶ Fig. 13.13). If some flow in varices still remains, sclerosing agents such as Sotradecol or absolute alcohol can be infused to accelerate variceal occlusion.

Postprocedural Management

After hemostasis of the jugular vein access is obtained, patients who received their TIPS for active bleeding are transferred to the intensive care unit. Patients who had their TIPS for ascites are monitored in a stepdown interventional radiology unit overnight. It is important to monitor central venous pressure because increased inflow from the portal circulation into the right atrium

When the follow-up portogram shows incomplete coverage of the entire TIPS tract, particularly at the hepatic vein origin, a second endoprosthesis should be added so that the entire hepatic vein is covered. At the end of deployment, the pigtail catheter is removed over the guidewire with care taken to not damage the

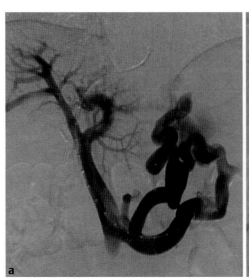

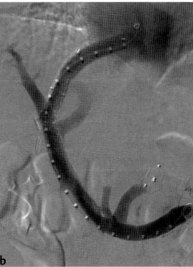

Fig. 13.13 Transjugular intrahepatic portosystemic shunt with embolization of gastric varices. (a) Portogram before embolization. (b) Follow-up portogram after embolization with Amplatzer occluders.

may lead to decompensation in patients with limited cardiac reserves. On the following day, the patients are returned to their hepatology wards to their referring physicians. The patients referred from other hospitals or clinics are often sent home. We schedule all patients for a 2- to 3-week follow-up visit in our outpatient clinic. At that time, we perform a baseline Doppler sonographic examination of the TIPS. Earlier examination does not give reliable results because of air trapped within the layers of the Viatorr endograft. Patients remain in the care of their primary physicians and are referred to us only for clinical suspicion of TIPS malfunction.

Periprocedural Complications and Their Prevention

When performed by experienced interventionalists, TIPS is safe and can be completed in 60 to 90 minutes. However, complications can occur, especially when contraindications to the procedure are neglected or proper procedural technique is not followed.[21,22] In patients with model for end-stage liver disease (MELD) scores exceeding 18 and short life expectancy, TIPS often accelerates liver failure. Patients with limited cardiac reserves can develop cardiac failure after TIPS. Neglect of preprocedural portal vein cross-sectional visualization makes the portal vein access completely blind with the attendant increased risk.

Jugular vein access with a micropuncture needle made under ultrasonic guidance almost eliminates complications experienced associated in the past with access guided by surface landmarks and carotid artery palpation. Similarly, advancement of the guidewire and the RUPS access set through the right atrium under fluoroscopic control prevents cardiac rhythm complications. With wedged hepatic venography, the use of a balloon occlusion catheter and moderate-pressure CO_2 injection reduces possible complications of peripheral catheter contrast medium injection such as hemorrhagic hepatic infarction and subcapsular hematoma. Numerous complications have been reported related to the transhepatic access of the portal vein, the most technically challenging aspect of the TIPS procedure. These include punctures of the intrahepatic biliary ducts and arteries; extrahepatic access of the portal vein; and extracapsular punctures with entrance into the peritoneum, gallbladder, and right kidney. These could lead to hemobilia, intrahepatic hemorrhage, hepatic infarction, and intraperitoneal bleeding. With good knowledge of hepatic and portal vein anatomy and cautious access and needle manipulation, most of these complications can be avoided except accidental entrance into intrahepatic biliary ducts or arteries (▶ Fig. 13.14). In these cases, it is imperative to recognize what has occurred during test injection with contrast material, and the trocar needle is removed for another attempt for portal vein access.

Close attention to selection of the endograft length and careful placement enables proper positioning with covering the entire intrahepatic tract from the portal vein wall to the IVC. When properly positioned, TIPS using endografts exhibits long-term patency and function in 80% to 90% of cases. No complications develop if 3 to 5 mm of the covered part of endograft extends into the portal vein and the IVC. Longer covered endograft extension into the portal vein, however, can decrease flow, limit liver perfusion, and lead to thrombosis of the intrahepatic portal vein. Similar flow problems may develop with long extension of the

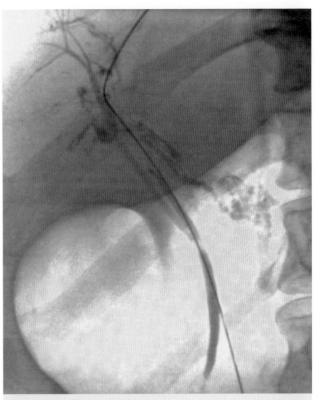

Fig. 13.14 Portal vein access complication with filling of biliary tree and lymphatics. A guidewire is in the portal vein.

endograft into the IVC. An extension of the bare part of the endograft above the portal vein wall into the liver parenchymal tract leads to early development of stenosis and shunt malfunction.

The occasionally reported endograft migration can be prevented by proper sizing, positioning during deployment, and using caution during exchange of catheters in the newly placed device. Particularly, the pigtail catheter should be straightened and balloon dilatation catheters completely deflated before their removal. During variceal embolization, selection of oversized occlusive devices prevents both their peripheral embolization and central migration.

The use of the smallest volume of contrast medium as possible should always be kept in mind because of many patients have compromised renal function. Patients with cirrhosis also have poor tolerance of infection. Therefore, the procedure must be performed under strict aseptic conditions and antibiotic coverage to prevent the occasionally reported sepsis after the procedure.

TIPS placement often results in exacerbation of old or development of new encephalopathy. Encephalopathy can be decreased by limiting the diameter of endoprosthesis, and underinflation of the placed endograft can preserve portal liver perfusion. In case of recurrence of a patient's bleeding or ascites, the endograft can be dilated to its original size. In patients with encephalopathy uncontrolled by medical treatment, reduction of TIPS diameter is necessary. The techniques of reduction are described in Chapter 18.

Conclusion

TIPS is a challenging procedure. However, in the hands of skillful, experienced interventionalists, it is performed safely in the overwhelming majority of cases. Careful evaluation of the indications for TIPS and careful adherence to good interventional technique are essential for prevention of TIPS complications.

Clinical Pearls

- The origin of TIPS can be traced to inadvertent entries into intrahepatic portal branches during transjugular cholangiography done in the late 1960s.
- The first clinical TIPS procedure using stents was performed in January 1988 in Freiburg, Germany, by Goetz Richter.
- TIPS is a challenging procedure. However, in the hands of skillful, experienced interventionalists, it is performed safely in the overwhelming majority of cases.
- Careful evaluation of the indications for TIPS and careful adherence to good interventional technique are essential for prevention of TIPS complications.
- Selection of the correct hepatic vein for access to the portal vein is critical for successful TIPS.
- Exact placement of the endograft is essential for long-term TIPS patency and function.
- Longer (>5 mm) covered endograft extension into the portal vein, however, can decrease flow, limit liver perfusion, and lead to thrombosis of the intrahepatic portal vein.

References

1. Rösch J, Hanafee W, Snow H, et al. Transjugular intrahepatic portacaval shunt. An experimental work. Am J Surg 1971;121:588–592.
2. Colapinto RF, Stronell RD, Gildiner M, et al. Formation of the intrahepatic portosystemic shunts using a balloon dilatation catheter: preliminary clinical experience. AJR Am J Roentgenol 1983;140:709–714.
3. Palmaz JC, Garcia F, Sibbitt RR, et al. Expandable intrahepatic portacaval shunt stents in dogs with chronic portal hypertension. AJR Am J Roentgenol 1986;147:1251–1254.
4. Richter GM, Palmaz JC, Nöldge G, et al. The transjugular intrahepatic portosystemic stentshunt (TIPSS): a new nonoperative transjugular percutaneous procedure. Radiology 1989;29:406–411.
5. Barton RE, Rösch J, Saxon RR, et al. TIPS: Short and long-term results: a survey of 1750 patients. Semin Intervent Radiol 1995;12:364–367.
6. Bromley PJ, Kaufman JA. Portal and hepatic veins. In: Kaufman JA, Lee MJ, editors. Vascular & Interventional Radiology: The Requisites. Philadelphia, Mosby, 2004, pp 377–406.
7. Funaki B. Transjugular intrahepatic portosystemic shunt. Semin Intervent Radiol 2008;25:168–174.
8. Haskal ZJ. Percutaneous management of portal hypertension. In Baum S, Pentecost M, editors. Abrams' Angiography Interventional Radiology, 2nd ed. Philadelphia, Lippincott Williams & Wilkins, 2006, pp 581–599.
9. Patel NY. The transjugular intrahepatic portosystemic shunt procedure. In Patel NH, Haskal ZJ, Kerlan, RK, editors. Portal Hypertension: Diagnosis and Interventions, 2nd ed. Fairfax, VA, Society of Cardiovascular & Interventional Radiology, 2001, pp 119–136.
10. LaBerge JM. Anatomy relevant to TIPS. Tech Vasc Intervent Radiol 1998;1:51–67.
11. Uflacker R, Reichert P, D'Albuquerque LC, de Oliveira e Silva A. Liver anatomy applied to the placement of transjugular intrahepatic portosystemic shunts. Radiology 1994;191:705–712.
12. Kerlan RK. TIPS technique. Tech Vasc Intervent Radiol 1998;1:68–79.
13. Saxon RR, Keller FS. Technical aspects of accessing the portal vein during the TIPS procedure. J Vasc Interv Radiol 1997;8:733–744.
14. Farsad K, Fuss C, Kolbeck KJ, et al. Transjugular intrahepatic portosystemic shunt creation using intravascular ultrasound guidance. J. Vasc Interv Radiol 2012;23(12):1594–1602.
15. Saugel B, Phillip V, Gaa J, et al. Advanced hemodynamic monitoring before and after transjugular intrahepatic portosystemic shunt: implications for selection of patients—a prospective study. Radiology 2012;262:343–352.
16. Riggio O, Ridola Ll, Angeloni S, et al. Clinical efficacy of transjugular intrahepatic shunt created with covered stents with different diameters: results of a randomized controlled trial. J Hepatology 2010;53:267–272.
17. Clark TW. Stepwise placement of a transjugular intrahepatic portosystemic shunt endograft. Tech Vasc Interv Radiol 2008;11:208–211.
18. Rössle M, Siegerstetter V, Olschewski M, et al. How much reduction in portal pressure is necessary to prevent variceal bleeding? A longitudinal study in 225 patients with transjugular intrahepatic portosystemic shunts. Am J Gastroenterol 2001;96:3379–3383.
19. Tesdal IK, Filser T, Weiss C, et al. Transjugular intrahepatic portosystemic shunts: adjunctive embolotherapy of gastroesophageal collateral vessels in the prevention of variceal rebleeding. Radiology 2005;236:360–367.
20. Bilbao JJT, Arias M, Longo JM, et al. Embolization of nonvariceal portosystemic collaterals in transjugular intrahepatic portosystemic shunts. Cardiovasc Intervent Radiol 1997;20:149–153.
21. Ripamonti R, Ferral H, Alonza M, Patel NH. Transjugular intrahepatic portosystemic shunt—related complications and practical solutions. Semin Intervent Radiol 2006;23:165–176.
22. Gaba RC, Khiatani VL, Knuttinen MG, et al. Comprehensive review of TIPS technical complications and how to avoid them. AJR Am J Roentgenol 2011;196:675–685.

Chapter 14: The Difficult Transjugular Portosystemic Shunt Procedure: Unconventional Techniques

Michael D. Darcy

Introduction

Although transjugular intrahepatic portosystemic shunts (TIPS) have become a mainstream procedure, they can still be technically challenging. Technical success rates are generally 90% to 100%,[1,2] although this tends to overestimate the ease with which these procedures are accomplished. This chapter covers anatomic problems that can increase the difficulty of a TIPS and strategies for achieving technical success despite these obstacles.

Indications and Contraindications

Indications for variations in standard tips technique include any case in which anatomic factors preclude performing TIPS in the standard way. These include but are not limited to:

- Venous access stenosis or occlusion
- Difficult angulation from the inferior vena cava (IVC) to the hepatic veins (HVs)
- HV occlusions
- Hepatic parenchymal problems (cysts, tumors, or fibrosis)
- Portal vein (PV) occlusions

Contraindications to specialized TIPS techniques include:

- The usual contraindications for any TIPS procedures (see other chapters)
- Lack of operator experience because some of these specialized techniques should not be attempted unless the operator is comfortable with standard TIPS procedures

Procedures

Access Problems

The initial step of any TIPS requires getting to the HVs from the venous access site. Occlusion of the right internal jugular (RIJ) vein can make TIPS more difficult right from the onset. It may be possible to puncture a thrombosed RIJ and recanalize the vein. Alternatively, a collateral vein may be useable if it communicates in a straight line down to the superior vena cava (SVC). If the right-sided access is not possible, the left IJ can be used. Hausegger et al[3] reported a 92% technical success rate for 12 TIPS done from a left IJ approach.

If the SVC is occluded, preventing access from above, performing the TIPS from a femoral approach has been described. One technique is to advance the puncture needle from an inferior HV into a portal branch.[4,5] Alternatively, a fine needle can be advanced percutaneously through a main portal branch into the IVC using CT or ultrasound guidance. A wire passed through this needle can then be snared from a femoral approach, and the rest of the case can then be done from the femoral access.[6]

Hepatic Vein Problems

The angle between the HV and the IVC can be very acute, particularly if the liver is small and pushed cephalad by significant ascites. This can make it difficult to advance the access needle into the HV. Adding some additional curve to the puncture needle can make it easier to advance the needle into the HV. The needle should be bent with a stiff wire in the lumen to avoid kinking the needle. Also, it is best to add the curve over several centimeters rather than trying to bend the needle too acutely in any one area. An acute angle from the IVC into the HV can also increase the chances that the needle may pop out into the IVC as the needle is positioned to make passes. Because breathing can cause caudal motion of the liver, light continuous pressure should be maintained on the needle to avoid the needle's popping out of the HV.

Hepatic vein occlusion can also present a major challenge. In Budd-Chiari syndrome, there is often still an HV stump. If this stump can be engaged with the access needle, passes toward the PV can be initiated from this stump (► Fig. 14.1). If no HV stump can be catheterized, needle passes can be made directly from the IVC. It is important to start in the upper 5 or 6 cm of the IVC because this is the intrahepatic segment. Puncturing from below this level risks starting from an extrahepatic location, raising the chance of hemorrhage. Because wedged hepatic venography cannot be performed, one may not know where to aim the needle. Boney landmarks can provide a rough guide. Using the patient's own vertebral body width as a unit of measure, 90% of right portal trunks are approximately one vertebral body width lateral to the spine.[7] Alternatively, the needle may be partially advanced to engage the liver parenchyma, and an intraparenchymal injection of CO_2 will often opacify the portal system (► Fig. 14.2).

Liver Parenchymal Problems

Because there is a higher incidence of hepatocellular carcinoma (HCC) in patients with cirrhosis, the radiologist may encounter patients with HCC who need TIPS. There are theoretic concerns about creating a TIPS tract through a tumor, including an increased risk of bleeding and hematogenous seeding of the tumor. Careful analysis of prior cross-sectional imaging may allow one to choose a path that does not transgress the tumor. This may mean using an atypical pathway such as the left HV to the left PV to avoid a large right lobe HCC.

Polycystic liver disease has been previously considered to be a contraindication to TIPS, presumably for fear of potential bleeding from the parenchymal tract into one of the cysts. However, several reports have described safe creation of TIPS in this setting.[8–11] Again, analysis of prior computed tomography or magnetic resonance imaging scans may help choose a path through a portion of liver that may be relatively free of cysts. As the access needle is advanced through the liver parenchyma, if a cyst is encountered, the needle may be redirected around the cyst, although it has never been proven that it is necessary to avoid going through cysts. With modern use of stent grafts for TIPS, the cyst would presumably be excluded from the blood flow through the shunt. The cysts cause expansion of the liver; thus, the tract from the HV to PV will be longer than for a TIPS in a liver without polycystic disease. Thus longer or overlapping stent grafts will be needed to line the tract.

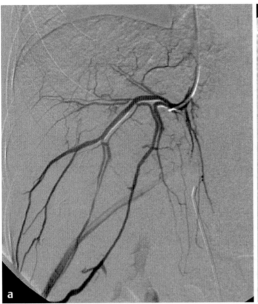
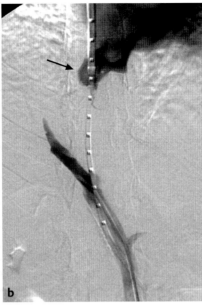

Fig. 14.1 Female patient with Budd-Chiari syndrome. **(a)** The hepatic venogram shows small spidery veins too small to accept the TIPS sheath and access needle. **(b)** Simultaneous portal and hepatic venograms after portal access was gained. The *arrow* points to the hepatic vein stump from which needle passes were initiated.

Portal Vein Problems

In small, shrunken, cirrhotic livers, the PV is more cephalad relative to the HV compared with the relationship seen in normal livers. In this situation, it is difficult to advance the access needle anteriorly enough, and the standard needle curve tends to pass caudal to the right portal trunk. Adding additional curve to the access needle can compensate and allow access into the PV. Alternatively, a long 21-gauge Chiba needle (Cook Inc., Bloomington, Indiana) can be advanced through the larger access needle, and this Chiba needle can be curved near its tip to provide additional curvature to the needle pass.[12]

If the PV is exceptionally high and cannot be punctured from the HV, the gunsight technique can be used.[13] With this technique,

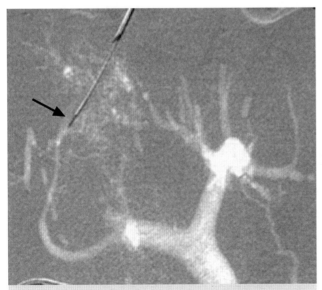

Fig. 14.2 CO_2 injection done through a long 21-gauge Chiba needle (*arrow*) advanced into the liver parenchyma. The portal system was well opacified which facilitated gaining access into the portal vein.

a snare is placed into the right PV via a percutaneous access, and a second snare is advanced from the jugular access into the HV. The two snares are fluoroscopically lined up by angling the image intensifier. A needle is then passed percutaneously through both of these snares. A wire passed through the percutaneous needle is pulled out the jugular access by the HV snare. This provides through-and-though wire access, which allows catheters to be passed from the jugular access across the tract into the PV.

Even with a normally positioned PV, accessing the PV is usually the most difficult aspect of a TIPS, and an inability to access the PV is a common cause of technical failure. Clearly, prior imaging should be reviewed before the case to determine if the PV is patent before starting TIPS.

If the PV is known to be patent and cannot be punctured, some attempt should be made to better localize the location of the PV. External ultrasonography can be used to identify the needle and its relationship to the right PV, but in the author's experience, this is difficult and requires a second operator to hold the ultrasound probe while the primary operator wields the transjugular needle.

One can replace the access needle with a balloon occlusion catheter in the HV for wedged venography if this was not already done at the start of the case. An easier step, if the needle is already in the liver parenchyma, is to do an intraparenchymal injection of CO_2, which will opacify the PV in the majority of cases.[14]

If one fails to find a PV that known to be patent, one should consider if he or she is searching in the wrong direction. Although the middle and right HVs can usually be easily distinguished, if the liver anatomy is distorted, it can be confusing as to which HV the operator is in. If the operator keeps turning the needle anteriorly thinking he or she is in the right HV but he or she is actually in the middle HV, gaining portal access will be unlikely, and continued needle passes are futile. In a number of cases, after multiple failed anterior needle passes from the presumed right HV, the author has found that turning the needle posteriorly allowed successful puncture of the PV. Even if the operator misjudges which HV he or she is in, a middle HV to PV shunt will still decompress the portal system.

If these maneuvers fail, more invasive means can be used. With ultrasound guidance, the left PV can usually be easily accessed for

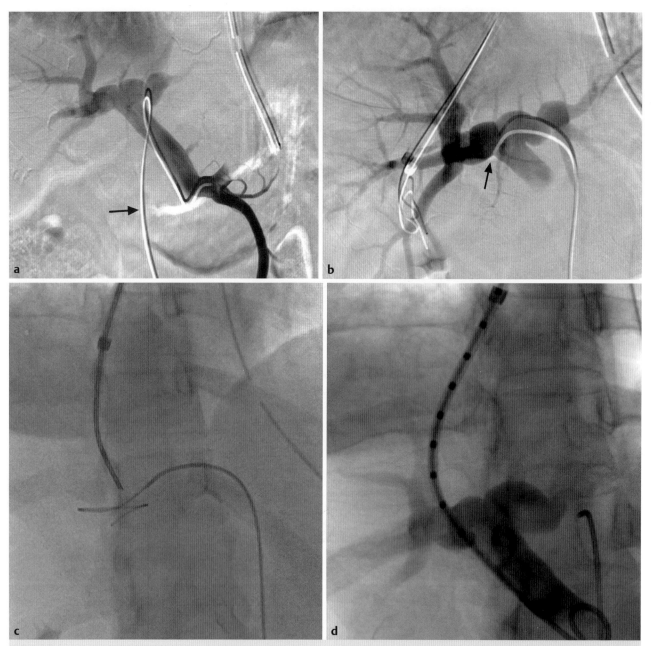

Fig. 14.3 (a) Portal venogram done via a catheter that has been advanced up the paraumbilical vein (*arrow*) into the main portal vein (PV). (b) The paraumbilical catheter has been manipulated so that the tip (*arrow*) is in the right portal trunk. (c) A wire passed through the paraumbilical catheter into the right PV acts as a fluoroscopically visible target for the puncture by the transjugular needle. (d) Portal venogram showing that access into the portal system was achieved precisely where the target wire had been positioned.

percutaneous placement of a wire or snare across into the right portal trunk. This can act as a live fluoroscopic target. The main risk this adds is the puncture of the liver capsule, and in a patient with ascites or coagulopathy, this increases the potential for intraperitoneal hemorrhage from the tract. However, if the percutaneous tract is embolized before this access is totally removed, the risk of hemorrhage is low. This can be done by pushing gelfoam pledgets or coils through the access sheath or catheter as it is withdrawn through the parenchyma.

Access into the portal system can also be obtained by paraumbilical vein puncture if the patient has a large recanalized paraumbilical vein. This access is obtained in the extraperitoneal portion of the anterior abdominal wall, and thus there is no violation of the liver capsule. Unfortunately, a recanalized paraumbilical vein large enough to puncture is only present in approximately 9% to 19% of cases.[15] If accessed, a catheter can be advanced up the recanalized paraumbilical into the portal system for venography and to place a wire or catheter as a target for the transjugular puncture attempts (▶ Fig. 14.3). Small vein size or tortuosity of the paraumbilical vein may prevent cannulation of the main PV even after successful access of a paraumbilical vein.

Rather than using invasive means to simply provide a target in the PV, a percutaneous approach can be used to actually create the tract between the HV and PV.[16] Using ultrasound guidance,

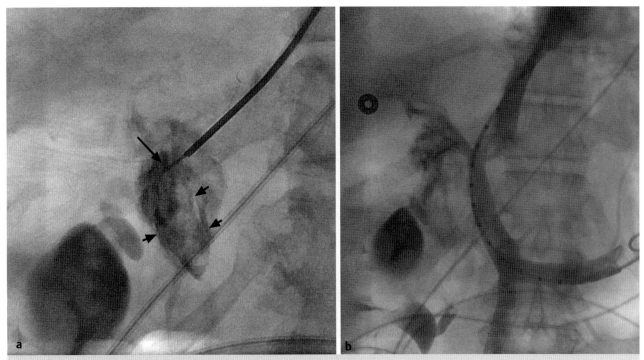

Fig. 14.4 (a) Despite having the portal vein (PV) outlined with contrast (*short arrows*), the Colapinto needle would not penetrate into the PV because of the dense periportal fibrosis. A 21-gauge Chiba needle (*long arrow*) advanced easily through the fibrosis into the PV. (b) Venogram after advancing a catheter into the PV over a stiff 0.018-inch guidewire.

a needle can be passed percutaneously through the right PV and on into the right HV. A wire fed through this needle can be snared and pulled out the jugular sheath. A catheter can then be fed over this wire from the jugular access down into the PV, providing the normal transjugular access route for stent deployment. This is similar to the gunsight technique but without using snares or the extra transhepatic access needed to get a snare into the PV.

Often the PV is surrounded by dense fibrous tissue. This can make it difficult to penetrate into the vein with a larger system such as a Colapinto needle (Cook Inc., Bloomington, Indiana). In fact, if the Colapinto needle flexes rather than penetrating farther into the liver, this is often a sign that the needle is indeed pointing at the PV. Decreasing the gauge of the needle used for the puncture allows better penetration through this dense tissue. A long 21-gauge Chiba needle can be introduced through the Colapinto needle and used to penetrate into the PV (▶ Fig. 14.4). The disadvantage of this is that this Chiba needle will only accept a 0.018-in wire over which it can be tough to advance larger catheters or sheaths. A stiff 0.018-in wire such as a Flex-T (Mallinckrodt Inc., St. Louis, Missouri) provides enough support that the Chiba needle can often be advanced over the wire down into the main PV. The Chiba needle can then be held steady like a guidewire over which the Colapinto needle and its outer 9-Fr catheter can then be advanced.

When access to the PV has been achieved, it is a good idea to keep the metal needle or cannula in place until the outer catheter is advanced into the PV. When this catheter is in the PV, a balloon can be advanced through it into the PV for tract dilatation. If the metal needle or cannula is pulled prematurely, leaving only the wire in the PV, it may be very difficult to advance a balloon catheter across the dense periportal fibrosis, and the catheter may instead buckle into the IVC.

Poral Vein Occlusion

Portal vein thrombosis can occur spontaneously and is seen in 10% to 25% of patients with cirrhosis.[17] PV thrombosis can greatly increase the complexity of TIPS, especially if the thrombus extends into the intrahepatic portal branches. The portal system may not readily opacify during wedged venography, so attempts to localize the PV before making needle passes may fail. During needle passes, it may be difficult to know when the PV has been entered because contrast may not readily flow away from the needle tip. If the portal thrombosis has progressed to cavernous transformation, the chance of technical success further decreases. In one large study,[18] the technical success rate was 99.5% when the PV was patent and 79% in patients with PV thrombosis but only 63% in those with cavernous transformation. TIPS can be created in the face of cavernous transformation if one of the periportal collateral vessels is large enough to be punctured and allow stent deployment.[19] Careful preprocedure vascular mapping can help plan such an approach.

When attempting TIPS in a patient with portal thrombosis, the initial needle passes can be attempted from the transjugular approach, but rather than attempting to aspirate blood, small contrast injections may opacify the PV branch. When a PV is entered, advancing a guidewire may then also be difficult because it may quickly run into thrombus. Using a hydrophilic coated wire may allow better penetration of the thrombus. If access is achieved, one then needs to be prepared to stent beyond the thrombus into a patent segment of the portal system. Mechanical thrombectomy devices can be used to remove some of the thrombus, but in the author's experience, that does not work well unless the thrombus is very acute.

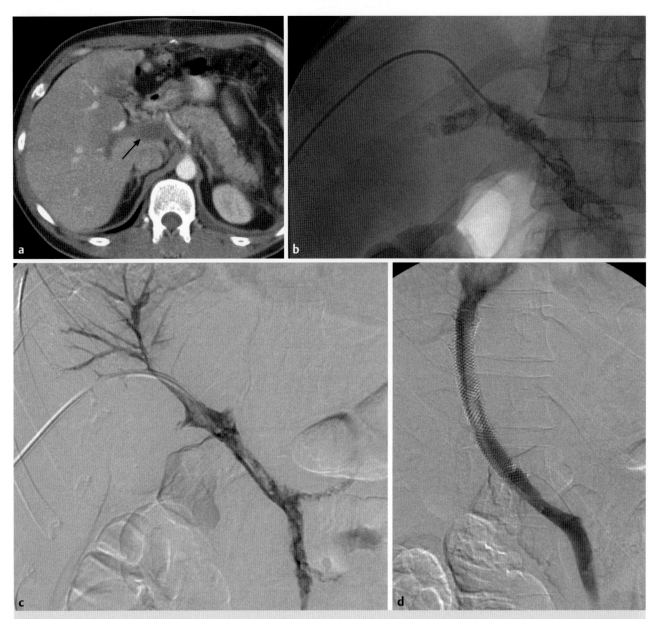

Fig. 14.5 (a) Computed tomography (CT) scan in a patient with variceal bleeding referred for transjugular intrahepatic portosystemic shunt (TIPS). The CT scan shows a thrombosed portal vein (PV) (*arrow*). (b) Portal venogram via a percutaneous transhepatic catheter confirming complete thrombosis of the PV. (c) After some mechanical thrombectomy, the portal system was slightly more patent, and transjugular access was successfully gained. (d) Final post-TIPS portogram after having cleared out the remaining portal clot with mechanical thrombectomy devices passed through the TIPS itself.

If access into the thrombosed PV cannot be achieved from the transjugular approach, an accessory percutaneous transhepatic access may be useful. From the percutaneous approach, it is possible to access more peripheral (and often patent) PV branches that cannot be entered from a transjugular approach. From the transhepatic access, wires can be passed across the PV; thrombus and thrombectomy devices or balloons can even be used to clear a path for the TIPS (▶ Fig. 14.5). The wire or balloons can be used as a target for the transjugular puncture. In a small series by Radosevich et al,[20] using a transhepatic approach improved the technical success rate to 100% compared with a 50% success rate in patients in whom TIPS was attempted purely from a transjugular approach.

Outcomes

This chapter has dealt with a variety of specialized and disparate techniques to overcome unique technical challenges. Most of these techniques have been reported in case reports or small series not amenable to overall outcomes analysis. However, TIPS created with these specialized techniques function similarly to standard TIPS with similar outcomes.

Conclusion

Multiple anatomic factors can make TIPS more challenging. Careful preprocedural assessment of the anatomy is critical. That plus knowledge of the ancillary techniques described in this chapter will allow clinicians to overcome many of these technical challenges.

Clinical Pearls

- Problems with access vein or HV occlusion can usually be solved with the techniques discussed in this chapter.
- Use of a 21-gauge needle can help penetrate into a PV surrounded by dense periportal fibrosis.
- Techniques to localize the PV can help prevent failure to access the PV.
- Although rarely needed, percutaneous access into the PV can be very useful to help localize difficult PVs or recanalize occluded PVs.

References

1. Gazzera C, Righi D, Doriguzzi Breatta A, et al. Emergency transjugular intrahepatic portosystemic shunt (TIPS): results, complications and predictors of mortality in the first month of follow-up. Radiologia Medica 2012;117(1):46–53.
2. Garcia-Pagan JC, Caca K, Bureau C, et al. Early use of TIPS in patients with cirrhosis and variceal bleeding. N Engl J Med 2010;362(25):2370–2379.
3. Hausegger KA, Tauss J, Karaic K, et al. Use of the left internal jugular vein approach for transjugular portosystemic shunt. AJR Am J Roentgenol 1998;171(6):1637–1639.
4. LaBerge JM, Ring EJ, Gordon RL. Percutaneous intrahepatic portosystemic shunt created via a femoral vein approach. Radiology 1991;181(3):679–681.
5. Sze DY, Magsamen KE, Frisoli JK. Successful transfemoral creation of an intrahepatic portosystemic shunt with use of the Viatorr device. J Vasc Interv Radiol 2006;17(3):569–572.
6. Bloch R, Fontaine A, Borsa J, et al. CT-guided transfemoral portocaval shunt creation. Cardiovasc Intervent Radiol 2001;24(2):106.
7. Darcy MD, Sterling DM. Comparison of portal vein anatomy and bony anatomic landmarks. Radiology 1996;200(3):707–710.
8. Bahramipour PF, Festa S, Biswal R, Wachsberg RH. Transjugular intrahepatic portosystemic shunt for the treatment of intractable ascites in a patient with polycystic liver disease. Cardiovasc Interv Radiol 2000;23(3):232–234.
9. Shin ES, Darcy MD. Transjugular intrahepatic portosystemic shunt placement in the setting of polycystic liver disease: questioning the contraindication. J Vasc Interv Radiol 2001;12(9):1099–102.
10. Sze DY, Strobel N, Fahrig R, et al. Transjugular intrahepatic portosystemic shunt creation in a polycystic liver facilitated by hybrid cross-sectional/angiographic imaging. J Vasc Interv Radiol 2006;17(4):711–715.
11. Spillane RM, Kaufman JA, Powelson J, et al. Successful transjugular intrahepatic portosystemic shunt creation in a patient with polycystic liver disease. AJR Am J Roentgenol 1997;169(6):1542–1544.
12. Kerns SR. Difficult portal vein access in transjugular intrahepatic portosystemic shunt placement [letter; comment]. J Vasc Interv Radiol 1995;6(6):985–986.
13. Haskal ZJ, Duszak R Jr, Furth EE. Transjugular intrahepatic transcaval portosystemic shunt: the gun-sight approach. J Vasc Interv Radiol 1996;7(1):139–142.
14. Hawkins IF Jr, Caridi JG. Fine-needle transjugular intrahepatic portosystemic shunt procedure with CO2. AJR Am J Roentgenol 1999;173(3):625–629.
15. Chin MS, Stavas JM, Burke CT, et al. Direct puncture of the recanalized paraumbilical vein for portal vein targeting during transjugular intrahepatic portosystemic shunt procedures: assessment of technical success and safety. J Vasc Interv Radiol 2010;21(5):671–676.
16. Yu SC. A double-wire technique for transjugular intrahepatic portosystemic shunt through a transabdominal-transjugular portosystemic approach. AJR Am J Roentgenol 2011;197(1):W181–W183.
17. Tsochatzis EA, Senzolo M, Germani G, et al. Systematic review: portal vein thrombosis in cirrhosis. Aliment Pharmacol Ther 2010;31(3):366–374.
18. Perarnau JM, Baju A, D'Alteroche L, et al. Feasibility and long-term evolution of TIPS in cirrhotic patients with portal thrombosis. Eur J Gastroenterol Hepatol 2010;22(9):1093–1098.
19. Wils A, van der Linden E, van Hoek B, Pattynama PM. Transjugular intrahepatic portosystemic shunt in patients with chronic portal vein occlusion and cavernous transformation. J Clin Gastroenterol 2009;43(10):982–984.
20. Radosevich PM, Ring EJ, LaBerge JM, et al. Transjugular intrahepatic portosystemic shunts in patients with portal vein occlusion. Radiology 1993;186(2):523–527.

Chapter 15: The Intravascular Ultrasound–Guided Direct Intrahepatic Portacaval Shunt

Bryan D. Petersen

Introduction

The transjugular intrahepatic shunt (TIPS) procedure is one of the most technically challenging and potentially hazardous procedures performed by interventional radiologists. As initially described, the TIPS is created from a "blind puncture" through the liver, generally from the right hepatic vein to the right portal vein (PV). When major complications arise, they are most often related to this step of the procedure.[1,2] Many techniques have been devised to identify and localize the PV to aid in the puncture.[3] Unfortunately, most of these methods have their limitations, and most interventionalists continue to use "blind puncture" through the liver when performing the TIPS procedure.

The intravascular ultrasound (IVUS)–guided direct intrahepatic portacaval shunt (DIPS) procedure was initially conceived as a modification of the TIPS procedure. The DIPS procedure was designed to replace the "blind puncture" step of the TIPS procedure, using a safer, image-guided (IVUS) approach.

The first DIPS were created using a homemade balloon-expandable Palmaz stent graft covered with polytetrafluoroethylene (PTFE).[4] Previous research at the Dotter Institute had demonstrated that a PTFE covering of the stent would dramatically increase the durability of a transhepatic portal caval shunt.[5,6] The use of a balloon-expandable stent graft also allowed for precise control of the diameter shunt and therefore the derived portosystemic gradient. This we termed *balloon-expandable gradients.*

The author has performed hundreds of DIPS procedures over the past 15 years. During this time period, the procedure has undergone only minor modifications. Since originally described, the greatest improvements have occurred in the IVUS imaging and development of stent grafts. Currently, we use the Acu-Nav IVUS system now from Biosense Webster (Johnson & Johnson Medical) and the VIATORR stent graft from W.L. Gore.

In the DIPS procedure, the IVUS is used to guide the PV puncture, and it is also a great aid in positioning and deployment of the stent graft. Today, with current equipment, the routine procedural time to perform the DIPS continues be just over 1 hour, with fluoroscopy times just over 10 minutes.

The DIPS procedure offers advantages over the conventional TIPS procedure because of guidance of the PV puncture, ease of stent graft placement, reduction of fluoroscopy times, and increased shunt durability. Also, in certain anatomic conditions, such as Budd-Chiari syndrome, and avoidance of hepatic masses, the DIPS may be preferable over the TIPS procedure.

I have previously described the "coaxial sheath" method for performing the DIPS procedure.[7] In some patients, the coaxial sheath method improves the alignment of the Rösch-Uchida liver access set (RUPS) puncture needle and Acu-Nav IVUS guidance. With this method, the needle and IVUS are essentially "locked" together, similar to a biopsy guide, and the alignment of these two devices remains stable. It also provides more support to the system during the transcaval puncture. This can be helpful in patients with extremely tough hepatic parenchyma (liver transplant) or extremely resistant PVs (PV thrombus).

The disadvantage is that the setup is longer and requires extra sheaths.

In general, the author now performs the procedure "freehand," as was first described, and uses the coaxial sheath method only in selective cases. The freehand method is simple, safe, and effective and will be presented here. The coaxial sheath method is described in some detail by Petersen.[7]

Equipment

Femoral Access

- 10-Fr sheath (Cook Medical)
- IVUS device (Biosense Webster, Johnson & Johnson)

Jugular Access

- RUPS (Cook Medical)
- 65-cm EchoTip Trocar needle (Cook Medical)
- 65-cm 4-Fr CXI catheter (Cook Medical)
- Platinum Plus 0.018 180-cm guidewire (Boston Scientific)
- Amplatz 0.035 180-cm guidewire (Boston Scientific)
- 5-Fr Marker Pigtail (Cook Medical)
- VIATORR stent graft (W.L. Gore)
- Powerflex 8 mm × 6 cm balloon catheter (Cordis, Johnson & Johnson)
- Two pressure transducers (Merit Medical Systems)

Equipment Modifications

Rösch-Uchida Liver Access Set

To facilitate the direct transcaval puncture, it is essential that the RUPS be modified by adding a secondary curve to the 14-gauge metal trocar (► Fig. 15.1) of the set. This will form a "cobra" shape to the device. The secondary curve of the cobra shape aids the transcaval puncture by giving support off the back wall of the inferior vena cava (IVC). To bend the device, the RUPS is assembled, complete with the standard 5-Fr catheter, and a 0.035-in guidewire is inserted through the lumen. With the guidewire in place, simple hand pressure is used to bend the device. The secondary curve is placed at or near the junction of the 10-Fr sheath and 10-Fr introducing catheter. The guidewire in the lumen protects the 14-gauge metal trocar of the system from being "kinked" or narrowed. Either kinking of the 14-gauge metal trocar or forming too acute an angle of the cobra curve will cause friction on the puncture needle set and should be avoided. The goal is to make the curve as acute as possible while also allowing for easy passage of the needle set. Care must be used when introducing the newly curved device into the patient and straightening this new shape. Be aware that regardless of attempts to maintain an acute angle of the cobra shape, the relatively narrow width of the IVC tends to straighten, or flatten, this angle.

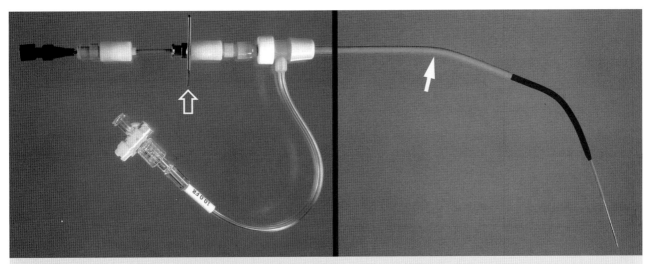

Fig. 15.1 Modified Rösch-Uchida liver access set (RUPS). Assembled modified RUPS with a modified puncture needle set. The *white arrow* marks an added secondary curve, creating a "cobra" shape. This image represents the most modest modification. Often both the secondary and primary curves of the set are made more acute. The secondary curve may be formed more toward the end of the 10-Fr sheath, attempting to form a near right angle. This curving or bending of the set is always performed with a 5-Fr catheter and guidewire in the set to prevent kinking of the lumen of the 14-gauge metal trocar. As an extreme angle as is allowable is generally best. The *open arrow* denotes the directional hub of the set.

Needle and Catheter (Puncture Needle Set)

The 5-Fr catheter and the 62.5-cm-long sharpened 0.038-in wire stylet of the RUPS is not used for the transcaval puncture in the DIPS procedure. The wire 0.038-in stylet is replaced with a 65-cm-long EchoTip Trocar needle (Cook Inc.). The original EchoTip Trocar needle had a sharpened diamond tip, facilitating straight passage through tough liver parenchyma. The tip of the needle is scored, making it extremely echogenic (▶ Fig. 15.2).

A 5-Fr catheter will slip over this needle with a very smooth transition between the needle and catheter. The author first replaced the standard 5-Fr catheter of the RUPS with a hydrophilic 5-Fr catheter with a marker tip (Slip Cath, Cook, Inc.). The hydrophilic material aids in passage through the liver, and the marker tip aids in fluoroscopic visualization. The drawback to this approach is that the hub of the hydrophilic catheter must be cut off to make the appropriate length to match the trocar needle. This 5-Fr catheter must be cut to length, such that it is approximately 1 cm shorter than the trocar needle, such that the echogenic tip of the needle is not covered.

More recently, the author has used 4-Fr crossing catheters, designed for peripheral vascular interventions, as a replacement for the 5-Fr hydrophilic catheter. These catheters are also manufactured at an inappropriate length for the procedure and must be cut to length as well. The 4 F CXI Support Catheter (Cook Inc.), placed over the 65-cm EchoTip Trocar needle has proven to be an excellent combination. Ideally, ultimately, a custom-made, crossing catheter of the appropriate length will be manufactured for this use.

After the PV puncture, the passage of a 0.035-in lumen catheter (as described earlier) into the PV is probably the most difficult step of the procedure. This is because of the tough nature of the PV and because of working at a mechanical disadvantage from the neck. The creation of this needle puncture set is a very important modification of the RUPS. It allows upsizing from the 0.018-in lumen of the EchoTip Trocar puncture needle to 0.035-in guidewires necessary for the remainder of the procedure.

Intravascular Ultrasonography

For the DIPS procedure, an IVUS catheter is introduced into the right femoral vein and then into the IVC to the level of the PV. The IVUS is first used to guide a needle puncture from the IVC to the PV. This transcaval puncture is performed directly through the caudate lobe of the liver by the modified RUPS, which has been introduced through the right internal jugular vein.

The IVUS catheter first used for the DIPS procedure was a 9-MHz mechanical probe from Boston Scientific. Similar to all other IVUS probes available at that time, it produced the typical 360-degree

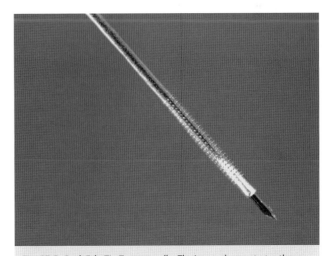

Fig. 15.2 Cook EchoTip Trocar needle. The image demonstrates the scored, echogenic tip of the 65-cm EchoTip Trocar needle (Cook Inc.). This needle has the preferred diamond tip stylet in place. The most recent iterations have a beveled Chiba stylet. Regardless, this needle is much more echogenic than the 0.038-in sharpened wire needle of the standard Rösch-Uchida liver access set (RUPS) and traverses the liver much easier. It accepts a 0.018-in guidewire.

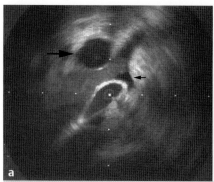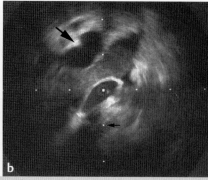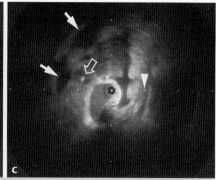

Fig. 15.3 Nine-MHz rotational 360-degree intravascular ultrasound (IVUS) image. A 9-MHz rotational IVUS mechanical rotational image produces 360-degree "axial" images oriented at 90 degrees from the tip of the transducer in the inferior vena cava (IVC). Although these images were made with an older Boston Scientific IVUS catheter, they are similar as to what may be achieved with the more modern Visions PV 8.2 9-Fr, 10-MHz rotational IVUS catheter from Volcano Corporation. **(a)** The transducer is at the center of the image in the IVC inferior to the portal vein (PV) bifurcation. The walls of the IVC appear echogenic. The *larger arrow* at the 11 o'clock position denotes the main PV. The *smaller arrow* at the 2 o'clock position denotes hypoechoic ascitic fluid. Flowing blood is also hypoechoic. The slightly echogenic material between the IVC and PV represents the caudate lobe of the liver. **(b)** The transducer has been positioned slightly more superiorly. The *larger arrow* at the 11 o'clock position now denotes the portal vein (PV) bifurcation. This is an excellent target for the direct intrahepatic portacaval shunt (DIPS) puncture. The *small black arrow* denotes a white dot on the screen. Each of these white dots, oriented in a crossing pattern, denotes 1 cm from the transducer at the epicenter. Note the close proximity of the IVC to the PV. The deepest penetration to be expected with this transducer is approximately 3 cm. **(c)** The transducer is again positioned slightly more superiorly than in part B. *Large white arrows* at the 9 and 11 o'clock structures denote hypoechoic left and right main PVs. The *outlined arrow* denotes the bright reflector of the EchoTip Trocar needle traversing the caudate lobe during the puncture. The needle follows an oblique course through the liver and will strike the PV bifurcation slightly more inferiorly. With this transducer, the entire course of the needle tract is not seen on the IVUS image. The orientation of the needle tip to the PV is similar to a jugular vein puncture using transcutaneous ultrasonography held transverse to the vein. The *larger arrowhead* denotes a 1-cm marker.

image oriented at 90 degrees from the transducer. When the DIPS was first performed, this probe was chosen because it was the lowest IVUS frequency probe available. Tissue penetration and visualization were adequate, and it was used successfully in the first 11 patients. Using this transducer, the average number of needle passes required to puncture the PV was from 1 to 3. With the "axial" type image produced by this transducer, the needle tip is visualized only by a bright reflector, crossing through the imaging plane, and as such, the entire needle path is not visualized (▶ Fig. 15.3). This imaging is similar to a jugular vein puncture performed under transcutaneous ultrasonography with the transducer held in a cross-sectional manner.

The author no longer uses this IVUS imaging system but performs the DIPS with the Acu-Nav IVUS described later. However, the images presented in ▶ Fig. 15.3 are important because they are very similar to the images created by the 10-MHz system available from Volcano Industries today. This Volcano IVUS system may be used for the DIPS procedure if an Acu-Nav system is not available.

The Acu-Nav IVUS device first became available more than 10 years ago. It was initially marketed by the Acuson Company, then acquired by Siemens Corporation, and now marketed by Johnson & Johnson. It has replaced all other IVUS systems used for the DIPS procedure. It has advantages of improved resolution, lower frequency (variable 5–10 MHz), and color Doppler. Most importantly, it has a "side fire vector," or sagittal imaging plane, such that the entire needle puncture tract through the liver may be visualized (▶ Fig. 15.4).

This device is designed for cardiac electrophysiology studies and interventions. It was originally manufactured as a 10-Fr device but is now available in both 8- and 10-Fr systems. The two catheters differ slightly in their sonic capabilities, but both give excellent imaging for the DIPS procedure. They are available only from Biosense Webster (Johnson & Johnson) but will connect to multiple different cardiac and traditional ultrasound units (Sequoia, Aspen, Cypress) all available from Siemens. Whereas the 10-Fr probe connected to the larger Sequoia unit has the most versatility, the smaller Cypress unit with the 8-Fr probe is more than adequate and is portable. The 8- and 10-Fr transducers are sold as single use only; however, the DIPS procedure is not taxing on either device, and if resterilized, they are capable of multiple uses.

The Procedure

The DIPS procedure requires both right internal jugular and right common femoral venous access. If required, a combination of either contralateral jugular or femoral vein may be used. Use of either left jugular or femoral vein it is not recommended for novice interventionalists because alignment of the IVUS and modified RUPS needle may be difficult.

Step 1: Femoral Venous Access and Intravascular Ultrasound Placement

Femoral vein access should be performed first. A 10-Fr, 40-cm sheath is placed into the access site. The Acu-Nav device should then be introduced into the IVC in a sterile fashion with the use of a cover over the handle. It is useful to support the cord of the transducer on the patient drape with the use of forceps, such that it will not be dislodged. The tip of the IVUS is placed near the intended site of puncture, the PV bifurcation. Next, all anatomy is verified with IVUS. The hepatic artery should be behind to the PV, which is anterior, because visualization is from the IVC. An aberrant replaced right hepatic artery may lie near the intended path

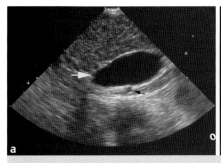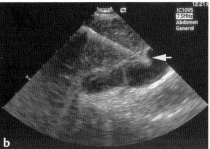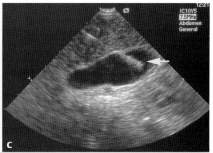

Fig. 15.4 Acu-Nav 5- to 10-MHz intravascular ultrasound (IVUS). Acu-Nav 5- to 10-MHz variable IVUS "side fire" image performed at 7.5 MHz. Much improved resolution is seen compared with a 9-MHz rotational mechanical probe. (**a**) The Acu-Nav catheter generates a sector image in a sagittal orientation. The inferior vena cava (IVC) is in the near field, obscured at this frequency. The patient's head (or the superior direction) is on the left of the image, and the patient's feet (or the inferior direction) are on the right of the image. The *white arrow* denotes the portal vein (PV) bifurcation, which is hypoechoic and ovoid in this IVUS orientation. Echogenic material between the near field and PV is the caudate lobe of the liver. The *small black arrow* denotes the hepatic artery, lying behind the PV (anterior direction). Color Doppler is available but not necessary. (**b,c**) Two sequential static images from transcaval puncture of portal vein (PV). The *white arrows* in both images denote the 21-gauge EchoTip Trocar needle. Note that the entire course of the needle puncture is seen in the images. Despite adequate curving of the Rösch-Uchida liver access set (RUPS), the course of the needle remains somewhat oblique, from superior to inferior in direction. This is because of flattening of the "cobra" shape by the relatively small diameter of the IVC. Inadequate curving of the RUPS may cause the needle course to be less acute, passing inferior to the PV. Flow disturbances in the PV may be detected by this high-resolution IVUS device, such as in the upper image. The tip of the needle set may indent the PV wall just before puncture (*white arrow*, **b**). Note the bright echogenic needle tip in the PV (*arrow*, **c**).

of puncture and should be avoided. Color Doppler may be helpful to establish the patency of the PV, absence of thrombus, and other abnormalities but is generally not required because visualization is quite good. At low frequencies, the Acu-Nav has the ability to penetrate quite deep into the liver (>15 cm). Adjustment of both the magnification and frequency is required to achieve an image similar to ▶ Fig. 15.4a. The Acu-Nav creates a sagittal image with cranial at the left-hand side of the image and caudal to the right. The ultrasound machines have the ability to invert left to right, so the operator should make sure that this is correct.

Step 2: Placement of the Modified RUPS

After right jugular venous access has been achieved, the gray polyethylene 10-Fr introducer of the RUPS is placed into the IVC over a stiff guidewire (Amplatz super stiff). A fully assembled, modified RUPS, complete with the 10-Fr sheath, and a standard 5-Fr introducing catheter should then be quickly introduced into the IVC over this stiff guidewire as a single unit. The tip of the 10-Fr catheter and metal trocar should be placed into the IVC inferior to the level of intended puncture below the PV bifurcation, and then the super stiff guidewire and 5-Fr catheter are quickly withdrawn. The tip of the 10-Fr catheter will impress upon the IVC and not introduce air or bleed. The 5-Fr catheter and super stiff wire may be left in the system as long as both are withdrawn into the straight portion of the metal 14-gauge trocar. Other methods of introduction of the device will result in flattening or straightening of the "cobra" shape of the device; the shape should be maintained.

With the IVUS centered on the site of intended puncture, the modified RUPS should then be gradually withdrawn from the neck, rotating the device, such that the tip of the 10-Fr catheter and metal trocar is oriented toward the PV. This is generally no more than 45 degrees off vertical. The direction arrow on the RUPS hub should be used as a general method of guidance. The distal tip of the RUPS may impact upon the IVUS probe and is of no consequence. Artifact will be seen in the IVUS image caused

by the metal trocar within the 10-Fr catheter, crossing the ultrasound beam. By retracting and rotating the modified RUPS, the tip of the 10-Fr catheter is oriented at the most cranial aspect of the image directed toward the target (▶ Fig. 15.5).

Step 3: The Transcaval Puncture

The puncture needle set is loaded into the modified RUPS with the EchoTip Trocar needle brought just to the end of the 10-Fr catheter but not protruding. Final adjustments can now be made before the needle set is thrust forward. The needle should be thrust fairly

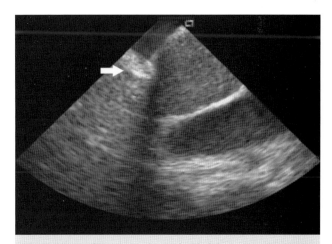

Fig. 15.5 Optimal positioning the Rösch-Uchida liver access set (RUPS) for the transcaval puncture. The RUPS has been withdrawn superiorly and rotated such that the tip of the 10-Fr catheter is directed at the portal vein (PV). The tip of the 10-Fr catheter with the metal trocar in the set is seen as a bright reflector in the near field (*arrow*). Note how the force of the RUPS has forced the inferior vena cava (IVC) wall away from the Acu-Nav transducer, such that the IVC wall can now be seen in the near field. Because the target (the PV) and RUPS are seen on the same image, this is the proper position to begin the puncture.

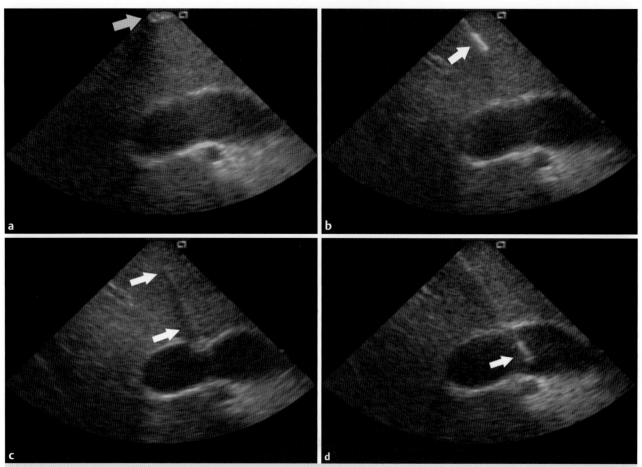

Fig. 15.6 Intravascular ultrasound–guided direct inferior vena cava (IVC) to portal vein (PV) puncture. (**a**) The freehand technique. This is a different patient than the one in Fig. 17.5A, with a less favorable anatomy. To achieve the proper angle for puncture, the Rösch-Uchida liver access set (RUPS) had to be retracted more superiorly (cephalad) than in Fig. 15.5a, just at the superior margin of the field of view (*arrow*). Compare this with Fig. 15.4, where the RUPS needed to be withdrawn even more superiorly off the field of view before initiation of the puncture, as described in the text. (**b**) The needle has been thrust through the IVC wall and into the caudate lobe. The bright reflector (*arrow*) of the EchoTip Trocar needle is readily visible when properly aligned with the ultrasound beam. (**c**) The path of the needle (*arrows*) is less apparent as it traverses slightly out of the path of the ultrasound. The needle tip deflects the PV wall as it passes through. (**d**) The reflective tip of the EchoTip Trocar needle has been advanced to the center of the PV (*arrow*). Note that the PV bifurcation has resumed the normal ovoid appearance.

briskly through the liver toward the PV. The reflective tip of the EchoTip Trocar needle is readily visible when in plane with the IVUS beam (▶ Fig. 15.6). The coaxial sheath technique maintains this alignment, but with a little practice, alignment of the two devices maybe maintained by freehand technique, and the coaxial method is not necessary. Generally, the needle tip pierces the PV fairly easily, although the needle may indent the PV just before puncturing the wall (▶ Fig. 15.4b).

If one senses that the needle is on a path to pass inferior to the PV, it indicates that the curve of the cobra shape on the RUPS was inadequate or at least straightened to some degree by a relatively small IVC. The operator has several choices. First, he or she may continue with the pass, hoping to strike the target lower than intended, such as in the main PV. Care must be taken not to puncture the PV in an extrahepatic region, or significant bleeding may occur. A second option is to remove the RUPS over a stiff guidewire, increase the curvature of the RUPS, and then try again. If adequate curvature cannot be obtained, the third option is to begin the puncture higher in the IVC, allowing the longer needle path to intersect the intended target.

To perform this "high puncture," one must retract the needle set superiorly, just at the margin of the IVUS image (▶ Fig. 15.6a). At times, the puncture may need to be initiated even higher, just off the field of view, before the needle is thrust forward. The caveat is to maintain the same left-to-right orientation of the set while withdrawing it in a cephalad direction. The coaxial sheath method was developed to maintain this alignment but is not routinely necessary. Unless there is some unforeseen difficulty, it is best to maintain the IVUS positioned on the intended target and bring the needle tip into the image rather than move the IVUS. In ▶ Fig. 15.4, the puncture was initiated much more superiorly, off the field of view seen on the IVUS.

Step 4: Upsizing the Guidewire

After the PV has been punctured, placement can then be confirmed with contrast injection (▶ Fig. 15.7), although there should be little doubt as the needle tip is readily visible on IVUS. Next, a stiff 0.018-in guidewire (Platinum Plus Boston Scientific) is advanced into the PV. Just as in TIPS, the author prefers that the

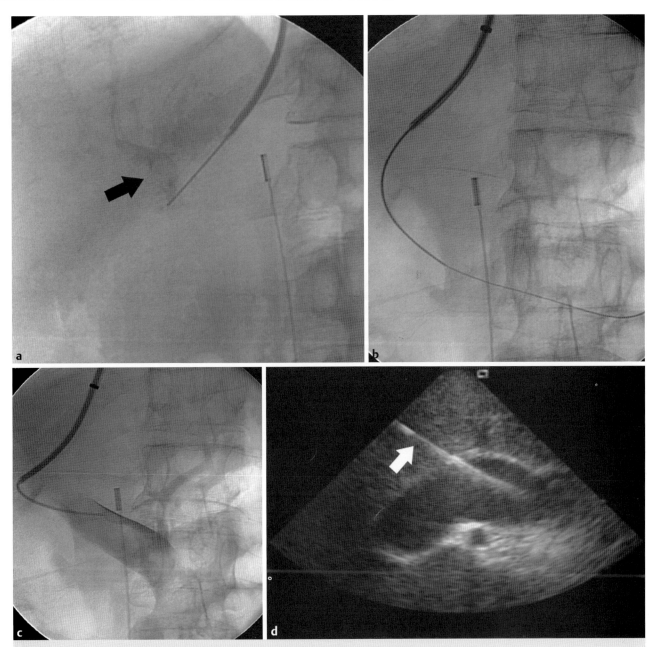

Fig. 15.7 Confirming portal vein (PV) puncture, upsizing the guidewire. (**a**) Although the echogenic tip of the needle is easily seen in the PV on intravascular ultrasound (IVUS), it is sometimes prudent to confirm its position by injecting a small amount of contrast through the hub (the *black arrow* denotes PV filling). Care must be taken in that if the needle tip is not cleanly in the PV, contrast injection into the adjacent liver parenchyma will obscure the IVUS images, hindering further efforts. Unlike the transjugular intrahepatic shunt procedure, because of the small lumen, it is difficult to aspirate blood through the needle for confirmation of PV access. (**b**) After confirmation of needle placement, the 0.018-in stiff guidewire is advanced into the PV. (**c**) Injection is through catheter of the puncture needle set, which has been advanced over EchoTip Trocar needle and 0.018-in guidewire into the PV. Contrast injection confirms placement. It is now time to upsize to a 0.035-in super stiff supportive wire for shunt portography and shunt placement. (**d**) Corresponding IVUS image of a 0.035-in Amplatz wire (*arrow*) crossing from the inferior vena cava and into the PV.

guidewire placement is deep into the splenic vein when possible. The catheter of the puncture needle set is advanced over both the needle and 0.018-in guidewire into the PV. Depending on the patient and the toughness of the PV, this can be the most difficult step of the procedure. To aid in passage of the 5-Fr catheter, the author changed the standard 5-Fr catheter of the RUPS to a 5-Fr hydrophylic catheter. With more recent changes in technology, the author now uses a 4-Fr crossing catheter (CXI Support

Catheter, Cook Medical), which has eliminated most of the difficulty with this step. Because the hydrophilic or crossing catheters must be "trimmed" to length (as described in Equipment Modifications earlier), they do lack the conventional connecting hub, which must be dealt with. Finally, a stiff Amplatz 0.035-in guidewire is placed into the PV through the modified 4- or 5-Fr catheter of the needle set, and the RUPS and catheters are removed, leaving the 10-Fr sheath in the neck.

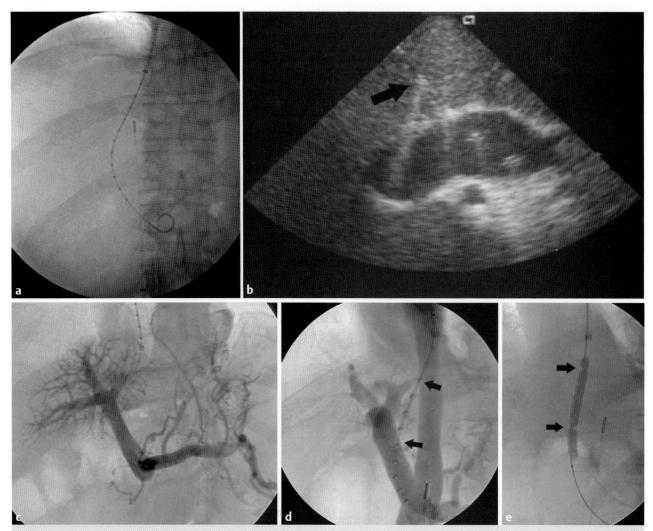

Fig. 15.8 Portography, manometry, and tract measurement. (**a**) The 5-Fr pigtail catheter, with sizing markers placed every 1 cm, has been placed into the portal vein (PV). (**b**) Note the excellent resolution of the intravascular ultrasound (IVUS) image with the metallic markers of the sizing catheter casting acoustic shadows in both the liver (*arrow*) and when in the PV. (**c**) Portography performed through marker pigtail catheter. Simultaneous pressure measurements are then performed through the 10-Fr sheath in the inferior vena cava (IVC) and 5-Fr pigtail in the PV, confirming the portosystemic gradient. (**d**) Magnified, slight left anterior oblique projection with simultaneous injection through 5-Fr pigtail in the PV and 10-Fr sheath in the IVC. A 40-cm-long, 10-Fr sheath in the common femoral aids in this study. A marker pigtail bridges the parenchymal tract from the IVC to the PV. *Arrows* denote approximate IVC and PV puncture sites. In this case, the distance approximates 4 cm between the veins. We generally place a VIATORR stent graft with the PTFE portion 1 cm longer than the measured distance (in this case, 5 cm). (**e**) Predilation of the tract may be performed to help advance the 10-Fr sheath into the PV. This is a 6-mm-diameter, 6-cm-long balloon catheter. The "waists" of the balloon denote the IVC and PV walls and may be used as a rough measurement of the length of the parenchymal tract. This should be performed with caution because fibrotic bands within the liver parenchyma may give similar impressions on the balloon, not reflecting the true length of the tract. In the event of an extrahepatic puncture of the PV, predilation may also cause significant bleeding.

Step 5: Portography, Manometry, and Tract Measurement

From this point, the procedure proceeds very similar to the TIPS. A 5-Fr marker pigtail is advanced over the stiff guidewire into the PV (▶ Fig. 15.8a and 15.8b), and portography with manometry is performed (▶ Fig. 15.8c). Tract measurements for stent graft placement are best judged by performing simultaneous injections in the IVC and PV using a marker catheter (▶ Fig. 15.8d). Similar to TIPS, the author uses a VIATORR device with the PTFE portion approximately 1 cm longer than the measured tract length. The length of the parenchymal tract may also be estimated with the

Acu-Nav IVUS and its internal calibration. Other methods include the use of a measuring wire or predilation of the tract with a balloon and measuring the distance between the "waists" of the IVC and PV impressions (▶ Fig. 15.8e).

Step 6: Intravascular Ultrasound–Guided Placement of the VIATORR Stent Graft

To deploy the VIATORR stent graft, the tip of the 10-Fr sheath of the RUPS must be advanced greater than 2 cm past the PV

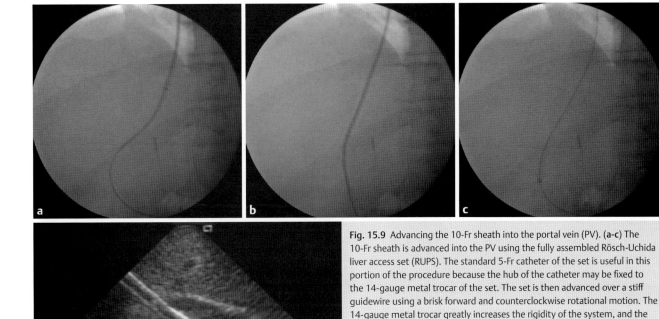

Fig. 15.9 Advancing the 10-Fr sheath into the portal vein (PV). **(a-c)** The 10-Fr sheath is advanced into the PV using the fully assembled Rösch-Uchida liver access set (RUPS). The standard 5-Fr catheter of the set is useful in this portion of the procedure because the hub of the catheter may be fixed to the 14-gauge metal trocar of the set. The set is then advanced over a stiff guidewire using a brisk forward and counterclockwise rotational motion. The 14-gauge metal trocar greatly increases the rigidity of the system, and the set will straighten the tract. This may cause significant patient discomfort. After the metal trocar and 10-Fr introducing catheter of the set are in the PV, the outer 10-Fr sheath should be quickly advanced over the set to establish secure access. It is best to quickly remove the trocar assembly, letting the 10-Fr sheath resume a gentle curve and leaving the guidewire in place. **(d)** Intravascular ultrasound image confirming 10-Fr sheath crossing from the inferior vena cava and into the PV.

puncture site. The best means to do this is to advance the assembled set (10-Fr sheath, 10-Fr catheter, 14-gauge trocar, 5-Fr introducing catheter) all into the PV over a stiff guidewire. Generally, a 0.035-in Amplatz super stiff wire is adequate. It is best to advance the whole set briskly into the PV, rotating the set in a counterclockwise direction, following the curve of the guidewire (▶ Fig. 15.9). If there is buckling or resistance to advancement, a stiffer guidewire, such as a 0.035-in Lunderquist (Cook Medical) may be used. The operator should make sure that all transitions to the RUPS are smooth because even minor irregularities to the edges of the sheath or catheter transitions can make this difficult.

Deployment of the VIATORR can be visualized by both fluoroscopy and IVUS; however, it is best seen by IVUS. The use of IVUS has improved accuracy and reduced the procedural and fluoroscopy time for this step of the procedure.

Just as in the TIPS procedure, with the 10-Fr sheath in the PV, the VIATORR stent graft is advanced to the tip of the sheath, and the sheath then is retracted, exposing the bare wire portion of the device, which expands. This bare wire portion of the stent graft is termed the PV "localizer," which in the TIPS procedure is intended to be drawn back against the PV wall under fluoroscopy. With the DIPS procedure, the positioning and deploying of the VIATORR can be observed with both fluoroscopy and IVUS. This greatly simplifies and improves accuracy of this portion of the procedure (▶ Fig. 15.10).

After the VIATORR has been deployed, it needs only balloon dilatation to fully open the device and establish the DIPS. Most commonly, a 10-mm VIATORR device of the appropriate length is deployed and then postdilated with an 8-mm-diameter balloon. Final portography and manometry are then performed (▶ Fig. 15.11). An 8-mm-diameter DIPS usually results in adequate portal decompression with a final portosystemic gradient between 4 and 8 mm Hg.

Control of the Extrahepatic Puncture

Portal vein access in the TIPS procedure is usually the main right PV or even more peripheral and in general is intrahepatic. The main target of the PV puncture in the DIPS procedure is the PV bifurcation. One might expect that the DIPS procedure, despite the IVUS guidance, could have more bleeding complications from the PV access because the PV bifurcation may be extrahepatic in up to 50% of patients.[8] When extrahepatic punctures of the PV occur in the TIPS procedure, we know that bleeding is often tamponaded by the dense fibrous connective tissue that surrounds the porta hepatis.[9,10] This may also explain why bleeding from an extrahepatic puncture is relatively uncommon in the DIPS procedure.

When intraperitoneal bleeding occurs during the DIPS procedure, it is most often caused by predilation of the tract, and PV, before placement of the VIATORR. If there is no tissue surrounding the PV puncture site and it is dilated, a catheter, sheath, or balloon must remain in the tract until the VIATORR can be deployed. This is why it is best to advance the 10-Fr sheath into the PV without predilation, as described in ▶ Fig. 15.9.

If for some reason the operator decides to predilate the tract before the 10-Fr sheath placement, he or she should be sure that the IVUS images that document the PV puncture is entirely

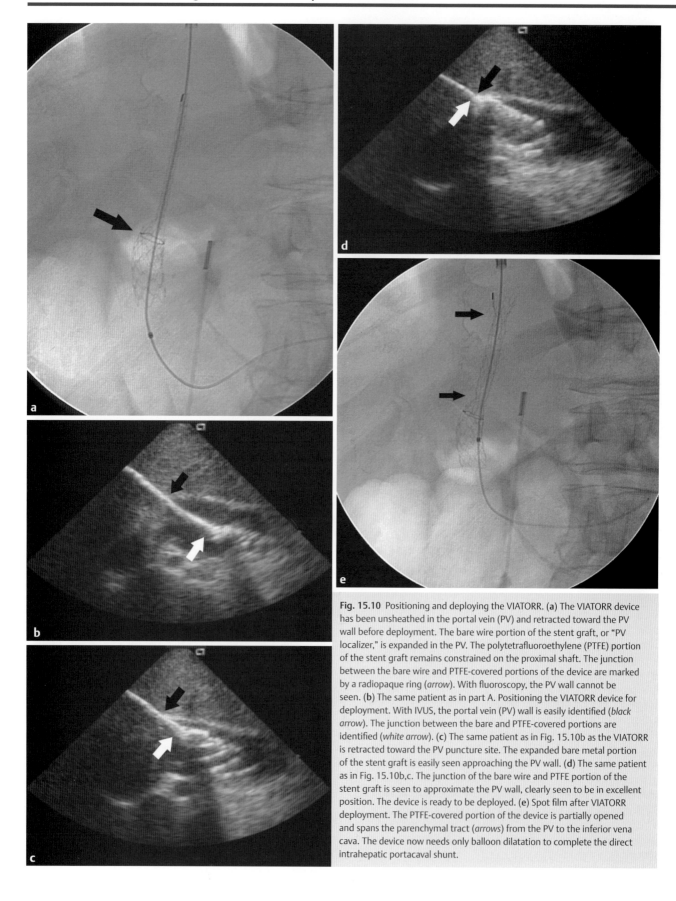

Fig. 15.10 Positioning and deploying the VIATORR. (a) The VIATORR device has been unsheathed in the portal vein (PV) and retracted toward the PV wall before deployment. The bare wire portion of the stent graft, or "PV localizer," is expanded in the PV. The polytetrafluoroethylene (PTFE) portion of the stent graft remains constrained on the proximal shaft. The junction between the bare wire and PTFE-covered portions of the device are marked by a radiopaque ring (*arrow*). With fluoroscopy, the PV wall cannot be seen. (b) The same patient as in part A. Positioning the VIATORR device for deployment. With IVUS, the portal vein (PV) wall is easily identified (*black arrow*). The junction between the bare and PTFE-covered portions are identified (*white arrow*). (c) The same patient as in Fig. 15.10b as the VIATORR is retracted toward the PV puncture site. The expanded bare metal portion of the stent graft is easily seen approaching the PV wall. (d) The same patient as in Fig. 15.10b,c. The junction of the bare wire and PTFE portion of the stent graft is seen to approximate the PV wall, clearly seen to be in excellent position. The device is ready to be deployed. (e) Spot film after VIATORR deployment. The PTFE-covered portion of the device is partially opened and spans the parenchymal tract (*arrows*) from the PV to the inferior vena cava. The device now needs only balloon dilatation to complete the direct intrahepatic portacaval shunt.

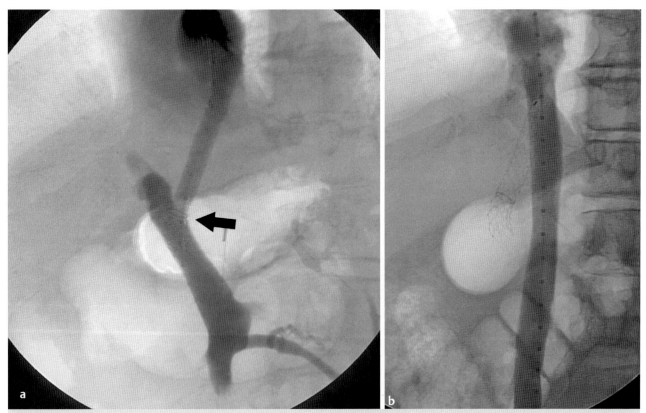

Fig. 15.11 Completion portography. (**a**) Completion portogram after VIATORR has been dilated to an 8-mm diameter. Compare with Fig. 15.8c before completion of the shunt. The small varices no longer fill, and there is significant shunting of flow from the portal circulation to the inferior vena cava (IVC). Note the straight course of the direct intrahepatic portacaval shunt (DIPS) directly to the IVC. The polytetrafluoroethylene (PTFE) portion of the VIATORR device begins at the portal vein (PV) wall (*arrow*), completely lining the parenchymal tract to the IVC. (**b**) Inferior vena cavagram performed after DIPS, anteroposterior projection. These are not routinely preformed after DIPS. The caval end of the VIATORR projects into the anterior wall of the IVC, not across the lumen, as suggested on this one projection. Note that the course of the DIPS begins inferior to the hepatic veins and relies on a longer segment of the patient's IVC than the TIPS procedure. In the hundreds of DIPS procedures the author has performed, he has not yet seen a case of IVC stenosis or shunt occlusion caused by projection of a stent graft into the IVC.

intrahepatic. The predilation balloon or sheath should also be no greater than 4 mm, such that if bleeding occurs, it may be controlled by placement of the sheath across the bleeding site and the VIATORR can be quickly deployed (▶ Fig. 15.12).

Direct Intrahepatic Portacaval Shunt Patency

The authors' reported series of the first 19 patients treated with the DIPS using the VIATORR stent graft demonstrated a 100% primary patency up to 30 months.[11] These patency figures were established using venography with manometry and are superior to published series of the TIPS procedure using either bare wire stents or the VIATORR stent graft. Although this is a small single-institution series with only midterm follow-up, no larger series of the DIPS procedure have been published.

Because of the deep position of the DIPS in the liver and the angle of the shunt, it is difficult to interrogate the shunt with ultrasound. There are no established ultrasound velocity criteria that correlate with degree of shunt stenosis and patency. As the authors have observed excellent patency and long-term durability of the DIPS, we have largely abandoned ultrasound surveillance of the shunt. We treat the patients clinically, and if there is

suspicion of shunt dysfunction, we proceed directly to venography to clarify.

Conclusion

The DIPS procedure has undergone little change since first described in 2001. There is no dedicated DIPS liver access set or needle, nor is there a dedicated IVUS device for the procedure. Perhaps with greater clinical demand, more dedicated equipment will become available. A purposely built needle of nitinol that is more flexible and echogenic and with a 0.035-in lumen would simplify the portal access portion of the procedure and obviate the need for trimming of the crossing catheters. One can also envision smaller IVUS devices with built-in guidance systems. If these were produced, perhaps the femoral puncture could be abandoned, and only a transjugular access would be necessary.

The DIPS procedure may be used as a replacement for the TIPS procedure or used selectively for TIPS failures and patients with unfavorable anatomy. The procedure is relatively easy to master, and after proficiency has been achieved, it proceeds quickly and safely. The procedure may ultimately find its role with interventional radiologists who are unfamiliar with performing

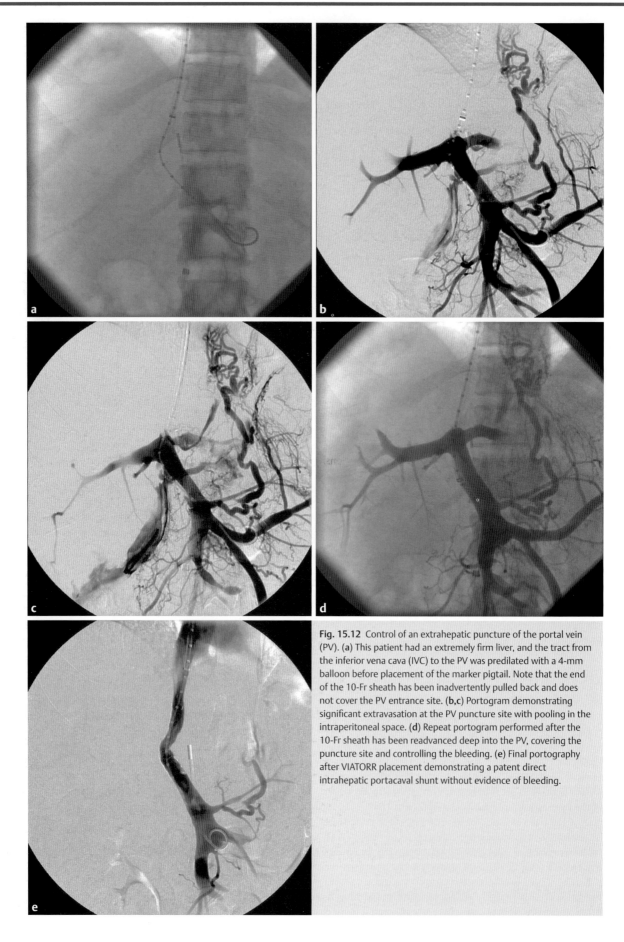

Fig. 15.12 Control of an extrahepatic puncture of the portal vein (PV). (**a**) This patient had an extremely firm liver, and the tract from the inferior vena cava (IVC) to the PV was predilated with a 4-mm balloon before placement of the marker pigtail. Note that the end of the 10-Fr sheath has been inadvertently pulled back and does not cover the PV entrance site. (**b,c**) Portogram demonstrating significant extravasation at the PV puncture site with pooling in the intraperitoneal space. (**d**) Repeat portogram performed after the 10-Fr sheath has been readvanced deep into the PV, covering the puncture site and controlling the bleeding. (**e**) Final portography after VIATORR placement demonstrating a patent direct intrahepatic portacaval shunt without evidence of bleeding.

the TIPS procedure and find the comfort and security of the image guidance aspects of the procedure more to their liking.

Clinical Pearls

- There are two guidance techniques for IVUS-guided TIPS: the coaxial sheath technique (needle and IVUS locked together) and the freehand technique.
- The advantages of the coaxial sheath technique is that it provides better needle support and thus is better in tough livers and the PV.
- The disadvantages of the coaxial sheath technique is that it requires extra sheaths and takes longer to set up.
- Jugular access is for the access needle, and femoral access is for the IVUS probe.
- An aberrantly replaced right hepatic artery may lie near the intended path of IVUS-guided DIPS and should be avoided.
- The portal target in IVUS-guided DIPS is the intrahepatic portal bifurcation.
- Pre-stent dilatation should not exceed 4 mm.
- The most common diameter for DIPS stents for adequate portal decompression is 8 mm; however, a 10-mm diameter VIATORR (self-expanding covered stent) is used and dilated to 8 mm.
- DIPS patency using the VIATORR stent has 100% patency up to 30 months.
- DIPS is difficult to interrogate by Doppler ultrasonography, and there are no standardized velocities indicative of DIPS dysfunction. As a result, follow-up is by clinical manifestations.

Acknowledgments

Special thanks to Ron Cook, CVT, of Providence Sacred Heart Medical Center, Spokane Washington.

References

1. Freedman A, Sanyal A, Tisnado J, et al. Complications of transjugular intrahepatic portosystemic shunts: a comprehensive review. Radiographics 1993;13:1185–1210.
2. Petersen B, Saxon R, Barton R, Lakin P. TIPS: management of major procedural complications. Semin Intervent Radiol 1998;12:355–363.
3. Saxon R, Keller F. Technical aspects of accessing the portal vein during the TIPS procedure. J Vasc Interv Radiol 1997;8:733–744.
4. Petersen B, Uchida B, Timmermans H, et al. Intravascular ultrasound (IVUS) guided direct intrahepatic portocaval shunt (DIPS) with PTFE covered stent-graft: feasibility in swine and initial clinical results. J Vasc Interv Radiol 2001;12:475–486.
5. Nishimine K, Saxon R, Kichikawa K, et al. Improved transjugular intrahepatic portosystemic shunt patency with PTFE-covered stent grafts: experimental results in swine. Radiology 1995;196:341–347.
6. Saxon R, Timmermans H, Uchida B, et al. Stent-grafts for revision of TIPS stenosis and occlusions: a clinical pilot study. J Vasc Interv Radiol 1997;8:539–548.
7. Petersen B. IVUS guided DIPS (intravascular ultrasound guided direct intrahepatic portocaval shunt): description of technique and technical refinements. J Vasc Interv Radiol 2003;14:21–32.
8. Schultz S, Laberge J, Gordon R, Warren R. Anatomy of the portal vein bifurcation: intra-versus extrahepatic location–implication for transjugular intrahepatic porto-systemic shunts. J Vasc Interv Radiol 1994;5:457–459.
9. Saxon R, Keller F. Technical aspects of accessing the portal vein during the TIPS procedure. J Vasc Interv Radiol 1997;8:733–744.
10. Davis A, Haskal Z. Extrahepatic portal vein puncture and intra-abdominal hemorrhage during transjugular intrahepatic portosystemic shunt creation. J Vasc Interv Radiol 1996;7:863–866.
11. Hoppe H, Wang S, Petersen B. Intravascular US-guided direct intrahepatic portocaval shunt with an expanded polytetraflouroethylene-coverd stent-graft. Radiology 2008;246(1):306–314.

Chapter 16: Hemodynamic Changes Following the Transjugular Intrahepatic Portosystemic Shunt

Deddeh Ballah and Timothy W.I. Clark

Introduction

Transjugular intrahepatic portosystemic shunt (TIPS) has become the standard of care for portal decompression for the treatment of complications of portal hypertension (PHT), including bleeding varices and diuretic-resistant ascites. The hemodynamic changes associated with TIPS creation are complex and affect the portomesenteric venous and arterial systems as well as the heart. This chapter focuses on the hemodynamic changes that occur after TIPS and their clinical significance.

Hemodynamics of Cirrhosis and Portal Hypertension in Brief

The hemodynamic changes caused by cirrhosis and PHTs result from a complex interplay of neuorhormonal and structural changes. Cirrhosis creates increased resistance to portal blood flow, inducing portal venous dilatation and congestion of portal venous flow. The increased resistance to portal blood flow leads to the development of portosystemic collaterals. Ultimately, there is an increase in portal venous inflow, creating a hyperdynamic circulation that maintains and exacerbates PHT.[1,2]

The intrahepatic resistance caused by cirrhosis has both static and dynamic components. Hepatic stellate cells can cause sinusoidal vasoconstriction via contractile cytoplasmic processes through paracrine effects of endothelin-1 (ET-1) and relaxation via interactions with sinusoidal endothelial and paracrine effects of nitrous oxide (NO). The quantity of hepatic stellate cells increases in cirrhosis and induces sinusoidal vasoconstriction with increased vascular resistance. Although there is decreased hepatic NO production, there is increased systemic and splanchnic NO production, causing decreased systemic vascular resistance (SVR).[1] This causes a decrease in central blood volume.[3] The systemic circulation attempts to compensate for the decrease in effective arterial blood volume by sympathetic activation, activation of the renin–angiotensin–aldosterone-system (RAAS), and an increase in antidiuretic hormone.[1] In response to the decreased SVR, cardiac output increases, producing a higher than normal cardiac index.[3] Chronic increases in flow with vasodilatation causes endothelial signaling that leads to chronic increase in vessel diameter.[3] Eventually, individuals experience cardiac insufficiency and are unable to maintain arterial pressure as vasodilatation progresses. The kidneys become underperfused, and patients go into renal failure.[3]

Similar to systemic circulation, the liver is equipped with an intrinsic mechanism to compensate for decreased total hepatic blood flow. When portal blood flow is decreased to the liver, the hepatic arterial buffer response (HABR) maintains hepatic perfusion by increasing hepatic artery flow. Cirrhotic patients have been observed via duplex Doppler ultrasound examination to have hepatofugal portal venous blood. Patients with hepatofugal portal venous blood flow have a statistically significant lower resistive index in their hepatic arteries compared with patients

with hepatopedal flow indicating an active HABR. Interestingly, resistive index does not correlate inversely with the portosystemic gradient. Patients with hepatofugal flow elicit the HABR, which is accompanied by a decrease in the resistive index of the hepatic artery.[4]

Intrahepatic Hemodynamic Changes After TIPS

TIPS is a high-volume conduit connecting the portal and caval systems that causes acute portal decompression.[2] This low-resistance portal outflow tract allows for an increase in portal blood flow[2,5] and portal vein (PV) diameter.[5] Low-dose galactose clearance and Doppler ultrasonography have been used to note the increase in portal venous flow to be 48% after TIPS placement. After TIPS placement, the velocities in the main PV increase up to 170%[2,5,6] and remain increased after shunt placement for at least up to 12 months.[6] After TIPS placement, velocity through shunts is high velocity. Although peak velocities through shunts decrease slightly over time, they remain higher than pre-TIPS velocities.[6] The low-resistance shunt also results in diversion of flow toward the shunt and away from the liver. Doppler ultrasonography demonstrates flow reversal in the right and left hepatic veins from hepatopedal flow to hepatofugal after TIPS insertion.[6] This is consistent with the finding that low-dose galactose clearance after TIPS demonstrates a 48% increase in portal blood flow but a 60% decrease in effective hepatic blood flow within 4 to 6 days after shunt. Color-flow Doppler measures that portal flow proximal to the TIPS increased with shunting. The increased portal flow is diverted through the stent and away from the hepatic parenchyma.[2] Rosemurgy et al point out that most portal flow after the TIPS is non-nutrient because it is preferentially shunted to the systemic venous system and does not supply the liver.[2] Dynamic computed tomography has been used to measure changes in perfusion of the liver parenchyma. Compared with control participants, patients with cirrhosis showed increased arterial hepatic perfusion, decreased portal blood hepatic perfusion, and decreased total hepatic perfusion. Post-TIPS measurements revealed a significant increase in arterial blood hepatic perfusion and total hepatic perfusion, but portal venous hepatic perfusion remained the same.[7] In contrast to other studies, liver scintigraphy evaluation after hepatic perfusion has shown portal venous blood flow velocity increased significantly as well as the contribution from portal venous blood flow for hepatic perfusion increased from 9.2% to 38.2%.[8]

TIPS creation does not only affect flow through the PVs but also affects flow through the hepatic arteries. Doppler ultrasound interrogation has found hepatofugal and hepatopedal portal venous flow in patients with cirrhosis. Gulberg et al[3] noted that the hepatic artery resistive index was lower in patients with hepatofugal flow compared with those with hepatopedal flow before TIPS. After TIPS creation, the hepatic artery resistive index decreased in patients with hepatopedal flow but did not change in patients with hepatofugal flow. Because TIPS creation in patients with hepatofugal flow does not cause a further decrease in the amount of hepatic blood supply originating from the PV, there is no further hepatic artery dilatation.[4] Twenty-four hours after TIPS placement, there is a statistically significant increase in hepatic artery peak systolic velocity (HAPSV). This increase in hepatic artery flow reflects the HABR because TIPS results in decreased portal venous flow delivered to the liver. The HAPSV decreases during 12-month follow-up but remains elevated above baseline.[6] Similarly, Patel et al[9] used Doppler ultrasonography to investigate hepatic arterial blood flow after TIPS. They found an increase in hepatic arterial peak systolic velocity and hepatic arterial blood flow after TIPS. Hepatic artery diameter did not change significantly after TIPS. There was no correlation between the change in average increase in hepatic arterial blood flow before and after TIPS and the change in portosystemic gradient before and after TIPS.[9] It is interesting to note that TIPS placement causes similar portosystemic gradient reductions in patients with cirrhosis with hepatofugal portal venous flow compared with those with hepatopedal portal venous flow.[4]

Direct measurements of hepatic artery blood flow with intravascular Doppler sonography to investigate real-time changes in velocity during TIPS insertion reveal the same results as studies using indirect measurement methods. As seen in other studies, the average arterial peak velocity and maximum arterial peak velocities increased significantly after TIPS. Balloon occlusion of the shunt has been performed to determine the reversibility of average arterial peak velocity. Balloon occlusion resulted in restoration of the arterial average peak velocity not only to pre-TIPS velocity, but it also decreased to below baseline. Deflation of the balloon resulted in an increase of average peak velocity to post-TIPS values.[10]

Itkin et al investigated a new method for direct measurement of intrahepatic blood flow.[11] Their study validated and optimized the use of a thermodilutional catheter with the ability to measure retrograde blood flow in a domestic swine model. The authors demonstrated a high correlation between portal venous flow measurements taken with a thermodilutional catheter versus a gold standard of a surgically placed perivascular Doppler probe ($r^2 = 0.96$; $P <0.001$). Thermodilutional catheter blood flow rates of the PV and hepatic artery were measured before TIPS and 2 weeks after TIPS. In the swine with greater blood flow in the TIPS compared with the PV, an arteriogram was performed and demonstrated filling of the left and right PV with hepatofugal flow toward the proximal end of the TIPS. An occlusion balloon inflated at the common origin of the hepatic artery demonstrated decreased flow through the TIPS. When the balloon was completely deflated, flow returned to baseline. Similar to the study by Radeleff et al, the significant increase in blood flow after TIPS has been demonstrated to be secondary to increased hepatic artery blood flow. This experiment demonstrated arterioportal shunting both angiographically and hemodynamically.[11]

A prospective clinical study quantified hepatic artery-to-PV shunting using a direct thermodilutional catheter-based technique and by measuring changes in blood oxygenation within the TIPS and PV in patients undergoing primary TIPS insertion or revision (▶ Fig. 16.1). The study quantified shunting assuming that flow in the TIPS (Q_{TIPS}) was the combination of main PV flow (Q_{portal}) plus the reversed intrahepatic portal flow from hepatic artery-to-portal shunting; that is, $Q_{TIPS} = Q_{portal}$ + reversed flow. There was a 64% increase in mean portal flow after TIPS. Mean Q_{TIPS} was a 44% increase from final Q_{portal} (▶ Fig. 16.2).

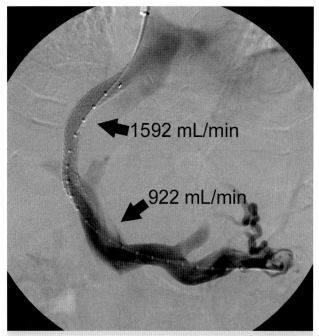

Fig. 16.1 Completion transjugular intrahepatic portosystemic shunt (TIPS) portogram showing the location of thermodilutional catheter during flow measurements in a patient with hepatitis C and alcoholic cirrhosis. Initial portosystemic gradient was 22 mm Hg; the final gradient was 8 mm Hg. Note the TIPS flow is higher than the main portal vein flow. *Reprinted with permission from Itkin M, Trerotola SO, Stavropoulos SW, et al. Portal flow and arterioportal shunting after transjugular intrahepatic portosystemic shunt creation. J Vasc Interv Radiol 2006;17(1):55–62.*

Given that only three of 26 patients had imaging evidence of an umbilical vein, it is highly unlikely that flow within a recanalized paraumbilical vein increased flow in the TIPS. This group hypothesized that shunting from the hepatic arterial system at

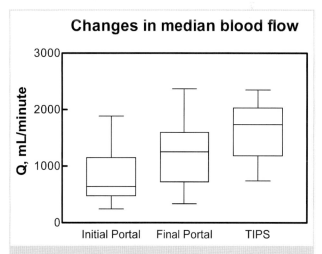

Fig. 16.2 Plot showing median (*middle of box*), 25th to 75th percentile (*edges of box*), and range (bars) of blood flows obtained during initial portal, final portal, and transjugular intrahepatic portosystemic shunt (TIPS) measurements in a prospective study of 26 TIPS patients. *Reprinted with permission from Itkin M, Trerotola SO, Stavropoulos SW, et al. Portal flow and arterioportal shunting after transjugular intrahepatic portosystemic shunt creation. J Vasc Interv Radiol 2006;17(1):55–62.*

the sinusoidal or presinusoidal level into the right and left PVs with hepatofugal flow into the TIPS. If arterioportal shunting occurs at the transvasal level, oxygen tension in the TIPS will be higher than in the PV. Conversely, if arterioportal shunting occurs via sinusoids where the efficient oxygen exchange of the periportal triad occurs, the oxygen tension will be lower in TIPS. Because there was only a small reduction in oxygen saturation when comparing the TIPS with the PV shunting, the study concluded that shunting occurs at the level of the sinusoid.[12]

The changes in hemodynamics after TIPS also have prognostic indications for patients. If one were to graph post-TIPS perfusion curves, they would appear "arterialized" because there is a loss of the portal augmentation phase. Interestingly, patients with arterialized waveforms but low total perfusion before TIPS had a significantly higher mortality rate than the groups with better total hepatic perfusion or a portal type waveform. Patients with portal-type flow curves do well after TIPS regardless of the total hepatic perfusion. Thus, perhaps the source of blood flow is not as important as the amount of blood flow to the liver.[13]

Systemic Hemodynamic Changes and Clinical Implications for Hepatorenal Syndrome and Ascites

The creation of a conduit connecting the systemic circulation to the portal circulation leads to a decrease in total peripheral resistance and allows for an increase of venous return to the heart. The combination of these two hemodynamic alterations has led some to postulate that TIPS worsens the hyperdynamic state of cirrhosis. Immediately after TIPS, the effects of increased preload drive the systemic hemodynamic changes. There are large increases of right atrial pressure and wedge pulmonary pressures immediately after TIPS indicating an increase in central venous return caused by splanchnic blood flow into the systemic circulation.[14-16] Despite the decrease in portal venous pressure and portosystemic gradient, the peripheral vasculature and pulmonary vasculature still remain vasodilated because vasodilatory substances from the splanchnic circulation are shunted to peripheral vascular beds by the newly created vascular communication.[14] This may explain why some studies do not observe an increase in mean arterial pressure (MAP) 1 hour after TIPS[16] but some note an increase in MAP that returns to baseline within 1 week of TIPS insertion.[17] Along with these changes, patients also experience an increase in end-diastolic volume, left ventricular ejection fraction, and left ventricular stroke volume.[15] Stanley et al noted that the decrease in portosystemic gradient had a significant correlation with the decrease in SVR and increase in cardiac output.[16] Post-TIPS magnetic resonance imaging of the heart reveals an increase in diastolic dimensions of the both the right and left cavities of the heart along with increased myocardial thickening during systole.[15]

Furthermore, there is increased myocardial thickening at the end of systole, signifying greater cardiac contractility.[15] As a result of the increasing preload and decrease in total peripheral resistance, there is also a significant increase in cardiac index immediately after TIPS. Several studies do not report a compensatory increase in heart rate in the setting of peripheral vasodilatation.[15,16] Elevated baseline epinephrine causes a decrease of β-adrenergic receptors on cardiac myocytes, leading to an attenuated cardiac stress response.[15] Whereas pulmonary artery pressure increases significantly after TIPS, pulmonary vascular resistance decreases nonsignificantly immediately after TIPS.[15] When using the azygous venous flow rate as a surrogate for gastrocollateral flow, one can conclude that the 30% decrease in flow rate over a 1-year after TIPS period—which is directly proportional to the decrease in changes in portal venous pressure—will decrease the risk of variceal bleed in cirrhotic patients.[17]

Follow-up of hemodynamic parameters reveals that patients undergo some adaptation to the hemodynamic changes caused by TIPS creation. Columbato et al noted that total peripheral resistance remained decreased at 2-month follow-up. Cardiac index, pulmonary capillary pressure, pulmonary arterial pressure, and right atrial pressure decreased during the 2 months after TIPS but were still elevated compared with pre-TIPS levels.[14] At 2 months, the decrease in cardiac index represents the beginning of cardiac adaptation to the increase in venous return to the heart.[14] Kovacs et al reported that at 4- to 6-month follow-up, stroke volume, cardiac dimension of the left ventricle, and total peripheral resistance returned to pre-TIPS values. However, these acute increases in preload resulted in mild left ventricular hypertrophy evidenced by an increase in left ventricular myocardial mass.[15] Lotterer et al studied the hemodynamic changes in patients for up to 1 year after TIPS creation and notably revealed that although cardiac output increased in the first 3 months after TIPS, it returned to baseline by 1 year after the procedure.[17]

TIPS creation does not result in systematic changes in cerebral perfusion in patients when comparing pre- and post-TIPS insertion. Patients may experience slight improvements in mental status in terms of reaction times and cirrhosis as evaluated by Child-Pugh score.[18]

TIPS has been seen to improve diastolic dysfunction. The ratio of early maximal ventricular filling velocity/late filling velocity (E/A) as a surrogate marker for diastolic dysfunction are those with a normal E/A ratio greater than 1. In the series of 32 TIPS patients reported by Cazzaniga et al, the number of patients with normal E/A increased after TIPS in eight patients (25%), and the number of patients with low E/A ratio decreased by eight (25%). Also, percent changes in E/A ratio were directly proportional to stroke volume, left ventricular end-diastolic volume, and atrial natriuretic peptide level.[19] Also, post-TIPS E/A was a predictor of mortality.[19]

Portal hypertension is often complicated by two entities that share pathophysiologic similarities: hepatorenal syndrome (HRS) and ascites. Ascites is caused by splanchnic vasodilatation, which increases portal venous flow coupled with increased hepatic resistance from PHT. The decrease in effective arterial blood volume results in activation of the RAAS and antinatriuretic factors that increase sodium retention and reabsorption. Changes in intestinal capillary pressure result in preferential fluid accumulation in the abdomen.[20] HRS is a progressive renal failure of otherwise normal kidneys caused by cirrhosis. Type I HRS has rapid onset with a high mortality rate. Liver transplant is the treatment of choice for HRS. Type II HRS is slower, progressive onset of renal failure. Because all patients with HRS are not good surgical candidates, TIPS offers another treatment option.[21]

Renal autoregulation ensures that the kidney receives constant blood flow regardless of fluctuation of blood pressure. However, the pathophysiology of cirrhosis affects this autoregulation in at least two ways. First, renal autoregulation only operates at a perfusion pressure of greater than 65 to 75 mm Hg. Renal blood flow decreases in proportion to this critical value, and autoregulation does not function properly. Thus, the systemic vasodilatation seen in cirrhosis impairs this renal mechanism. Second, the chronic increase in sympathetic tone observed in patients with cirrhosis negatively impacts the effects of renal autoregulation. As mentioned earlier, this vasodilatation results in a reflexive increase in systemic sympathetic tone. This causes a rightward shift of renal autoregulation and causes renal blood flow and renal function to be highly dependent on blood pressure. In a patient with a baseline normal sympathetic tone, this acute increase in sympathetic tone would activate the RAAS cascade and allow for adequate renal perfusion. However, in a cirrhotic, vasodilated patient, the pressures produced by patients with cirrhosis are not sufficient to maintain renal function and rather exacerbates renal underperfusion.[22]

Investigating the changes in renal vasoactive substances along with hemodynamic parameters elucidates physiologic changes that lead to improved renal function after TIPS. Stadlbauer et al closely examined the effect of TIPS on hemodynamics 3 to 4 weeks after TIPS placement in patients with no ascites, diuretic-responsive ascites, intractable ascites, type II HRS, and refractory ascites requiring TIPS. This study demonstrated the relationships between hemodynamic parameters and hormone imbalances in patients with increasing levels of fluid retention. At baseline, they noted that patients with type II HRS had higher creatinine than other groups. Stadlbauer et al noted that creatinine clearance decreased as patients' severity of fluid retention increased. Based on what we know from renal autoregulation and liver cirrhosis, it is not surprising that patients with refractory ascites and type II HRS had lower MAP and SVR and increased cardiac output compared with the other groups of patients. Similarly, patients with HRS and refractory ascites have higher plasma norepinephrine compared with the other groups of patients. Although all groups had decreased renal blood flow and renal perfusion pressure, patients with type II HRS and refractory ascites had much lower values. MAP, urine sodium excretion, creatinine clearance, and SVR positively correlated with renal blood flow. Cardiac output, hepatic venous pressure gradient, and norepinephrine serum levels had negative correlations with renal blood flow. Insertion of TIPS led to a decrease in hepatic venous pressure gradient and serum norepinephrine levels, leading to an increase in renal blood flow without a significant change in blood pressure.[22]

Brensing et al investigated effects of TIPS placement on renal function in patients with type I and type II HRS. The study found that patients with type I and type II HRS had very different glomerular filtration rates (GFRs) but had similar decreases in urine sodium excretion and serum sodium.[21] Similar to the study by Stadlbauer et al., within the first month of TIPS placement, there is a significant improvement of renal function markers such as serum creatine, creatinine clearance, serum urea, sodium excretion, and urine volume. Four of seven (57%) hemodialysis-dependent patients had restored kidney function, allowing for withdrawal of hemodialysis and reintroduction of diuretics. Portal and systemic activation of the renin–angiotensin system were both decreased after TIPS. After TIPS placement, ET-1 decreased in the portal system.[21] TIPS insertion leads to improved central venous filling, leading to decrease in systemic vasoconstrictors, leading to increased sodium excretion and increased GFR.[23] A decrease in sinusoidal pressure after TIPS may also decrease sympathetic-mediated renal proximal tubule sodium retention.[21]

It is interesting to note that although there are immediate changes in hemodynamic parameters, TIPS does not provide an acute increase in renal blood flow.[16] Guevara et al demonstrated that the suppression of hormones closely linked to volume status in cirrhotic patients, such as renin, aldosterone, and epinephrine, did not occur 1 week after TIPS in their series of seven patients with type I HRS.[24] One month after TIPS, patients had improved hemodynamics, with decreased creatinine and blood urea nitrogen, but GFR and renal plasma flow (RPF) increased but were still below normal. There was also significant increase in urine volume but a nonsignificant increase in free water clearance and sodium excretion. As a result, the positive sodium balance resulted in all patients experiencing ascites. And although the RAAS and sympathetic nervous systems were significantly decreased from pre-TIPS values, they still remained abnormal. Furthermore, arterial pressure did not change after TIPS. However, because the patients were able to maintain their blood pressure to pre-TIPS levels in the setting of RAAS suppression, this suggests that patients may be restoring their renal autoregulation curve to normal.[24]

The aforementioned studies discussed the use of TIPS in patients without adjunctive medical therapy to optimize their hemodynamic status. Wong et al explored the utility of TIPS in treating patients with type I HRS in conjunction with midodrine, octreotide, and albumin to optimize hemodynamic function before TIPS. Ten of the 14 patients (71%) in this series responded to medical therapy with a significant increase in GFR, renal plasma flow, urinary volume, and urine sodium and a decrease in renal vascular resistance, serum creatinine, and serum urea. These patients benefitted from TIPS creation. As in other series, these patients demonstrated an increasing hyperdynamic state with increased cardiac output and reduction in SVR that was associated with increased MAP and increase in central blood volume. However, after 6 months, systemic hemodynamics trended toward normal with a decrease in central blood volume, again demonstrating the resolution of the worsened hyperdynamic state after TIPS. Patients also had a decrease in renin, aldosterone, and norepinephrine during their 12-month follow-up period.[25]

The results of several studies show that HRS patients benefit from TIPS, but some evidence suggests that some patients benefit significantly more than others. Anderson et al revealed a significant correlation between the amount of renal dysfunction and the amount of renal improvement.[26] In other words, patients with worse kidney function benefit the most from TIPS creation. In patients with increased creatinine, there was a decrease in creatinine level after TIPS. The authors found that indication for TIPS placement can also effect a change in creatinine. Only patients who had TIPS for variceal bleeding and had poor kidney function had an improvement in renal function after TIPS, but patients who had TIPS for variceal bleeding and normal creatinine did not see improvement in renal function. Furthermore, patients who had refractory ascites or hepatohydrothorax had an improvement in renal function after TIPS. Interestingly, patients without renal dysfunction before TIPS had an increase in model for end-stage liver disease (MELD) score after TIPS, but patients with renal dysfunction showed a decrease in MELD score after TIPS.[26]

Several series have shown the success of TIPS in the treatment of ascites. The hormonal changes crucial to restoration of renal function in patients with HRS are also those necessary to improve ascites. A study by Wong et al revealed patients with ascites who had improved natriuresis and hormonal profile did not have increased renal blood flow or improved MAP. In fact, it occurred in the setting of vasodilatation.[23] Thus, it would seem that the neurohormonal changes are more important in the treatment of ascites as opposed to return to a normal hemodynamic profile. A subsequent study by Wong et al noted that with normalization of sinusoidal pressure below the critical value of 8 mm Hg, natriuresis begins at 2 weeks. This 2-week natriuresis is related to normal plasma renin activity and a decrease of aldosterone. However, a negative sodium balance was achieved at 4 weeks, which is consistent with other studies. At 1 month after TIPS, there is already a marked increase in serum sodium consistent with improvement of hyponatremia. At 12 months, there is a marked decrease in RAAS hormones and norepinephrine corresponding to a decrease in sodium reabsorption and increase in natriuresis. As ascites is increasingly controlled by restoration of normal neurohormonal substances that cause natriuresis, patients require fewer diuretics and paracenteses.[27]

Long-term follow-up studies have demonstrated that TIPS is effective in the treatment of ascites. At 6 months after TIPS, all patients in this 14-patient series had complete resolution. Fourteen months after TIPS, patients had markedly improved renal hemodynamics with a decrease in renal vascular resistance along with a significant increase in renal blood flow and GFR. They also demonstrate the ability to maintain sodium balance. Sodium balance was maintained in most patients except four of 14 (29%) with mild pedal edema. Sodium loading at 14 months showed the appropriate physiologic responses with increased sodium excretion and suppression of the RAAS.[28]

Conclusion

Portal hypertension can produce a multitude of hemodynamic changes that can have life-threatening complications. TIPS is a minimally invasive procedure that has proven effectiveness in the treatment of varices, HRS, and ascites. The portal, cardiovascular, and renal changes that occur after TIPS are complex and interdependent; an improved understanding of these effects can improve patient selection, risk stratification, and follow-up protocols.

Clinical Pearls

- Post-TIPS hemodynamics are complex and involve not only the portomesenteric venous system but the arterial circulation and heart as well.
- Liver cirrhosis causes increased peripheral vascular resistance. Neurohormonal and structural changes, including portosystemic shunt creation, lead to hyperdynamic portal circulation.
- Liver cirrhosis leads to reduced NO production by the liver and increased systemic and splanchnic NO production, which leads to systemic vasodilation and hyperdynamic circulation, decreased cardiac index, reduced intravascular volume, and increased antidiuretic hormone and leads to eventual cardiac insufficiency, renal hypoperfusion, and renal failure.
- Because of decreased inline portal blood flow to the liver, there is decreased hepatic arterial resistive index and compensatory increase in hepatic arterial flow mediated by the HABR.

- TIPS is a high-velocity conduit that bridges the portal vein with the hepatic vein and thus shunts from the PV to the hepatic vein. This leads to an approximate 50% increase in main portal flow but a decrease inline portal perfusion.
- The reduced portal hepatic perfusion after TIPS leads to increased arterial peak systolic velocity and increased arterial flow.

References

1. Kim MY, Baik SK, Lee SS. Hemodynamic alterations in cirrhosis and portal hypertension. Korean J Heptal 2010;16(4):347–352.
2. Iwakiri Y, Groszmann RJ. The hyperdynamic circulation of chronic liver diseases: from the patient to the molecule. Hepatology 2006;43(2 suppl 1):S121–S131.
3. Gulberg V, Haag K, Rossle M, Gerbes AL. Hepatic arterial buffer response in patients with advanced cirrhosis. Hepatology 2002;35(3):630–634.
4. Rosemurgy AS, Zervos EE, Goode SE, et al. Differential effects on portal and effective hepatic blood flow. A comparison between transjugular intrahepatic portasystemic shunt and small-diameter H-graft portacaval shunt. Ann Surg 1997;225(5):601–607; discussion 7–8.
5. Lafortune M, Martinet JP, Denys A, et al. Short- and long-term hemodynamic effects of transjugular intrahepatic portosystemic shunts: a Doppler/manometric correlative study. AJR Am J Roentgenol 1995;164(4):997–1002.
6. Foshager MC, Ferral H, Nazarian GK, et al. Duplex sonography after transjugular intrahepatic portosystemic shunts (TIPS): normal hemodynamic findings and efficacy in predicting shunt patency and stenosis. AJR Am J Roentgenol 1995;165(1):1–7.
7. Weidekamm C, Cejna M, Kramer L, et al. Effects of TIPS on liver perfusion measured by dynamic CT. AJR Am J Roentgenol 2005;184(2):505–510.
8. Menzel J, Schober O, Reimer P, Domschke W. Scintigraphic evaluation of hepatic blood flow after intrahepatic portosystemic shunt (TIPS). Eur J Nucl Med 1997;24(6):635–641.
9. Patel NH, Sasadeusz KJ, Seshadri R, et al. Increase in hepatic arterial blood flow after transjugular intrahepatic portosystemic shunt creation and its potential predictive value of postprocedural encephalopathy and mortality. J Vasc Interv Radiol 2001;12(11):1279–1284.
10. Radeleff B, Sommer CM, Heye T, et al. Acute increase in hepatic arterial flow during TIPS identified by intravascular flow measurements. Cardiovasc Intervent Radiol 2009;32(1):32–37.
11. Itkin M, Trerotola SO, Kolff JW, Clark TW. Measurement of portal blood and transjugular intrahepatic portosystemic shunt flow with use of a retrograde thermodilutional catheter. J Vasc Interv Radiol 2004;15(10):1105–1110.
12. Itkin M, Trerotola SO, Stavropoulos SW, et al. Portal flow and arterioportal shunting after transjugular intrahepatic portosystemic shunt creation. J Vasc Interv Radiol 2006;17(1):55–62.
13. Walser EM, DeLa Pena R, Villanueva-Meyer J, et al. Hepatic perfusion before and after the transjugular intrahepatic portosystemic shunt procedure: impact on survival. J Vasc Interv Radiol 2000;11(7):913–918.
14. Colombato LA, Spahr L, Martinet JP, et al. Haemodynamic adaptation two months after transjugular intrahepatic portosystemic shunt (TIPS) in cirrhotic patients. Gut 1996;39(4):600–604.
15. Kovacs A, Schepke M, Heller J, et al. Short-term effects of transjugular intrahepatic shunt on cardiac function assessed by cardiac MRI: preliminary results. Cardiovasc Intervent Radiol 2010;33(2):290–296.
16. Stanley AJ, Redhead DN, Bouchier IA, Hayes PC. Acute effects of transjugular intrahepatic portosystemic stent-shunt (TIPSS) procedure on renal blood flow and cardiopulmonary hemodynamics in cirrhosis. Am J Gastroenterol 1998;93(12):2463–2468.
17. Lotterer E, Wengert A, Fleig WE. Transjugular intrahepatic portosystemic shunt: short-term and long-term effects on hepatic and systemic hemodynamics in patients with cirrhosis. Hepatology 1999;29(3):632–639.
18. Iversen P, Keiding S, Mouridsen K, et al. Transjugular intrahepatic portosystemic shunt does not alter cerebral blood flow. Clin Gastroenterol Hepatol 2011;9(11):1001–1003.
19. Cazzaniga M, Salerno F, Pagnozzi G, et al. Diastolic dysfunction is associated with poor survival in patients with cirrhosis with transjugular intrahepatic portosystemic shunt. Gut 2007;56(6):869–875.
20. Senzolo M, Cholongitas E, Tibballs J, et al. Transjugular intrahepatic portosystemic shunt in the management of ascites and hepatorenal syndrome. Eur J Gastroenterol Hepatol 2006;18(11):1143–1150.

21. Brensing KA, Textor J, Perz J, et al. Long term outcome after transjugular intrahepatic portosystemic stent-shunt in non-transplant cirrhotics with hepatorenal syndrome: a phase II study. Gut 2000;47(2):288–295.

22. Stadlbauer V, Wright GA, Banaji M, et al. Relationship between activation of the sympathetic nervous system and renal blood flow autoregulation in cirrhosis. Gastroenterology 2008;134(1):111–1119.

23. Wong F, Sniderman K, Liu P, et al. Transjugular intrahepatic portosystemic stent shunt: effects on hemodynamics and sodium homeostasis in cirrhosis and refractory ascites. Ann Intern Med 1995;122(11):816–822.

24. Guevara M, Gines P, Bandi JC, et al. Transjugular intrahepatic portosystemic shunt in hepatorenal syndrome: effects on renal function and vasoactive systems. Hepatology 1998;28(2):416–422.

25. Wong F, Pantea L, Sniderman K. Midodrine, octreotide, albumin, and TIPS in selected patients with cirrhosis and type 1 hepatorenal syndrome. Hepatology 2004;40(1):55–64.

26. Anderson CL, Saad WE, Kalagher SD, et al. Effect of transjugular intrahepatic portosystemic shunt placement on renal function: a 7-year, single-center experience. J Vasc Interv Radiol 2010;21(9):1370–1376.

27. Quiroga J, Sangro B, Nunez M, et al. Transjugular intrahepatic portal-systemic shunt in the treatment of refractory ascites: effect on clinical, renal, humoral, and hemodynamic parameters. Hepatology 1995;21(4):986–994.

28. Wong W, Liu P, Blendis L, Wong F. Long-term renal sodium handling in patients with cirrhosis treated with transjugular intrahepatic portosystemic shunts for refractory ascites. Am J Med 1999;106(3):315–322.

Chapter 17: Budd-Chiari Syndrome: Transjugular Intrahepatic Portosystemic Shunt and Hepatic Vein Recanalization

Sundeep Punamiya and Hector Ferral

Introduction

Budd-Chiari syndrome (BCS) refers to hepatic venous outflow obstruction, occurring at any level from hepatic veins to the suprahepatic segment of the inferior vena cava (IVC). The obstruction may be caused by hepatic lesions such as a tumor, cyst, or abscess and is termed "secondary BCS," but this accounts for only a small number of cases. In most cases, it occurs from thrombosis of the hepatic veins or the IVC and is termed "primary BCS." Several prothrombotic risk factors are known to cause primary BCS (▶ Table 17.1), one or more of which are detected in almost 90% of cases.[1]

Primary BCS begins with acute thrombosis of the hepatic vein outflow over a variable length of the hepatic vein, IVC, or both. This later evolves toward fibrous sequelae, forming stenosis, webs, or membranes.[2] The resultant venous obstruction causes an increase in hepatic sinusoidal pressure that leads to a cascade of events in the liver, beginning with hepatocellular congestion, necrosis, and finally cirrhosis. Over a period of time, venous collaterals develop in an attempt to spontaneously decongest the liver. Extrahepatic portal vein thrombosis is seen in 15% of patients with BCS, likely secondary to flow stasis within the portal vein and preexisting prothrombotic diatheses.[3]

Budd-Chiari syndrome is classified according to the level of hepatic venous outflow obstruction (▶ Table 17.2). Endovascular treatment of BCS is based on the level of obstruction, chronicity of disease, and morphology of the obstructive lesion.[4,5]

Treatment of Budd-Chiari Syndrome

Anticoagulation and, if possible, treatment of underlying disorders (e.g., myeloproliferative disease, paroxysmal nocturnal hemoglobinuria) form the cornerstone of therapy in BCS and should be initiated as early as possible in the disease.[4] Anticoagulation alone succeeds in controlling liver disease in 10% of patients.[5]

Next, whenever possible, recanalization of the hepatic venous outflow by angioplasty and stenting should be attempted because it restores physiological blood flow and decongests the liver with minimal risk. This is offered in both symptomatic and asymptomatic patients and is feasible if the stenosis or occlusion of the hepatic veins or IVC is of short segment.[6]

A transjugular intrahepatic portosystemic shunt (TIPS) is recommended in symptomatic patients with BCS when (1) the hepatic vein occlusive segment is long, (2) there is failure to recanalize the hepatic veins, or (3) there is no clinical benefit from hepatic vein recanalization.[7–10] Surgery is considered only when radiologic procedures fail to resolve the symptoms or if the liver dysfunction is very severe, warranting an urgent liver transplantation.

Hepatic Venous Recanalization

Strategies to Recanalize Hepatic Venous Outflow

The first step involves angiographic assessment of the venous outflow. If the IVC lumen is compromised at or above the level of insertion of hepatic veins, it should be recanalized first. Caval recanalization would suffice if the hepatic veins are patent or if there is a prominent inferior right hepatic vein that contributes to the hepatic venous outflow. Hepatic vein recanalization is required in absence of any single, dominant hepatic outflow channel. For this, restoring flow to the largest of the three hepatic veins is usually sufficient for relief of symptoms.

Table 17.1 Common Causes of Thrombotic Diathesis Associated with Budd-Chiari Syndrome, with Recommended Investigations[1]

Common Causes	Recommended Investigations
Myeloproliferative disorders	Complete blood cell count, bone marrow biopsy, total red blood cell mass, and serum erythropoietin after correction for iron deficiency, endogenous erythrocyte colonies, and *V617F JAK2* mutation
Antiphospholipid syndrome	Anticardiolipin antibodies, lupus anticoagulant, anti-β_2-glycoprotein-1 antibodies, antinuclear antibodies
Paroxysmal nocturnal hemoglobinuria	Flow cytometry for CR55- and CD59-deficient cells
Hyperhomocysteinemia	Serum folate, vitamin B_{12}, and homocysteine levels, MTHFR polymorphism
Factor V Leiden mutation	Activated Protein C resistance, DNA analysis for G1691A substitution in factor V gene
Prothrombin gene mutation	DNA analysis for G20210A substitution in factor II gene
Protein C deficiency	Protein C plasma level
Protein S deficiency	Protein S plasma level
Antithrombin III deficiency	Antithrombin III plasma level
Behçet's disease	History and clinical examination
Oral contraceptive use	History
Pregnancy and postpartum status	History and clinical examination

MTHFR: methylene tetrahydrofolate reductase.

Table 17.2 Classification of Budd-Chiari Syndrome According to Site of Obstruction[4,5]

Site of Obstruction	Frequency According to Imaging Techniques (%)	Criteria
Small hepatic veins	NA	Involvement of veins that cannot be clearly shown on hepatic venography or ultrasonography, including terminal hepatic veins and intercalated and interlobular veins
Large hepatic veins	50	Involvement of veins that are regularly seen on hepatic venography or ultrasonography, including segmental branches of hepatic veins
Inferior vena cava	2	Involvement of one segment of the IVC, which extends from the entry level of the right, middle, and left hepatic veins to the junction between the IVC and the right atrium
Combined obstruction	47	Involvement of the large hepatic veins and IVC

IVC: inferior vena cava.

Technique of Inferior Vena Cava Recanalization

Recanalization is usually attempted from a femoral transvenous approach using a catheter and hydrophilic guidewire to cross the lesion. An IVC web or stenosis is generally traversable and can be easily dilated and stented with a large-diameter self-expandable or balloon-expandable stent (▶ Fig. 17.1).

An IVC membrane, however, cannot be crossed easily with a guidewire and often requires fenestration. This can be achieved with the stiff back end of a guidewire or with a Rösch-Uchida or Ring needle, at times accompanied by a coaxial long 22-gauge needle advanced carefully toward the patent suprahepatic IVC. A suitable entry point can be identified with a pigtail catheter placed in the suprahepatic IVC from a jugular approach (▶ Fig. 17.2). After successful fenestration, the membrane is sequentially dilated with angioplasty balloons of increasing diameter before deployment of a large-diameter stent.

Technique of Hepatic Vein Recanalization

The hepatic vein can be recanalized from a transvenous approach or a transhepatic approach, either alone or in combination.

1. **Transvenous approach** (▶ **Fig. 17.3**): The hepatic vein ostium is accessed from a jugular or femoral access, after which the hepatic vein lesion is traversed with a guidewire or fenestrated with a TIPS puncture needle. The lesion is then dilated and stented, usually with a balloon-expandable stent.
2. **Transhepatic approach** (▶ **Fig. 17.4**): This is generally used when the transvenous approach fails. A peripheral hepatic vein branch is accessed with an Accustick or Neff set under ultrasound guidance, and a 6- to 8-Fr sheath is inserted. An appropriately angled angiographic catheter and guidewire are then used to cross the hepatic vein lesion. If the lesion cannot be traversed with a guidewire, a Chiba needle can be used for fenestration. After it is crossed, the lesion is dilated

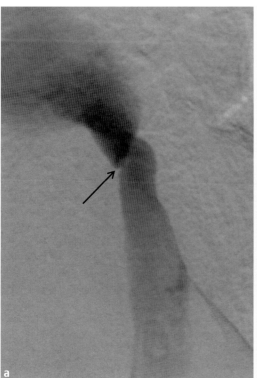
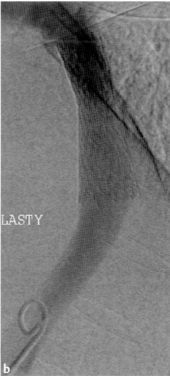

Fig. 17.1 A 54-year-old man with Budd-Chiari syndrome from an occult myeloproliferative disorder. (a) Cavogram shows a weblike narrowing (*arrow*) in the suprahepatic inferior vena cava with a 30–mm Hg pressure gradient across it. (b) The lesion could be crossed with a hydrophilic wire, dilated sequentially with 10- and 16-mm angioplasty balloons, and stented with a 20-mm diameter nitinol stent.

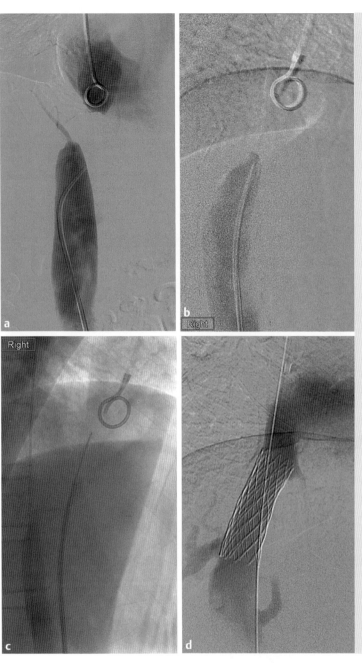

Fig. 17.2 Inferior vena cava (IVC) membrane in a 43-year-old man with systemic lupus erythematosus. (**a**) Cavogram shows a 2-cm-long IVC occlusion. (**b**) A Rösch-Uchida liver access set (RUPS) cannula was introduced, with its tip directed superiorly and anteriorly toward the patent suprahepatic segment. (**c**) Fenestration done with a 22-gauge coaxial Chiba needle, using a pigtail catheter placed in the suprahepatic IVC as a target. (**d**) Cavogram after balloon dilatation and deployment of a Palmaz XL balloon-expandable stent.

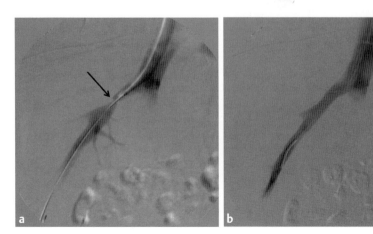

Fig. 17.3 Transvenous recanalization of a hepatic vein stenosis in a 35-year-old man with Budd-Chiari syndrome caused by polycythemia vera and presenting with a large hepatic hydrothorax. (**a**) The middle hepatic vein was cannulated with a multipurpose catheter introduced from a jugular access, and the venogram shows a focal stenosis of the middle hepatic vein (*arrow*). The right and left hepatic veins were occluded. (**b**) The stenosis could be crossed with a guidewire and primarily stented with a 9-mm Palmaz stent.

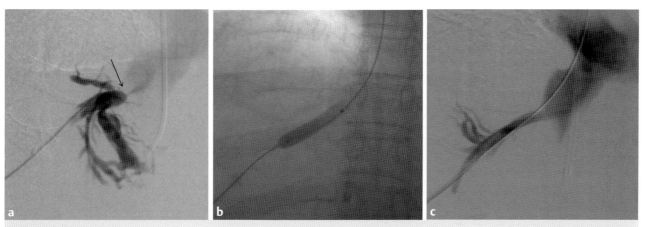

Fig. 17.4 Transhepatic recanalization of a hepatic vein stenosis in a 36-year-old man with Budd-Chiari syndrome presenting with ascites. (**a**) The hepatic vein could not be cannulated from the jugular vein and had to be accessed percutaneously from an ultrasound-guided transhepatic puncture after large-volume paracentesis. Venogram through a percutaneous 7-Fr sheath shows a weblike narrowing at the ostium of the right hepatic vein (*arrow*). (**b**) The stenosis was crossed with a guidewire and dilated with an 8-mm angioplasty balloon. (**c**) Posttreatment venography shows a satisfactory result, after which the parenchymal tract was occluded with embolization coils and Gelfoam slurry.

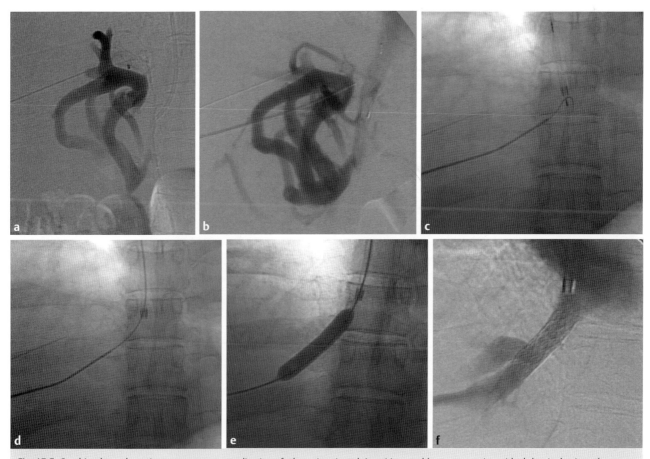

Fig. 17.5 Combined transhepatic–transvenous recanalization of a hepatic vein web in a 44-year-old man presenting with abdominal pain and large-volume ascites. (**a**) Hepatic venography shows the occluded right hepatic vein, which could not be accessed from the jugular vein and had to be accessed from a percutaneous transhepatic approach. (**b**) The occlusion could not be traversed with a wire and required fenestration with a sheathed needle. (**c,d**) After needle fenestration, the wire was snared from the jugular sheath. (**e**) Subsequent balloon angioplasty and stenting were performed from the jugular access. (**f**) Patency of vein was restored after implantation of a 10-mm Palmaz stent. The percutaneous needle tract was embolized.

and stented from the transhepatic route itself, after which the tract is embolized with coils or glue. It is common for patients with BCS to have large-volume ascites; therefore, a peritoneal drain may be required when this approach is being used.

3. **Combined transhepatic–transvenous approach** (▶ Fig. 17.5): This alternative could be used if there is concern for upsizing the parenchymal tract in patients having significant ascites. With this method, the hepatic vein lesion is crossed from a transhepatic approach as outlined earlier. When the guidewire enters the IVC, it is snared and removed from the jugular access. Subsequent balloon dilatation and stent placement are then continued from the jugular approach.

Technique of Combined Inferior Vena Cava and Hepatic Vein Recanalization

If the IVC is obstructed at the level of the hepatic vein insertion, it often requires restoration of flow through the IVC as well as the hepatic vein. This can be performed in two different ways:

1. **Kissing stent approach** (▶ Fig. 17.6): The IVC and hepatic veins are each recanalized as explained earlier, after which "kissing" self-expandable stents are deployed across the hepatic vein and IVC.

2. **T-stent approach** (▶ Fig. 17.7): The IVC is first recanalized and stented. Next, the hepatic vein obstruction is crossed from a transhepatic approach, and the IVC lumen is entered through the stent wall. An angioplasty balloon is then used to dilate the hepatic vein lesion and caval stent interstices followed by deployment of a balloon-expandable stent, ensuring that the hepatic vein stent protrudes slightly into the caval lumen.

Results and Complications of Hepatic Venous Outflow Recanalization

Hepatic venous outflow recanalization has a technical success rate of up to 97%, with failures reported mostly in patients with long segment occlusion.[6–10] In a large retrospective study, cumulative 1-, 5-, and 10-year primary and secondary patency rates of 95%, 77% and 58%, and 97%, 90% and 86%, respectively, have been achieved.[8] Predictably, reocclusion rates were higher in patients undergoing balloon angioplasty than stenting (31% vs. 7.7%). Interestingly, one fourth of these patients remained asymptomatic despite the occlusion, presumably from development of

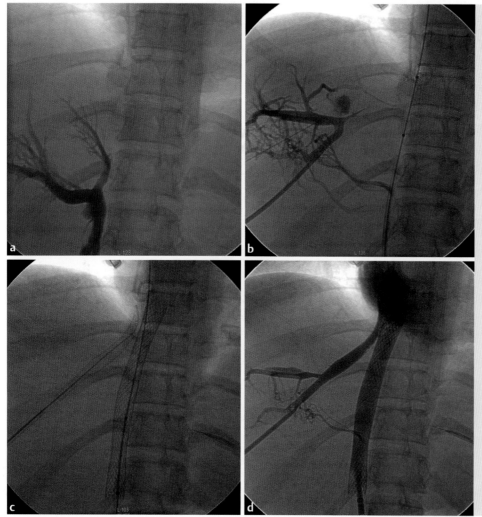

Fig. 17.6 Combined hepatic and caval recanalization with kissing stents in a 28-year-old woman having chronic occlusion at the hepatocaval confluence. (**a**) Cavogram from the femoral approach shows an 8-cm-long occlusion of the juxta hepatic inferior vena cava (IVC). (**b**) Percutaneous hepatic venogram shows an occlusion 4 cm in length of the right hepatic vein. (**c**) The caval occlusion could be recanalized with the stiff back end of the guidewire, but the hepatic vein occlusion required needle fenestration, after which 8- and 16-mm-diameter Wallstents were deployed side by side in the hepatic vein and IVC, respectively. (**d**) Final venogram shows patency restored to the IVC and right hepatic vein.

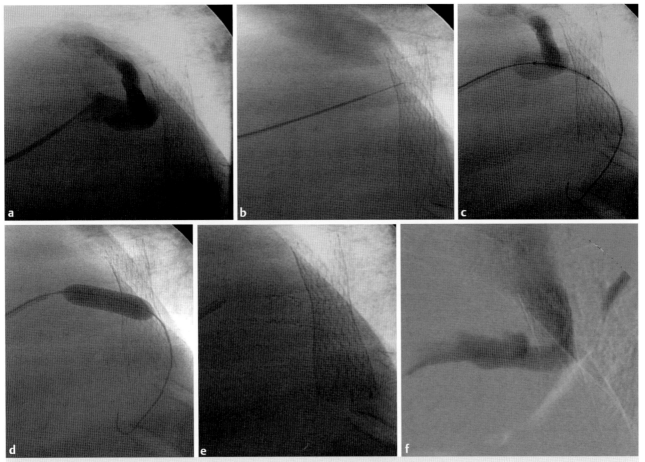

Fig. 17.7 T-stenting for a 54-year-old man with Budd-Chiari syndrome from an occult myeloproliferative disorder who had undergone stenting of an inferior vena cava (IVC) web, with no clinical response. (**a**) Percutaneous hepatic venogram showing membranous occlusion at the ostium of the middle hepatic vein. (**b**) Needle fenestration of the hepatic vein membrane was done with a 22-gauge Chiba needle, penetrating the IVC stent. (**c-e**) The stent was fenestrated with an angioplasty balloon after which a 10-mm Palmaz stent was deployed across the IVC stent fenestration. (**f**) Posttreatment venography shows good flow across the hepatic vein and IVC stents.

more venous collaterals. Recanalization procedures are fairly safe, with no reported deaths in most case series. However, severe complications such as hepatic laceration, capsular perforation, and venous rupture have been reported in fewer than 2% of patients, requiring prompt surgical intervention.[8] Long-term outcomes of hepatic outflow recanalization are excellent, with cumulative 1-, 5-, and 10-year survival rates of 96%, 83%, and 73%, respectively.

Transjugular Intrahepatic Portosystemic Shunt

The use of TIPS in the management of BCS was first reported in 1993.[11] This report included the description of two patients: one with fulminant BCS and the other with subacute BCS. The procedure was successful in both patients, and it established the possibility of managing this condition with a percutaneously created shunt.[11] The ability to manage BCS with a minimally invasive procedure represented a significant progress mainly because surgical options may be limited.[12–14] Several reports have now been published, and for the most part, all have demonstrated that TIPS is a valid therapeutic option in patients with BCS.[12,15–22]

Technique of Transjugular Intrahepatic Portosystemic Shunt in Budd-Chiari Syndrome

Creation of a TIPS in a patient with BCS may be technically difficult because there is either stenosis or absence of hepatic veins. The technical difficulties associated with TIPS creation in these patients may make the procedure lengthy and increase the risk for a technical failure or a major complication.[15,21] Technical modifications such as intraparenchymal puncture, transcaval puncture, and ultrasound-guided TIPS may be necessary to create a successful track between the IVC and the portal vein.[21,23–25] In addition, because these patients usually have enlarged livers, the creation of the track usually requires more than one stent to cover the entire length properly.[21]

Hepatic venous occlusion often requires a transcaval puncture for the TIPS. The cava can be most safely punctured in its retrohepatic or "safe" zone within 6 cm of the right atrium.[26] At this site, however, the puncture needle tends to slide down the IVC during the transcaval puncture because of lack of anchorage. A left internal jugular vein approach is useful in such cases because

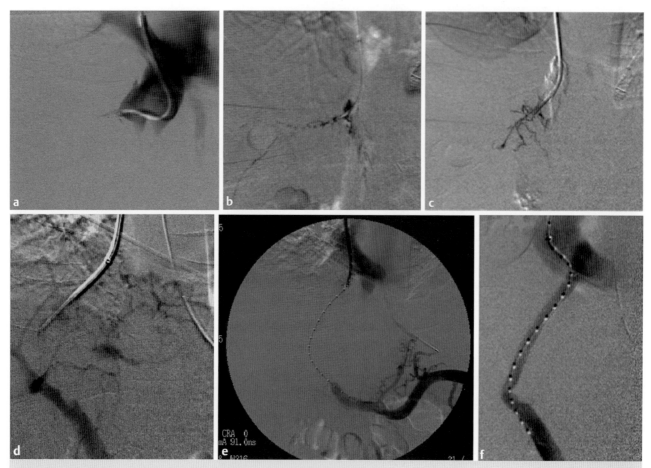

Fig. 17.8 A 29-year-old man, previously healthy, presented to the hospital with fulminant liver failure. The initial workup with an emergency transjugular liver biopsy (not shown) showed signs of severe congestion, consistent with the diagnosis of fulminant Budd-Chiari syndrome (BCS). The images were obtained during an emergency transjugular intrahepatic portosystemic shunt (TIPS) procedure. (**a**) Image obtained during TIPS creation in a patient with BCS. The spot film shows an Amplatz left coronary catheter advanced from the left internal jugular vein. A small "nipple" is identified, corresponding to the stump of the occluded hepatic vein. (**b**) The angiographic catheter has now been advanced into the liver parenchyma, and contrast injection demonstrates atretic hepatic veins. (**c**) The guiding cannula has been gently buried within the liver parenchyma. Contrast has been injected via the tip of the Rösch-Uchida system (Cook, Bloomington, Indiana). The classic "spider-web" appearance is demonstrated. (**d**) The needle has been carefully advanced into the liver parenchyma. The spot film was obtained during CO_2 injection into the liver parenchyma via the Rösch-Uchida system. The portal vein is clearly demonstrated. (**e**) Image obtained after successful entry into the portal system. The portogram was performed using a measuring catheter. Notice the long track through the liver parenchyma. (**f**) Direct portogram performed after successful shunt creation shows a widely patent shunt from the right portal vein, directly into the inferior vena cava. This shunt was created with two overlapping VIATORR stent grafts.

the angle of entry into the right side of the liver coming from a left IJV approach is usually very direct, and in the authors' opinion, makes it easier to "bury" the trocar or puncture system into the liver parenchyma. A gentle but firm forward pressure needs to be applied into this area to perform the transparenchymal puncture. Most patients will have a small hepatic vein "stump" (▶ Fig. 17.8) corresponding to the occluded hepatic vein, and the operator should attempt to anchor the needle system within this small stump.

Many operators prefer a coaxial access system for these cases such as the RUPS-100 (Cook, Bloomington, Indiana), Transjugular Access Set (AngioDynamics, Queensbury, New York), or a coaxial 21-gauge needle (Chiba biopsy needle, Cook) because this kind of access system allows the operator to anchor the guiding trocar into the stump and advance the puncture needle through the parenchyma. After the trocar is firmly placed in this position, the needle may be advanced into the liver parenchyma. When the puncture needle is within the parenchyma, a gentle CO_2 injection

can be performed (▶ Fig. 17.8d). Access into the portal vein will be easier if a roadmap is established. The operator needs to be careful with needle passes in patients with BCS because these livers are usually soft and not hard as typically seen in patients with cirrhosis. The technical challenge in BCS cases is the occlusion of the hepatic veins, not the traversal of the liver parenchyma. After access into the portal vein is obtained, a portogram must be performed to confirm good position within the portal venous system. The authors recommend the use of a measuring catheter to determine the length of the transparenchymal tract with precision because these patients usually have long transparenchymal tracts because the liver is usually enlarged from liver congestion. After the length of the tract is confirmed, the tract is lined with self-expandable metallic stents. The use of VIATORR stent grafts improves the long-term patency, and the use of this stent is recommended in these cases. The ideal stent position is within the main portal vein; the stented segment needs to be extended all the way into the IVC as shown in ▶ Fig. 17.8f.

Results and Complications of Transjugular Intrahepatic Portosystemic Shunt

Results of TIPS procedures in patients with BCS have been encouraging with a more than 90% technical success rate and more than 75% clinical success rate.[19,21,27] TIPS can be created with bare-metal stents and recently with stent grafts.[21] TIPS creation with bare-metal stents has the disadvantage of reduced patency rates compared with TIPS created with covered stents.[12,19,21,28] Gandini and coworkers found improved shunt patency rates in patients undergoing TIPS with expanded polytetrafluoroethylene (ePTFE)–covered stents. The mean patency duration was 4.4 months for patients treated with bare stents compared with 22.2 months for patients treated with stent grafts.[19] The 6- and 12-month patency rates were 100% and 85.7%, respectively, for stent grafts compared with 16.7% and 0% for bare stents ($P < 0.001$).[19] TIPS in patients with BCS is technically challenging, and this increases the risk of having a technical failure or a major complication during the procedure.[21] Garcia-Pagan et al reported a technical failure rate of 7% and a complication rate of 17.7%.[21] Fatal complications were seen in only two patients and included IVC injury and IVC occlusion by the stent.[21] Nonfatal complications were subcapsular hematoma, hemoperitoneum, hemobilia, heart failure, infection, supraventricular tachycardia, IVC compression, and hemolysis in 133 patients with BCS in whom a TIPS was attempted.[21]

In Garcia-Pagan et al's series, 13% of patients died after TIPS, and 6.5% required a liver transplant[21]; the causes of death were liver failure, sepsis, hematologic disorders, stroke, and gastrointestinal bleeding of unknown cause.[21] TIPS dysfunction was seen in 41% of patients in Garcia-Pagan et al's series.[21] Dysfunction was managed with additional stent placement in 35 patients, balloon angioplasty in 20, and thrombolysis in 6. As mentioned previously, these authors found that patency rates were better in patients treated with stent grafts as opposed to bare-metal stents.[21] The transplant-free survival rates in this group of patients at 1, 5, and 10 years were 88%, 78%, and 69%, respectively.[21]

Conclusion

Budd-Chiari syndrome is a heterogenous and complex disease, management of which requires a multidisciplinary approach involving teams from hepatology, hematology, transplant surgery, and interventional radiology (IR). IR forms the core of this group, with image-guided endovascular procedures being accepted as the principle modality to treat almost all forms of BCS. Strategies for the endovascular treatment of BCS should be individualized, depending on clinical condition and morphology of the venous obstruction. Anticoagulation and recanalization of the hepatic vein or IVC are favored as first-line therapy for both symptomatic and asymptomatic patients because they maintain physiological blood flow and arrest progression of liver disease, with excellent safety, efficacy, and survival outcomes. Failure of hepatic venous outflow recanalization, either technical or clinical, would benefit from a TIPS shunt. Reported technical and clinical results of TIPS have been very good, with transplant-free survival rates significantly better than for those treated with medical therapy alone. The use of stent grafts is recommended to improve the long-term patency of these shunts.

References

1. Bittencourt PL, Couto CA, Ribeiro DD. Portal vein thrombosis and Budd-Chiari syndrome. Clin Liver Dis 2009;13:127–144.
2. Okuda K. Inferior vena cava thrombosis at its hepatic portion (obliterative hepatocavopathy). Semin Liver Dis 2002;22:15–26.
3. Murad SD, Valla DC, de Groen PC, et al. Pathogenesis and treatment of Budd-Chiari syndrome combined with portal vein thrombosis. Am J Gastroenterol 2006;101:83–90.
4. Janssen HLA, Garcia-Pagan JC, Elias E, et al. Budd-Chiari syndrome: a review by an expert panel. J Hepatol 2003;38:364–371.
5. Plessier A, Denninger MH, Casadevall N, et al. Relevance of the criteria commonly used to diagnose myeloproliferative disorder in patients with splanchnic vein thrombosis. Br J Haematol 2005;129:553–560.
6. Zhang CQ, Fu LN, Xu L, et al. Long-term effect of stent placement in 115 patients with Budd-Chiari syndrome. World J Gastroenterol 2003;9:2587–2591.
7. Eapen CE, Velissaris D, Heydtmann M, et al. Favourable medium term outcome following hepatic vein recanalization and/or transjugular intrahepatic portosystemic shunt for Budd Chiari syndrome. Gut 2006; 55:878–884.
8. Han G, Qi X, Zhang W, et al. Percutaneous recanalization for Budd-Chiari syndrome: an 11-year retrospective study on patency and survival in 177 Chinese patients from a single centre. Radiology 2013;266:657–667.
9. Plessier A, Sibert A, Consigny Y, et al. Aiming at minimal invasiveness as a therapeutic strategy for Budd-Chiari syndrome. Hepatology 2006;44:1308–1316.
10. Amarapurkar DN, Punamiya SJ, Patel ND. Changing spectrum of Budd-Chiari syndrome in India with special reference to non-surgical treatment. World J Gastroenterol 2008;14:278–285.
11. Ochs A, Sellinger M, Haag K, et al. Transjugular intrahepatic portosystemic stent-shunt (TIPS) in the treatment of Budd-Chiari syndrome. J Hepatol 1993; 18:217–225.
12. Murad SD, Plessier A, Hernandez-Guerra M, et al. Etiology, management, and outcome of the Budd-Chiari syndrome. Ann Intern Med 2009;151:167–175.
13. Bachet JB, Condat B, Hagege H, et al. Long-term portosystemic shunt patency as a determinant of outcome in Budd-Chiari syndrome. J Hepatol 2007;46:60–68.
14. Cauchi JA, Oliff S, Baumann U, et al. The Budd-Chiari syndrome in children: the spectrum of management. J Pediatr Surg 2006;41:1919–1923.
15. Abujudeh H, Contractor D, Delatorre A, et al. Rescue TIPS in acute Budd-Chiari syndrome. Am J Roentgenol 2005;185:89–91.
16. Akoum R, Mahfoud D, Ghaoui A, et al. Budd-Chiari syndrome and heparin-induced thrombocytopenia in polycythemia vera: successful treatment with repeated TIPS and interferon alpha. J Cancer Res Ther 2009;5:305–308.
17. Corso R, Intotero M, Solcia M, et al. Treatment of Budd-Chiari syndrome with transjugular intrahepatic portosystemic shunt (TIPS). Radiol Med 2008;113: 727–738.
18. Cura M, Haskal Z, Lopera J. Diagnostic and interventional radiology for Budd-Chiari syndrome. Radiographics 2009;29:669–681.
19. Gandini R, Konda D, Simonetti G. Transjugular intrahepatic portosystemic shunt patency and clinical outcome in patients with Budd-Chiari syndrome: covered versus uncovered stents. Radiology 2006;241:298–305.
20. Ganger DR, Klapman JB, McDonald V, et al. Transjugular intrahepatic portosystemic shunt (TIPS) for Budd-Chiari syndrome or portal vein thrombosis: review of indications and problems. Am J Gastroenterol 1999;94:603–608.
21. Garcia-Pagan JC, Heydtmann M, Raffa S, et al. TIPS for Budd-Chiari syndrome: long-term results and prognostics factors in 124 patients. Gastroenterology 2008;135:808–815.
22. Hernandez-Guerra M, Turnes J, Rubinstein P, et al. PTFE-covered stents improve TIPS patency in Budd-Chiari syndrome. Hepatology 2004;40:1197–1202.
23. Peynircioglu B, Shorbagi AI, Balli O, et al. Is there an alternative to TIPS? Ultrasound-guided direct intrahepatic portosystemic shunt placement in Budd-Chiari syndrome. Saudi J Gastroenterol 2010;16:315–318.
24. Boyvat F, Aytekin C, Harman A, et al. Transjugular intrahepatic portosystemic shunt creation in Budd-Chiari syndrome: percutaneous ultrasound-guided direct simultaneous puncture of the portal vein and vena cava. Cardiovasc Intervent Radiol 2006;29:857–861.
25. Boyvat F, Harman A, Ozyer U, et al. Percutaneous sonographic guidance for TIPS in Budd-Chiari syndrome: direct simultaneous puncture of the portal vein and inferior vena cava. Am J Roentgenol 2008;191:560–564.
26. Soares GM, Murphy TP. Transcaval TIPS: Indications and anatomic considerations. J Vasc Interv Radiol 1999;10:1233–1239.
27. Lopez-Mendez E, Chavez-Tapia NC, Avila-Escobedo L, et al. Early experience of Budd-Chiari syndrome treatment with transjugular intrahepatic portosystemic shunt. Ann Hepatol 2006;5:157–160.
28. Cejna M. Should stent-grafts replace bare stents for primary transjugular intrahepatic portosystemic shunts? Semin Intervent Radiol 2005;22:287–299.

Chapter 18: Transjugular Intrahepatic Portosystemic Shunt Reduction for Post-TIPS Hepatic Encephalopathy

Adam D. Talenfeld and David C. Madoff

Indications for Transjugular Intrahepatic Portosystemic Shunt Reduction

Hepatic encephalopathy (HE) is a known complication of transjugular intrahepatic portosystemic shunt (TIPS) creation. The most widely used system for grading the severity of HE is the West Haven criteria (▶ Table 18.1). The incidence of new or newly worsened hepatic encephalopathy (HE) after transjugular intrahepatic portosystemic shunt (TIPS) creation has traditionally been reported as 20% to 31%, although some series have reported this figure to be as high as 44%, and a recent randomized multicenter study reported a rate of HE after TIPS of 33%.[1–5] The rate of post-TIPS HE refractory to medical management has traditionally been established at 4% to 7%, although more recently this number has been reported to approach 8%.[6–8] Despite initial concerns, rates of HE with covered TIPS appear to be the same or slightly less than as seen with bare-metal TIPS,[9] although whether this reflects a difference in the design of TIPS shunt materials or a refinement of TIPS technique is uncertain. Although liver transplant is an option for a small subset of these patients, most will need endovascular TIPS revision. ▶ Table 18.2 outlines the indications and relative contraindications for TIPS reduction.

Reduction's Predecessor: Transjugular Intrahepatic Portosystemic Shunt Occlusion

Ligation of surgically created portosystemic shunts was reported by Hanna et al in 1981 for the treatment of HE refractory to medical therapies.[10] In 1984, Potts et al reported endovascular deployment of a detachable balloon within a surgically created splenorenal shunt that resulted in complete shunt occlusion and substantially improved liver function.[11] Use of coil embolization for surgical shunt occlusion was reported in 1987 via transfemoral and percutaneous transhepatic approaches,[12] and a variety of techniques were subsequently implemented by surgeons and interventional radiologists for TIPS occlusion in the setting of refractory HE. These included various combinations of coil embolization and intra-TIPS Greenfield filter deployment.[13,14] Also described was temporary transjugular inflation of latex occlusion balloons, left in place for up to 48 hours on a guidewire or with a supporting transjugular sheath to achieve shunt thrombosis without permanent indwelling foreign material, so as to allow subsequent recanalization.[7,8]

Results

The proliferation of shunt occlusion procedures was limited by reports of rapidly ensuing hemodynamic instability, and death thought to be due to suddenly and severely reduced cardiac preload and renal perfusion as well as reports of recurrent variceal bleeding.[12,13,15] A retrospective single-center analysis of 38 TIPS occlusion and reduction procedures performed over a 14-year period reported a high rate of TIPS occlusion-related complications, including a procedure-related death rate of 9% (3 of 29 TIPS occlusion patients). From these data, the authors strongly recommended newer reduction techniques over TIPS occlusion for refractory HE.[14] Central embolization of the balloon or of the induced TIPS thrombus into the pulmonary circulation, either periprocedurally or during any subsequent recanalization attempt, has been an additional theoretical concern raised with all balloon-mediated TIPS occlusion techniques.[13,16]

Early Transjugular Intrahepatic Portosystemic Shunt Reduction Techniques: Reducing Stents

The first report of a technique for intentionally narrowing without occluding a TIPS was described in 1994 by Haskal and Middlebrook.[17] This technique involved weaving a 3-0 silk suture circumferentially through the interstices of the midportion of a Wallstent (Boston Scientific, Natick, MA), which was partially deployed on a sterile back table, achieving a constrained stent diameter of 5 mm. The stent was then resheathed in a long 9-Fr sheath and deployed by unsheathing the stent from a transjugular approach coaxially within a long 12-Fr sheath. The authors acknowledged that the technique was more involved than many contemporary occlusion techniques but noted that the sutures could be broken with angioplasty if wider shunt patency is later desired. Reduced flow within the revised shunt was thought to be due to increased turbulence of flow because contrast was seen passing through the interstices of the newly placed constrained stent immediately after placement.

Various other techniques for deploying reducing stents within existing TIPS shunts were described. One of these made use of a coaxial smaller balloon-expanded stent to constrain a larger self-expanding stent.[18] Another technique comprised partially deploying one end of a larger balloon-expanded stent and fully deploying the other.[19] The narrow, partially deployed end of the stent reduced flow through the TIPS, and the wider fully deployed end fixed the new stent to the walls of the shunt.

Table 18.1 West Haven Criteria for Grading of Hepatic Encephalopathy

Grade	Clinical Signs
I	Trivial lack of awareness Euphoria or anxiety Shortened attention span Impaired performance of addition
II	Lethargy or apathy Minimal disorientation to time or place Subtle personality change Inappropriate behavior Impaired performance of subtraction
III	Somnolence to semi-stupor but responsive to verbal stimuli Gross disorientation
IV	Coma (unresponsive to verbal or noxious stimuli)

Table 18.2 Indications and Contraindications for Transjugular Intrahepatic Portosystemic Shunt Reduction

Indications	Relative Contraindications*
Refractory post-TIPS hepatic encephalopathy (strong indication)	Patient is candidate for liver transplant (can be bridge to transplant)
Post-TIPS hepatic insufficiency (weak indication; transplant is preferred)	Patient cannot tolerate risk of rebleeding or recurrent ascites

*There are no absolute contraindications.
TIPS: transjugular intrahepatic portosystemic shunt.

A premanufactured reducing stent was made commercially available in Europe in the mid-1990s. Preloaded in a 7-Fr delivery sheath, the self-expanding nitinol Memotherm stent (Angiomed, Karlsruhe, Germany) expanded to a predesigned hourglass shape. Postdeployment angioplasty with 10-, 12-, or 14-mm balloons would enlarge the ends of the stent for fixation, and smaller balloons could be used to open the midportion of the reducing stent to either 4 or 6 mm. A polyethylene terephthalate (PET, or Dacron polyester) fiber net was woven through the interstices of the narrow portion of the stent to induce thrombosis of the space between the original and reducing shunts.

Results

Similar to all literature reporting TIPS modification procedures, the literature describing use of reducing stents is composed of case reports and small single-center series. However, probably because they allowed both a partial and more gradual elevation in portosystemic gradient (PSG), reducing stents were much less often associated with fatal hemodynamic complications, and TIPS reduction quickly replaced TIPS occlusion in the 1990s.[14] Haskal and Middlebrook[17] reported their first stent immediately increased the patient's PSG by 3 mm Hg, decreased shunt velocity by one third, and restored hepatopetal flow in portal branches as well as markedly reducing the patient's HE. It remained patent through 8 months of follow-up. Results reported in small series describing other reducing stent techniques noted better success in treating patients with HE than those with more fulminant hepatic insufficiency.[20,21] It was hypothesized that either the procedure itself or the maximum hemodynamic effect of shunt reduction took place too long after hepatic insufficiency ensued to reverse the cascade of hepatic necrosis. In contrast to their TIPS occlusion predecessors, there were no procedure-related complications described with these TIPS reduction techniques.

When stent-based TIPS reduction techniques were found inadequately to decrease flow, embolization of spaces between the reducing stents and original TIPS was advocated, either with an emulsion of iodized oil and hydroxylated corn protein derivative (Ethibloc; Ethicon, Norderstedt, Germany) or with coils.[19,22]

The investigators who initially described use of the Memotherm prefabricated reducing stent reported clinical response in 4 of 7 patients.[20] Subsequently, however, other researchers found clinical improvement in only 2 of 6 patients treated with the Memotherm stent. It is no longer commercially available.[21]

Modern Techniques: Reducing Stent Grafts

Several covered stents have become commercially available in the past decade, allowing development of a multitude of new TIPS reduction techniques. Roughly, these techniques can be categorized into five categories, as follow.

Balloon-Expanded Stent Graft Sculpting Techniques

Quaretti et al first described use of a covered stent in TIPS reduction, making use of an extended polytetrafluoroethylene (ePTFE)–covered balloon-expanded stainless steel stent (Jostent; Jomed, Rangendingen, Germany).[23] The procedure requires deploying the stent graft on a sterile back table. A 48-mm-long Jostent, balloon-expandable from 6 to 12 mm in diameter is tightly crimped onto a 12 × 40-mm balloon catheter (Opta; Cordis, Roden, The Netherlands), such that the balloon lies half within and half outside what will be the inferior third of the reducing stent graft (with the stent crimped only to the superior half of the balloon). The stent graft is then deployed through a 10-Fr-long sheath placed within the original TIPS by inflating the balloon where loaded in the inferior third of the stent graft, deflating the balloon, repositioning it halfway within the superior third of the stent graft and reinflating, leaving the middle third of the covered stent at its factory minimum 6-mm diameter. Gastroesophageal varices were embolized with coils and 3% Polidocanol detergent sclerosant before reducing the shunt.

Another technique using covered Jostents for TIPS reduction was described by Fanelli et al using a 3-0 polyglactin suture tied around the midportion of a 10 × 40-mm balloon catheter (Wanda, Boston Scientific).[24] The covered Jostent is then deployed on a back table, hand mounted on the balloon catheter, and advanced into the midportion of the TIPS via a 10-Fr jugular sheath. The balloon is insufflated to nominal pressure, deflated, and removed. A 5-mm balloon is then insufflated in the midportion of the newly deployed reducing stent graft. Larger balloons can be used as needed to achieve the desired hemodynamic response. ▶ Fig. 18.1 illustrates this constraining suture concept.

Kroma et al[25] described direct deployment of iCast stent grafts to reduce TIPS using either 10 × 38-mm or 10 × 59-mm devices. Intentionally incomplete insufflation of the factory-installed deployment balloon is used to create a centrally narrowed configuration of the iCast stent graft, conceptually outlined in ▶ Fig. 18.2. Serially larger angioplasty balloons were used in the midportion of the deployed iCast to decrease as needed the amount of shunt flow reduction. The authors emphasize that other ePTFE-covered balloon-expanded stents may not expand with the same symmetry.

Results

Quaretti et al[23] found both technical and clinical success intervening in a patient developing liver failure 1 week after TIPS. The PSG increased from 10 to 25 cm H_2O. Peak velocity in the reduced shunt increased from 130 to 195 cm/s, and flow in the shunt, as measured

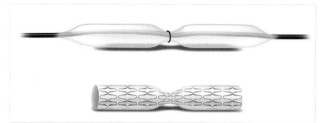

Fig. 18.1 Suture-constrained deployment balloon technique. A Jostent stainless steel balloon-expandable polytetrafluoroethylene (PTFE)-covered stent graft has been removed from its factory-mounted balloon and a suture tied around the midportion of another balloon. The balloon has been insufflated on a back table to illustrate this constraint. The stent graft, having been hand crimped to the deflated, sutured balloon, is then deployed by insufflating and again deflating the balloon. The suture-constrained balloon has been removed from the ex vivo–deployed reducing stent graft in this diagram.

by Doppler, decreased from 2.6 to 1.8 L/min. Serum bilirubin fell from 23 to 3.5 mg/dL 7 days after reduction and 1.5 mg/dL at 7-month follow-up. There were no procedure-related complications, and the patient remained free of recurrent bleeding through the follow-up period.

Fanelli et al[24] claimed technical, hemodynamic, and clinical success in all 12 patients described in their case series. They reported no difficulties with deployment and found a mean increase in PSG from 6.6 to 15.1 mm Hg. Doppler examinations performed 1 day after reduction revealed an average decrease in velocity of shunt flow from 85 to 25 cm/s. To raise the PSG to desired levels, use of 5-mm balloons to angioplasty the center of the shunt was required in 2 of 12 cases, but most patients (9 of 12) required 6-mm angioplasty, and one required balloon expansion to 7 mm. Mean serum ammonia levels decreased from 168 to 73 mcg per 100 mL. Although not directly reported, mean pre- and post-TIPS reduction West Haven HE grade calculated from the data presented in their report declined from 2.9 to 0.4. Similarly calculated mean serum bilirubin level was 1.9 mg/dL before and 1.6 mg/dL after TIPS reduction. Mean model for end-stage liver disease (MELD) scores were 13 before and 12 after reduction. No analysis was performed of correlation between these values and survival or between other variables on which data were collected and outcomes, including Child-Pugh class, age, or indication for the

original TIPS, although the raw data themselves were presented. The authors reported that at 1-year follow-up, 6 patients were alive and well, 4 had died of cardiac or multiorgan failure (2 during the first 30 days after reduction), 1 received a liver transplant and did well, and 2 were lost to follow-up. Although they did not report prereduction embolization of gastroesophageal varices, the group also did not report rebleeding during follow-up.

Kroma et al[25] reported technical difficulty in deploying each of the 4 iCast PTFE-covered reducing stents in the series describing their technique of partial factory-mounted i-Cast balloon insufflation to achieve a narrow, reducing waist. Each reducing stent graft was inadvertently partially withdrawn on removal of its deploying balloon, the authors suspected, because of friction of the balloon on the narrow, incompletely deployed portion of the reducing stent graft and lack of sufficient friction between the more completely deployed ends of the reducing stent graft. In 3 of 4 cases, the ends of the iCast were more completely apposed to the walls of the original TIPS using a separate 6-mm-diameter balloon. In one case, despite this additional maneuver, the iCast stent graft moved cephalad on withdrawal of the access sheath, so a bare-metal 10 × 26-mm balloon-expanded stent (Lifestent; Edwards Lifesciences, Irvine, CA) was deployed, overlapping the cephalad edge of the iCast as an anchor. The authors measured final PSG but used angiographic demonstration of return of minimal antegrade portal branch flow as their determinant of sufficiency of TIPS flow reduction. Coil embolization of recurrent flow within large gastric varices was performed as needed in one case. A mean increase of PSG of 8 mm Hg (59%) was noted. Serum ammonia levels changed from a mean of 60 to a mean of 51 in the three subjects for whom it was calculated. Bilirubin changed from 26 to 18. Mean MELD scores were 24 both before and after the reducing procedures. HE grades were 1.8 before and 2.2 after the reduction procedures in this small series. Mean survival time after TIPS reduction was 148 days when including 1 patient who received a transplant and 68 days excluding that patient. None of the deaths was found to be procedure related.

Purse-String Suture–Mediated Reduction Technique

Madoff et al[26] described the first TIPS reduction to make use of a Wallgraft (Boston Scientific, Natick, MA), a PET-covered Wallstent. In their permutation of the reducing stent technique, either a 10- or 12-mm-diameter Wallgraft is fully deployed on a sterile back table. A 6- or 8-mm angioplasty balloon or corresponding dilator is used to appropriately size the narrow portion of the stent graft, which is then constrained with a purse-string 3-0 silk suture woven between the graft's interstices approximately one-third the distance from its leading end. A scalpel may be used to cut the covering from the trailing half of the Wallgraft so as to prevent inadvertent occlusion of the hepatic vein. The modified Wallgraft is then loaded into the tip of a long 9- or 10-Fr sheath and deployed within the TIPS shunt by unsheathing the reducing stent graft while pinning it in place using the sheath's dilator with its tip cut off to serve as a pusher. Variations of the technique were subsequently described by several groups, one of which described coil embolization of a large esophageal varix before shunt reduction.[27,28] An illustration of a reducing stent graft deployed using this type of technique is illustrated in ▶ Fig. 18.3. An example of such a reducing stent graft seen in vivo is shown in ▶ Fig. 18.4.

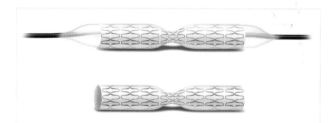

Fig. 18.2 Incomplete iCast insufflation. An iCast polytetrafluoroethylene (PTFE)-covered balloon-expandable stainless steel stent graft is incompletely insufflated on its factory-mounted balloon catheter. Unlike as depicted in Fig. 18.1, there is no constraining suture or other constraining device used with this technique. The balloon catheter is removed, leaving the covered stent graft in place. This technique has been limited in vivo by cephalad migration of the reducing stent graft during withdrawal of its deployment balloon.

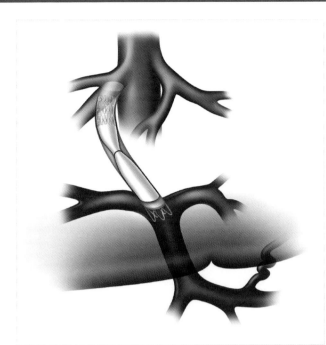

Fig. 18.3 Purse-string technique. Diagram of a purse-string–reducing stent graft technique. A Wallgraft (polyethylene terephthalate [PET]-covered Wallstent) with a purse-string suture constricting its midportion is deployed within the original transjugular intrahepatic portosystemic shunt (TIPS). The narrow midportion of the Wallgraft reduces flow through the shunt. There is no need for adjunctive coil or other embolization of the dead space between the Wallgraft and the original TIPS.

Results

Madoff et al[26] achieved technical and hemodynamic success in all 6 patients, with a mean increase of PSG from 8.3 to 17.6 mm Hg. Five of 6 patients had reduction in HE within 72 hours. One patient who did not respond clinically and died within 30 days of the reduction procedure was known also to have thrombotic

thrombocytopenic purpura. Although no mechanism of death was described, the authors speculated that HE might have been at least partly a manifestation of the comorbid condition rather than or in addition to HE. None of the three patients receiving TIPS for variceal bleeding experienced rebleeding after reduction. Although no periprocedural complications occurred, 1 patient developed recurrent large volume ascites 2 months after TIPS reduction and was found to have shunt occlusion. This patient was treated with mechanical thrombectomy (Angiojet; Possis, Minneapolis, MN and Arrow-Trerotola; Arrow International, Reading, PA) followed by angioplasty of the shunt to 10 mm. HE did not return. Another patient developed recurrent HE at 6 months, which was treated with a second purse-string–constrained Wallgraft reduction. Two months later, this patient experienced an episode of melena with significant blood loss. Although no varices were seen endoscopically, shunt occlusion was seen on Doppler interrogation. Given prior studies of Wallgrafts for TIPS in animal models, it was hypothesized that the PET polymer might have played a prothrombotic role in the patients with poor outcomes.[29-31]

In their case report, Cox et al[27] showed technical and hemodynamic success, with an increase in the PSG from 1 to 7 mm Hg. They claimed significant improvement in HE and shunt patency by Doppler follow-up at 11 months after reduction. The case report by Clarke et al[28] documented technical, hemodynamic, and clinical success as uncomplicated deployment, increase in PSG from 7 to 12 mm Hg, and resolution of HE at 3 months' follow-up.

Coaxial Constraining Stent-Over-Stent-Graft Technique

Jacquier et al[32] adapted the technique of a constricting stent using a Wallgraft in lieu of the originally described Wallstent and a smaller, balloon-expanded Uni Wallstent in place of the originally described constraining Palmaz stent (▶ Fig. 18.5). This technique uses a 10- or 11-Fr-long sheath via jugular access and crosses the TIPS with an Amplatz wire (Cook Medical, Bloomington, IN). A 6 × 20-mm Uni Wallstent (Boston Scientific, Natick, MA) is deployed in the inferior aspect of the TIPS and is pinned to the

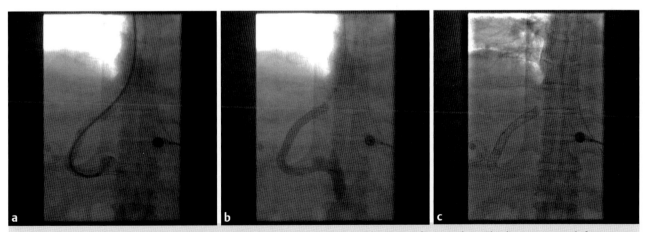

Fig. 18.4 Purse-string suture technique. (**a**) Prereduction angiogram demonstrating wide patency of existing shunt. The shunt is composed of two overlapping VIATORR stent grafts connecting the right hepatic and a branch of the right portal. There is no flow demonstrated in other portal branches. (**b**) Postreduction angiogram demonstrating restoration of antegrade flow in the main portal branches and narrowing of the diameter of the transjugular intrahepatic portosystemic shunt. (**c**) Postreduction radiograph demonstrating the constrained Wallgraft within the hepatic parenchymal portion of the original VIATORR.

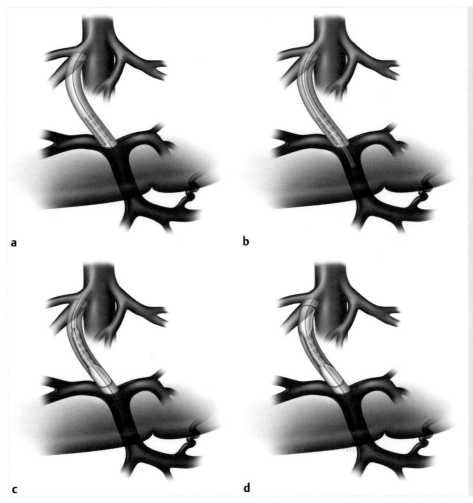

Fig. 18.5 Coaxial stents technique. (a) A 6-mm Uni Wallstent is deployed over an Amplatz wire in the caudal third of the original transjugular intrahepatic portosystemic shunt and its deployment balloon catheter removed. (b) A Wallgraft is then inserted over the same wire through the Uni Wallstent. (c) The Wallgraft is then deployed until just before the "point of no return," and the entire system is pulled back, ensuring appropriate alignment of the reducing stent graft system. (d) The remainder of the Wallgraft is deployed, its midportion constricted by the coaxial balloon-expanded Uni Wallstent.

wall of the TIPS by the tension in the Amplatz wire within the curved original TIPS, preventing cephalad migration. The Uni Wallstent is itself then canalized in vivo over the Amplatz wire by a 10 × 50-mm Wallgraft until the Uni Wallstent lies around the midportion of the Wallgraft. The caudal 2 cm of the Wallgraft are then deployed, and the entire system is pulled back until the end of the Wallgraft lines up with the end of the hepatic parenchymal tract of the original TIPS. The Wallgraft is then completely deployed and its caudal and cephalad aspects angioplastied with a 10-mm balloon.

A permutation of this technique was reported by Weintraub et al[33] using a 4-cm-long iCast PTFE-coated stainless steel balloon-expanded stent graft (Atrium Medical, Hudson, NH) to constrain a 10 × 94-mm Wallstent. On a back table, the tip of a 10-Fr TIPS sheath (Cook Medical) is cut off approximately halfway along its taper to allow room for delivery of the hybrid Wallstent-iCast system. The Wallstent delivery system is loaded through the sheath and partially deployed (to the limit marker band). The iCast stent graft is loaded onto the midportion of the closed Wallstent and hand crimped onto the Wallstent. The tip of the Wallstent delivery system is then also cut off to prevent the system from catching during delivery, and the entire system is pulled back into the 10-Fr sheath. TIPS access is secured with a 12-Fr sheath and an Amplatz wire. The 10-Fr sheath and preloaded reducing stent graft assembly is passed through the

12-Fr sheath into position inside the TIPS and the 10-Fr sheath is withdrawn, deploying the majority of the Wallstent-iCast graft system. After ensuring appropriate placement, the remainder of the Wallstent is deployed in standard fashion. A 4 × 40-mm balloon is then insufflated within the iCast stent graft, and the ends of the graft are flared to 8 mm with another balloon to appose the ends of the iCast graft to the walls of the original TIPS. Larger balloons may be used to widen the waist of the iCast-covered stent.

Results

Jacquier et al[32] noted technical, hemodynamic, and clinical success in all patients, with 0% 30-day periprocedural morbidity. One patient had episodes of upper gastrointestinal (GI) bleeding at 3 and 9 months after reduction and was found angiographically to have pseudointimal hyperplasia of the narrowed Wallgraft. Another patient died 16 months after reduction from severe liver failure; 2 months before death, he was found to have TIPS occlusion. A correlation between the Dacron graft material covering the Wallgraft and shunt thrombosis was suspected. Although not reported in this series, others have criticized this technique as also posing a significant, if theoretical, risk of intraprocedural stent migration.[30]

In their case report, Weintraub et al[33] described technical and hemodynamic success, with a PSG increase from 1 to 28 mm Hg and a postreduction angiogram demonstrating antegrade flow in portal vein branches. A positive clinical response was reported but not quantified; however, the patient experienced an episode of hematemesis several weeks later and died shortly thereafter of cardiac arrest.

Parallel Constraining Stent and Stent Graft Technique

In 2004, Saket et al[34] published the initial use of parallel stents to reduce a TIPS. Included with their report of 5 TIPS reduction cases using 5 distinct techniques, these investigators described the first side-by-side placement of a stent and stent graft inside a TIPS to reduce flow. An esophageal varix and splenorenal shunt were coil-embolized before shunt reduction. With this technique, a long 10-Fr sheath and 2 guidewires are used to gain access through the TIPS. A 10 × 50-mm Viabahn ePTFE-covered self-expanding nitinol stent graft (W.L. Gore & Associates, Flagstaff, AZ) is deployed within the TIPS over one wire. A 7-Fr-long sheath is then advanced coaxially through the 10-Fr sheath and used to deliver a 6 × 37-mm balloon-expanded Express stent (Boston Scientific). The 7-Fr sheath is partially withdrawn, and the balloon-expanded stent is deployed adjacent the superior aspect of the Viabahn, externally compressing and narrowing the more compliant stent graft. Six- and 8-mm-diameter balloons are then insufflated within the Express stent and the Viabahn stent graft, respectively, to achieve an appropriate PSG. The authors point out that flow within the reduced TIPS can be further reduced or increased by subsequent balloon angioplasty of either the Express or Viabahn stents, respectively.

Holden et al[35] later reduced a TIPS with a 10-mm-diameter VIATORR stent graft (W.L. Gore & Associates, Flagstaff, AZ) via a 10-Fr-long sheath and a 5 × 12-mm Palmaz Genesis balloon-expanded stent (Cordis, Miami Lakes, FL) through a 6-Fr-long sheath, each sheath being positioned within the original TIPS from a separate jugular access. ▶ Fig. 18.6 illustrates this parallel reduction technique.

Maleux et al[36] described a variation of the parallel technique using access gained from jugular and femoral veins, with 10-Fr and flexible 8-Fr-long sheaths placed over Amplatz wires into the TIPS from jugular and femoral approaches, respectively. A 6 × 17-mm balloon-expanded stent (Express Vascular LD, Boston Scientific) is then positioned in the midportion of the original TIPS from the femoral approach. A 10-mm-diameter VIATORR stent graft is then positioned in the TIPS from the jugular approach such that its ends exactly overlap the ends of the original TIPS shunt. The balloon-expanded stent is then deployed and its balloon left insufflated while the parallel VIATORR stent graft is deployed using standard technique. The balloon is then deflated and carefully removed, leaving both newly deployed stents in place, side by side within the original shunt. Embolization was performed of esophagogastric varices visualized on postreduction angiography in 4 patients.

Sze et al[37] later reported refinement of the original parallel stent technique in which placement of the balloon-expanded stent at the cephalad end of the TIPS rather than in the middle to allow for not only intraprocedural but future access to this stent if additional shunt narrowing is desired. With this method, the self-expanding stent graft component is deployed first, and a sheath is not used in deployment of the balloon-expanded stent unless it is inadvertently passed beyond the caudal edge of the already deployed stent graft and needs to be pulled back without catching. Four of 6 reductions in the series published with report of the modified technique make use of 10 × 50-mm Wallgrafts alongside bare-metal stents, 1 used a VIATORR, and 1 used a Viabahn.

Results

Saket et al[34] reported technical and hemodynamic success, with an increase in the PSG from 12 to 20 mm Hg and an increase of the maximum flow velocity in the shunt from 178 to 218 cm/s measured by Doppler ultrasonography. There were no periprocedural complications. They measured a decrease in plasma ammonia from 57 to 45 μmol/L, a decrease in serum bilirubin from 12.6 to 4.9 mg/dL, a decrease in the MELD score from 18 to 14,

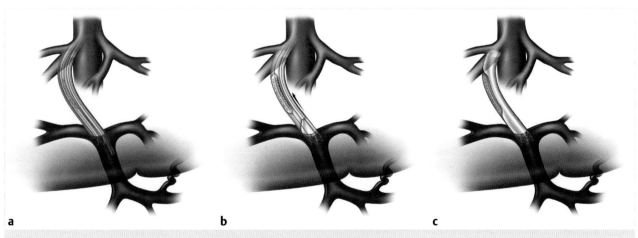

a   b   c

Fig. 18.6 Parallel stent and stent graft technique. (**a**) Via separate jugular punctures, a 6-Fr-long sheath containing a 5-mm-diameter balloon-expandable stent is passed alongside a 10-Fr-long sheath containing a 10-mm-diameter VIATORR stent graft within the original transjugular intrahepatic portosystemic shunt. (**b**) The 6-Fr sheath has been removed and the balloon-expanded stent deployed. The balloon remains insufflated. The VIATOR stent graft used for reduction has been partially deployed by unsheathing. (**c**) The reduction procedure complete; the reducing VIATORR stent graft is constrained in its midportion by the balloon-expanded stent.

and a decrease in West Haven HE grade from 3 to 1. The patient survived to receive a liver transplant and was alive at follow-up 2 months after reduction.

Holden et al[35] reported an increase of PSG from 4 to 10 mm Hg in their case report using the parallel technique without technical difficulty or immediate periprocedure complication. They reported increased velocity in the narrowed segment of the reduced TIPS by Doppler and clinically improved HE without reaccumulation of ascites (which had been the indication for TIPS placement); however, hepatic function continued to deteriorate, and the patient died 4 weeks after reduction of multiorgan failure.

In their report of 15 patients receiving new parallel TIPS reduction procedures and 2 patients receiving parallel TIPS reduction for failed primary reduction procedures, Maleux et al[36] documented technical success in all patients and a mean increase of the PSG from 6.3 to 11.9 mm Hg in the 15 primary reduction patients. There was reopacification of intrahepatic portal vein branches in postreduction angiograms for 12 patients. Resolved or decreased symptoms of HE were found in 13 patients. Four patients demonstrated no improvement at all, and each died shortly after shunt reduction. None of the patients who failed to improve clinically had restoration of hepatopetal portal vein branch flow seen angiographically despite increases in PSG. Although they could not prove statistical significance, the authors thought that angiographic restoration of hepatopetal flow was a better prognostic indicator of clinical response to shunt reduction than increase in the PSG. The investigators reported a 6-month mortality rate of 41%, with 3 deaths from multiorgan failure, 3 of septicemia thought to be unrelated to the TIPS interventions, and 1 of complications of end-stage lymphoma. They speculated that the high mortality rate seen in this series reflected the poor general condition of the TIPS reduction patient population. There were 3 occlusions documented in this series, 1 occurring during 1 of 3 repeat shunt reduction procedures and the other 2 found after recurrence of large-volume ascites and hepatic hydrothorax. All were treated by endovascular means.

Sze et al[37] in a series of 6 patients receiving parallel reduction with a variety of stents, stent lengths and stent grafts reported technical and hemodynamic success in all patients, the latter being defined as reestablishment of hepatopetal flow in portal vein branches. The mean PSG increase was from 9 to 17 mm Hg. There were no rebleeds in patients who had received TIPS for ruptured esophagogastric varices. (All patients with this indication for TIPS received embolization or sclerosis of the varices at the time of reduction.) None of 3 patients having received TIPS for refractory large-volume fluid accumulation required reintervention for this indication. One patient died within 30 days of the reduction procedure from multiorgan failure complicating small bowel obstruction. Three other patients died within 3 months of TIPS reduction, 1 each from liver failure, sepsis, and intracranial hemorrhage after a fall. Mean West Haven HE grade decreased from 3.0 to 0.8. Patients getting reduction procedures for HE did better than patients needing reduction for hepatic insufficiency. One patient died after 9 months from heart failure. The last patient received a liver transplant 6 months after reduction and was alive and well at 4-year follow-up.

In the same publication, Sze et al also studied various parallel reducing stent grafts ex vivo and noted the only stent graft to preserve an oval cross-section alongside a balloon-expanded constraining stent was the Wallgraft. They further showed that the Wallgraft's original oval cross-section was better preserved when deployed after the balloon-expanded stent, not before it. The ePTFE-covered stents all assumed concave, crescent configurations alongside the balloon-expanded stents. The authors argue in favor of using Wallgrafts for reductions due to their better preserved oval cross-sectional configuration and because of more reliable and significant reductions in flow with easier subsequent wire access, should that be required. They speculated that use of ePTFE-lined VIATORR stent grafts in creation of the original TIPS in this small series shielded their reducing Wallgrafts from the pseudointimal hyperplasia that may be associated with thrombosis of Wallgrafts as primary TIPS and in reductions of primary Wallgraft TIPS.

In 2010, Cookson et al[38] described a slightly modified version of the parallel technique using Palmaz Blue and Genesis balloon-expanded stents (Cordis, Warren, NJ). Technical and hemodynamic success was achieved in all 8 patients, with a mean PSG rise from 4.9 to 10.5 mm Hg after reduction. Increased portal branch opacification was seen in postreduction angiograms in 3 patients, but there was no correlation appreciated between antegrade portal branch flow or degree of PSG increase and reduction in grade of HE. Gastroesophageal varices were visible in 1 patient before reduction but were not embolized. The mean HE grade decreased from 2.6 to 1.5, and HE improved or resolved in 5 of 8 patients. No adverse events occurred in these 5 patients, with a mean follow-up duration of 4.5 months. Three patients' HE did not improve. These same 3 patients also had episodes of recurrent GI hemorrhage. Two of 3 died, 1 of renal failure and 1 of hepatorenal syndrome.

Lasso Technique

Monnin-Bares et al[39] described a "lasso" technique of customized reducing stent graft placement (► Fig. 18.7). The lasso catheter is assembled on a back table using a 0.021-in guidewire folded on itself and loaded into a 6-Fr guide catheter. Over a stiff 0.035-in wire placed through a 12-Fr sheath inserted in the jugular, a 10×40-mm, 10×50-mm or 10×60-mm ePTFE-covered balloon-expandable stent graft (Advanta V12; Atrium Medical, Hudson, NH) is positioned within the TIPS with its inferior half inserted through the open lasso. The covered stent and lasso system are then centered within the covered portion of the TIPS and the balloon-expanded stent graft deployed. The lasso is tightened around the covered stent with the deployment balloon of the balloon-expanded stent still inflated. The back end of an Amplatz wire is advanced internally to the end of the lasso catheter to provide support while the balloon is deflated and withdrawn to the cephalad end of the newly deployed stent. Angioplasty is performed to fix the new stent in place before further withdrawing the balloon. The PSG can be increased by tightening the lasso around the covered stent or further reduced by reintroducing and insufflating a balloon in the midportion of the covered stent. Upon final withdrawal of the lasso catheter, a balloon is again insufflated in the superior aspect of the covered stent to prevent migration from the lasso catching on the outside of the reduced stent graft.

Results

Technical and hemodynamic success was seen in all 5 patients, with a mean PSG increasing from 4.0 to 14.4 mm Hg and

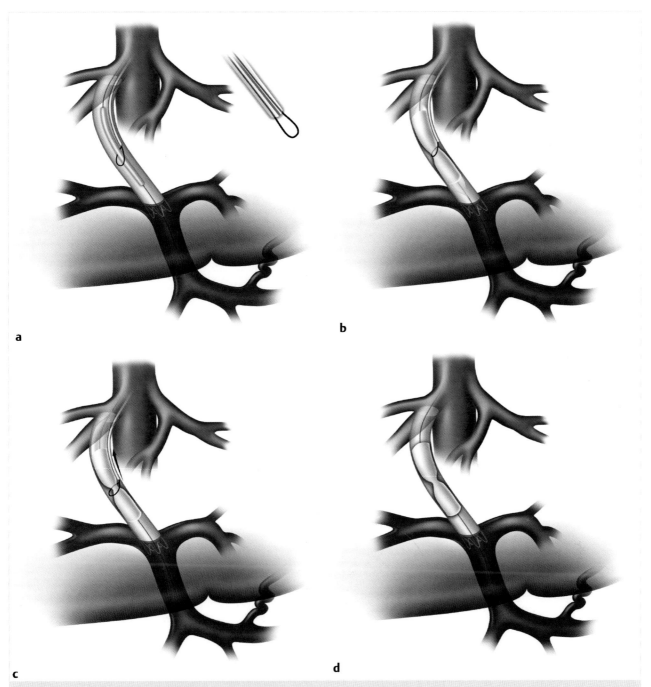

Fig. 18.7 Lasso technique. (**a**) In the first step of the lasso catheter–reducing stent graft technique described by Monnin-Bares et al,[39] a 10-mm-diameter Advanta V12 polytetrafluoroethylene (PTFE)-covered balloon-expandable stent is passed through the loop of a homemade lasso catheter lying alongside it inside the transjugular intrahepatic portosystemic shunt to be reduced. The inset here shows a magnified view of the lasso–catheter assembly in which the back end of a stiff 0.035-in wire provides support to a 6-Fr guide catheter. A 0.021-in guidewire has been folded in half and both ends fed backward through the guide catheter on a sterile back table, creating an adjustable snare or lasso with which to control the size of the waist on the reducing Advanta stent graft. (**b**) The stent graft has been deployed by insufflating its factory-mounted balloon. The ends of the 0.021-in wire have been pulled back through the guide catheter, closing the lasso and constricting the midportion of the stainless steel stent graft to a desired diameter. (**c**) The lasso is maintained in position around the stent graft while the balloon is deflated and pulled back into the cephalad aspect of the newly deployed Advanta covered stent. The balloon is then reinflated in the cephalad aspect of the stent graft to ensure full apposition to the original transjugular intrahepatic portosystemic shunt. The balloon is left inflated here while the lasso is opened, and the lasso–catheter system withdrawn over the newly deployed reducing stent graft (*arrow*). (**d**) The balloon is again deflated and withdrawn (not shown), leaving the reducing stent graft in place.

restoration of antegrade flow in portal vein branches in all patients after reduction with their lasso technique.[39] There was immediate, complete resolution of HE in 4 of 5 patients. The fifth patient showed initial partial improvement but then experienced deterioration in mentation and overall clinical status and died 1 week after reduction. One patient developed recurrent large-volume ascites and hydrothorax 8 months after reduction and found to have shunt occlusion and was treated with endovascular recanalization and angioplasty. Another patient developed recurrent ascites and pleural effusion but was found to have a patent shunt. The last 2 patients were free of adverse events, with a mean follow-up of 8 months after reduction. There was no mention of whether adjunctive variceal embolization was performed in the 1 patient who had received TIPS for GI hemorrhage.

Other Transjugular Intrahepatic Portosystemic Shunt Reduction Studies, Products, and Techniques

Kochar et al[14] reviewed outcomes related to 38 TIPS modifications; however, interpretation of their results is difficult because 75% of the modifications were occlusions and 6 of 9 reductions were with Memotherm reducing stents (3 were with "other devices"). Technical success was not reported. Hemodynamic failure was confirmed with Doppler studies when there was lack of clinical response. The study highlighted a high periprocedure complication rate associated with occlusion techniques and a strong direct correlation between clinical response to reduction treatment and survival.

Maleux et al[21] reported 16 patients with refractory HE treated with a variety of reducing techniques, including 6 Memotherm reducing stents; 4 self-expanding factory-shaped hourglass, polyurethane-covered stent grafts (Optimed, Ettlingen, Germany); and 6 VIATORR stent grafts constrained coaxially within Memotherm reducing stents. There were no immediate periprocedural complications. The authors reported no technical failures or difficulties with deployment. PSGs were approximately doubled on average for patients receiving both reducing stents and reducing stent grafts, although the absolute initial gradients and

absolute increases in gradients were about half that in the reducing stent group compared with the stent graft reduction group. HE improved in 8 of 10 stent graft TIPS reduction patients but in only 2 of 6 patients treated with the reducing stents. Two of 4 patients treated with Optimed polyurethane-covered stents were treated for recurrence of pre-TIPS symptoms. One of these 2 patients was found angiographically to have severe stenosis of the reduced shunt; the other had occlusion, leading the authors to suggest superior patency of PTFE over polyurethane. Two patients in each of the VIATORR ePTFE-covered stent group needed additional reduction procedures performed. The authors speculated that a lower increase in PSG and uncertainty as to thrombosis of the space between reducing stent and original TIPS were likely causes of a significantly worse response in patients receiving the Memotherm. They pointed out that very little data existed on the efficacy of adjunctive "dead-space" embolization procedures.

Conclusion

Development or worsening of HE is a common complication of TIPS creation. Most patients with post-TIPS HE respond well to medical management, but a significant minority require endovascular intervention. TIPS reduction, originally performed with bare stents, seeks to reduce but not eliminate flow within TIPS shunts so as to prevent the sudden and profound hemodynamic shifts and mortality associated with intentional complete TIPS occlusion.

The advent of commercially available stent grafts beginning around the year 2000 has led to many new techniques that allow more immediate, effective, and precise TIPS flow reduction, with improved clinical outcomes. ▶ Table 18.3 highlights the relative advantages and disadvantages of the dominant contemporary TIPS reduction techniques.

Although the patient population requiring TIPS reductions is small and the literature is composed mostly of case reports and small case series, trends can be noted. These are detailed in the Clinical Pearls section at the end of the chapter. The majority of patients with post-TIPS HE but stable liver function experience substantial or complete recovery after TIPS reduction with one of these modern techniques. In the stent graft era, HE that does

Table 18.3 Pros and Cons of Types of Transjugular Intrahepatic Portosystemic Shunt Reduction Procedures

Procedure Type	Pros	Cons
"Sculpting" of balloon-expanded stent grafts	Less instrumentation Less costly Allows for serial dilation of reducing waist	Some versions of technique liable to stent graft migration Cannot reconstrict waist
Purse-string suture constraint of Wallgraft	Straightforward, reliable deployment	Fixed diameter of reducing waist Reports of Wallgraft-related TIPS thrombosis (possibly less frequent if original TIPS is PTFE lined)
Coaxial stent-constrained Wallgrafts	Serial dilatation of reducing waist	Some techniques theoretically liable to intraprocedural stent migration Cannot reconstrict waist Reports of Wallgraft-related TIPS thrombosis
Parallel stent and reducing stent graft deployment	Allows for easy intraprocedural and subsequent increase or decrease in TIPS diameter	Technically more complex
Parallel lasso catheter and stent graft	Allows easy intraprocedural increase or decrease in TIPS diameter	Does not allow for easy subsequent reduction of TIPS diameter Technically more complex

PTFE: polytetrafluoroethylene; TIPS: transjugular intrahepatic portosystemic shunt.

not improve after shunt reduction, similar to post-TIPS fulminant liver failure, is associated with a poor prognosis.

Clinical Pearls

- Most post-TIPS encephalopathy can be treated medically.
- Literature describing the efficacy of various TIPS-reducing techniques and their efficacy is composed of case series and case reports.
- TIPS reduction has replaced TIPS occlusion because of sudden, often fatal hemodynamic changes associated with the latter technique.
- Covered stents have replaced bare-metal stents for TIPS reduction because of their immediate and more predictable ability to decrease flow.
- TIPS reduction with covered stents is highly effective in the treatment of medicine-refractory hepatic encephalopathy.
- There are many different TIPS reduction techniques, each possessing individual risks and benefits. Dominant techniques tend to fall into 5 broad categories: stent-in-a-stent coaxially constrained stent grafts; purse-string–constrained stent-grafts; parallel-constrained stent grafts; balloon-expanded, "sculpted" single ePTFE-covered reducing stent grafts; and the lasso catheter–constrained stent grafts.
- Several reports have linked reduction with polyurethane- or -covered stents (Wallgrafts) and TIPS occlusion from pseudo-intimal hyperplasia. One recent study, however, suggests that reducing Wallgrafts may be safely used if a PTFE-covered stent was placed as the original TIPS.
- Partial insufflation of ePTFE-covered balloon-expanded stent grafts on their factory-mounted balloons as stand-alone reduction devices appears to carry a high risk of device migration.
- Angiographic reappearance of hepatopetal flow in portal vein branches may be a better indicator of clinical response to TIPS reduction than absolute or relative increases in portosystemic pressure gradients.
- Embolization of gastroesophageal varices at the time of TIPS reduction is advised and is routinely performed by a majority of authors. An increase in portosystemic gradient post-TIPS reduction to greater than 12 mm Hg is often necessary but is unlikely to result in recurrent variceal bleeding, possibly because of frequent use of adjunctive varix embolization during the reduction procedure.
- Lack of improvement in encephalopathy has been correlated with poor survival after TIPS reduction.
- Unlike encephalopathy, liver failure after TIPS may not respond to reduction procedures. Although many patients are not candidates, liver transplant remains the only effective long-term treatment of post-TIPS hepatic insufficiency. TIPS reduction may potentially serve as a bridge to transplant in this severely ill patient population with otherwise uniformly poor outcomes.

References

1. Sanyal AJ, Freedman AM, Shiffman ML, et al. Portosystemic encephalopathy after transjugular intrahepatic portosystemic shunt: results of a prospective controlled study. Hepatology 1994;20:46–55.
2. Jalan R, Elton RA, Redhead DN, et al. Analysis of prognostic variables in the prediction of mortality, shunt failure, variceal rebleeding and encephalopathy following the transjugular intrahepatic portosystemic stent-shunt for variceal haemorrhage. J Hepatol 1995;23:123–128.
3. Somberg KA, Riegler JL, LaBerge JM, et al. Hepatic encephalopathy after transjugular intrahepatic portosystemic shunts: incidence and risk factors. Am J Gastroenterol 1995;90:549–555.
4. Eesa M, Clark T. Transjugular intrahepatic portosystemic shunt: state of the art. Semin Roentgenol 2011;46:125–132.
5. Bureau C, Pagan JC, Layrargues GP, et al. Patency of stents covered with polytetrafluoroethylene in patients treated by transjugular intrahepatic portosystemic shunts: long-term results of a randomized multicentre study. Liver Int 2007;27:742–747.
6. Riggio O, Angeloni S, Salvatori FM, et al. Incidence, natural history, and risk factors of hepatic encephalopathy after transjugular intrahepatic portosystemic shunt with polytetrafluoroethylene-covered stent grafts. Am. J. Gastroenterol 2008;103: 2738–2746.
7. Haskal ZJ, Cope C, Soulen MC, et al. Intentional reversible thrombosis of transjugular intrahepatic portosystemic shunts. Radiology 1995;195:485–488.
8. Kerlan RK Jr, LaBerge JM, Baker EL, et al. Successful reversal of hepatic encephalopathy with intentional occlusion of transjugular intrahepatic portosystemic shunts. J Vasc Interv Radiol 1995;6:917–921.
9. Yang Z, Hang G, Wu Q, et al. Patency and clinical outcomes of transjugular intrahepatic portosystemic shunt with polytetrafluoroethylene-covered stents versus bare stents: a meta-analysis. J Gastroenterol Hepatol 2010;25: 1718–1725.
10. Hanna SS, Smith RS, Henderson JM, et al. Reversal of hepatic encephalopathy after occlusion of total portasystemic shunts. Am J Surg 1981;142:285–289.
11. Potts JR 3rd, Henderson JM, Millikan WJ Jr, et al. Restoration of portal venous perfusion and reversal of encephalopathy by balloon occlusion of portal systemic shunt. Gastroenterology 1984;87:208–212.
12. Uflacker R, Silva Ade O, d'Albuquerque LA, et al. Chronic portosystemic encephalopathy: embolization of portosystemic shunts. Radiology 1987;165:721–725.
13. Paz-Fumagalli R, Crain MR, Mewissen MW, et al. Fatal hemodynamic consequences of therapeutic closure of a transjugular intrahepatic portosystemic shunt. J Vasc Interv Radiol 1994;5:831–834.
14. Kochar N, Tripathi D, Ireland H, et al. Transjugular intrahepatic portosystemic stent shunt (TIPSS) modification in the management of post-TIPSS refractory hepatic encephalopathy. Gut 2006;55:1617–1623.
15. Jalan R, Hayes P. Risk of intentional reversible thrombosis of transjugular intrahepatic portosystemic shunt. Radiology 1995;197:587–588.
16. Madoff DC, Wallace MJ. Reduced stents and stent-grafts for the management of hepatic encephalopathy after transjugular intrahepatic portosystemic shunt creation. Semin Intervent Radiol 2005;22:316–328.
17. Haskal ZJ, Middlebrook MR. Creation of a stenotic stent to reduce flow through a transjugular intrahepatic portosystemic shunt. J Vasc Interv Radiol 1994;5:827–830.
18. Forauer AR, McLean GK. Transjugular intrahepatic portosystemic shunt constraining stent for the treatment of refractory postprocedural encephalopathy: a simple design utilizing a Palmaz stent and Wallstent. J Vasc Interv Radiol 1998;9:443–446.
19. Gerbes AL, Waggershauser T, Holl J, et al. Experiences with novel techniques for reduction of stent flow in transjugular intrahepatic portosystemic shunts. Z Gastroenterol 1998;36:373–377.
20. Hauenstein KH, Haag K, Ochs A, et al. The reducing stent: treatment for transjugular intrahepatic portosystemic shunt-induced refractory hepatic encephalopathy and liver failure. Radiology 1995;194:175–179.
21. Maleux G, Verslype C, Heye S, et al. Endovascular shunt reduction in the management of transjugular portosystemic shunt-induced hepatic encephalopathy: preliminary experience with reduction stents and stent grafts. Am J Roentgenol 2007;188:659–664.
22. Madoff DC, Wallace, MJ, Ahrar K, et al. TIPS-related hepatic encephalopathy: management options with novel endovascular techniques. Radiographics 2004;24:21–37.
23. Quaretti P, Michieletti E, Rossi S. Successful treatment of TIPS-induced hepatic failure with an hourglass stent-graft: a simple new technique for reducing shunt flow. J Vasc Interv Radiol 2001;12:887–890.
24. Fanelli F, Salvatori FM, Rabuffi P, et al. Management of refractory encephalopathy after insertion of TIPS: long-term results of shunt reduction with hourglass-shaped balloon-expandable stent-graft. Am J Roentgenol 2009; 193:1696–1702.
25. Kroma G, Lopera J, Cura M, et al. Transjugular intrahepatic portosystemic shunt flow reduction with adjustable polytetrafluoroethylene-covered balloon-expandable stents. J Vasc Interv Radiol 2009;20:981–986.
26. Madoff DC, Perez-Young IV, Wallace MJ, et al. Management of TIPS-related refractory hepatic encephalopathy with reduced Wallgraft endoprostheses. J Vasc Interv Radiol 2003;14:369–374.

27. Cox MW, Soltes GD, Lin PH, et al. Reversal of transjugular intrahepatic porto-systemic shunt (TIPS)-induced hepatic encephalopathy using a strictured self-expanding covered stent. Cardiovasc Intervent Radiol 2003;26:539–542.

28. Clarke G, Patal R, Tsao S, et al. Treatment of refractory post-transjugular porto-systemic stent-shunt encephalopathy: a novel case of stent luminal reduction. Eur J Gastroenterol Hepatol 2004;16:1387–1390.

29. Haskal ZJ, Brennecke LH. Transjugular intrahepatic portosystemic shunts formed with polyethylene terephthalate-covered stents: experimental evaluation in pigs. Radiology 1999;213:853–859.

30. Otal P, Rousseau H, Vinel J-P, et al. High occlusion rate in experimental trans-jugular intrahepatic portosystemic shunt created with a Dacron-covered nitinol stent. J Vasc Interv Radiol 1999;10:183–188.

31. Cejna M, Thurnher S, Pidlich J, et al. Primary implantation of polyester-covered stent-grafts for transjugular intrahepatic portosystemic stent shunts (TIPSS): a pilot study. Cardiovasc Interv Radiol 1999;22:305–310.

32. Jacquier A, Vidal V, Monnet O, et al. A modified procedure for transjugular intrahe-patic portosystemic shunt flow reduction. J Vasc Interv Radiol 2006;17:1359–1363.

33. Weintraub JL, Mobley DG, Weiss ME, et al. A novel endovascular adjusta-ble polytetrafluoroethylene-covered stent for the management of hepatic encephalopathy after transjugular intrahepatic portosystemic shunt. J Vasc Interv Radiol 2007;18:563–566.

34. Saket RR, Sze DY, Razavi MK, et al. TIPS reduction with use of stents or stent-grafts. J Vasc Interv Radiol 2004;15:745–751.

35. Holden A, Ng R, Gane E, et al. A technique for controlled parallel closure of a transjugular intrahepatic portosystemic shunt tract in a patient with hepatic encephalopathy. J Vasc Interv Radiol 2006;17:1957–1961.

36. Maleux G, Heye S, Verslype C, et al. Management of transjugular intrahepatic portosystemic shunt-induced refractory hepatic encephalopathy with the parallel technique: results of a clinical followup study. J Vasc Interv Radiol 2007;18:986–993.

37. Sze DY, Hwang GL, Kao JS, et al. Bidirectionally adjustable TIPS reduction by par-allel stent and stent-graft deployment. J Vasc Interv Radiol 2008;19:1653–1658.

38. Cookson DT, Zaman Z, Gordon-Smith J, et al. Management of transjugular intrahepatic portosystemic shunt (TIPS)-associated refractory hepatic enceph-alopathy by shunt reduction using the parallel technique: outcomes of a retro-spective case series. Cardiovasc Intervent Radiol 2011;34:92–99.

39. Monnin-Bares V, Thony F, Sengel C, et al. Stent-graft narrowed with lasso catheter: an adjustable TIPS reduction technique. J Vasc Interv Radiol 2010;21:275–280.

Chapter 19: Patency Outcomes of Transjugular Intrahepatic Portosystemic Shunts in the Stent-Graft Era

Bogdan Iliescu, Ziv J. Haskal, and Bertrand Janne d'Othée

Introduction

Twenty years elapsed between the original animal description of the transjugular intrahepatic portosystemic shunt (TIPS) in 1969 and the first human case. Those early human shunts were created with balloon expandable Palmaz stents, later moving to self-expanding stents. In 1992, the Wallstent became the first FDA-approved device for TIPS; thousands of patients were treated thereafter as the procedure became widely disseminated.[1–9] With these cases came increasing reports documenting frequent TIPS stenoses and occlusions, developing in as many as 25% to 50% of patients within 6 months of shunt creation.[3,10–13] This shunt dysfunction was associated with recurrent variceal bleeding, affecting 9.8% to 24% of patients in controlled trials.[14–21] Extensive literature developed, validating sonographic means of follow-up, the need for follow-up programs and repeated shunt revisions.[22–28] The patency question clouded the wider application of TIPS, particularly in 'healthier' Childs A patients.

These issues spurred a decade of investigations into both characterizing the histopathologic processes causing stenoses and solving them. Approaches included anticoagulation and antiplatelet regimens, radiation, and brachytherapy.[29–34] In the late1990's, both animal and human feasibility studies described marked patency improvements in TIPS lined with expanded polytetraflouoroethylene (ePTFE).[35–39] These led to commercial development of an FDA-approved TIPS ePTFE endograft, the VIATORR (W. L. Gore & Associates, Flagstaff, AZ). With this, most TIPS patency issues were resolved, and TIPS research turned increasingly to reassessment of prior clinical outcomes, with covered stents. Shunt creation for portal hypertension remains the mainstay treatment, with reduced mortality, morbidity, and hospitalization secondary to their creation in many patients electively rather than emergently.[40,41] This chapter reviews this history, as well as the current state of TIPS patency in the era of covered stents.

Histopathology of Shunt Stenosis

LaBerge et al reported the first human histology of seven TIPS explants in 1991.[42] Within a week of TIPS creation, metal stent wires were shown pressing back the surrounding liver tract, lined with clot and fibrin. By 3 weeks, pseudointimal tissue composed of myofibroblasts grew from the surrounding liver, enveloping the stents. By 3 months, dense collagen layers lined the lumina of the TIPS, with shunt stenoses (▶ Fig. 19.1). Subsequent post mortem and transplant donors further confirmed these findings.[42–46] This pseudo-endothelium appeared to be derived from the liver parenchyma (rather than dropout endothelialization).[47] In contrast, TIPS lined with stent-grafts only develop a thin pseudo-endothelium (▶ Fig. 19.2).

The outflow hepatic vein represents a second site of distinct shunt stenosis (▶ Fig. 19.3). After TIPS formation, its caliber has been shown to reduce to half its original diameter.[3] These stenoses appeared as early as 90 to 180 days after initial shunt placement (▶ Fig. 19.4). This intimal hyperplasia appears similar to that seen in other veins or anastomoses, as with dialysis graft venous stenoses or other surgical vascular anastomoses.[10,48,49]

A third, unique cause of TIPS failure is the biliary-to-TIPS fistula. As part of creating the shunt, biliary structures can be naturally traversed. In some cases, a sufficiently large bile duct may be punctured in close proximity to the eventual TIPS tract, allowing bile leakage into the tract. The thrombotic effect of bile can lead to recurring shunt occlusion within hours after creation.[50] The phenomenon is unique to bare stents. The inhibitory effect of

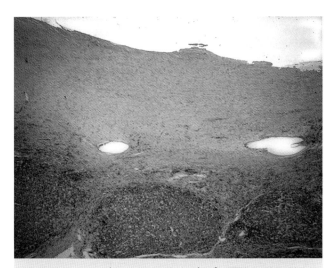

Fig. 19.1 Human explant specimen 9 months after TIPS creation using a Wallstent demonstrates a thick layer of fibroblasts that has grown through the stent wires, narrowing the shunt lumen. (Reprinted with permission of the SIR.)

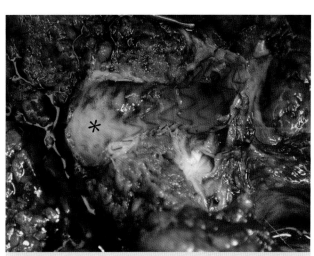

Fig. 19.2 Photograph of a gross specimen with a VIATORR-lined TIPS. This 14-month explant post liver transplant demonstrates only a thin white pseudo-endothelium (*asterisk*) lining parts of the stent, with no tract thrombus or stenosis.

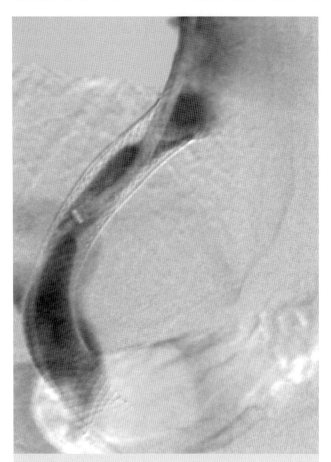

Fig. 19.3 Four-month venogram of a bare stent TIPS demonstrates diffuse stenosis of both the intraparenchymal and hepatic vein outflow portions of the TIPS. (Reprinted with permission of the SIR.)

bile on smooth muscle cells formation prevents the gradual pseudoendothelial proliferation that encompasses the bare stent's wires and leads to "TIPS healing."[51,52] This issue was resolved with ePTFE TIPS endografts that were designed to be relatively bile impermeable due to an outer fluoroethylene polymer wrap.

Medical Approaches to Inhibit Shunt Stenosis

Adjunct medical therapy has been studied for its potential to reduce TIPS occlusion in bare stent shunts. In a randomized trial of 49 TIPS patients treated for acute and subacute variceal hemorrhage, there were no shunt occlusions in the anticoagulation group compared with the control group, which had 5 shunt occlusions within the first 3 months.[29] The role of biliary leaks was not described. Subsequent follow-up demonstrated no significant difference in shunt dysfunction between the treated and control groups. Further, the routine use of anticoagulation in patients treated for variceal hemorrhage can create therapeutic dilemmas. Ultimately, anticoagulation has, in the stent graft era, little role in TIPS, with the exception of patients requiring anticoagulation because of underlying hypercoagulable syndromes. The majority of these patients are ones treated for Budd-Chiari syndrome or noncirrhotic patients treated for acute porto-spleno-mesenteric thrombosis.

In another trial, Siegerstetter et al randomized 84 patients to antiplatelet-derived growth factors and anti-aggregation agents vs. controls.[30] While they reported some evidence of reduced hepatic outflow vein stenosis in the experimental group, the therapy has not found widespread approval, partly presumably due to the development of endografts, the lack of widespread availability of some of the agents tested, and reluctance to expose patients with prior bleeding to prolonged clotting times.

The Development of TIPS Endografts

Animal Studies

The search for an alternative to the bare metal stent for lining the TIPS tract began with animal TIPS models. The porcine model proved to be an excellent substrate because it allowed the creation of shunts using human tools and techniques. Further, porcine TIPS histology mimics that seen in humans, with both intra-shunt and hepatic vein stenosis, though at a very accelerated rate: within a few weeks of TIPS creation.[35] These reliable effects are seen without the need for inducing portal hypertension or cirrhosis in the animal, a daunting task in growing swine.[53,54]

Multiple materials have been studied within this model, among them polyethylene terephthalate (PET), silicone, polycarbonate urethanes, and expanded polytetrafluoroethylene (ePTFE).[55–57] In 1995, Nishimine et al described the results of the first studies of ePTFE in swine TIPS.[35] Shunts created with handmade PTFE-lined stent grafts demonstrated a 69% patency rate at 4 weeks, compared to 8% for shunts utilizing bare stents. Additionally, stenoses in the patent PTFE-lined stents were less than 50%. At 3 months, 46% of the stent grafts were still patent. Shunt occlusion was attributed to draining vein stenosis in 38% of the failed shunts. This was echoed in a subsequent study by Haskal et al in 1997, using an encapsulated PTFE-stent graft designed for TIPS.[36] In 8 shunts, seven demonstrated wide patency by 5 months, while 85% of the bare stent control group demonstrated occlusions and stenoses by 4 weeks. Histologic reports of the explants paralleled the appearance of those described in prior human studies.[44,45] In contrast, TIPS created with silicone-covered endografts,[57] polycarbonate urethanes,[56] and polyethylene terephthalate/polyester,[58] showed no improvement or worse results, compared with bare stent controls (▶ Fig. 19.5).

Early Human Experience

With the promising animal results of TIPS, early human feasibility studies in both revision and de novo TIPS applications were reported (▶ Fig. 19.6).[38,49] In 1997, a Dotter Institute pilot study reported the use of a handmade ePTFE endograft used in revising failing TIPS.[49] Six patients were treated with a custom-made PTFE graft mounted on a Z-stent. This stent graft was dilated to 14 mm and held in place within the endothelial layer by Wallstents. Some shunts remained patent to 315 days. The results of this preliminary study indicated that the PTFE coating of the revised grafts was effective in prolonging shunt patency in patients with failing TIPS.

Ferral et al reported a series of 13 TIPS created with polyester fabric-covered nitinol stents (modified Cragg Endopro System I

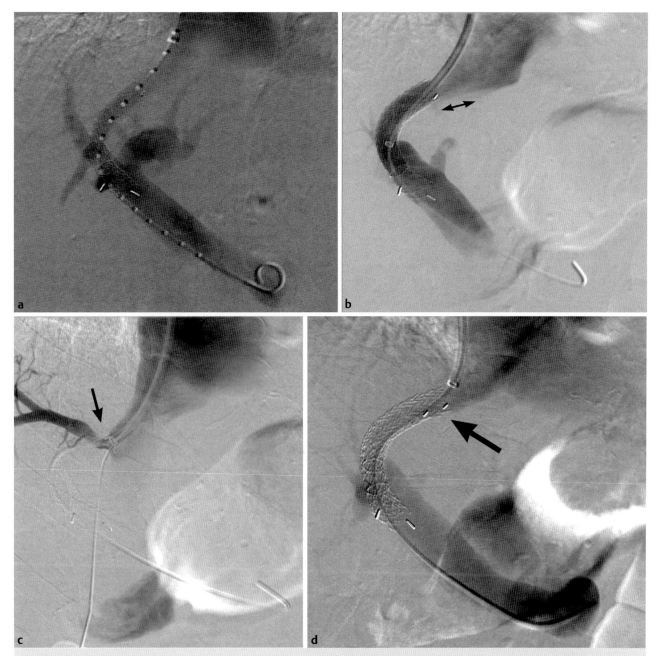

Fig. 19.4 A 60-year-old woman with nonalcoholic liver cirrhosis who underwent VIATORR TIPS creation for treatment of portal gastropathy and refractory ascites. (a) Digital subtraction portal venography after TIPS creation. The portosystemic gradient dropped from 21 mm Hg to 10 mm Hg. Her ascites resolved over several weeks. (b) Fourteen months later, she returned with recurrent ascites requiring frequent paracenteses and diuretic therapy. TIPS venography demonstrates an unstented segment of outflow hepatic vein (*double arrow*). The shunt is otherwise widely patent. In retrospect, the hepatic vein was incompletely covered at the time of initial shunt creation. (c) Hepatic venogram with catheters in both the TIPS and the inferior vena cava demonstrates the secondary stenosis of the outflow vein (*arrow*). (d) After placement of a coaxial VIATORR, the portosystemic gradient was reduced from 18 mm Hg to 12 mm Hg. At the 4-week follow-up, her ascites had spontaneously diuresed.

stent graft).[59] While the long-term follow-up and shunt patency assessments were mixed and somewhat incompletely described, this study focused on the technical success of shunt creation with nondedicated stent grafts and the immediate patency results. The thrombotic effect of polyethylene terephthalate graft material within the TIPS tracts, as with swine, was confirmed in a subsequent series using PET-covered Wallstents.[58] This series described salvage of PET-lined TIPS using PTFE-covered stent grafts. The

reason for the thrombogenic effect of polyester in the de novo TIPS tract is specific to acute shunt creation and its exposure to a fresh parenchymal tract. Luo et al described similar findings with higher 1-year and 2-year patency rates of 91% and 85% for PTFE stents versus 78% and 63% for PET-covered stents.[60] Later studies and experience have shown that PET is not as thrombotic, when used to reduce mature endothelialized bare stent or ePTFE-lined shunts.

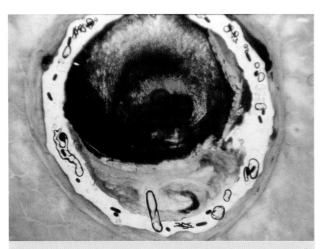

Fig. 19.5 Two-week explant from a porcine TIPS created with a non-porous prototype polycarbonate urethane endograft demonstrates shunt thrombosis without evidence of endothelialization.

Outcomes of Bare Versus Commercially Available Covered Stents

The encouraging animal and preliminary human study data led to numerous reports of custom-made PTFE stent grafts. These further confirmed the marked shunt patency improvements.[37,38,58,61-64] A commercially designed TIPS endograft was manufactured by W. L. Gore and Associates and was marketed as the "VIATORR TIPS endoprosthesis." The randomized multicenter U.S. trial comparing it to the Wallstent was begun in 1999, and led to FDA on label approval of the device for both de novo and revision TIPS applications. This study enrolled 253 patients and shunt stenosis was evaluated by venography. There was a marked decrease in shunt stenosis at 6 months in the VIATORR group, to only 16% as compared to 42% (p < 0.001) in the Wallstent

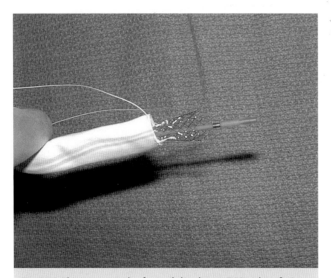

Fig. 19.6 This is an example of an early hand-sewn TIPS endograft. Pre-expanded ePTFE was sutured onto the leading end of a Wallstent. It was then compressed into a loading cartridge using a surrounding lacing suture (not shown).[38]

group, with an associated significantly longer time to revision in the stent-graft group.

These findings fostered the exponential growth in use of TIPS stent grafts (► Table 19.1). Hausegger et al utilized sonography and venography for follow-up evaluation of such patients, reporting patency rates at 6 months and 12 months of 87% and 80%, respectively.[65] In the subgroup of patients evaluated by venography, the portosystemic gradient remained essentially unchanged at 6 months. In 2007, Bureau et al reported a multicenter study in France, Spain, and Canada in which 80 patients were randomized to VIATORR or bare stents.[66] Patients were followed by ultrasound every 3 months and angiography every 6 months, or at the time of dysfunction. At 2 years, the VIATORR group patency rate was 76% versus 36% in the bare stent group (p = 0.001), and absence of encephalopathy in 67% and 51% (p < 0.05), respectively. The probability of survival at 2 years for VIATORR and bare stent patients was not statistically significant at 58% and 45%, respectively. Ultrasound surveillance was deemed insufficiently accurate enough to predict shunt dysfunction in this study. However, a retrospective review of 126 patients post TIPS surveillance with ultrasound demonstrated that shunt dysfunction detection rates are equivalent for stent graft and bare stent shunts.[67] In 2003, Angermayr et al confirmed improved survival in a retrospective comparative review of patients treated with stent grafts versus bare stents in the creation of TIPS, reporting a survival rate of 88% versus 73% at 1 year and 76% versus 62% at 2 years, respectively (p = 0.01).[68]

The new predictable durability of shunts fostered further comparisons with different shunt diameters. In 2010, Riggio et al reported randomization of cirrhotic patients with variceal bleeding and/or refractory ascites to 8-mm or 10-mm diameter VIATORR stent grafts.[69] Evaluated outcomes included recurrent symptoms and encephalopathy. The trial was stopped after enrolling 45 patients, as patients treated with the 8-mm device were found to have persistent ascites or varices after TIPS. The overall decrease in pressure gradient was significantly lower in the 10-mm group, explaining the observed differences, without decreased hepatic encephalopathy. While the findings are notable, it is arguable that the question of optimizing stent diameters has not been resolved, as ascites and hemorrhage cohorts were mixed together. The goal is to create the smallest portosystemic shunt that will treat the given indication in a patient (► Fig. 19.7). To that end, a diametrically adjustable TIPS endograft could be a great advantage to patients. At present, this is achieved by deployment of a 10-mm VIATORR without balloon expansion, or initial dilation only to 8-mm. Later, continued radial expansion of the endograft can be performed, as needed, and may lead to a fully expanded stent graft in many patients.

In a 2010 New England of Journal Medicine study, Garcia-Pagan et al reported a randomized comparison of patients with acute variceal hemorrhage treated with early TIPS (with endografts) compared with continued endoscopic therapy.[70] Sixty-three patients were included: 32 patients treated with TIPS, 31 with pharmacologic and endoscopic therapy. At a mean 16 months follow-up, rebleeding or inability to control bleeding was far lower in the TIPS group vs. endoscopic therapy (3% vs. 50%, p < 0.001) and 1-year survival was 86% and 61%, respectively (p < 0.001). Days in intensive care units were 8.6 ± 9 vs. 3.6 ± 4 in TIPS patients (p = 0.01) and overall hospitalization time (median 15 vs. 4 days, p = 0.014) were significantly higher in the non-TIPS group. This study was the first to show that early TIPS

Table 19.1 Multiple Studies Evaluating Patency of ePTFE Stent-Grafts Versus Bare Stents in the Creation of Transjugular Intrahepatic Portosystemic Shunts Confirm the Higher Patency Rates of PTFE-Lined Shunts

Author	Year	Study Type	Patient Number		Patency	
			Bare Stent	Endograft	Bare Stent	Endograft
					1 YEAR	1 YEAR
Angeloni et al[89]	2004	Prospective Nonrandomized	87	32	57.5%	87%
Bureau et al[91]	2004	Prospective Randomized	39	41	56%	87%
Charon et al[100]	2004	Retrospective	0	100	NA	84%
Barrio et al[93]	2005	Retrospective	20	50	18%	100%
Rossle et al[101]	2006	Retrospective	0	100	NA	90%
Tripathi et al[96]	2006	Retrospective	316	157	46%	92%
Gandini et al[102]	2006	Retrospective	6	7	0%	85.7%
Wu et al[103]	2010	Retrospective	30	30	70%	100%
Maleux et al[104]	2010	Retrospective	126	96	51%	81%
					2 YEAR 1 YEAR	2 YEAR 1 YEAR
Perarnau et al[74]	2014	Prospective Randomized	67	62	37.4%	66%
Lauermann et al[75]	2016	Retrospective	80	83	83.3%	93.1%
				Range	18–83.3%	81–100%

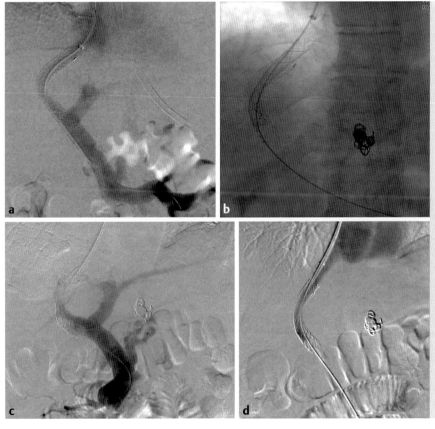

Fig. 19.7 Excessive encephalopathy after VIATORR TIPS creation. A 47-year-old male with cirrhosis presented with life-threatening esophageal variceal hemorrhage and hydrothorax. (**a**) After TIPS, the portosystemic gradient pressure decreased from 23 mm Hg to 11 mm Hg. (**b**) Three months post TIPS, he presented with persistent encephalopathy despite maximal medical therapy (xifaxan and lactulose). A 6-0 PTFE suture-constrained Wallgraft was placed within the shunt, raising the portosystemic gradient from 12 to 18 mm Hg. His encephalopathy resolved and his hydrothorax remained controlled. (**c**) Five months after TIPS reduction, he returned with recurrent hydrothorax. Venography demonstrated TIPS occlusion. (**d**) A VIATORR was deployed within the occluded shunt but left at the smaller caliber. The portosystemic gradient decreased from 28 mm Hg to 17 mm Hg. One year later, he continued to remain encephalopathy free and without recurrent hydrothorax.

creation with endografts led to prolonged transplant-free survival, reduced bleeding, and shorter hospitalization.

The utilization of other ePTFE stent grafts has been reported, although they were not "purpose-built" for TIPS. In 2011, Xue et al reported the results of 80 patients treated with TIPS from a total of 137 between 2002 and 2009; no follow-up was available for the remaining 57 patients.[71] Thirty-seven Fluency (Bard Peripheral Vascular, Tempe AZ) patients and 43 bare stent patients were described, with reduced re-bleeding rates in the endograft patients (13.5% vs. 32.6%). The higher rates of encephalopathy in patients treated with larger diameter devices led to their recommendation of 8-mm stents in Child A and C patients.

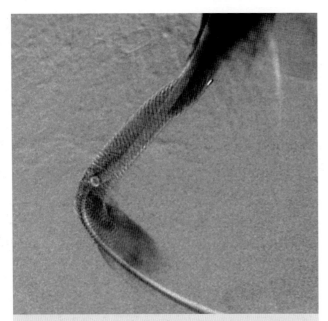

Fig. 19.8 Five-year follow-up venogram of a bare stent TIPS, which was later revised using a VIATORR. Three prior revisions had been performed due to recurrent stenoses and variceal hemorrhage. The shunt remained widely patent at 8-year sonographic follow-up (not shown).

The results of a trial comparing TIPS outcomes in a total of 128 patients by Gaba et al were reported in 2012, where 58 shunts were created using Wallstents, and 70 using a VIATORR stent graft.[72] The findings confirmed the previously reported greater dysfunction rates in bare stent shunts; however, they found a significant reduction in rebleeding rates in patients who received concomitant variceal embolization (5% vs. 25% in the nonembolized group; p = 0.013). They confirmed much longer shunt patency in the VIATORR patients (▶ Fig. 19.8).

Stent grafts have improved patency in de novo TIPS, as well as shunt revisions. In 2011, Jirkovsky et al reported the results of a retrospective study of 121 patients with bare metal TIPS dysfunction who were treated with angioplasty alone, new bare stent placement, or PTFE endografts.[73] The stent graft patency of 88.1% and 80.8% at 12 and 24 months, respectively, was significantly higher than angioplasty alone (49.7% at 12 months and 25.3% at 24 months; p = 0.0001) as were the bare stent revised patients (patency of 74.9% at 12 months and 64.9% at 24 months; p = 0.005). These significantly prolonged patency rates mimic those seen in de novo TIPS created with endografts.

The results of a prospective, randomized clinical trial to evaluate TIPS patency were reported by Perarnau et al in 2014.[74] A total of 137 patients were randomized into two groups: shunt creation with stent grafts and bare stents. They reported a significantly lower dysfunction of stent grafts compared to bare stents, with similar hepatic encephalopathy and death rates, confirming the superior patency rate of stent grafts. These findings were confirmed by Lauermann et al in 2016, who reported significantly higher patency rates in TIPS created with covered stents versus bare stents, with no difference in technical success rate, encephalopathy, or death rates (▶ Table 19.1).[75]

A retrospective review of 262 patients treated with ePTFE-lined shunts created over a 10-year period was reported by Weber et al

in 2015.[76] Patency rates of 74%, 62%, and 50% were found at 2-, 4-, and 6-year follow-up, respectively. The secondary patency rates were reported as 99%, 91%, and 84% for 2, 4, and 6 years, respectively, with 30% of revisions needed past 2 years from placement. This data confirms long-term patency of stent grafts, with the need for close follow-up and monitoring beyond 2 years post shunt creation. The multitude of retrospective as well as randomized studies clearly favor the stent graft patency over bare stents for the de novo as well as revision of transjugular intrahepatic portosystemic shunts.

Patency Outcomes of Endograft Use in Budd-Chiari Patients

Patients with Budd-Chiari Syndrome (BCS) represent a unique group of individuals with obstruction of the hepatic venous outflow (▶ Fig. 19.9). The creation of TIPS in these patients is complicated by their hypercoagulability as well as their predilection to shunt stenosis and thrombosis, frequently requiring multiple shunt revisions. In 2008, Darwish Murad et al reported a 2-year patency rate of 56% in PTFE-covered TIPS vs. 12% in those created with bare stents (p = 0.09).[77]

The prolonged patency of stent grafts was further confirmed by a multicenter study of 124 BCS patients treated with TIPS. There was a significantly lower rate of shunt dysfunction in patients treated with PTFE grafts compared to those with bare stents (p = 0.001), concluding that long-term survival for patients with BCS treated by TIPS is excellent.[78] With the advent of stent graft use the durability of the shunts has increased, associated with a decrease in revision rates and excellent clinical outcome.[79-84]

The presence of jaundice in patients with BCS may prevent the creation of TIPS in some patients. He et al reported the successful placement of a transjugular intrahepatic portosystemic shunt in 21 patients with severe hyperbilirubinemia secondary to BCS, with 100% technical success rate and no complications.[85] At 8 weeks post shunt creation, there was a significant decrease in total bilirubin from 266.24+/−122.03 to 40.11+/−3.52 μmol/L (p < 0.01), with no jaundice present in all patients at 1-year follow-up.

Pediatric TIPS and Endografts

The number of pediatric patients who require TIPS is much smaller, but patency issues are similar to those in adults. Smaller series have reported the benefits of use of endografts in this population. In a series of 9 patients less than 18 years of age (including an infant less than 18 months old) with varices, Vo et al reported in 2012 a TIPS patency rate of 100%, up to a mean follow-up duration of 20 months (range: 4 days to 32 months), utilizing PTFE endografts. There were no major complications associated with the shunt creation.[86]

In 2012, Di Giorgio et al further confirmed the feasibility of TIPS creation in the pediatric population, for patients who did not respond to medical and endoscopic treatment of ascites or bleeding varices.[87] Of the 13 children treated with VIATORR stent grafts, the portosystemic gradient was successfully decreased in 11 children, with 10 children experiencing complete resolution of the portal hypertension symptoms. They reported no cases of encephalopathy and shunt patency to 20.4 months (range 0.2-67 months). Subsequently, results of a retrospective review of

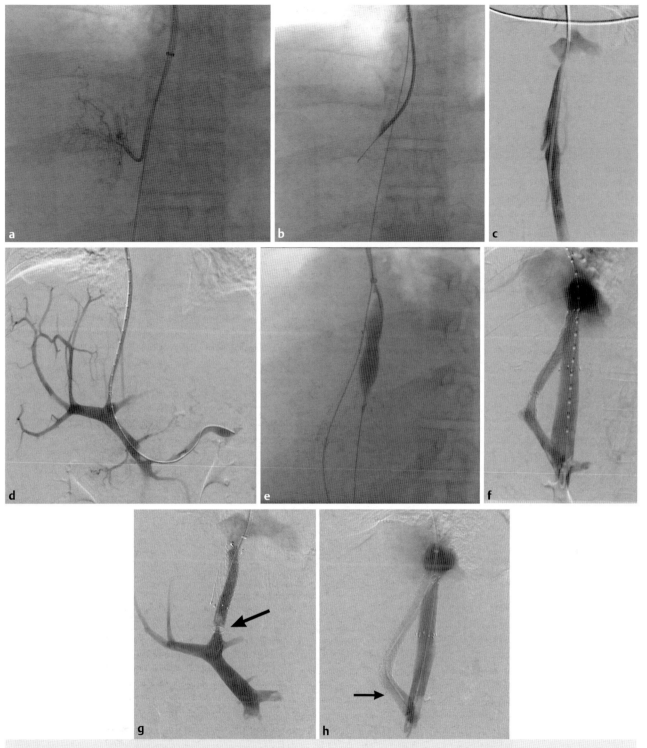

Fig. 19.9 A 37-year-old man with massive ascites due to subacute Budd-Chiari Syndrome. While ePTFE stent grafts have minimized shunt thromboses, these patients have proven prone to development of early or late hyperplastic stenoses at both portal and caval anastomoses. (**a**) Venogram of a remnant small hepatic vein demonstrates the typical spider web appearance of hepatic vein collaterals. (**b**) Trans-caval hepatic biopsy revealed hepatic congestion and sinusoidal dilatation (not shown). (**c**) Inferior vena cavagram demonstrates typical compression of the cephalic portion of the IVC from hepatic congestion. The trans-caval gradient was 12 mm Hg. (**d**) Trans-caval portography during shunt creation demonstrates splaying of the intrahepatic portal vein branches and thrombus at the spleno-portal junction. The initial portal vein pressure was 42 mm Hg. The portosystemic gradient was 29 mm Hg. (**e**) After shunt creation, the VIATORR impinged upon the IVC lumen. A bare metallic stent was placed and balloon expanded within the cava, adjacent to the VIATORR. (**f**) Final simultaneous TIPS and caval venography. Final portosystemic gradient was 10 mm Hg. The trans-caval gradient was 4 mm Hg. (**g**) His ascites rapidly resolved after TIPS. However, it recurred 2 months later and repeat venography demonstrated that a stenosis had developed at the uncovered portal end of the TIPS endograft (*arrow*). (**h**) This was treated with additional stent graft placement (Fig. 19.4b) (*arrow* showing leading end of newer VIATORR). At 1.5 years of follow up, he remains ascites free and liver function tests are normal.

outcomes in children with ePTFE-covered shunts, placed to treat gastrointestinal bleeding, were reported by Zurera et al in 2015 in a series of 12 children with a mean age of 9.[88] There were 2 stenoses found, at 9 and 54 months, and 2 graft occlusions at 7 and 12 months, all successfully treated with coaxial stent placement.

Finally, due to different ages of the pediatric patient, although adult-sized endografts have been utilized, some will require smaller, balloon expandable endografts.

Rationale for Use of Uncovered Stents in Some TIPS

With the widespread utilization of stent grafts for the creation of modern TIPS, there remains a population of cases where the use of uncovered stents to line the transhepatic tract may be desirable. Bare metal stents may be indicated during emergent TIPS creation in patients with high risk or known bacteremia, in order to minimize the risk of seeding prosthetic graft material. The TIPS can be revised with a stent graft at a later date once the infections are resolved.

Another subgroup that may benefit from bare stent TIPS includes patients with higher risk of encephalopathy. In these, the progressive narrowing of the bare metal TIPS can provide an "auto-titration" of the shunt luminal diameter, balancing encephalopathy vs. control of bleeding or ascites. At a later date, an endograft can be placed into the narrowed lumen to stabilize it at that diameter.

Bare stents may be of benefit for patients in whom there is desired obsolescence of their TIPS. In acute porto-spleno-mesenteric thrombosis and occlusion, in which lysis and therapy is achieved by the presence of a TIPS, there may not be a need for lifelong diversion and self-closure of the TIPS may be desirable.

Finally, living donor liver transplant recipients with small for size livers, in whom early portal hypertension results in ascites, may be treated with the creation of TIPS. As the organ hypertrophies over time to compensate for the hepatic function required in the recipient, there may not be a need for continued decompression; thus, a bare stent tract would eventually stenose and occlude, and additional intervention may not be required.

Conclusion

The development and widespread utilization of PTFE stent-grafts have resulted in TIPS reaching a decade of durability and patency for treatment of patients with stigmata of portal hypertension. Despite the multiple reports of prolonged patency and durability of PTFE shunts compared to the bare stents, there are many unanswered questions that remain to be investigated.

The widespread utilization of PTFE stent grafts in the creation of TIPS has resulted in a dramatic and noticeable increase in shunt patency, both in de novo and revised grafts, with a reduction in the need for further interventions and frequency of surveillance. Currently it is estimated that more than 8 of 10 shunts created worldwide are lined with a PTFE endograft. Further studies must continue to revisit the early control trials of bare stents with the now commonly used stent grafts.[39,69,70,74–76,89–96]

The optimal shunt diameter remains to be confirmed, and is unlikely to be universally optimal for all patients. Gaba et al[97] and Pieper et al[98] found that placing a self-expanding ePTFE stent graft such as the VIATORR or a bare stent, within a newly created shunt, results in a shunt diameter close to the stent's native size, even in cases where the stent was under-dilated at the time of placement. The ability to customize and tailor the ideal diameter for individual patients and indication will be a necessity in order to provide prime response and symptomatic outcome, while minimizing complications and encephalopathy. Shunt design technology investigation needs to parallel the clinical investigation, perhaps by the creation of devices that allow diametric adjustment of shunt size.[99]

References

1. Tesdal IK, Jaschke W, Buhler M, et al. Transjugular intrahepatic portosystemic shunting (TIPS) with balloon-expandable and self-expanding stents: technical and clinical aspects after 3 1/2 years' experience. Cardiovasc Intervent Radiol 1997;20(1):29–37.
2. Rossle M, Siegerstetter V, Huber M, Ochs A. The first decade of the transjugular intrahepatic portosystemic shunt (TIPS): state of the art. Liver 1998;18(2):73–89.
3. Haskal ZJ, Pentecost MJ, Soulen MC, Shlansky-Goldberg RD, Baum RA, Cope C. Transjugular intrahepatic portosystemic shunt stenosis and revision: early and midterm results. AJR Am J Roentgenol 1994;163(2):439–44.
4. Haskal ZJ, Rees CR, Ring EJ, Saxon R, Sacks D. Reporting standards for transjugular intrahepatic portosystemic shunts. Technology Assessment Committee of the SCVIR. J Vasc Interv Radiol 1997;8(2):289–97.
5. Hebbard GS, Fitt G, Thomson KR, et al. Transjugular intrahepatic portal-systemic shunts (TIPS)–initial experience and clinical outcome. Australian and New Zealand Journal of Medicine 1994;24(2):141–8.
6. Lau LD, Wong LL, Tsai NC, Kon KN, Wong LM. Transjugular intrahepatic portosystemic shunt (TIPS): treatment of esophageal variceal bleeding. Hawaii Med J 1995;54(1):382–5.
7. Lind CD. Transjugular intrahepatic portosystemic shunt (TIPS) in the management of esophageal variceal hemorrhage. Compr Ther 1995;21(4):189–94.
8. Rousseau H, Vinel JP, Bilbao JI, et al. Transjugular intrahepatic portosystemic shunts using the Wallstent prosthesis: a follow-up study. Cardiovasc Intervent Radiol 1994;17(1):7–11.
9. Rosch J. Development of transjugular intrahepatic portosystemic shunt. J Vasc Interv Radiol 2015;26(2):220–2.
10. Saxon RS, Ross PL, Mendel-Hartvig J, et al. Transjugular intrahepatic portosystemic shunt patency and the importance of stenosis location in the development of recurrent symptoms. Radiology 1998;207(3):683–93.
11. LaBerge JM, Somberg KA, Lake JR, et al. Two-year outcome following transjugular intrahepatic portosystemic shunt for variceal bleeding: results in 90 patients. Gastroenterology 1995;108(4):1143–51.
12. Sterling KM, Darcy MD. Stenosis of transjugular intrahepatic portosystemic shunts: presentation and management. AJR Am J Roentgenol 1997;168(1):239–44.
13. Nazarian GK, Ferral H, Castaneda-Zuniga WR, et al. Development of stenoses in transjugular intrahepatic portosystemic shunts. Radiology. 1994;192(1):231–4.
14. Jalan R, Forrest EH, Stanley AJ, et al. A randomized trial comparing transjugular intrahepatic portosystemic stent-shunt with variceal band ligation in the prevention of rebleeding from esophageal varices. Hepatology. 1997;26(5):1115–22.
15. Cello JP, Ring EJ, Olcott EW, et al. Endoscopic sclerotherapy compared with percutaneous transjugular intrahepatic portosystemic shunt after initial sclerotherapy in patients with acute variceal hemorrhage. A randomized, controlled trial. Ann Intern Med 1997;126(11):858–65.
16. Merli M, Salerno F, Riggio O, et al. Transjugular intrahepatic portosystemic shunt versus endoscopic sclerotherapy for the prevention of variceal bleeding in cirrhosis: a randomized multicenter trial. Gruppo Italiano Studio TIPS (G.I.S.T.). Hepatology 1998;27(1):48–53.
17. Rossle M, Deibert P, Haag K, et al. Randomised trial of transjugular-intrahepatic-portosystemic shunt versus endoscopy plus propranolol for prevention of variceal rebleeding. Lancet 1997;349(9058):1043–9.
18. Sauer P, Theilmann L, Stremmel W, Benz C, Richter GM, Stiehl A. Transjugular intrahepatic portosystemic stent shunt versus sclerotherapy plus propranolol for variceal rebleeding. Gastroenterology 1997;113(5):1623–31.
19. Sanyal AJ, Freedman AM, Luketic VA, et al. Transjugular intrahepatic portosystemic shunts compared with endoscopic sclerotherapy for the prevention of recurrent variceal hemorrhage. A randomized, controlled trial. Ann Intern Med 1997;126(11):849–57.

20. Cabrera J, Maynar M, Granados R, et al. Transjugular intrahepatic portosystemic shunt versus sclerotherapy in the elective treatment of variceal hemorrhage. Gastroenterology 1996;110(3):832–9.

21. Garcia-Villarreal L, Martinez-Lagares F, Sierra A, et al. Transjugular intrahepatic portosystemic shunt versus endoscopic sclerotherapy for the prevention of variceal rebleeding after recent variceal hemorrhage. Hepatology 1999;29(1):27–32.

22. Haskal ZJ, Carroll JW, Jacobs JE, Arger PH, Yin D, Coleman BG, et al. Sonography of transjugular intrahepatic portosystemic shunts: detection of elevated portosystemic gradients and loss of shunt function. J Vasc Interv Radiol 1997;8(4):549–56.

23. Lake D, Guimaraes M, Ackerman S, Hannegan C, Schonholz C, Selby JB, et al. Comparative results of Doppler sonography after TIPS using covered and bare stents. AJR Am J Roentgenol 2006;186(4):1138–43.

24. Middleton WD, Teefey SA, Darcy MD. Doppler evaluation of transjugular intrahepatic portosystemic shunts. Ultrasound Quarterly 2003;19(2):56–70; quiz 108–10.

25. Zizka J, Elias P, Krajina A, Michl A, Lojik M, Ryska P, et al. Value of Doppler sonography in revealing transjugular intrahepatic portosystemic shunt malfunction: a 5-year experience in 216 patients. AJR Am J Roentgenol 2000;175(1):141–8.

26. Puttemans T, Agneessens E, Mathieu J. T.I.P.S.: follow-up imaging and revision procedure. Acta Gastroenterol Belg 2000;63(2):174–8.

27. Furst G, Malms J, Heyer T, Saleh A, Cohnen M, Frieling T, et al. Transjugular intrahepatic portosystemic shunts: improved evaluation with echo-enhanced color Doppler sonography, power Doppler sonography, and spectral duplex sonography. AJR Am J Roentgenol 1998;170(4):1047–54.

28. Kanterman RY, Darcy MD, Middleton WD, Sterling KM, Teefey SA, Pilgram TK. Doppler sonography findings associated with transjugular intrahepatic portosystemic shunt malfunction. AJR Am J Roentgenol 1997;168(2):467–72.

29. Sauer P, Theilmann L, Herrmann S, Bruckner T, Roeren T, Richter G, et al. Phenprocoumon for prevention of shunt occlusion after transjugular intrahepatic portosystemic stent shunt: a randomized trial. Hepatology 1996;24(6):1433–6.

30. Siegerstetter V, Huber M, Ochs A, Blum HE, Rossle M. Platelet aggregation and platelet-derived growth factor inhibition for prevention of insufficiency of the transjugular intrahepatic portosystemic shunt: a randomized study comparing trapidil plus ticlopidine with heparin treatment. Hepatology 1999;29(1):33–8.

31. Hausegger KA, Portugaller H, Macri NP, Tauss J, Schedlbauer P, Deutschmann J, et al. Covered stents in transjugular portosystemic shunt: healing response to non-porous ePTFE covered stent grafts with and without intraluminal irradiation. Eur Radiol 2003;13(7):1549–58.

32. Dvorak J, Hulek P, Raupach J, Vanasek T, Petera J, Krajina A, et al. Endovascular brachytherapy of transjugular intrahepatic portosystemic shunt. Cardiovasc Radiat Med 2000;2(1):3–6.

33. Pokrajac B, Cejna M, Kettenbach J, Schamp S, Fellner C, Seitz W, et al. Intraluminal 192Ir brachytherapy following transjugular intrahepatic portosystemic shunt revision: long-term results and radiotherapy parameters. Cardiovasc Radiat Med 2001;2(3):133–7.

34. Lessie T, Yoon HC, Nelson HA, Fillmore DJ, Baldwin GN, Miller FJ. Intraluminal irradiation for TIPS stenosis: preliminary results in a swine model. J Vasc Interv Radiol 1999;10(7):899–906.

35. Nishimine K, Saxon RR, Kichikawa K, Mendel-Hartvig J, Timmermans HA, Shim HJ, et al. Improved transjugular intrahepatic portosystemic shunt patency with PTFE-covered stent-grafts: experimental results in swine. Radiology 1995;196(2):341–7.

36. Haskal ZJ, Davis A, McAllister A, Furth EE. PTFE-encapsulated endovascular stent-graft for transjugular intrahepatic portosystemic shunts: experimental evaluation. Radiology 1997;205(3):682–8.

37. DiSalle RS, Dolmatch BL. Treatment of TIPS stenosis with ePTFE graft-covered stents. Cardiovasc Intervent Radiol 1998;21(2):172–5.

38. Haskal ZJ. Improved patency of transjugular intrahepatic portosystemic shunts in humans: creation and revision with PTFE stent-grafts. Radiology 1999;213(3):759–66.

39. Cejna M, Peck-Radosavljevic M, Thurnher S, et al. ePTFE-covered stent-grafts for revision of obstructed transjugular intrahepatic portosystemic shunt. Cardiovasc Intervent Radiol 2002;25(5):365–72.

40. Perry BC, Kwan SW. Portosystemic shunts: stable utilization and improved outcomes, two decades after the transjugular intrahepatic portosystemic shunt. J Am Coll Radiol 2015.

41. Deltenre P, Trepo E, Rudler M, et al. Early transjugular intrahepatic portosystemic shunt in cirrhotic patients with acute variceal bleeding: a systematic review and meta-analysis of controlled trials. Eur J Gastroenterol Hepatol 2015;27(9):e1–9.

42. LaBerge JM, Ferrell LD, Ring EJ, et al. Histopathologic study of transjugular intrahepatic portosystemic shunts. J Vasc Interv Radiol 1991;2(4):549–56.

43. Sanyal AJ, Contos MJ, Yager D, Zhu YN, Willey A, Graham MF. Development of pseudointima and stenosis after transjugular intrahepatic portasystemic shunts: characterization of cell phenotype and function. Hepatology 1998;28(1):22–32.

44. Terayama N, Matsui O, Kadoya M, et al. Transjugular intrahepatic portosystemic shunt: histologic and immunohistochemical study of autopsy cases. Cardiovasc Intervent Radiol 1997;20(6):457–61.

45. Ducoin H, El-Khoury J, Rousseau H, et al. Histopathologic analysis of transjugular intrahepatic portosystemic shunts. Hepatology 1997;25(5):1064–9.

46. Teng GJ, Bettmann MA, Hoopes PJ, Ermeling BL, Yang L, Wagner RJ. Transjugular intrahepatic portosystemic shunt in a porcine model: histologic characteristics at the early stage. Acad Radiol 1998;5(8):547–55.

47. Sanyal AJ, Mirshahi F. Endothelial cells lining transjugular intrahepatic portasystemic shunts originate in hepatic sinusoids: implications for pseudointimal hyperplasia. Hepatology 1999;29(3):710–8.

48. Clark TW, Agarwal R, Haskal ZJ, Stavropoulos SW. The effect of initial shunt outflow position on patency of transjugular intrahepatic portosystemic shunts. J Vasc Interv Radiol 2004;15(2 Pt 1):147–52.

49. Saxon RR, Timmermans HA, Uchida BT, et al. Stent-grafts for revision of TIPS stenoses and occlusions: a clinical pilot study. J Vasc Interv Radiol 1997;8(4):539–48.

50. Saxon RR, Mendel-Hartvig J, Corless CL, et al. Bile duct injury as a major cause of stenosis and occlusion in transjugular intrahepatic portosystemic shunts: comparative histopathologic analysis in humans and swine. J Vasc Interv Radiol 1996;7(4):487–97.

51. Teng GJ, Lu Q. Bile leakage during transjugular intrahepatic portosystemic shunt creation: in vitro effect of bile on growth and function of human umbilical vein endothelium. Radiology 2005;235(3):867–71.

52. Teng GJ, Bettmann MA, Hoopes PJ, et al. Transjugular intrahepatic portosystemic shunt: effect of bile leak on smooth muscle cell proliferation. Radiology 1998;208(3):799–805.

53. Kichikawa K, Saxon RR, Nishimine K, Nishida N, Uchida BT. Experimental TIPS with spiral Z-stents in swine with and without induced portal hypertension. Cardiovasc Intervent Radiol 1997;20(3):197–203.

54. Pavcnik D, Saxon RR, Kubota Y, et al. Attempted induction of chronic portal venous hypertension with polyvinyl alcohol particles in swine. J Vasc Interv Radiol 1997;8(1 Pt 1):123–8.

55. Haskal ZJ, Brennecke LH. Transjugular intrahepatic portosystemic shunts formed with polyethylene terephthalate-covered stents: experimental evaluation in pigs. Radiology 1999;213(3):853–9.

56. Haskal ZJ, Brennecke LJ. Porous and nonporous polycarbonate urethane stent-grafts for TIPS formation: biologic responses. J Vasc Interv Radiol 1999;10(9):1255–63.

57. Tanihata H, Saxon RR, Kubota Y, et al. Transjugular intrahepatic portosystemic shunt with silicone-covered Wallstents: results in a swine model. Radiology 1997;205(1):181–4.

58. Haskal ZJ, Weintraub JL, Susman J. Recurrent TIPS thrombosis after polyethylene stent-graft use and salvage with polytetrafluoroethylene stent-grafts. J Vasc Interv Radiol 2002;13(12):1255–9.

59. Ferral H, Alcantara-Peraza A, Kimura Y, Castaneda-Zuniga WR. Creation of transjugular intrahepatic portosystemic shunts with use of the Cragg Endopro System I. J Vasc Interv Radiol 1998;9(2):283–7.

60. Luo XF, Nie L, Wang Z, et al. Stent-grafts for the treatment of TIPS dysfunction: fluency stent vs Wallgraft stent. World J Gastroenterol 2013;19(30):5000–5.

61. Petersen B, Uchida BT, Timmermans H, Keller FS, Rosch J. Intravascular US-guided direct intrahepatic portacaval shunt with a PTFE-covered stent-graft: feasibility study in swine and initial clinical results. J Vasc Interv Radiol 2001;12(4):475–86.

62. Andrews RT, Saxon RR, Bloch RD, et al. Stent-grafts for de novo TIPS: technique and early results. J Vasc Interv Radiol 1999;10(10):1371–8.

63. Sze DY, Vestring T, Liddell RP, et al. Recurrent TIPS failure associated with biliary fistulae: treatment with PTFE-covered stents. Cardiovasc Intervent Radiol 1999;22(4):298–304.

64. LaBerge JM, Kerlan RK. Liver infarction following TIPS with a PTFE-covered stent: is the covering the cause? Hepatology 2003;38(3):778–9; author reply 9.

65. Hausegger KA, Karnel F, Georgieva B, et al. Transjugular intrahepatic portosystemic shunt creation with the Viatorr expanded polytetrafluoroethylene-covered stent-graft. J Vasc Interv Radiol 2004;15(3):239–48.

66. Bureau C, Pagan JC, Layrargues GP, et al. Patency of stents covered with polytetrafluoroethylene in patients treated by transjugular intrahepatic portosystemic shunts: long-term results of a randomized multicentre study. Liver Int 2007;27(6):742–7.

67. Engstrom BI, Horvath JJ, Suhocki PV, et al. Covered transjugular intrahepatic portosystemic shunts: accuracy of ultrasound in detecting shunt malfunction. AJR Am J Roentgenol 2013;200(4):904–8.

68. Angermayr B, Cejna M, Koenig F, et al. Survival in patients undergoing trans-jugular intrahepatic portosystemic shunt: ePTFE-covered stentgrafts versus bare stents. Hepatology 2003;38(4):1043–50.

69. Riggio O, Ridola L, Angeloni S, et al. Clinical efficacy of transjugular intrahepatic portosystemic shunt created with covered stents with different diameters: results of a randomized controlled trial. J Hepatol 2010;53(2):267–72.

70. Garcia-Pagan JC, Caca K, Bureau C, et al. Early use of TIPS in patients with cir-rhosis and variceal bleeding. N Engl J Med 2010;362(25):2370–9.

71. Xue H, Yuan J, Chao-Li Y, Palikhe M, Wang J, Shan-Lv L, et al. Follow-up study of transjugular intrahepatic portosystemic shunt in the treatment of portal hypertension. Dig Dis Sci 2011;56(11):3350–6.

72. Gaba RC, Omene BO, Podczerwinski ES, et al. TIPS for treatment of variceal hem-orrhage: clinical outcomes in 128 patients at a single institution over a 12-year period. J Vasc Interv Radiol 2012;23(2):227–35.

73. Jirkovsky V, Fejfar T, Safka V, Hulek P, Krajina A, Chovanec V, et al. Influence of the secondary deployment of expanded polytetrafluoroethylene-covered stent grafts on maintenance of transjugular intrahepatic portosystemic shunt patency. J Vasc Interv Radiol 2011;22(1):55–60.

74. Perarnau JM, Le Gouge A, Nicolas C, et al. Covered vs. uncovered stents for transjugular intrahepatic portosystemic shunt: a randomized controlled trial. J Hepatol 2014;60(5):962–8.

75. Lauermann J, Potthoff A, Mc Cavert M, et al. Comparison of technical and clinical outcome of transjugular portosystemic shunt placement between a bare metal stent and a PTFE-stentgraft device. Cardiovasc Intervent Radiol 2016;39(4):635–6.

76. Weber CN, Nadolski GJ, White SB, et al. Long-term patency and clinical analysis of expanded polytetrafluoroethylene-covered transjugular intrahepatic porto-systemic shunt stent grafts. J Vasc Interv Radiol 2015;26(9):1257–65; quiz 65.

77. Darwish Murad S, Luong TK, Pattynama PM, Hansen BE, van Buuren HR, Janssen HL. Long-term outcome of a covered vs. uncovered transjugular intrahepatic portosystemic shunt in Budd-Chiari syndrome. Liver Int 2008;28(2):249–56.

78. Garcia-Pagan JC, Heydtmann M, Raffa S, et al. TIPS for Budd-Chiari syndrome: long-term results and prognostics factors in 124 patients. Gastroenterology 2008;135(3):808–15.

79. Cura M, Haskal Z, Lopera J. Diagnostic and interventional radiology for Budd-Chiari syndrome. Radiographics 2009;29(3):669–81.

80. Molmenti EP, Segev DL, Arepally A, et al. The utility of TIPS in the management of Budd-Chiari syndrome. Ann Surg 2005;241(6):978–81; discussion 82–3.

81. Eapen CE, Velissaris D, Heydtmann M, Gunson B, Olliff S, Elias E. Favourable medium term outcome following hepatic vein recanalisation and/or transjug-ular intrahepatic portosystemic shunt for Budd Chiari syndrome. Gut 2006; 55(6):878–84.

82. Lopez-Mendez E, Chavez-Tapia NC, Avila-Escobedo L, Cabrera-Aleksandrova T, Uribe M. Early experience of Budd-Chiari syndrome treatment with transjug-ular intrahepatic portosystemic shunt. Ann Hepatol 2006;5(3):157–60.

83. Corso R, Intotero M, Solcia M, Castoldi MC, Rampoldi A. Treatment of Budd-Chiari syndrome with transjugular intrahepatic portosystemic shunt (TIPS). Radiol Med 2008;113(5):727–38.

84. Fitsiori K, Tsitskari M, Kelekis A, Filippiadis D, Triantafyllou K, Brountzos E. Transjugular intrahepatic portosystemic shunt for the treatment of Budd-Chiari syndrome patients: results from a single center. Cardiovasc Intervent Radiol 2014;37(3):691–7.

85. He FL, Wang L, Zhao HW, et al. Transjugular intrahepatic portosystemic shunt for severe jaundice in patients with acute Budd-Chiari syndrome. World J Gas-troenterol 2015;21(8):2413–8.

86. Vo NJ, Shivaram G, Andrews RT, Vaidya S, Healey PJ, Horslen SP. Midterm follow-up of transjugular intrahepatic portosystemic shunts using polytet-rafluoroethylene endografts in children. J Vasc Interv Radiol 2012;23(7): 919–24.

87. Di Giorgio A, Agazzi R, Alberti D, Colledan M, D'Antiga L. Feasibility and efficacy of transjugular intrahepatic portosystemic shunt (TIPS) in children. J Pediatr Gastroenterol Nutr 2012;54(5):594–600.

88. Zurera LJ, Espejo JJ, Lombardo S, Gilbert JJ, Canis M, Ruiz C. Safety and efficacy of expanded polytetrafluoroethylene-covered transjugular intrahepatic por-tosystemic shunts in children with acute or recurring upper gastrointestinal bleeding. Pediatr Radiol 2015;45(3):422–9.

89. Angeloni S, Merli M, Salvatori FM, et al. Polytetrafluoroethylene-covered stent grafts for TIPS procedure: 1-year patency and clinical results. Am J Gastroen-terol 2004;99(2):280–5.

90. Rossi P, Salvatori FM, Fanelli F, et al. Polytetrafluoroethylene-covered nitinol stent-graft for transjugular intrahepatic portosystemic shunt creation: 3-year experience. Radiology 2004;231(3):820–30.

91. Bureau C, Garcia-Pagan JC, Otal P, et al. Improved clinical outcome using polytetrafluoroethylene-coated stents for TIPS: results of a randomized study. Gastroenterology 2004;126(2):469–75.

92. Ockenga J, Kroencke TJ, Schuetz T, et al. Covered transjugular intrahepatic por-tosystemic stents maintain lower portal pressure and require fewer reinter-ventions than uncovered stents. Scand J Gastroenterol 2004;39(10):994–9.

93. Barrio J, Ripoll C, Banares R, et al. Comparison of transjugular intrahepatic por-tosystemic shunt dysfunction in PTFE-covered stent-grafts versus bare stents. Eur J Radiol 2005;55(1):120–4.

94. Echenagusia M, Rodriguez-Rosales G, Simo G, Camunez F, Banares R, Echena-gusia A. Expanded PTFE-covered stent-grafts in the treatment of transjugu-lar intrahepatic portosystemic shunt (TIPS) stenoses and occlusions. Abdom Imaging 2005;30(6):750–4.

95. Vignali C, Bargellini I, Grosso M, et al. TIPS with expanded polytetrafluoroeth-ylene-covered stent: results of an Italian multicenter study. AJR Am J Roentge-nol 2005;185(2):472–80.

96. Tripathi D, Ferguson J, Barkell H, Macbeth K, Ireland H, Redhead DN, et al. Improved clinical outcome with transjugular intrahepatic portosystemic stent-shunt utilizing polytetrafluoroethylene-covered stents. Eur J Gastroen-terol Hepatol 2006;18(3):225–32.

97. Gaba RC, Parvinian A, Minocha J, et al. Should transjugular intrahepatic porto-systemic shunt stent grafts be underdilated? J Vasc Interv Radiol 2015;26(3): 382–7.

98. Pieper CC, Sprinkart AM, Nadal J, et al. Postinterventional passive expansion of partially dilated transjugular intrahepatic portosystemic shunt stents. J Vasc Interv Radiol 2015;26(3):388–94.

99. Haskal ZJ. Transjugular intrahepatic portosystemic shunt endografts: a decade in and due for revision? J Vasc Interv Radiol 2015;26(3):395–7.

100. Charon JP, Alaeddin FH, Pimpalwar SA, et al. Results of a retrospective mul-ticenter trial of the Viatorr expanded polytetrafluoroethylene-covered stent-graft for transjugular intrahepatic portosystemic shunt creation. J Vasc Interv Radiol 2004;15(11):1219–30.

101. Rossle M, Siegerstetter V, Euringer W, Olschewski M, Kromeier J, Kurz K, et al. The use of a polytetrafluoroethylene-covered stent graft for transjugular intra-hepatic portosystemic shunt (TIPS): Long-term follow-up of 100 patients. Acta Radiolog 2006;47(7):660–6.

102. Gandini R, Konda D, Simonetti G. Transjugular intrahepatic portosystemic shunt patency and clinical outcome in patients with Budd-Chiari syndrome: covered versus uncovered stents. Radiology 2006;241(1):298–305.

103. Wu X, Ding W, Cao J, et al. Favorable clinical outcome using a covered stent fol-lowing transjugular intrahepatic portosystemic shunt in patients with portal hypertension. J Hepatobiliary Pancreat Sci 2010;17(5):701–8.

104. Maleux G, Perez-Gutierrez NA, Evrard S, et al. Covered stents are better than uncovered stents for transjugular intrahepatic portosystemic shunts in cir-rhotic patients with refractory ascites: a retrospective cohort study. Acta Gas-troenterol Belg 2010;73(3):336–41.

Chapter 20: Doppler Surveillance of Transjugular Intrahepatic Portosystemic Shunts in the Stent-Graft Era

Nirvikar Dahiya, Michael F. Lin, and Christine O. Menias

Introduction

A transjugular intrahepatic portosystemic shunt (TIPS) is an artificially created conduit within the liver that diverts portal flow into the systemic circulation. Normally reserved as the last treatment for decompensated liver disease before liver transplantation, it aims to control variceal bleeding and refractory ascites. As the name suggests, this procedure is performed through a percutaneous access site in the jugular vein, usually on the right side, and provides a much less invasive option to open surgery. First described by Rosch in 1969,[1] the TIPS procedure began to exert its role in end-stage liver disease management in the mid-1980s upon the introduction of endovascular stents. In 1988, Rössle et al reported the first successful TIPS deployment in humans.[2] Since then, it has gained widespread recognition as the mainstay treatment for portal hypertension (PHT) refractory to medical therapy.[2]

To clarify the appropriate indications for TIPS placement, the American Association for the Study of Liver Diseases (AASLD) has compiled a comprehensive practice guideline for this procedure[3] available at www.aasld.org. The contraindications and common indications for TIPS and their recommended use outlined by AASLD are summarized in ► Table 20.1 and ► Table 20.2.

The success of the TIPS procedure largely stems from the advent of endovascular stent grafts, which prevent tract closure. The first-generation stent grafts were bare-metal stents, mainly Wallstents (Boston Scientific, Natick, Massachusetts), which were prone to thrombosis or stenosis because of pseudointimal hyperplasia. Stent patency is characterized as either primary or secondary. *Primary stent patency* refers to the duration a stent remains patent from the time of deployment to first intervention. *Secondary stent patency* refers to the lifespan of a stent to complete loss of function despite interventions. The primary stent patency rate for earlier generation stents is highly variable but generally low. Two studies cited 2-year primary patency rates of 5%[4] and 26%.[5] The secondary patency rate can be quite high, with 83% patency

at 5 years reported by one study that monitored long-term stent patency rate.[6] Stenosis usually occurs within the stent or at the hepatic venous outflow.

Subsequent development of expanded-polytetrafluoroethylene (PTFE)-covered endoprostheses (VIATORR Gore-Tex vascular graft, W.L. Gore and Associates) significantly improved stent patency. The covered stent graft is a self-expanding high-radial-strength nitinol stent graft that has a proximal region lined internally by a thin layer of expanded PTFE, which is impermeable to bile and mucin. One end of the stent has an uncovered region. The uncovered region placed in the portal system allows normal blood flow at the portal confluence, and the covered region placed intrahepatically provides an impermeable interface with the hepatic parenchyma. The expanded PTFE lining also reduces in-stent neointimal hyperplasia.[7] The stent patency rate is even higher if the stent is extended to the level of the inferior vena cava (IVC).[8] Ample data show clear survival benefit offered by covered stents compared with bare-metal stents.[9–11] Surprisingly and against intuition, covered stents are also associated with a decreased incidence of hepatic encephalopathy (HE),[12] which was initially expected to be higher given the improved stent patency rate.

Variceal bleeding occurs in the setting of advanced liver cirrhosis complicated by PHT. First-line therapy for variceal bleeding consists of a combination of pharmacologic and endoscopic treatments, including vasoactive medication, prophylactic antibiotics, and endoscopic band ligation or injection sclerotherapy. In severe cases, transfusion may also be needed. Patients with hepatic venous pressure gradients (HVPGs) of 20 mm Hg or more are at high risk for treatment failure.[13] TIPS is highly effective in controlling acute variceal bleeding, including the high-risk patient population, and can be used as rescue therapy if first-line treatments fail. Hemostasis is generally achieved when the HVPG is reduced to 12 mm Hg or less. This conventional treatment algorithm is now under challenge by recent data from a multicenter study, which found significant survival benefit in high-risk patients with cirrhosis when TIPS was deployed early.[14]

In addition to controlling variceal bleeding, TIPS effectively reduces ascites refractory to diuretic therapy. Left untreated, refractory ascites often progresses to hepatorenal syndrome and hydrothorax. Although these conditions are treatable by large-volume paracentesis (LVP) and pleurodesis, reaccumulation of fluid can be expected. These procedures also carry the risk of progressive circulatory dysfunction, eventually leading to hepatorenal syndrome. Each procedure also carries inherent technical risks. Assuming there are no stent graft complications, ascites resolves within 1 month after TIPS placement. Patients are able to enjoy a longer ascites-free window than that offered by LVP. With amelioration of total body fluid shift, the renal function also improves.

Post-TIPS HE is a common occurrence, reported to occur in 5% to 35% of patients.[15] The nitrogenous compounds from the gastrointestinal tract, in particular ammonia, gain direct systemic access through a patent TIPS. A decrease in the caliber of the stent

Table 20.1 Contraindications to Placement of a Transjugular Intrahepatic Portosystemic Shunt

Absolute
Primary prevention of variceal bleeding
Congestive heart failure
Multiple hepatic cysts
Uncontrolled systemic infection or sepsis
Unrelieved biliary obstruction
Severe pulmonary hypertension

Relative
Hepatoma especially if central
Obstruction of all hepatic veins
PV thrombosis
Severe coagulopathy (INR > 5)
Thrombocytopenia of <20,000/cm³
Moderate pulmonary hypertension

INR: international normalized ratio; PV: portal vein.

Table 20.2 Common Indications for Transjugular Intrahepatic Portosystemic Shunt Recommendation

Efficacy Determined by Controlled Trials	
Secondary prevention of variceal bleeding	TIPS is effective; not recommended for primary prophylactic prevention of bleeding for varices that never bled.
Refractory cirrhotic ascites	TIPS is effective; reserve for patients intolerant of repeated large LVPs.
Efficacy Assessed in Uncontrolled Series	
Refractory acutely bleeding varices	TIPS is effective in controlling variceal bleeding that is refractory to medical therapy and should be used in preference to surgery.
Portal hypertensive gastropathy	Limit use of TIPS to those who have recurrent bleeding despite beta-blocker therapy.
Bleeding gastric varices	TIPS is effective and is the preferred approach.
Gastric antral vascular ectasia	TIPS is ineffective in patients with cirrhosis; not recommended.
Refractory hepatic hydrothorax	TIPS is effective; reserve for effusions uncontrollable by diuretics and sodium restriction.
Hepatorenal syndrome	Investigatory use of TIPS pending publication of controlled trials
Budd-Chiari syndrome	TIPS is recommended for those who fail anticoagulation therapy.
Veno-occlusive disease	TIPS is not recommended.
Hepatopulmonary syndrome	TIPS is not recommended.

LVP: large-volume paracentesis; TIPS: transjugular intrahepatic portosystemic shunt.

(available in 8-, 10-, and 12-mm diameters) theoretically reduces the risk of HE. However, this is not well supported by current data, and a recent study[16] found no difference in the rate of HE when comparing 8- and 10-mm stents. Furthermore, the 8-mm stent was ineffective in portal decompression. Fortunately, the vast majority of patients with post-TIPS HE are successfully treated with conservative management. A small percentage of patients are refractory to these treatments and require further intervention, including shunt occlusion, size reduction, or even emergent liver transplantation. A host of other complications related to TIPS placement include TIPS infection, intraperitoneal hemorrhage, stent stenosis or migration, fistula formation, hemobilia, and sepsis, as well as the dreaded hepatic infarction leading to fulminant liver failure.

Current AASLD practice guideline recommends imaging the liver before the TIPS procedure to assess hepatic vascular patency and exclude masses.[17] Imaging modalities may include Doppler ultrasonography, computed tomography (CT), or magnetic resonance imaging (MRI). Both MRI and ultrasonography are highly accurate for depicting portal venous flow direction, and MRI is more sensitive than Doppler for detecting collateral vessels.[18] In general, Doppler ultrasonography is most commonly used

because it is more readily available. In patients with large ascites, the liver may be deeply displaced, complicating Doppler evaluation of hepatic vessels. Difficulty in acoustic penetration secondary to deep location of the vessel of interest (▶ Fig. 20.1) may lead to a false diagnosis of vascular thrombosis. In these patients, contrast-enhanced CT or MRI is helpful in clarifying equivocal Doppler findings.

Sonographic Terminology

Sonographic terminologies used in TIPS evaluation are standardized mostly based on the direction of blood flow with respect to a reference structure. *Hepatofugal flow* describes flow away from the liver, and *hepatopedal flow* describes blood flow toward the liver. *Antegrade flow* is a term used for the direction of blood flow under normal physiologic conditions. Conversely, *retrograde flow* is in the opposite direction as antegrade flow. TIPS stents are evaluated in their proximal, mid, and distal segments. The proximal segment is the portion closest to the portal vein (PV). The distal segment is the portion closest to the hepatic vein. Again, these terminologies are with respect to the expected blood flow

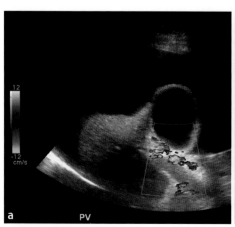
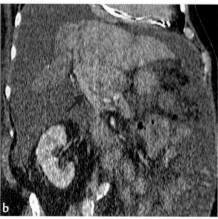

Fig. 20.1 Pseudothrombosis of the main portal vein (PV) secondary to its deep location. **(a)** Routine liver Doppler evaluation before the transjugular intrahepatic portosystemic shunt (TIPS) procedure showing a lack of flow in the main PV. **(b)** Computed tomography performed later the same day definitively demonstrated opacification of the main PV (*red arrow*).

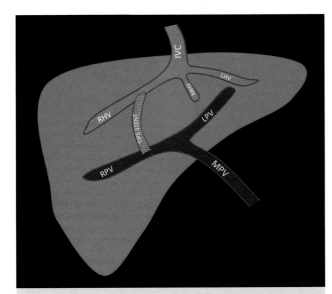

Fig. 20.2 Illustration showing the expected transjugular intrahepatic portosystemic shunt stent position bridging the right portal vein (RPV) and the right hepatic vein (RHV). IVC: inferior vena cava; LHV: left hepatic vein; LPV: left portal vein; MHV: middle hepatic vein; MPV: main portal vein. (*Used with permission from Patel N, ed. SCVIR Syllabus: Portal Hypertension: Diagnosis & Interventions, 2nd ed. Fairfax, VA: Society of Interventional Radiology; 2001: ©SIR, 2001. All rights reserved.*)

direction through a properly functioning stent shunting blood from portal to systemic circulation.

Normal Transjugular Intrahepatic Portosystemic Shunt Examination

Ultrasonography Technique

TIPS stents are deeply embedded in the liver, usually connecting the right portal and hepatic veins (▶ Fig. 20.2). To optimally visualize the stent, low-frequency transducers such as the 3.5-MHz curved array or a 2.5-MHz phased array transducers are superior for depth penetration. The preferred scanning position is using an intercostal window with the patient turned slightly to the left while lying supine. In some patients, a subcostal approach with superior probe angulation may provide better visualization (▶ Fig. 20.3). The latter approach is especially helpful for assessment of the distal end of the stent. Decreasing the dynamic range helps to improve contrast between the stent and surrounding liver parenchyma. Doppler scale should be optimized for measuring the relatively high flow velocity within the stent and may need to be decreased when evaluating slower flow in the portal and hepatic veins. Velocity should be measured at a Doppler angle of less than 60 degrees. Ideally, Doppler measurements should be taken at a resting stage of the respiratory cycle, preferably at end expiration, because flow velocity within the stent can be decreased by 22 cm/s on average during deep inspiration.[19] This pattern in velocity change can be extrapolated to include the portal venous system, which is also preferably evaluated at end expiration.

Normal Gray-Scale and Doppler Findings

On ultrasonography, the wire mesh of the stent wall appears as two parallel echogenic white lines that are slightly corrugated (▶ Fig. 20.4). With appropriate angulation, flow within the entire stent can be easily displayed on color Doppler (▶ Fig. 20.5). Sonographically, bare-metal stents and covered stents cannot be distinguished. The latter may have gas embedded in the fabric, which produces a well-known acoustic barrier that precludes Doppler sampling of this region in the immediate post–stent deployment period.[20] This acoustic barrier usually resolves within 1 week.

In a cirrhotic liver, TIPS provides a low-pressure channel for diverting portal venous flow to the IVC. Changes to the intrahepatic flow dynamics are immediate after stent placement. Such changes include reversal of flow in the right and left PVs (▶ Fig. 20.6). Flow volume and velocity increase throughout the main PV. Acceptable flow velocities within the TIPS differ slightly across institutions but are generally considered normal within a range of 90 to 190 cm/s.[21] Doppler and gray-scale evaluations of the stent and hepatic vessels should be followed by a survey of the abdomen for collaterals and ascites. The presence of either may indicate inadequate portal decompression. The hepatic parenchyma must be thoroughly evaluated in post-TIPS patients who are also at increased risk for hepatocellular carcinoma.

Abnormal Transjugular Intrahepatic Portosystemic Shunt Examination

Stent Thrombosis

Doppler ultrasonography has been shown to be very effective for diagnosing stent thrombosis.[19,22-27] Provided that the Doppler parameters have been set accurately, lack of flow in the stent lumen on color or pulsed Doppler (▶ Fig. 20.7) is diagnostic of

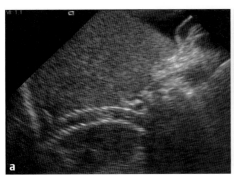
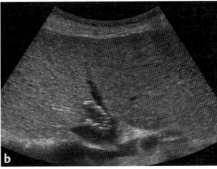

Fig. 20.3 Acoustic windows used for stent visualization. (a) Longitudinal view of a normal TIPS stent through an intercostal acoustic window. (b) Transverse subcostal view with superior angulation showing the distal end of the stent in the right hepatic vein.

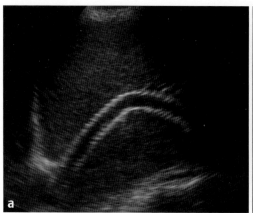
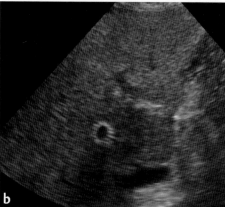

Fig. 20.4 Sonographic appearance of a transjugular intrahepatic portosystemic shunt (TIPS) stent. Longitudinal (a) and transverse (b) views demonstrating the echogenic walls of the TIPS stent with a corrugated appearance. The lumen is normally anechoic on gray scale.

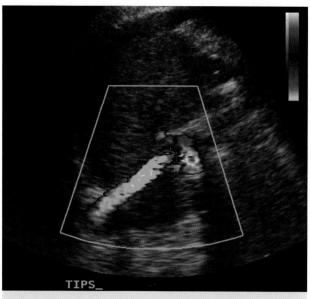

Fig. 20.5 Color Doppler evaluation of a normal transjugular intrahepatic portosystemic shunt stent. Flow is seen within the entire stent heading toward the hepatic vein. By convention, flow away from the transducer is coded blue.

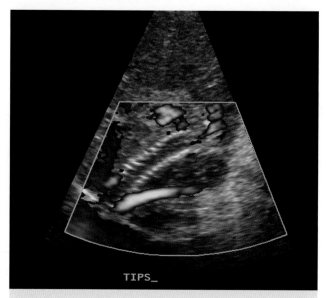

Fig. 20.7 Power Doppler evaluation of the transjugular intrahepatic portosystemic shunt stent. No flow is noted throughout the entire stent consistent with an occluded stent secondary to thrombosis. The Doppler parameters are appropriate because normal flow is seen in the adjacent hepatic veins.

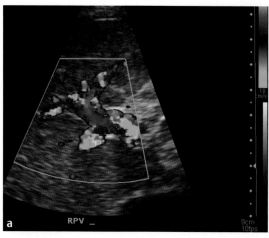
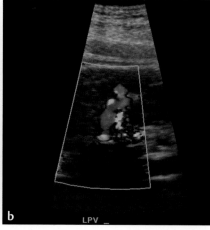

Fig. 20.6 Expected retrograde flow in the right (a) and left (b) portal veins after transjugular intrahepatic portosystemic shunt creation.

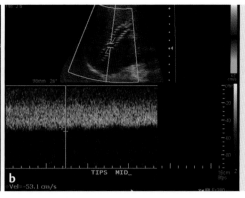

Fig. 20.8 Doppler evaluation of the transjugular intrahepatic portosystemic shunt (TIPS) stent with distal stenosis. (a) Elevated peak systolic velocity (262 cm/s) is detected at the distal end of the stent. (b) Peak systolic velocity is decreased (53 cm/s) in the mid segment of the TIPS stent proximal to the stenosis.

stent thrombosis. With inappropriate Doppler settings, slow flow through the stent can imitate thrombosis. When slow flow in the stent is suspected, augmenting flow within the portal venous system by compressing the periumbilical region of the abdomen is occasionally helpful.

Shunt Stenosis

Multiple parameters have been investigated for diagnosing shunt stenosis. The most common of these include the following.

Intrastent Flow Velocity

Flow velocity within a hemodynamically significant stenosis is elevated. Conversely, velocity is expected to be low in the nonstenotic segments (▶ Fig. 20.8; Fig. 20.9). Multiple studies have attempted to define TIPS stenosis by sets of flow velocities, with varying results.[23,24,26] At the authors' institution, the 90- to 190-cm/s flow velocity range used to define a patent, functioning stent has comparable sensitivity and specificity of 82% and 72%, respectively.[28]

An intrastent velocity gradient, or the difference between the upper and lower limits of normal velocity range, of more than 100 cm/s has a positive predictive value of 82% for detecting stenosis. However, this gradient may not be present in diffuse stenosis in which velocities are increased throughout the stent. Studies have also shown an increase of more than 50 cm/s on successive TIPS follow-up examinations to be a sensitive predictor of stent stenosis.[27] This underscores the importance of serial follow-ups and monitoring for temporal change in velocities in addition to analyzing absolute flow velocities on individual examinations.

The follow-up intervals differ among institutions. At the authors' institution, the first examination is done within 24 hours for uncovered stents or at 1 month for covered stents after TIPS placement. Subsequent follow-up examinations are performed at 3, 6, and 12 months. After the first year, yearly follow-up examinations are sufficient unless clinical manifestations of stent dysfunction dictate otherwise.

Main Portal Vein Velocity

After portal venous decompression by TIPS, the main PV velocity increases.[23,24] TIPS malfunction is reflected as a decrease in portal venous flow. Velocity below 30 to 40 cm/s in the main PV and a 20% reduction in peak velocities between successive examinations are associated with TIPS malfunction.[28,29]

Intrahepatic Portal Vein Flow Direction

TIPS provides a low-resistance outflow for the portal system. Assuming lack of collateral vessels, reversal of flow (hepatofugal) within the left and right PVs is normally expected with a patent TIPS. Interval change from the expected hepatofugal direction to hepatopedal within a branch of the PV between successive TIPS evaluations is highly suggestive of stent malfunction,[28] although this is a relatively late finding.

Hepatic Artery Velocity

Hepatic arterial flow increases after TIPS placement because of diverted portal venous flow from the liver. This phenomenon has been studied in the past with variable success.[24,28]

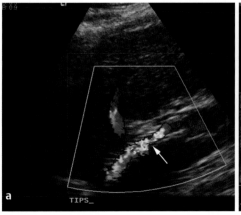

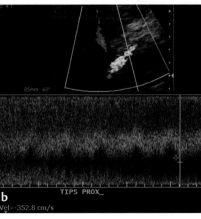

Fig. 20.9 Doppler evaluation of transjugular intrahepatic portosystemic shunt (TIPS) stent with proximal stenosis. (a) Focal aliasing (arrow) on color Doppler in the proximal TIPS stent suggests elevated velocities caused by stenosis. (b) Spectral waveform analysis reveals an elevated peak systolic velocity of 352 cm/s in the region of focal aliasing, confirming stenosis.

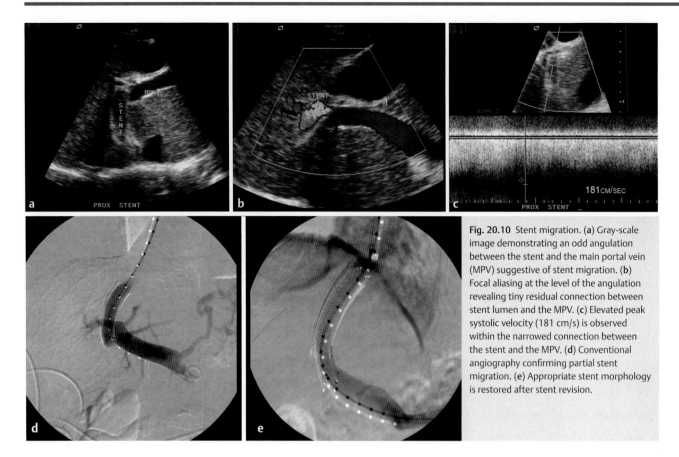

Fig. 20.10 Stent migration. (**a**) Gray-scale image demonstrating an odd angulation between the stent and the main portal vein (MPV) suggestive of stent migration. (**b**) Focal aliasing at the level of the angulation revealing tiny residual connection between stent lumen and the MPV. (**c**) Elevated peak systolic velocity (181 cm/s) is observed within the narrowed connection between the stent and the MPV. (**d**) Conventional angiography confirming partial stent migration. (**e**) Appropriate stent morphology is restored after stent revision.

Hepatic Venous Flow

Stenosis between the distal end of the stent and IVC may direct some flow back into the draining hepatic vein toward the liver. This flow abnormality has been reported[30] but is not well studied. Angle-corrected intrastent flow velocities and temporal velocity change are good indicators for detecting stent malfunction. However, combining multiple parameters can increase overall sensitivity and positive predictive value for diagnosing shunt stenosis.[31]

Other Complications

Rarely, TIPS stents may encounter complications that are morphologic in nature. These complications tend to be more readily noticeable than flow abnormalities. Stent migration wherein the stent dislodges from its hepatic or portal venous insertion site and embeds within the liver parenchyma is easily seen (▶ Fig. 20.10). A kink in the stent may also cause stent dysfunction (▶ Fig. 20.11). Occasionally, thrombus within the stent may be apparent on gray-scale imaging (▶ Fig. 20.12).

Pitfalls and Artifacts

Transjugular Intrahepatic Portosystemic Shunt Stent

When evaluating TIPS by Doppler ultrasonography, one should bear in mind the myriad artifacts that mimic stent abnormalities. In a large patient, deep location of the stent may give a false impression of stent occlusion caused by a faint Doppler signal. The highly reflective lung–diaphragm interface commonly responsible for the mirror image artifact may generate a "virtual stent," which is the mirror image of the TIPS, extending above the diaphragm. Occasionally, only the "virtual stent" is seen, creating the illusion of stent migration. A simple chest radiograph will confirm true stent position and resolve any ambiguity. The morphology of the TIPS also poses inherent pitfalls for Doppler signal sampling. Shaped like an arch, the Doppler angle almost invariably approaches 90 degrees along certain segments within the stent regardless of the acoustic window. Within these segments, focal Doppler signal void may be confused for thrombus despite patent flow (▶ Fig. 20.13).

Changing the angle of insonation may help to eliminate this artifact. Along the same lines, the distal stent is often displayed in an orientation such that the Doppler angle approaches zero degrees. This can manifest as focal color aliasing and be confused for stenosis. Correcting the pulse repetition frequency may help minimize this artifact, and it is also important to analyze the peak flow velocity on the Doppler waveform sampled in this region to distinguish this artifact from true stenosis.[32] The nature of the stent may also impact analysis. Bare-metal stents allow intrastent permeation of adjacent portal and hepatic venous blood, occasionally causing color aliasing, which may be confused for a stenosis. Therefore, knowledge of the type of stent placed is helpful when performing Doppler evaluation of a TIPS stent.

Portal Vein

Peak velocity in the PV should be sampled in the proximal to mid segment of the main PV, closer to the portosplenic confluence. If measured near the main PV bifurcation, retrograde blood volume

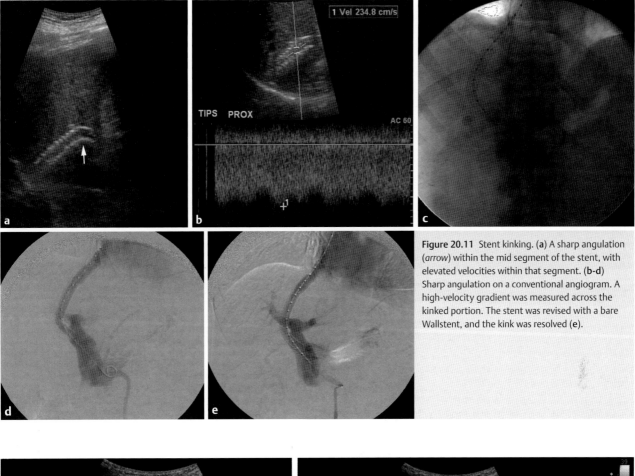

Figure 20.11 Stent kinking. **(a)** A sharp angulation (*arrow*) within the mid segment of the stent, with elevated velocities within that segment. **(b-d)** Sharp angulation on a conventional angiogram. A high-velocity gradient was measured across the kinked portion. The stent was revised with a bare Wallstent, and the kink was resolved **(e)**.

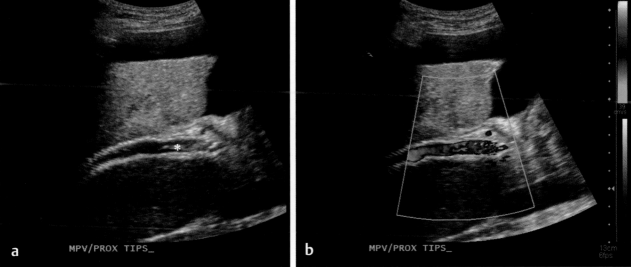

Fig. 20.12 (a) Echogenic thrombus (*asterisk*) within the proximal stent. **(b)** Color Doppler image demonstrating the nonocclusive nature of the thrombus with flow seen around the thrombus.

from the left PV into the TIPS may spuriously accelerate flow and may mask underlying stent malfunction that would otherwise be reflected as decreased velocity in the main PV.

When identifying the right and left PVs, one should not rely solely on color Doppler. The hepatic arterial system is often hypertrophied in cirrhosis and dilates even more after TIPS placement.

Conversely, the portal venous system is typically atretic in cirrhosis. On color Doppler, robust flow within a hypertrophied hepatic artery can be mistaken for portal venous flow. Spectral waveform analysis of the vessel in question will help distinguish PV from the adjacent hepatic artery. A well-recognized artifact in the PVs, particularly the right PV, is helical flow (▶ Fig. 20.14).[33]

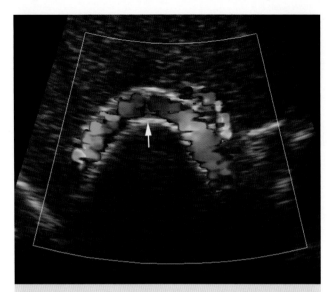

Fig. 20.13 Partial loss of Doppler signal in the mid segment of the transjugular intrahepatic portosystemic shunt stent (*arrow*) where the Doppler angle is at 90 degrees.

This represents flow turbulence within focally ectatic segment of the PV and can be confused with flow reversal in the PV. In these instances, interrogation of more distal portal venous branches would help establish true flow direction.

One of the late signs of critical stent stenosis is hepatopedal flow in the intrahepatic PVs. However, during deep inspiration this may temporarily be hepatofugal. This happens when the negative intrathoracic pressure generated during deep inspiration is large enough to overcome the flow obstruction by stent stenosis. Recognition of this phenomenon should alert readers to presence of potential stent stenosis.

Conclusion

TIPS is highly effective in management of end-stage liver disease. Patients should be closely monitored by serial ultrasound Doppler

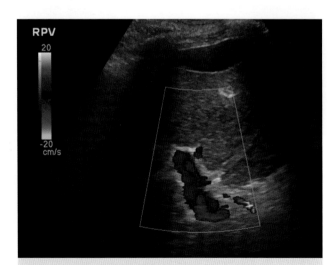

Fig. 20.14 Helical flow in the right portal vein. This is a clinically insignificant finding and should not be misinterpreted as bidirectional flow.

examinations to assess stent patency. Properly performed, ultrasonography is highly sensitive in detecting stent malfunction.

Clinical Pearls

- The goal of TIPS is to reduce HVPG to less than 12 mm Hg.
- Cover stents are superior to bare-metal stents in their long-term stent patency rate.
- Optimizing Doppler parameters is critical for accurate evaluation of stent function.
- Normal intrastent flow velocity range is 90 to 190 cm/s.
- Normal intrahepatic right and left portal vein flow direction should be hepatofugal (retrograde) in a patent, functioning stent.
- Main portal vein velocity is above 30 to 40 cm/s in a patent, functioning stent.
- Suggested serial ultrasound follow-up interval (for newer covered stents) is 1, 3, 6, and 12 months after stent deployment and annually thereafter.

References

1. Rosch J, Hanafee WN, Snow H. Transjugular portal venography and radiologic portacaval shunt: an experimental study. *Radiology* 1969;92(5):1112–1114.
2. Rössle M, Richter GM, Nöldge G, et al. New non-operative treatment for variceal haemorrhage. Lancet 1989;2(8655):153.
3. Boyer TD, Haskal ZJ; American Association for the Study of Liver Diseases. The role of transjugular intrahepatic portosystemic shunt (TIPS) in the management of portal hypertension: update 2009. Hepatology 2010;51:306.
4. Saxon RR, Ross PL, Mendel-Hartvig J, et al. Transjugular intrahepatic portosystemic shunt patency and the importance of stenosis location in the development of recurrent symptoms. Radiology 1998;207:683–693.
5. Sterling KM, Darcy MD. Stenosis of transjugular intrahepatic portosystemic shunts: presentation and management. AJR Am J Roentgenol 1997;168:239–244.
6. ter Borg PC, Hollemans M, Van Buuren HR, et al. Portosystemic shunts: long-term patency and clinical results in a patient cohort observed for 3–9 years. Radiology 2004;231:537–545.
7. Gandini R, Konda D, Simonetti G. Transjugular intrahepatic portosystemic shunt patency and clinical outcome in patients with Budd-Chiari syndrome: covered versus uncovered stents. Radiology 2006;241:298–305.
8. Hausegger KA, Karnel F, Georgieva B, et al. Transjugular intrahepatic portosystemic shunt creation with the Viatorr expanded polytetrafluoroethylene-covered stent-graft. J Vasc Interv Radiol 2004;15(3):239–248.
9. Yang Z, Han G, Wu Q, et al. Patency and clinical outcomes of transjugular intrahepatic portosystemic shunt with polytetrafluoroethylene-covered stents versus bare stents: a meta-analysis. J Gastroenterol Hepatol 2010;25(11):1718–1725.
10. Mittal S, Kasturi KS, Sood G. Metaanalysis of comparison of shunt patency and clinical outcomes between bare and polytetrafluroethylene (PTFE) stent in transjugular intrahepatic portosystemic shunt (TIPS). Gastroenterology 2010;138(suppl):S816.
11. Angermayr B, Cejna M, Koenig F, et al. Survival in patients undergoing transjugular intrahepatic portosystemic shunt: ePTFE-covered stentgrafts versus bare stents. Hepatology 2003;38:1043–1050.
12. Bureau C, Pagan J, Layrargues GP, et al. Patency of stents covered with polytetrafluoroethylene in patients treated by transjugular intrahepatic portosystemic shunts: long-term results of a randomized multicenter study. Liver Int 2007;27(6):742–747.
13. Moitinho E, Escorsell A, Bandi JC, et al. Prognostic value of early measurements of portal pressure in acute variceal bleeding. Gastroenterology 1999;117:622–631.
14. Garcia-Pagan JC, Caca K, Bureau C, et al. Early use of TIPS in patients with cirrhosis and variceal bleeding. N Engl J Med 2010;362:2370–2379.
15. Zuckerman DA, Darcy MD, Bocchini TP, et al. Encephalopathy after transjugular intrahepatic portosystemic shunting: analysis of incidence and potential risk factors. AJR Am J Roentgenol 1997;169:1727–1731.
16. Riggio O, Ridola L, Angeloni S, et al. Clinical efficacy of transjugular intrahepatic portosystemic shunt created with covered stents with different diameters: results of a randomized controlled trial. J Hepatology 2010;53:267–272.

17. Boyer T, Haskal Z; American Association for the Study of Liver Disease (AASLD). AASLD practice guidelines: the role of transjugular intrahepatic portosystemic shunt (TIPS) in the management of portal hypertension. Hepatology 2010;51(1):1–16.

18. Kraus BB, Ros PR, Abbitt PL, et al. Comparison of ultrasound, CT, and MR imaging in the evaluation of candidates for TIPS. J Magn Reson Imaging 1995;5(5):571–578.

19. Kiewer MA, Hertzberg BS, Heneghan JP, et al. Transjugular intrahepatic portosystemic shunts (TIPS): effects of respiratory state and patient position on the measurement of Doppler velocities. AJR Am J Roentgenol 2000;175:149–152.

20. Otal P, Smayra T, Bureau C, et al. Preliminary results of a new expanded-polytetrafluoroethylene-covered stent-graft for transjugular intrahepatic portosystemic shunt procedures. Am J Roentgenol 2002;178:141–147.

21. Middleton, WD, Teefey SA, Darcy MD. Doppler evaluation of transjugular intrahepatic portosystemic shunts. Ultrasound Q 2003;19(2):56–70.

22. Fung Y, Glajchen N, Shapiro RS, et al. Portal vein velocities measured by ultrasound: usefulness for evaluating shunt function following TIPS placement and TIPS revision. Abdom Imaging 1998;23:511–514.

23. Surratt RS, Middleton WD, Darcy MD, et al. Morphologic and hemodynamic findings at sonography before and after creation of a TIPS shunt. AJR Am J Roentgenol 1993;160:627–630.

24. Foshager MC, Ferral H, Nazarian GK, et al. Duplex sonography after TIPS shunt: normal hemodynamic findings and efficacy in predicting shunt patency and stenosis. AJR Am J Roentgenol 1995;165:1–7.

25. Chong WK, Malisch TA, Mazer MJ, et al. TIPS shunt: US assessment with maximum flow velocity. Radiology 1993;189:789–793.

26. Feldstein VA, Patel MD, LaBerge JM. TIPS shunts: accuracy of Doppler US in determination of patency and detection of stenoses. Radiology 1996;201:141–147.

27. Dodd GD, Zajko AB, Orons PD, et al. Detection of TIPS shunt dysfunction: value of duplex Doppler sonography. AJR Am J Roentgenol 1995;164:1119–1124

28. Kanterman RY, Darcy MD, Middleton WD, et al. Doppler sonographic findings associated with TIPS shunt malfunction. AJR Am J Roentgenol 1997;168:467–472.

29. Haskal ZJ, Carroll JW, Jacobs JE, et al. Sonography of transjugular intrahepatic portosystemic shunts: detection of elevated portosystemic gradients and loss of shunt function. J Vasc Interv Radiol 1997;8:549–556.

30. Feldstein VA, Laberge JM. Hepatic vein flow reversal at duplex sonography: sign of TIPS shunt malfunction. AJR Am J Roentgenol 1994;162:839.

31. Zizka J, Elias P, Krajina A, et al. Value of Doppler sonography in revealing transjugular intrahepatic portosystemic shunt malfunction: a 5-year experience in 216 patients. AJR Am J Roentgenol 2000;175:141–148.

32. Wachsberg RH. Doppler ultrasound evaluation of transjugular intrahepatic portosystemic shunt function: pitfalls and artifacts. Ultrasound Q 2003;19(3):139–148.

33. Middleton WD. Color Doppler: image interpretation and optimization. Ultrasound Q 1996;14:194–208.

Chapter 21: Transjugular Intrahepatic Shunts for Variceal Bleeding: Results of Clinical Studies

Kunal V. Shah and Timothy W.I. Clark

Introduction

Variceal hemorrhage is a well-recognized and frequently lethal complication of portal hypertension (PHT). In nearly 50% of patients with cirrhosis, gastroesophageal varices are present at the time of diagnosis.[1] These varices grow at a rate of 7% per year, and the 1-year rate of sentinel bleeding is 12%.[2,3] When bleeding occurs, patients have an 80% chance of rebleeding within 1 year and a mortality rate of bleeding episodes approaching 33%.[4] Since its inception the transjugular intrahepatic shunt (TIPS) procedure has evolved in portal access techniques, shunt technology, image guidance, and shunt surveillance. Because of these refinements, TIPS has largely supplanted most surgical shunting procedures as a means of long-term portal decompression. This chapter summarizes our current understanding of the role of TIPS for variceal bleeding.

Prevention of Variceal Rebleeding: Early Clinical Studies

Over the past 20 years, TIPS has increasingly become a vital tool in reducing PHT for preventing variceal rebleeding. Rosch et al initially described this conduit as a durable means for treating variceal bleeding while avoiding open surgery.[5] More than 10 randomized prospective trials have compared TIPS with endoscopic therapy (ET) in the prevention of variceal rebleeding.[6] The initial trials conducted in the mid to late 1990s with bare-metal stents (BMS) demonstrated that patients treated with TIPS rebled at a lower frequency than those treated with ET (18.9% vs. 46.6%,

respectively).[7] This benefit was juxtaposed by a higher rate of hepatic encephalopathy in TIPS patients (34% vs. 19%, respectively).[7] Most of the trials also indicated no difference in overall mortality rate between the two procedures, yet there were consistently fewer deaths caused by rebleeding in the TIPS group (2.4% vs. 7.7%).[7–11] A recent meta-analysis that collected data from 12 randomized controlled trials (RCTs) and four previous meta-analyses confirmed these results (decreased rebleeding rates, increased encephalopathy, no change in overall mortality rate with TIPS) and reported no difference in the number of hospital days between the two treatment arms.[12] Escorsell et al compared TIPS with pharmacologic therapy (propanolol + isosorbide-5-mononitrate) and found similar results as endoscopy trials. The TIPS arm had lower rebleeding probability (13% vs. 49%), higher rates of encephalopathy (38% vs. 14%), and no difference in survival probability.[13] Each of these trials was limited by high rates of crossover from the endoscopic or medical arms to rescue therapy with TIPS, which may have masked differences in mortality rate as patients who would have died from recurrent variceal bleeding in the endoscopic arm were shunted with TIPS. These initial RCTs also raised recognition that the BMS used for TIPS were prone to dysfunction, which led to the recurrence of PHT and subsequent bleeding (▶ Fig. 21.1).

These recurrences developed in 25% to 50% of patients after 6 to 12 months.[14–17] Dysfunction rates accumulated over time and were reported as high as 70% after 2 years in several trials.[12,18] The etiology of dysfunction was hypothesized to be multifactorial. Potential causes included thrombosis from stent migration or biliary fistula (▶ Fig. 21.2), parenchymal stenosis from fibrotic

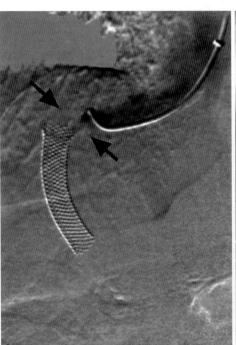
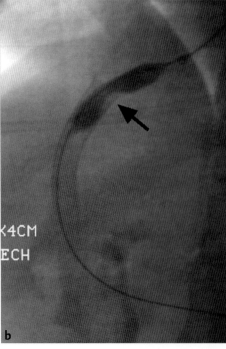

Fig. 21.1 A 51-year-old man with alcoholic cirrhosis and previous transjugular intrahepatic portosystemic shunt (TIPS) for recurrent variceal bleeding. **(a)** The TIPS was created with a bare stent 4 months earlier, and the stent has retracted into the hepatic parenchymal tract. Catheter advanced to the area of stenosis (*arrows*) where TIPS joins hepatic vein. **(b)** Additional stent placed across shunt stenosis and dilated with balloon catheter.

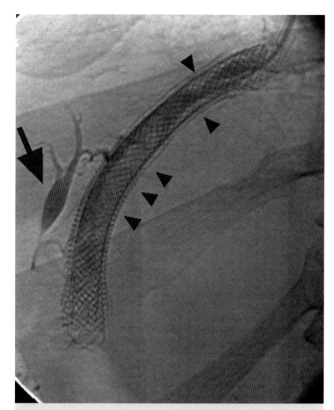

Fig. 21.2 Biliary fistula producing transjugular intrahepatic portosystemic shunt (TIPS) occlusion. Ultrasonography in this 52-year-old patient (not shown) revealed absent flow through the TIPS. Injection of contrast through a catheter placed into the occluded TIPS reveals a biliary fistula (*arrow*) and filling defects throughout the shunt (*arrowheads*) consistent with stenosis and thrombotic occlusion.

healing, and intimal hyperplasia from chronic injury.[14,15,19–21] These technical problems mandated more intense clinical and imaging follow-up, with frequent reinterventions and higher costs.[21] Although TIPS was proven to be superior to ET in the prevention of rebleeding, the drawbacks of greater encephalopathy, stent complications, and lack of demonstrable survival benefit led

to the recommendation that ET remain the standard of care as first-line therapy for patients with variceal bleeding.

The Era of Stent Grafts

The need for better stents for TIPS with longer patency rates drove the innovation of polytetrafluoroethylene (PTFE)-covered stent grafts. In 1995, Nishimine et al reported the first use of these stent grafts in pig studies with subsequent improvement in patency rates.[22] Saxon et al reported initial clinical results in 1997 of the use of stent grafts for revision of TIPS. They reported an initial mean primary patency of 50 days compared with a mean of 229 days after graft placement.[15] Haskal achieved similar results in 1999 and showed a mean patency duration of 19 months in a series of 13 patients.[19] These initial PTFE grafts appropriately blunted physiologic responses such as myofibroblast invasion and extracellular collagen deposition while also preventing bile leaks.[19] In 1999, W. L. Gore & Associates developed the first commercially available stent graft using expanded PTFE (ePTFE) marketed as VIATORR (▶ Fig. 21.3). Before its approval by the United States Food and Drug Administration (FDA), several European series confirmed the ability of the device to maintain patency for mean follow-up times of 282 to 387 days.[21,23]

In 2003, Angermayr et al performed the first large retrospective study comparing BMS with stent graft patency rates and survival data. Three-month, 1-year, and 2-year survival rates were reported as 93%, 88%, and 76% for the ePTFE group and 83%, 73%, and 62% for the BMS group ($n = 89$ for stent graft, $n = 419$ BMS).[24] This represented the first case-control study that not only supported the increased technical patency of TIPS stent grafts but also indicated improved survival with stent grafts. However, studies by Hausegger et al and Charon et al did not support these claims of improved mortality rates. They reported 1-year survival rates of 72% and 65%, respectively, for stent grafts with no statistical difference between groups.[25,26] Stent grafts were expected to have higher rates of encephalopathy, but most retrospective studies showed no significant difference between the two types of stents.[25,26,27] The reported incidence of recurrent bleeding with stent grafts was 3.7% to 7%, compared with rebleeding rates of 18% to 20% in the BMS.[7,25,26]

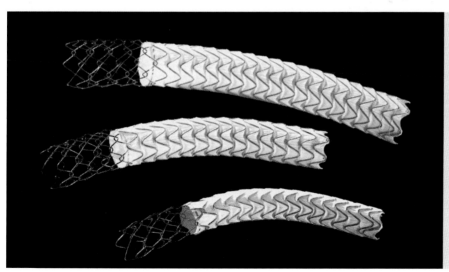

Fig. 21.3 The VIATORR (W. L. Gore, Flagstaff, Arizona) device is a polytetrafluoroethylene (PTFE) conduit supported by a nitinol stent skeleton. The portal venous end of the device is uncovered to permit unimpeded portal blood flow through the stent interstices.

Although there are only a minimal number of RCTs comparing stent grafts with BMS, the results of these trials are concordant with earlier retrospective studies (► Table 21.1). The clinical study performed for PMA (premarket approval) by the FDA of the VIATORR device for TIPS was a multicenter RCT with 253 subjects who underwent de novo TIPS procedure with either VIATORR or a commercially available bare-metal endoprosthesis (Boston Scientific Wallstent). Variceal bleeding was the primary indication in 35% to 36% of these patients. Primary patency success was defined as portosystemic pressure gradient (PSG) of less than 12 mm Hg and percent diameter stenosis less than 50%. At 6 months, primary patency rates were 60% and 22.7% for the VIATORR and control group, respectively. There was no significant difference between time to return of symptoms, but the VIATORR group had significantly fewer shunts with stenosis and reduced need for shunt revisions.[28] Bureau et al performed a smaller RCT with 80 patients that also demonstrated better patency, less reintervention, decreased encephalopathy, and similar long-term survival with TIPS stent grafts.[29,30] Primary patency of covered and BMS groups were 86% and 47%, respectively, at 1 year, and 80% and 19% at 2 years. A more recent meta-analysis by Yang et al also confirmed previous reports

and indicated a trend toward better survival with PTFE stent grafts.[31]

Current Practice Guidelines

It is clear that ePTFE-covered stents are superior to their bare-metal precursors. The convincing data led the American Association for the Study of Liver Diseases to update their TIPS practice guidelines in 2009 to recommend the use of stent grafts for TIPS.[33]

Primary Prevention of Variceal Bleeding

It is well known that the standard of care for primary prevention of variceal bleeding remains β-blockers because surgical shunts or TIPS pose significant incremental risks.[33] No studies have been completed to assess the efficacy of TIPS for primary prevention.

Acute Bleeding

Acute hemorrhage from ruptured varices represents a clinical emergency. If not adequately treated, the mortality rate can

Table 21.1 Summary of Clinical Studies of Transjugular Intrahepatic Shunt Stent Grafts*

Study PI	Year	Study	Bare-Metal Stent (n)	Stent Graft (n)	Patency	HEN	Survival	Comments
Saxon et al[15]	1997	CS	6	6	229 d	NA	NA	Shunt revision with stent graft (vs. 50 d for BM)
Haskal[19]	1999	CS	NA	14	570 d	NA	NA	Seven de novo, seven revision
Cejna et al[23]	2001	CS	NA	16	82%	NA	NA	Percent at 6 mo; patency defined as > 50% stenosis or PPG > 12
Otal et al[21]	2002	CS	NA	20	80%	5%	NA	Patency at 387 d, 100% secondary patency rate
Angermayr et al[24]	2003	RS	419	89	NA	NA	88%	Survival: 93%, 88%, 76% vs. 83%, 73%, 62% (3 mo, 1 y, 2 y)
Angeloni et al[32]	2004	RS	87	32	83%	Similar	Similar	Stenosis in hepatic or PV greater in stent graft group: 33% vs. 3%
Hausseger[25]	2004	RS	NA	71	81%	31%	NA	Recurrent bleeding rate of 3.7%
Charon et al[26]	2004	RS	NA	100	84%	14%	65%	Recurrent bleeding rate of 8.0%
FDA Trial[28]	2004	RCT	128	125	58%	Similar	Similar	Percent at 6 mo (vs. 29.8% [per protocol]); patency defined as PPG < 12 mm Hg and percent diameter stenosis < 50%
Bureau et al[29]	2004	RCT	41	31	76%	33%	Similar	Percent reported at 2 y; clinical relapse 10.2% vs. 29.3% (SG vs. BM)
Lau et al[55]	2005	RS	NA	16	90%	13%	NA	Dacron stent graft (PET)
Barrio et al[56]	2005	RS	50	20	>90%	Similar	Similar	0% dysfunction at 12 mo (vs. 82%); dysfunction defined as PPG > 12 mm Hg
Tripathi et al[43]	2006	RS	316	157	92%	22%	Similar	Shunt insufficiency defined as PPG > 12 mm Hg or > 20% of immediate post-TIPS value or radiologic evidence of shunt occlusion
Jung et al[27]	2009	RS	41	40	38%	Similar	Similar	Only 3-mo patency rates were statistically different (94% vs. 63%), survival difference in ascites group (87% vs. 45%)
Garcia-Pagan et al[40]	2010	RCT	31 (drugs + EBL)	32	NA	28%	86%	1-y free of failure to control bleeding and rebleeding: 97% vs. 50% (TIPS vs. drugs)

*Data presented are at 1 year unless otherwise specified in the comments section.
BM: bare metal, CS: case series; EBL: endoscopic band ligation; HEN: hepatic encephalopathy; NA: not studied or assessed; PET: polyethylene terephthalate; PPG: portosystemic pressure gradient; PV: portal vein; RCT: randomized controlled trial; RS: retrospective; SG: stent graft (covered stents); TIPS: transjugular intrahepatic shunt.

approach 80%.[34] Patients must be immediately stabilized and treated with pharmacologic therapy and ET. Spontaneous hemostasis only occurs in 50% of patients.[35] If bleeding persists despite initial therapy, emergent TIPS is recommended for portal decompression. The effectiveness of TIPS in controlling refractory bleeding is tempered by a high mortality rate. The urgency of the procedure along with the worse clinical status of patient (model for end-stage liver disease [MELD] score, Acute Physiology and Chronic Health Evaluation [APACHE] II score, and Child-Pugh class) account for this higher mortality. Specifically, Child-Pugh class C; elevated hepatic venous pressure gradient (HPVG, greater than 20 mm Hg); hemodynamic instability; and other comorbidities such as heart failure, sepsis, and multiorgan failure contribute to poor outcomes.[36,37] Vangeli et al compiled data from 15 studies in which TIPS was used to control refractory bleeding. Immediate control was achieved in 94% with rebleeding seen in 12%, but the mortality rate was high at 6 weeks, approaching 36% to 50%.[38] A large case series published by Gazzera et al further supported this high first month mortality rate seen in emergent TIPS patients. These investigators correlated mortality to Child class C, elevated creatinine and prolonged prothrombin time and not to TIPS technique.[34]

Early TIPS

More recent studies have challenged the notion of waiting for medical and endoscopic failure before initiating TIPS. The idea of "early" TIPS performed within 24 to 72 hours of a sentinel bleed was first described by Monescillo et al in 2004. They performed an RCT on 116 patients with acute variceal bleeding and stratified the patients into low- and high-risk groups for uncontrolled bleeding or rebleeding based on HPVG (greater than 20 mm Hg considered high risk). Among the high-risk group, they randomly allocated one group to receive TIPS within 24 hours and one group to receive continued medical therapy ($n = 26$ for both groups). Patients receiving TIPS had fewer treatment failures (12% vs. 50%), reduced transfusional requirements (2.2% vs. 3.7%), decreased need for intensive care (3% vs. 16%), and lower 1-year mortality rate (31% vs. 65%).[39] Of note, the Monescillo et al trial did not use the current standard of care in the medical arm and used BMS for the TIPS group.

In 2010, Garcia-Pagan et al expanded on this paradigm of early TIPS by reporting an RCT with 63 patients comparing continued pharmacologic therapy and endoscopic band ligation (EBL) with TIPS with ePTFE stent grafts. Rather than using HPVG as a stratification tool, this study used clinical status as inclusion criteria (Child-Pugh class C and class B with persistent bleeding at endoscopy were included). The results of this study showed a higher 1-year probability of successful control of bleeding and of variceal rebleeding for the TIPS group (97% and 50%). Even more significantly, the data indicated a higher 1-year survival rate for the TIPS group (86% vs. 61%).[40] Interestingly, there was no statistical difference in hepatic encephalopathy between the two groups.

These data contrast previous studies mentioned earlier in the chapter that showed TIPS reduces rebleeding rate but without improving survival. These older studies led to the current recommendations for TIPS as rescue or salvage therapy. Although these newer trials by Garcia-Pagan and Monescillo have smaller sample sizes, they may represent a paradigm shift in the treatment of patients with advanced liver disease as a result of improved shunt

technology. TIPS could eventually be considered as adjuvant therapy as opposed to second line.

Gastric Varices

Gastric varices (GVs), although more rare than their esophageal counterparts, do represent a treatment challenge in patients with PHT. Approximately 10% to 36% of variceal hemorrhage cases arise from GVs.[41] These varices may have a lower overall bleeding risk than esophageal varices, but they can bleed more profusely and be more difficult to control after hemorrhage occurs.[41,42]

The use of TIPS to control rebleeding from these varices has been shown to be effective in a few small series.[41–44] In 1998, Chau et al reported the first series analyzing the effectiveness of TIPS in treating GV. This retrospective study analyzed 112 patients (84 with esophageal varices [EV], 28 with GV) receiving emergency TIPS. There were no significant differences between the groups in regard to disease severity, bleeding, portal hemodynamics, or mortality.[41] Rees et al reported similar clinical results in a retrospective study of 64 patients (52 with EV and 12 with GV) undergoing emergency TIPS. This study also found no difference in portosystemic pressure gradients (PPGs) between the two types of varices, challenging the notion that GV bleed at lower pressures.[42] Tripathi et al supported the previous studies in their retrospective trial of 272 patients (232 with EV and 40 with GV); however, they reported a significantly lower mortality rate in the GV group (30.7% vs. 38.7% at 1 year and 49.5% vs. 74.9% at 2 years), which they attribute to lower overall PPG (unlike Rees et al's study).[43] Lo et al performed an RCT comparing cyanoacrylate glue via endoscopy ($n = 37$) and TIPS ($n = 35$) in the treatment of bleeding GVs. TIPS was shown to have less rebleeding (11% vs. 34%) but similar frequencies of complications and survival.[45] Despite the limited data, TIPS remains an important treatment modality for GV, although the amount of decompression needed may be lower compared with EV.

A newer treatment modality for GV is the use of balloon-occluded retrograde transvenous obliteration (BRTO). This procedure is the treatment of choice in many institutions in Japan in patients with GVs and a gastrosystemic shunt. Data are limited to a few small case series, but it may be a viable option for patients who are not good TIPS candidates or those with isolated GVs and splenic vein thrombosis.[46] Further discussion is beyond the scope of this chapter; please see Chapters 28 to 31 of this book.

Ectopic Varices

Ectopic varices (EcV) are rare but can cause up to 5% of variceal bleeding and be very difficult to treat.[47,48] Locations of these varices include the small bowel, rectum, stomas, umbilicus, retroperitoneum, and nearly anywhere else along the gastrointestinal tract.[48] A few series of analyzing the use of TIPS in refractory ectopic bleeding have been reported.[47,49,50] Kochar et al performed the largest, single-center retrospective study and indentified 28 patients with EcV treated with TIPS (eight of the 28 received VIATORR stents with the remaining receiving BMS; these groups were not analyzed separately). Six of nine patients who underwent emergency TIPS for acute bleeding achieved hemostasis. A 21% rebleeding rate at a median duration of 101 days was reported. Cumulative survival rates were 81%, 72%, and 61% at 1, 3, and 6 months, respectively.[47] Interestingly, this study did show that three of the patients did have recurrent bleeding despite a functioning, patent stent. The authors hypothesized that EcVs have larger diameters than EVs, which leads to increased wall tension by LaPlace's law and therefore higher chances of rebleeding. TIPS remains a viable, first-line option for acute and chronic treatment of bleeding EcVs, especially when the location is inaccessible by endoscopy.

Variceal Embolization

Variceal embolization (VE) has been used to control bleeding even before the use of TIPS became widespread.[51,52] Currently, is it used alongside TIPS to help prevent rebleeding, especially in the acute setting. Tesdal et al performed a nonrandomized, prospective trial of 95 patients to compare TIPS alone ($n = 42$) with TIPS plus VE ($n = 53$). BMS were used for TIPS, and VE was performed when varices continued to fill and PPG was greater than 12 mm Hg using sclerosing agents and coils. The 2- and 4-year rates of patients free of rebleeding were 61% and 53% in the TIPS-only group and 84% and 81% in the VE group, respectively. There was no statistical difference between the groups in terms of survival; however, the authors noted a potential survival benefit after 48 months of treatment in the VE group.[53] Several years later, Gaba et al performed a retrospective study that also compared TIPS alone ($n = 37$) with TIPS plus VE ($n = 15$), but these data were compiled using ePTFE stent grafts. In this study, VE was performed at the discretion of the operator based on the number and size of varices and degree of filling after TIPS placement. Coil embolization was used, and the two vessels included were the coronary vein or gastrosplenic varix. A total of 21.6% of the TIPS-only patients rebled, but only 6.7% of the VE patients rebled during median follow-up periods of 199 and 252 days, respectively. Notably, this difference was not statistically significant. However, in patients who presented with emergent hemorrhage, a statistical significance in rebleeding rates was seen between the two groups (25% in the TIPS-only and 0% in the VE group).[54]

The data for concomitant VE during TIPS is not overwhelmingly powered, but it does warrant further large-scale prospective studies. VE remains an important treatment option in patients with severe variceal bleeding and can be used on a case-by-case basis.

Conclusion

The use of TIPS for variceal bleeding has clearly evolved since its inception. Once considered only as salvage therapy or a bridge to transplantation, it now has a growing role in preventing rebleeding. More data are needed to compare new stent grafts with current endoscopic techniques, but the initial results are promising especially in patients with more severe liver disease (Child class B or C; elevated MELD score).[39,40] TIPS also serves an important role in controlling acute bleeding refractory to medical therapy and preventing rebleeding in gastric and EcVs. Patients with PHT and its sequelae will continue to benefit from our investigation and understanding of TIPS and other treatment modalities.

Clinical Pearls

- Approximately 50% of patients with cirrhosis have gastroesophageal varices at the time of diagnosis.

- When bleeding occurs, patients have an 80% chance of rebleeding within 1 year and a mortality rate of bleeding episodes approaching 33%.
- The effectiveness of TIPS in controlling refractory bleeding in the acute or emergent setting is tempered by a high mortality rate.
- No studies have been completed to assess the efficacy of TIPS for primary prevention. TIPS remains for use as a secondary prevention.
- ePTFE-covered stents are clearly superior to their bare-metal precursors from a patency standpoint and may have improved patient survival rates.
- Recent studies with small sample sizes in very selected groups of patients show reduced rebleeding and improved survival for patients undergoing TIPS versus those managed with combined pharmaceutical and endoscopic therapy.
- TIPS could eventually be considered as adjuvant therapy as opposed to second-line therapy.
- TIPS remains an important treatment modality for GVs, although the amount of decompression needed may be lower compared with EVs.
- BRTO is the treatment of choice in many institutions in Japan in patients with GVs and a gastrosystemic shunt.
- The data for concomitant variceal embolization during TIPS is not overwhelmingly powered, but it does warrant further large-scale prospective studies. VE remains an important treatment option in patients with severe variceal bleeding and can be used on a case-by-case basis.

References

1. Kovalak M, Lake J, Mattek N, et al. Endoscopic screening for varices in cirrhotic patients: data from a national endoscopic database. Gastrointest Endosc 2007;65(1):82–88.
2. Merli M, Nicolini G, Angeloni S, et al. Incidence and natural history of small esophageal varices in cirrhotic patients. J Hepatol 2003;38(3):266–72.
3. D'Amico G, Pagliaro L, Bosch J. Pharmacological treatment of portal hypertension: an evidence-based approach. Semin Liver Dis 1999;19(4):475–505.
4. Pagliaro L, D'Amico G, Luca A, et al. Portal hypertension: diagnosis and treatment. J Hepatol 1995;23(suppl 1):36–44.
5. Rosch J, Hanafee WN, Snow H. Transjugular portal venography and radiologic portacaval shunt: an experimental study. Radiology 1969;92(5):1112–1114.
6. LaBerge JM. Transjugular intrahepatic portosystemic shunt—role in treating intractable variceal bleeding, ascites, and hepatic hydrothorax. Clin Liver Dis 2006;10(3):583–598, ix.
7. Papatheodoridis GV, Goulis J, Leandro G, et al. Transjugular intrahepatic portosystemic shunt compared with endoscopic treatment for prevention of variceal rebleeding: a meta-analysis. Hepatology 1999;30(3):612–622.
8. Cabrera J, Maynar M, Granados R, et al. Transjugular intrahepatic portosystemic shunt versus sclerotherapy in the elective treatment of variceal hemorrhage. Gastroenterology 1996;110(3):832–839.
9. Sanyal AJ, Freedman AM, Luketic VA, et al. Transjugular intrahepatic portosystemic shunts compared with endoscopic sclerotherapy for the prevention of recurrent variceal hemorrhage. A randomized, controlled trial. Ann Intern Med 1997;126(11):849–857.
10. Sauer P, Theilmann L, Stremmel W, et al. Transjugular intrahepatic portosystemic stent shunt versus sclerotherapy plus propranolol for variceal rebleeding. Gastroenterology 1997;113(5):1623–1631.
11. Sauer P, Hansmann J, Richter GM, et al. Endoscopic variceal ligation plus propranolol vs. transjugular intrahepatic portosystemic stent shunt: a long-term randomized trial. Endoscopy 2002;34(9):690–697.
12. Zheng M, Chen Y, Bai J, et al. Transjugular intrahepatic portosystemic shunt versus endoscopic therapy in the secondary prophylaxis of variceal rebleeding in cirrhotic patients: meta-analysis update. J Clin Gastroenterol 2008;42(5):507–516.

13. Escorsell A, Banares R, Garcia-Pagan JC, et al. TIPS versus drug therapy in preventing variceal rebleeding in advanced cirrhosis: a randomized controlled trial. Hepatology 2002;35(2):385–392.

14. Haskal ZJ, Davis A, McAllister A, Furth EE. PTFE-encapsulated endovascular stent-graft for transjugular intrahepatic portosystemic shunts: experimental evaluation. Radiology 1997;205(3):682–688.

15. Saxon RR, Timmermans HA, Uchida BT, et al. Stent-grafts for revision of TIPS stenoses and occlusions: a clinical pilot study. J Vasc Interv Radiol 1997;8(4):539–548.

16. Saxon RS, Ross PL, Mendel-Hartvig J, et al. Transjugular intrahepatic portosystemic shunt patency and the importance of stenosis location in the development of recurrent symptoms. Radiology 1998;207(3):683–693.

17. Chopra S, Dodd GD 3rd, Chintapalli KN, et al. Transjugular intrahepatic portosystemic shunt: accuracy of helical CT angiography in the detection of shunt abnormalities. Radiology 2000;215(1):115–122.

18. Casado M, Bosch J, Garcia-Pagan JC, et al. Clinical events after transjugular intrahepatic portosystemic shunt: correlation with hemodynamic findings. Gastroenterology 1998;114(6):1296–1303.

19. Haskal ZJ. Improved patency of transjugular intrahepatic portosystemic shunts in humans: creation and revision with PTFE stent-grafts. Radiology 1999;213(3):759–766.

20. Sze DY, Vestring T, Liddell RP, et al. Recurrent TIPS failure associated with biliary fistulae: treatment with PTFE-covered stents. Cardiovasc Intervent Radiol 1999;22(4):298–304.

21. Otal P, Smayra T, Bureau C, et al. Preliminary results of a new expanded-polytetrafluoroethylene-covered stent-graft for transjugular intrahepatic portosystemic shunt procedures. AJR Am J Roentgenol 2002;178(1):141–147.

22. Nishimine K, Saxon RR, Kichikawa K, et al. Improved transjugular intrahepatic portosystemic shunt patency with PTFE-covered stent-grafts: experimental results in swine. Radiology 1995;196(2):341–347.

23. Cejna M, Peck-Radosavljevic M, Thurnher SA, et al. Creation of transjugular intrahepatic portosystemic shunts with stent-grafts: initial experiences with a polytetrafluoroethylene-covered nitinol endoprosthesis. Radiology 2001;221(2):437–446.

24. Angermayr B, Cejna M, Koenig F, et al. Survival in patients undergoing transjugular intrahepatic portosystemic shunt: ePTFE-covered stentgrafts versus bare stents. Hepatology 2003;38(4):1043–1050.

25. Hausegger KA, Karnel F, Georgieva B, et al. Transjugular intrahepatic portosystemic shunt creation with the Viatorr expanded polytetrafluoroethylene-covered stent-graft. J Vasc Interv Radiol 2004;15(3):239–248.

26. Charon JP, Alaeddin FH, Pimpalwar SA, et al. Results of a retrospective multicenter trial of the Viatorr expanded polytetrafluoroethylene-covered stent-graft for transjugular intrahepatic portosystemic shunt creation. J Vasc Interv Radiol 2004;15(11):1219–1230.

27. Jung HS, Kalva SP, Greenfield AJ, et al. TIPS: comparison of shunt patency and clinical outcomes between bare stents and expanded polytetrafluoroethylene stent-grafts. J Vasc Interv Radiol 2009;20(2):180–185.

28. Summary of Safety and Effectiveness Data: Gore Viatorr TIPS Endoprosthesis; 2011. http://www.accessdata.fda.gov/cdrh_docs/pdf4/P040027b.pdf.

29. Bureau C, Garcia-Pagan JC, Otal P, et al. Improved clinical outcome using polytetrafluoroethylene-coated stents for TIPS: results of a randomized study. Gastroenterology 2004;126(2):469–475.

30. Bureau C, Pagan JC, Layrargues GP, et al. Patency of stents covered with polytetrafluoroethylene in patients treated by transjugular intrahepatic portosystemic shunts: long-term results of a randomized multicentre study. Liver Int 2007;27(6):742–747.

31. Yang Z, Han G, Wu Q, et al. Patency and clinical outcomes of transjugular intrahepatic portosystemic shunt with polytetrafluoroethylene-covered stents versus bare stents: a meta-analysis. J Gastroenterol Hepatol 2010;25(11):1718–1725.

32. Angeloni S, Merli M, Salvatori FM, De Santis A, Fanelli F, Pepino D, Attili AF, Rossi P, Riggio O. Polytetrafluoroethylene-covered stent grafts for TIPS procedure: 1-year patency and clinical results. Am J Gastroenterol 2004 Feb;99(2):280–5.

33. Boyer TD, Haskal ZJ. The role of transjugular intrahepatic portosystemic shunt (TIPS) in the management of portal hypertension: update 2009. Hepatology 2010;51(1):306.

34. Gazzera C, Righi D, Doriguzzi Breatta A, et al. Emergency transjugular intrahepatic portosystemic shunt (TIPS): results, complications and predictors of mortality in the first month of follow-up. Radiol Med 2012;117(1):46–53.

35. Prandi D, Rueff B, Roche-Sicot J, et al. Life-threatening hemorrhage of the digestive tract in cirrhotic patients. An assessment of the postoperative mortality after emergency portacaval shunt. Am J Surg 1976;131(2):204–209.

36. Kalva SP, Salazar GM, Walker TG. Transjugular intrahepatic portosystemic shunt for acute variceal hemorrhage. Tech Vasc Interv Radiol 2009;12(2):92–101.

37. Augustin S, Gonzalez A, Genesca J. Acute esophageal variceal bleeding: current strategies and new perspectives. World J Hepatol 2010;2(7):261–274.

38. Vangeli M, Patch D, Burroughs AK. Salvage tips for uncontrolled variceal bleeding. J Hepatol 2002;37(5):703–704.

39. Monescillo A, Martinez-Lagares F, Ruiz-del-Arbol L, et al. Influence of portal hypertension and its early decompression by TIPS placement on the outcome of variceal bleeding. Hepatology 2004;40(4):793–801.

40. Garcia-Pagan JC, Caca K, Bureau C, et al. Early use of TIPS in patients with cirrhosis and variceal bleeding. N Engl J Med 2010;362(25):2370–2379.

41. Chau TN, Patch D, Chan YW, et al. "Salvage" transjugular intrahepatic portosystemic shunts: gastric fundal compared with esophageal variceal bleeding. Gastroenterology 1998;114(5):981–987.

42. Rees CJ, Nylander DL, Thompson NP, et al. Do gastric and oesophageal varices bleed at different portal pressures and is TIPS an effective treatment? Liver 2000;20(3):253–256.

43. Tripathi D, Therapondos G, Jackson E, et al. The role of the transjugular intrahepatic portosystemic stent shunt (TIPSS) in the management of bleeding gastric varices: clinical and haemodynamic correlations. Gut 2002;51(2):270–274.

44. Barange K, Peron JM, Imani K, et al. Transjugular intrahepatic portosystemic shunt in the treatment of refractory bleeding from ruptured gastric varices. Hepatology 1999;30(5):1139–1143.

45. Lo GH, Liang HL, Chen WC, et al. A prospective, randomized controlled trial of transjugular intrahepatic portosystemic shunt versus cyanoacrylate injection in the prevention of gastric variceal rebleeding. Endoscopy 2007;39(8):679–685.

46. Ferral H. Balloon-occluded retrograde transvenous occlusion. Tech Vasc Interv Radiol 2008;11(4):225–229.

47. Kochar N, Tripathi D, McAvoy NC, et al. Bleeding ectopic varices in cirrhosis: the role of transjugular intrahepatic portosystemic stent shunts. Aliment Pharmacol Ther 2008;28(3):294–303.

48. Norton ID, Andrews JC, Kamath PS. Management of ectopic varices. Hepatology 1998;28(4):1154–1158.

49. Vidal V, Joly L, Perreault P, et al. Usefulness of transjugular intrahepatic portosystemic shunt in the management of bleeding ectopic varices in cirrhotic patients. Cardiovasc Intervent Radiol 2006;29(2):216–219.

50. Vangeli M, Patch D, Terreni N, et al. Bleeding ectopic varices—treatment with transjugular intrahepatic porto-systemic shunt (TIPS) and embolisation. J Hepatol 2004;41(4):560–566.

51. Smith-Laing G, Scott J, Long RG, et al. Role of percutaneous transhepatic obliteration of varices in the management of hemorrhage from gastroesophageal varices. Gastroenterology 1981;80(5 pt 1):1031–1036.

52. Takase Y, Shibuya S, Chikamori F, et al. Recurrence factors studied by percutaneous transhepatic portography before and after endoscopic sclerotherapy for esophageal varices. Hepatology 1990;11(3):348–352.

53. Tesdal IK, Filser T, Weiss C, et al. Transjugular intrahepatic portosystemic shunts: adjunctive embolotherapy of gastroesophageal collateral vessels in the prevention of variceal rebleeding. Radiology 2005;236(1):360–367.

54. Gaba RC, Bui JT, Cotler SJ, et al. Rebleeding rates following TIPS for variceal hemorrhage in the Viatorr era: TIPS alone versus TIPS with variceal embolization. Hepatol Int 2010;4(4):749–756.

55. Lau CT, Scott M, Stavropoulos SW, et al. Dacron-covered stent-grafts in transjugular intrahepatic portosystemic shunts: initial experience. Radiology 2005;236(2):725–759.

56. Barrio J, Ripoll C, Bañares R, et al. Comparison of transjugular intrahepatic portosystemic shunt dysfunction in PTFE-covered stent-grafts versus bare stents. Eur J Radiol 2005;55(1):120–124.

Chapter 22: Transjugular Intrahepatic Portosystemic Shunts for Ascites and Hepatic Hydrothorax: Results of Clinical Studies

Jeanne M. LaBerge, Kanti Pallav Kolli, and Robert K. Kerlan Jr.

Introduction

The transjugular intrahepatic portosystemic shunt (TIPS) procedure is a useful treatment option in the management of patients with ascites caused by liver disease. Indeed, at tertiary referral centers with active liver transplantation programs, refractory ascites may be the most common indication for TIPS.[1] Yet ascites remains a controversial indication for TIPS, and this procedure is less commonly performed outside of tertiary referral centers or in patients who are not candidates for liver transplantation. This chapter reviews the current approach to TIPS for ascites with an emphasis on the evidence to support the use of TIPS in patients with refractory ascites.

Ascites by definition is the accumulation of more than 25 cc of fluid in the peritoneal cavity. Ascites is characterized by amount according to grade as follows: grade 1 is minimal fluid detectable by ultrasonography only, grade 2 is moderate fluid usually detectable on physical examination and symptomatic, and grade 3 is severe or tense ascites.[2] Although there are many causes of ascites, in the United States, more than 85% of patients with ascites have an underlying cause related to liver dysfunction. Because the etiology of liver disease in the context of ascites is usually cirrhosis, we refer in this chapter chiefly to "cirrhotic ascites." But it is well to keep in mind that, uncommonly, ascites may be the sequelae of noncirrhotic liver disease such as Budd-Chiari syndrome.

Cirrhotic ascites occurs in patients with portal hypertension (PHT). It is one of the four clinical manifestations of PHT, which include variceal bleeding, ascites, hypersplenism, and encephalopathy. However, the onset of ascites requires more than just elevation of portal pressure. Ascites develops in patients with PHT when arterial vasodilation results in a hyperdynamic circulation stimulating renal vasoconstriction and sodium retention.

Pathophysiology and Pressures

Therapies aimed at lowering portal pressure have long been known to ameliorate the clinical sequelae of variceal bleeding and ascites. For variceal bleeding, Garcia-Tsao et al[3] have established a clear threshold value below which variceal bleeding does not occur (hepatic venous pressure gradient [HVPG] <12 mm Hg). When the portal pressure is lowered below this threshold, bleeding stops. However, the relationship of portal pressure to the occurrence of ascites is not so clear-cut. Although cirrhotic ascites is dependent on PHT, the exact threshold for its occurrence is not well established. Authors have suggested thresholds ranging from 8 to 12 mm Hg.[4,5] More important, the development of ascites is also due to two additional important factors, sodium balance and the hyperdynamic circulation.[2,6] This means that therapeutic interventions that lower portal pressure may not completely resolve ascites when the other two causes are not ameliorated.

Thus it is important to note from a pathophysiologic perspective that the effect of TIPS on patients with ascites is much less predictable than the effect of TIPS on patients with variceal bleeding. Moreover, although the effect of TIPS on variceal bleeding is immediate and bleeding usually stops within days, the effect of TIPS on ascites may take months to 1 year to show full effect. Because this is a fairly long time interval, the patient's behavior during this interval may influence results. In particular, noncompliance with a sodium-restricted diet or lack of abstinence from alcohol may influence the outcome of TIPS in follow-up.

In the early 1990s, numerous clinical trials were conducted to evaluate the use of TIPS for patients with variceal bleeding. In many of these trials, it was observed that some patients who also had ascites responded well to TIPS. But the response was not predictable. By the mid-1990s, numerous investigators began to more carefully study the effect of TIPS in patients with ascites who did not have variceal bleeding. In general, investigators postulated that TIPS would be as effective as a surgical side-to-side portocaval at treating ascites but hopefully with less upfront operative morbidity and mortality.

Before discussing TIPS outcomes in greater detail, it is worthwhile to review general approaches to the treatment of ascites and some definitions. Readers can find a more comprehensive coverage of current management strategies in the American Association for the Study of Liver Diseases (AASLD) Guidelines just updated in 2013[7,8] and the European Association for the Study of the Liver (EASL) Guidelines.[9]

Treatment Options

First-Line Therapy

After a diagnosis of cirrhotic ascites is secured by analysis of the ascitic fluid, dietary salt restriction (<2000 mg/day of sodium) is the initial treatment. For patients with grade 2 or 3 ascites, if sodium restriction alone fails to control ascites, then diuretics are initiated. Spironolactone, an aldosterone antagonist, is initiated at a dosage of 100 mg/day and can be increased to a dosage of 400 mg/day. Loop diuretics such as furosemide are added up to a dosage of 160 mg/day as necessary.[6]

Patients on diuretic therapy for ascites are monitored carefully for electrolyte abnormalities and renal failure. Complications of diuretics include hyponatremia (serum sodium <120 mmol/L), hypo- or hyperkalemia (K <3 mmol/L or >6 mmol/L), and renal failure (increase in creatinine by 100% to a value >2 mg/dL). Approximately 5% to 10% of patients with ascites cannot be adequately managed with diuretics and salt restriction.[2]

Second-Line Therapy

Patients whose ascites does not respond to maximal diuretic therapy or that recurs rapidly are deemed to have "refractory ascites," and such patients are candidates for second-line therapy. As well, patients who have a clinically significant complication from diuretics such as renal impairment or hyponatremia are also candidates for second-line therapy.

Second-line treatment options include large-volume paracentesis (LVP), TIPS, and peritoneovenous shunts. Peritoneovenous shunts have largely been abandoned because of their poor patency and high morbidity. This procedure is now only performed when the other second-line therapies are not possible and transplantation is not feasible.[6]

Large-volume paracentesis is defined as removal of more than 5 L of ascites.[2,7] In this procedure, all abdominal ascites is usually removed (i.e., total paracentesis), and albumin is infused intravenously (8 g albumin per liter of fluid removed) to minimize the circulatory effects of the procedure. LVP may be performed every 2 weeks. If LVP is needed more often than every 2 weeks, patients are probably not adhering to sodium restriction.

TIPS has been performed widely throughout the world since the early 1990s, and the technique is well established. Briefly, a needle is advanced from the hepatic vein into the portal vein (PV), and a channel is created to decompress the PV. The channel is lined by a metal stent to maintain patency. The desired portal pressure gradient after shunt formation is 8 to 12 mm Hg. However, the precise post-TIPS pressure gradient cannot usually be accurately controlled prospectively by the operator.

It is important to recognize that a significant modification in TIPS technique occurred in the early 2000s. Most of the clinical trials that are summarized in this chapter were carried out before that time using "bare-metal" TIPS. But in the early 2000s, the polytetrafluoroethylene (PTFE)-covered stent was introduced for TIPS, and this innovation has resulted in significant improvements in patency. Another potential difference between bare-metal TIPS and covered TIPS is that with covered stent TIPS, the stent extends all the way into the inferior vena cava, and most operators measure postprocedure gradient from the PV to the right atrium.

Results of Clinical Studies: TIPS for Refractory Ascites

Outcome Variables

The endpoints of interest in evaluating patients treated by TIPS for refractory ascites are:

- **The amount of ascites:** This result is most often treated as a categorical variable with three categories, complete resolution, improvement, or no improvement.
- **Survival:** This endpoint is calculated using actuarial analysis either up to time of transplantation (transplant-free survival) or including transplantation (overall survival).
- **Complications:** Encephalopathy, variceal bleeding, spontaneous bacterial peritonitis (SBP), renal failure, liver failure
- **Quality of life and cost**

Because patients treated for refractory ascites generally have more severe liver disease than those treated for variceal bleeding alone, survival is a particularly important endpoint. In general, the development of ascites in patients with cirrhosis confers a poor prognosis with a 1-year survival rate of 85% dropping to 50% at 2 years.[6] The development of refractory ascites confers an even worse prognosis.

The most significant complications from TIPS performed to treat refractory ascites in most published trials are encephalopathy and liver failure. Encephalopathy is the most frequent serious complication. Liver failure is the most serious complication and one that can precipitate the need for liver transplantation.

Table 22.1 Indications and Contraindications for Transjugular Intrahepatic Portosystemic Shunt to Treat Ascites

Indications
- Refractory ascites
- Diuretic refractory ascites
- Complications of LVP
- Hepatic hydrothorax

Contraindications
- Absolute
  - Uncontrolled encephalopathy
  - Congestive heart failure (ejection fraction <50%)
  - Severe pulmonary artery hypertension
  - Unrelieved biliary obstruction
- Relative
  - Age older than 70 years
  - Severe liver dysfunction (bilirubin > 5 mg/dL, CP > 12, MELD score >18)
  - Significant encephalopathy
  - INR > 2

CP: Child-Pugh score; INR: international normalized ratio; LVP: large-volume paracentesis; MELD: model for end-stage liver disease.

Indications and Contraindications

The indications and contraindications for TIPS in the setting of refractory ascites are shown in ▸ Table 22.1.

Prospective Cohort Trials: TIPS for Ascites

During the first decade of TIPS research in the 1990s, a number of cohort series focused on the use of TIPS to control ascites. The results of nine of these studies[10–18] are summarized in ▸ Table 22.2. Note that in these uncontrolled studies, improvement in ascites varied widely (47% to 97%) as did the severity of liver disease in the patient populations studied with the percentage of patients with severe liver disease (Child's class C) ranging from 41% to 75%.

Careful study of the effects of TIPS on patients with ascites has shown that urinary sodium excretion and serum creatinine improve steadily within 4 weeks of the procedure and can normalize in 6 month to 1 year of the procedure.[1] As well, the circulatory dysfunction that accompanies PHT is ameliorated by TIPS, thus improving ascites. Detailed studies evaluating nutritional status after successful TIPS have shown positive improvement in nitrogen balance, dry weight, and total body fat.[19–21] These beneficial effects can lead to improved quality of life.

Table 22.2 Transjugular Intrahepatic Portosystemic Shunt for Ascites: Early Cohort Studies[10–18]

Studies (n)	9
Patients (n)	295
Mean follow-up time	6–17 months
Technical success rate (%)	93–100
Ascites improvement rate (%)	47–96
Child's C disease (%)	14–90
1-year survival rate (%)	41–75

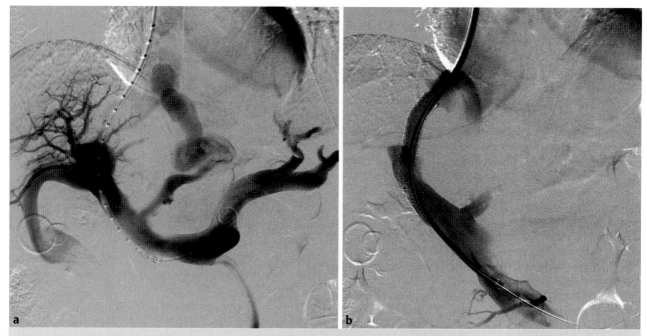

Fig. 22.1 Transjugular intrahepatic portosystemic shunt (TIPS) for refractory ascites. A 62-year-old man with cryptogenic cirrhosis and esophageal varices presented with ascites refractory to diuretic therapy. Despite large-volume paracenteses up to twice weekly, he developed leakage of ascitic fluid from an umbilical hernia (Flood syndrome), and a TIPS procedure was performed. In follow-up, leakage from the umbilical hernia ceased, the patient lost 40 to 50 lbs. in the ensuing year, and ascites was well controlled with diuretics. (**a**) Transjugular portal venogram before TIPS completion showing portal hypertension with hepatofugal flow in splenic and inferior mesenteric veins and filling of coronary vein and recanalized umbilical vein. Pre-TIPS portosystemic gradient (PSG) was 15 mm Hg. (**b**) Post-TIPS venogram demonstrating portal decompression. Note the use of a VIATORR-covered stent. Post-TIPS PSG was 7 mm Hg.

A typical example of a successful TIPS performed to treat refractory ascites is shown in ▸ Fig. 22.1.

Randomized Trials: TIPS versus Large-Volume Paracentesis

Because the initial cohort study results were quite heterogeneous, largely because of variations in the patient populations studied, there was no consensus among experts on the role of TIPS in the management of patients with refractory ascites. Randomized controlled trials (RCTs) have been conducted in an attempt to more accurately distinguish the differences in outcome of the two second-line therapies—TIPS and LVP—for refractory

ascites. The results of the first five of these RCTs[22-26] are shown in ▸ Table 22.3.

Of note, the patient populations studied in these RCTs were carefully controlled but different in each trial. In the majority of the studies, patients with advanced liver disease were excluded (bilirubin >3–5 mg/dL) as were patients with significant encephalopathy (grade 2 or refractory). In these studies, only 40% to 60% of the patients screened were enrolled in the study. Also of note, these five studies spanned a wide time period from 1996 to 2004. Technical success varied from 77% to 100%. During most of this period, the TIPS procedure was performed with bare-metal stents, and consequently secondary patency rates were fairly low, ranging from 46% to 93%.

Table 22.3 Randomized Controlled Trials: Transjugular Intrahepatic Portosystemic Shunt versus Large-Volume Paracentesis for Refractory Ascites

Authors, year	Patients (n)	Tx-Free Survival		Ascites Improvement		Encephalopathy		TIPS Technical Success (%)	TIPS Assisted Patency (%)
		%TIPS	%LVP	%TIPS	%LVP	%TIPS	%LVP		
Lebrec et al, 1996	25	29	56	38	0	15	6	77	46
Rossle et al, 2000	60	58	32	79*	24*	23	13	100	93
Gines et al, 2002	70	26	30	51*	17*	60*	34*	97	91
Sanyal et al, 2003	109	35	33	58*	16*	38	21	94	NA
Salerno et al, 2004	66	59*	29*	79*	42*	61	39	89	82

*Statistically significant difference.
LVP: large-volume paracentesis; TIPS: transjugular intrahepatic portosystemic shunt; Tx: treatment.

Outcomes

Reduction in Ascites

In all five studies, TIPS was shown to be superior to LVP in control of ascites. The percentage of patients with improved ascites after TIPS ranged widely from 38% to 84% and those improved with LVP ranged from 0 to 43%.

Encephalopathy

In all five studies, encephalopathy was worse in the TIPS patients (15% to 61%) than in the LVP patients (6% to 39%).

Survival

Survival over the period of follow-up in these studies was not significantly different in the two groups in all but one study (TIPS: 29% to 59%; LVP: 29% to 60%). It is interesting to review the results of these studies with respect to publication date. The earliest study by Lebrec and colleagues[22] published in 1996 appears to be an outlier possibly because of the early nature of the investigation. The authors showed very poor results with TIPS, and this is the only study demonstrating a survival superiority with LPV. However, the technical success reported in this study (77%) is markedly lower than that demonstrated in the other four studies. As well, in the Lebrec study patency was only 46%.

Meta-Analyses of Randomized Controlled Trials

Based on these five RCTs, the role of TIPS compared with LVP continued to be uncertain. Although TIPS was more effective at control of ascites, TIPS appeared to be associated with a greater risk of encephalopathy. Accordingly, many experts and guidelines continued to recommend LVP over TIPS.

Meta-analyses have been performed to more closely evaluate the results of these five studies and to identify patient subgroups that are more likely to benefit from TIPS.[27-30] One problem with pooling the five studies for the purpose of meta-analysis is heterogeneity of data and differences in endpoint definitions. For example, in terms of screening, although in four studies,[22,23,25,26] 40% to 60% of screened patients were enrolled, in the Sanyal North American Study for the Treatment of Ascites (NASTRA) study[24] only 21% of screened patients were enrolled. Such degree of patient exclusion during screening brings into question selection bias and compromises the widespread applicability of the pooled results.

Heterogeneity in data has been accounted for in some of these meta-analyses using statistical modeling and reassessment of the raw results. D'Amico and colleagues[27] noted that heterogeneity in survival results can be eliminated by removing the Lebrec study from the analysis. When looking at the remaining four studies only, D'Amico found that survival significantly favored TIPS.

In another attempt to overcome study heterogeneity, Salerno and colleagues[31] performed a data analysis using individual patient data rather than pooling study results. Looking at transplant-free survival at 1 and 2 years, Salerno found a survival advantage in the TIPS patients. This was true even in patients with severe liver disease (model for end-stage liver disease [MELD] score, 10–20).

Complications

In addition to encephalopathy, the three most common complications seen in the patients with refractory ascites were gastrointestinal bleeding, SBP, and renal failure. In a meta-analysis of the complications from the RCTs based on individual patient data, Salerno et al[31] found that the overall rate of PHT-related complications was lower in the TIPS group than in the LVP group (15% vs. 28%; $P = 0.05$).

Overall Efficacy for Management of Ascites

Overall one may expect that 68% to 76% of patients treated by TIPS for refractory ascites will have a complete or partial response. In an analysis of 16 cohort studies, Russo and colleagues[32] noted on average 51% complete and 68% complete or partial response. In the five randomized trials described, a mean positive response after TIPS was observed in 76% of patients. Whereas 42% of patients treated by TIPS eventually required LVP for tense ascites, 89% of those treated with LVP required repeat LVP for tense ascites.

Current Ongoing Studies

Because of the promising results published by Salerno et al showing a survival advantage of TIPS in the meta-analysis of individual patient data, there is enthusiasm for evaluating TIPS versus LVP in the era of covered stents. The improved patency afforded with covered stents may tip the balance in favor of TIPS. An industry-sponsored trial is currently underway in which 250 patients will be randomized to TIPS or LVP. Of note, the inclusion criteria for the ongoing trial are less strict than prior RCTs, and the study aims to evaluate TIPS when performed early after the diagnosis refractory ascites.

TIPS for Hepatohydrothorax

Hepatohydrothorax is an indication for TIPS that bears separate discussion because of the unique presentation of these patients and their limited treatment options. By definition, hepatohydrothorax is the accumulation of at least 500 cc of fluid in the pleural space in patients with cirrhosis who do not have any other cause for pleural effusion such as primary cardiac, pulmonary, or pleural disease.[33] Effusions are transudative and demonstrate laboratory characteristics similar to cirrhotic ascites in the abdomen. Hydrothorax occurs in patients with congenital or acquired rents or defects in the diaphragm. Abdominal ascites pass through such defects into the chest. The pleural fluid is most commonly localized to the right chest (80%) but may also occur on the left side only (17%) or bilaterally (3%). Interestingly, approximately 20% of patients with hydrothorax do not have detectable abdominal ascites.

Patients usually present with shortness of breath, and the diagnosis is secured by diagnostic thoracentesis. Pleural fluid is evaluated to determine if it is a transudate. It is also analyzed for infection because SBP may also affect the pleural fluid.

Hepatohydrothorax is observed in 5% to 10% of patients with cirrhotic ascites, and the initial treatment is salt restriction and diuretics.[33] Few effective options are available to treat patients who are refractory to medical management. Thoracentesis with

Table 22.4 Transjugular Intrahepatic Portosystemic Shunt for Ascites: Early Cohort Studies

Authors, year	Patients (n)	% Response	% Total	% Partial
Gordon et al, 1997	24	78	58	20
Siegerstetter et al, 2001	40	82	71	11
Spencer et al, 2002	21	74	63	11
Dhanasekaran et al, 2010	73	75	60	15

removal of 1 to 2 L of fluid can be performed, but repetitive thoracentesis is an uncomfortable prospect for patients and is not as well tolerated as serial abdominal LVP. Generally, a limit of 1 to 2 L is recommended per thoracentesis procedure to minimize the occurrence of reexpansion pulmonary edema.[34] However, some authors do not agree with this "2-L rule" and recommend that a total thoracentesis be performed.[33]

Surgical attempts at obliterating the pleural space via video-assisted thoracoscopic surgery (VATS) pleurodesis and/or repair of diaphragmatic defects have been associated with a low success rate and high morbidity. Surgical morbidity may be as high as 57% for diaphragmatic repair. Talc pleurodesis performed during VATS may only be successful in approximately 50% of cases.[33]

Given the paucity of effective treatment options, TIPS appears to be an attractive therapy for the management of hydrothorax. One might expect that TIPS would improve or eliminate hydrothorax with the same efficacy as is seen when the procedure is performed for refractory abdominal ascites.

Data on TIPS for hydrothorax come only from cohort studies. Because there is no other effective therapy, an RCT is not possible. Results of the four largest cohort studies[35–38] are summarized in ▶ Table 22.4. Improvement was observed in 74% to 82% with complete resolution in 58% to 71%. Note that TIPS in three of these four studies was performed before the era of covered stents, and consequently, the rate of shunt stenosis was high—50% at 1 year in the Siegerstetter series.[36]

The largest cohort series by Dhanasekaran et al[38] bears further comment. Seventy-three patients were treated by TIPS for refractory hepatohydrothorax. Initially, after 1 month, 79.4% of patients responded to TIPS: 58.9% experienced complete resolution, and 20.5% had a partial response. After 6 months, 75% of patients demonstrated a persistent response (60% complete; 15% partial). Despite this good response to therapy, the overall survival rate at 1 year was only 48%, reflecting the severity of the underlying medical condition. As well, complications from the procedure were not insignificant. Fourteen patients died within 30 days, 43% from liver failure, 29% from respiratory distress, and 14% from renal failure. The major long-term complications were encephalopathy (15%) and infection (8%).

An example of a typical successful TIPS in a patient with hepatohydrothorax is shown in ▶ Fig. 22.2. A rare example of reexpansion pulmonary edema after total thoracentesis before TIPS is shown in ▶ Fig. 22.3.

In sum, TIPS appears to be the treatment of choice for patients with refractory hepatohydrothorax, but as with TIPS for ascites, the procedure is contraindicated in those with uncontrolled encephalopathy and should be used sparingly in patients with advanced liver dysfunction.

Conclusion

Several conclusions are warranted based on the clinical data published to date. TIPS is an important second-line treatment for patients with ascites refractory to sodium restriction and diuretics. At present, guidelines in the United States and in Europe support the use of TIPS as second-line therapy but only after failed LVP in most cases. Meta-analysis of individual data from five RCTs comparing TIPS and LVP for management of refractory ascites suggests a trend toward improved survival with TIPS. If these data are borne out by ongoing prospective trials using covered stents, then TIPS may supplant LVP as a second-line therapy in patients without contraindication to the procedure. Hepatohydrothorax is a special subset of ascites in which TIPS is indicated to treat symptomatic patients refractory to medical management. Although improvement in symptoms can be expected in 75% of patients, overall survival may be limited by the severity of the underlying disease and approaches 50% at 1 year.

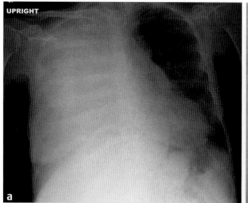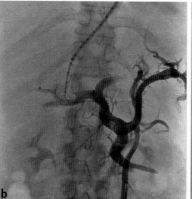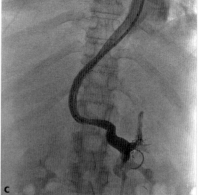

Fig. 22.2 Transjugular intrahepatic portosystemic shunt (TIPS) for hepatohydrothorax. A 54-year-old woman with primary biliary cirrhosis, ascites, and hepatohydrothorax developed renal insufficiency on diuretic therapy and required frequent paracentesis and thoracentesis. TIPS was performed. Ascites and hepatohydrothorax were subsequently controlled with diuretics. (a) Chest radiograph before TIPS showing a large right pleural effusion with shift of the mediastinum to the left. (b) Transjugular portal venogram before TIPS completion showing portal hypertension. Pre-TIPS portosystemic gradient (PSG) was 33 mm Hg. (c) Post-TIPS venogram demonstrating portal decompression. Post-TIPS PSG was 17 mm Hg.

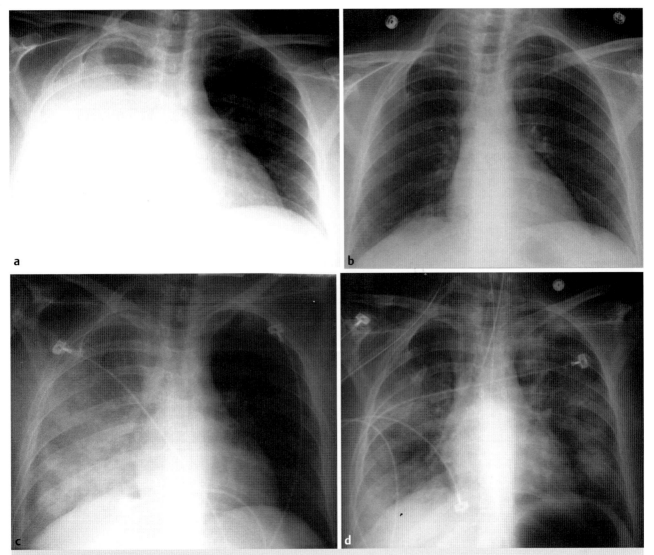

Fig. 22.3 Reexpansion pulmonary edema, a complication of large-volume thoracentesis. A middle-aged man with cirrhosis and a large right pleural effusion underwent thoracentesis before transjugular intrahepatic portosystemic shunt (TIPS). All of the pleural fluid was drained. After the procedure, he developed marked shortness of breath and signs and symptoms of reexpansion pulmonary edema. Increased right atrial pressures after TIPS may have also contributed to the pulmonary compromise. (a) Chest radiograph before TIPS demonstrating a large right pleural effusion. (b) Chest radiograph after total thoracentesis before TIPS. (c) Chest radiograph after TIPS showing unilateral pulmonary edema. (d) Chest radiograph 24 hours later showing bilateral pulmonary edema.

Clinical Pearls

- TIPS is an important second-line treatment for patients with ascites refractory to sodium restriction and diuretics.
- At present, guidelines in the United States and Europe support the use of TIPS as second-line therapy but only after failed LVP in most cases.
- RCTs comparing TIPS and LVP for management of refractory ascites suggests a trend toward improved survival with TIPS.
- If improved patient survival TIPS compared with LVP is confirmed, then TIPS may supplant LVP as a second-line therapy.
- Hepatohydrothorax is a special subset of ascites where TIPS is indicated to treat symptomatic patients refractory to medical management.

- Unlike ascites, although improvement in hepatohydrothorax symptoms can be expected in 75% of patients, overall survival may be limited.

References

1. Rössle M, Gerbes AL. TIPS for the treatment of refractory ascites, hepatorenal syndrome and hepatic hydrothorax: a critical update. Gut 2010;59(7):988–1000.
2. Møller S, Henriksen JH, Bendtsen F. Ascites: pathogenesis and therapeutic principles. Scand J Gastroenterol 2009;44(8):902–911.
3. Garcia-Tsao G, Groszmann RJ, Fisher RL, et al. Portal pressure, presence of gastroesophageal varices and variceal bleeding. Hepatology 1985;5(3):419–424.
4. Nair S, Singh R, Yoselewitz M. Correlation between portal/hepatic vein gradient and response to transjugular intrahepatic portosystemic shunt creation in refractory ascites. J Vasc Interv Radiol 2004;15(12):1431–1434.

5. Thalheimer U, Leandro G, Samonakis DN, et al. TIPS for refractory ascites: a single-centre experience. J Gastroenterol 2009;44(10):1089–1095.

6. Wong F. Management of ascites in cirrhosis. J Gastroenterol Hepatol 2012; 27(1):11–20.

7. Runyon BA. Introduction to the revised American Association for the Study of Liver Diseases Practice Guideline management of adult patients with ascites due to cirrhosis 2012. Hepatology 2013;57(4):1651–1653.

8. Boyer TD, Haskal ZJ; American Association for the Study of Liver Diseases. The role of transjugular intrahepatic portosystemic shunt (TIPS) in the management of portal hypertension: update 2009. Hepatology 2010;51(1):306.

9. European Association for the Study of the Liver. EASL clinical practice guidelines on the management of ascites, spontaneous bacterial peritonitis, and hepatorenal syndrome in cirrhosis. J Hepatol 2010;53(3):397–417.

10. Ferral H, Bjarnason H, Wegryn SA, et al. Refractory ascites: early experience in treatment with transjugular intrahepatic portosystemic shunt. Radiology 1993;189:795–801.

11. Somberg KA, Lake JR, Tomlanovich SJ, et al. Transjugular intrahepatic portosystemic shunts for refractory ascites: assessment of clinical and hormonal response and renal function. Hepatology 1995;21:709–716.

12. Quiroga J, Sangro B, Nunez M, et al. Transjugular intrahepatic portal-systemic shunt in the treatment for refractory ascites: effect on clinical, renal, humoral, and hemodynamic parameters. Hepatology 1995;21:986–994.

13. Ochs A, Rössle M, Haag K, et al. The transjugular intrahepatic portosystemic stent-shunt for refractory ascites. N Engl J Med 1995;332:1192–1197.

14. Crenshaw WB, Gordon FD, McEniff NJ, et al. Severe ascites: efficacy of the transjugular intrahepatic portosystemic shunt in treatment. Radiology 1996; 200:185–192.

15. Forrest EH, Stanley AJ, Redhead DN, et al. Clinical response after transjugular intrahepatic portosystemic stent shunt insertion for refractory ascites in cirrhosis. Aliment Pharmacol Ther 1996;10:801–806.

16. Martinet JP, Fenyves D, Legault L, et al. Treatment of refractory ascites using transjugular intrahepatic portosystemic shunt (TIPS): a caution. Dig Dis Sci 1997;42:161–166.

17. Trotter JF, Suhocki PV, Rockey D. Transjugular intrahepatic portosystemic shunt in patients with refractory ascites: effect on body weight and Child-Pugh score. Am J Gastroenterol 1998;93:1891–1894.

18. Deschaenes M, Dufresne M, Bui B, et al. Predictors of clinical response to TIPS in cirrhotic patients with refractory ascites. Am J Gastroenterol 1999;94:1361–1365.

19. Trotter JF, Suhocki PV, Rockey DC. Transjugular intrahepatic portosystemic shunt (TIPS) in patients with refractory ascites: effect on body weight and Child-Pugh score. Am J Gastroenterol 1998;93(10):1891–1894.

20 Plauth M, Schütz T, Buckendahl DP, et al. Weight gain after transjugular intrahepatic portosystemic shunt is associated with improvement in body composition in malnourished patients with cirrhosis and hypermetabolism. J Hepatol 2004;40(2):228–233.

21. Allard JP, Chau J, Sandokji K, et al. Effects of ascites resolution after successful TIPS on nutrition in cirrhotic patients with refractory ascites. Am J Gastroenterol 2001;96(8):2442–2447.

22. Lebrec D, Giuily N, Hadengue A, et al. Transjugular intrahepatic portosystemic shunts: comparison with paracentesis in patients with cirrhosis and refractory ascites: a randomized trial. French Group of Clinicians and a Group of Biologists. J Hepatol 1996;25:135–144.

23. Rossle M, Ochs A, Gulberg V, et al. A comparison of paracentesis and transjugular intrahepatic portosystemic shunting in patients with ascites. N Engl J Med 2000;342:1701–1707.

24. Sanyal AJ, Genning C, Reddy KR, et al. North American Study for the Treatment of Refractory Ascites Group. The North American Study for the Treatment of Refractory Ascites. Gastroenterology. 2003;124(3):634–641.

25. Gines P, Uriz J, Calahorra B, et al. Transjugular intrahepatic portosystemic shunting versus paracentesis plus albumin for refractory ascites in cirrhosis. Gastroenterology 2002;123(6):1839–1847.

26. Salerno F, Merli M, Riggio O, et al. Randomized controlled study of TIPS versus paracentesis plus albumin in cirrhosis with severe ascites. Hepatology 2004;40(3):629–635.

27. D'Amico G, Luca A, Morabito A, et al. Uncovered transjugular intrahepatic portosystemic shunt for refractory ascites: a meta-analysis. Gastroenterology 2005;129(4):1282–1293.

28. Deltenre P, Mathurin P, Dharancy S, et al. Transjugular intrahepatic portosystemic shunt in refractory ascites: a meta-analysis. Liver Int 2005;25(2): 349–356.

29. Albillos A, Banares R, Gonzalez M, et al. A meta-analysis of transjugular intrahepatic portosystemic shunt versus paracentesis for refractory ascites. J Hepatol 2005;43(6):990–996.

30. Saab S, Nieto JM, Ly D, et al. TIPS versus paracentesis for cirrhotic patients with refractory ascites. Cochrane Database Syst Rev 2004;(3):CD004889.

31. Salerno F, Cammà C, Enea M, et al. Transjugular intrahepatic portosystemic shunt for refractory ascites: a meta-analysis of individual patient data. Gastroenterology 2007;133(3):825–834.

32. Russo MW, Sood A, Jacobson IM, et al. Transjugular intrahepatic portosystemic shunt for refractory ascites: an analysis of the literature on efficacy, morbidity, and mortality. Am J Gastroenterol 2003;98(11):2521–2527.

33. Krok KL, Cárdenas A. Hepatic hydrothorax. Semin Respir Crit Care Med 2012; 33(1):3–10.

34. Porcel JM, Light RW. Pleural effusions. Dis Mon 2013;59(2):29–57.

35. Gordon FD, Anastopoulos HT, Crenshaw W, et al. The successful treatment of symptomatic, refractory hepatic hydrothorax with transjugular intrahepatic portosystemic shunt. Hepatology 1997;25:1366–1369.

36. Siegerstetter V, Deibert P, Ochs A, et al. Treatment of refractory hepatic hydrothorax with transjugular intrahepatic portosystemic shunt: long-term results in 40 patients. Eur J Gastroenterol Hepatol 2001;13(5):529–534.

37. Spencer EB, Cohen DT, Darcy MD. Safety and efficacy of transjugular intrahepatic portosystemic shunt creation for the treatment of hepatic hydrothorax. J Vasc Interv Radiol 2002;13(4):385–390.

38. Dhanasekaran R, West JK, Gonzales PC, et al. Transjugular intrahepatic portosystemic shunt for symptomatic refractory hepatic hydrothorax in patients with cirrhosis. Am J Gastroenterol 2010;105(3):635–641.

Chapter 23: The Transjugular Intrahepatic Portosystemic Shunt as a Prelude to and After Liver Transplantation

Bill S. Majdalany and Wael E.A. Saad

Introduction

Transjugular intrahepatic portosystemic shunt (TIPS) is an artificial conduit between the systemic and portal venous systems. This percutaneous procedure is commonly performed in patients with portal hypertension (PHT) for the management of variceal hemorrhage, refractory ascites, hepatic hydrothorax, and Budd-Chiari syndrome. TIPS creation has largely supplanted surgical portosystemic shunts for the decompression of PHT because it is less invasive and can be placed in patients with advanced hepatic failure.[1] Although portosystemic shunts can mitigate the complications of PHT, they are not a definitive treatment of what is usually irreversible and progressive hepatic disease. Ultimately, liver transplantation, if the patient is an appropriate candidate, is generally the optimal long-term therapeutic option. With respect to liver transplantation, TIPS has an additional major advantage over surgical portosystemic shunts, namely its wholly intrahepatic location and potential for *en bloc* removal with the native liver at the time of recipient hepatectomy. In contradistinction, surgical portosystemic shunts such as the Warren shunt, Drapanas shunt, portocaval anastomosis, or splenorenal shunts and others all require additional surgery for their takedown or ligation.[2]

The demand for liver transplants has been consistent with approximately 15,000 patients on the waiting list at any particular time. Given a slowly worsening donor shortage, median pretransplant wait times increased from 12.9 months in 2009 to 18.5 months in 2011, which may also increase rates of drop-off from the transplant list.[3] For these patients, TIPS routinely serves as "a bridge to transplantation," ameliorating the symptoms and risk of PHT in the meantime.

Aside from the accepted indications of TIPS placement, several studies have evaluated TIPS before transplantation, not as a temporizing measure for the management of portal hypertensive sequela but as a pretransplant prelude with the premise that decompression of the portal circulation would decrease portosystemic collateral engorgement, resulting in a reduction of intraoperative bleeding during liver transplantation.[2,4–22] However, these studies, mostly in the transplant literature, have been equivocal from an intraoperative and posttransplant clinical outcome standpoint.

Additionally, TIPS creation in liver transplant recipients is equally worthy of discussion because there has been a debate about whether liver transplantation increases the technical difficulty of the TIPS procedure. Several recent studies evaluating the outcomes of TIPS in liver transplant recipients are reviewed.[23–30] This chapter discusses the results of TIPS as a preoperative prelude to liver transplantation and the technical and clinical outcomes of TIPS in liver transplant recipients.

TIPS as a Preoperative Prelude to Liver Transplantation

Careful selection of liver transplant candidates and medical optimization of those at higher risk has been found to reduce hospital resource utilization and improve outcomes.[31–33] Specifically, intraoperative blood product administration serves as a surrogate marker directly related to hospital resource utilization and inversely related to clinical outcomes.[2,31] Given that the typical liver transplant candidate has PHT, it follows that portal vein engorgement and increased portosystemic collateral flow are present. Redirecting portal venous flow through a shunt alters the pressure gradient across the portal system, thereby collapsing the portosystemic collaterals and presumably reducing the risk of intraoperative bleeding and use of blood products.

Before the improvements in endoscopic therapeutics and the development of TIPS, the complications of PHT were managed surgically. As TIPS began to be performed more commonly than surgical shunts, comparisons between orthotopic liver transplants with surgical portosystemic shunts versus TIPS emerged. Patients with surgical portosystemic shunts have shunt reversal or take-down performed at the time of transplantation. However, because surgical shunts are often adhesed, discerning the surgical anatomy and performing the surgical dissection can be difficult. Ultimately, the higher operative complexity results in longer operative time, requiring more blood transfusions at transplantation and more hospital resources.

In comparison, TIPS has the potential for complete in situ removal with the recipient's hepatectomy adding little technical complexity to the transplant surgery. However, it is notable that TIPS malposition or migration can complicate liver transplantation. Multiple published cases have reported the presence of the TIPS stent in the inferior vena cava, right atrium, pulmonary artery, extrahepatic portal vein, and superior mesenteric vein with or without vascular incorporation.[34–44] Although these reports have noted a malpositioned TIPS stent, all technical surgical difficulties that were encountered were overcome. While the exact incidence is not accurately known, improvements in stent technology have decreased stent migration, and medical centers with greater expertise and higher volume of TIPS likely have fewer problems with accurate and appropriate placement. Generally, the placement of TIPS has become safer and more routine over time and should not preclude transplant listing or complicate the transplantation, provided the availability of high quality preoperative imaging.[45]

Multiple comparative analyses between patients who have had a TIPS performed before liver transplant and patients who have not had a TIPS before liver transplant have been performed evaluating parameters such as intraoperative blood loss, recipient hepatectomy time, total operative time, patient survival, graft survival, postoperative complication rates, mean intensive care unit stay, and hospital stays.[2,10,20–22,44,46–54] Across all parameters, in particular with respect to intraoperative transfusion of blood products, conflicting results have been published with no consistent difference emerging. Saad and coworkers published the only study comparing adult right lobe living related liver transplants with or without intentional TIPS 48 to 72 hours before transplant surgery.[2] This case-controlled retrospective study also showed no significant value in performing TIPS before living related liver transplantation. However, the authors did conclude that TIPS may reduce the risk of poor outcomes in patients with high APACHE II (Acute Physiology and Chronic Health Evaluation II) scores and coagulopathy.

Development of partial portal vein thrombosis is not uncommon in patients with liver failure and may herald full portal vein thrombosis, which develops in up to 26% of patients awaiting liver transplant. Similar to portal venous engorgement, portal vein thrombosis can technically complicate the transplant graft anastomosis and increase morbidity and mortality post-transplant.[55,56] In most clinical scenarios, anticoagulation is the mainstay of therapy for venous thromboses. However, patients with PHT have an elevated risk of life-threatening bleeding on a background of intrinsic liver dysfunction, which typically precludes this as a long-term therapeutic strategy. TIPS creation has been used to prevent complete portal venous thrombosis and to improve portal vein recanalization in both patients with and without cirrhosis.[57,58] Additionally, D'Avola et al[59] and Gaba et al[60] collectively documented 19 cases of partial portal vein thrombosis in patients who first underwent TIPS and then ultimately liver transplantation. None of the patients in these publications had residual thrombus at the time of transplant. In comparison, D'Avola et al noted that only 50% of the control group with partial portal vein thrombosis maintained portal patency until the time of transplant. Theoretically, clot resolution and portal patency may be attributable to the resultant improved anterograde flow dynamics. Although this has only been observed in a relatively small subset of patients, partial portal vein thrombosis may ultimately represent an evolving indication for TIPS in pretransplant candidates.

TIPS in Liver Transplant Recipients

The first human liver transplant was performed in 1963, but 1-year survival was not achieved until 1967. Cumulative improvements and evolution of surgical techniques and medications have made the practice of liver transplantation more successful. Liver transplant recipients are living longer, and because of sheer longevity, there is a higher likelihood of developing primary allograft failure or recurrence of the initial underlying cause of their liver disease, most commonly hepatitis C. These two etiologies are the leading cause of recurrent PHT in liver transplant recipients who undergo TIPS, but in reviewing the published literature, the cause varies among institutions.[23,24] In the United Sates, TIPS is performed in 1% to 4% of the liver transplant recipient population.[24,27,28] In three studies involving four institutions in the United States, a total of 81 liver transplant recipients underwent a TIPS procedure out of a total of 3785 liver transplant recipients (2.1%, n = 81 of 3785).[24,27,28] Reversely, 5.5% of TIPS procedures performed at two of these institutions were found to be in transplant recipients.[24]

Reports by Nolte et al[61] of 1 patient (1998), Lerut et al[26] of 8 patients (1999), and Amesur et al[25] of 12 patients (1999) were the initial publications on placement of TIPS after liver transplantation. In total, these reports comprised 21 patients in whom the etiology of recurrent PHT was recurrent hepatitis C in 76% (16 of 21 patients) and recurrent hepatitis B, recurrent primary biliary cirrhosis, hepatic veno-occlusive disease, and lymphoproliferative disease each in single cases. The etiology was not reported

or was unknown in 1 patient. Refractory ascites or hepatic hydrothorax was the presenting symptom in 62% (13 of 21 patients), variceal hemorrhage in 33% (7 of 21 patients), and 1 case was performed in the setting of redo biliary surgery.

In the years 2000 to 2009, six additional reports were published comprising an additional 57 patients with the three largest series by Kim et al[27] of 11 patients, Choi et al[30] of 18 patients, and Finkenstedt et al[62] of 10 patients. Again, the predominant cause of recurrent PHT was recurrent hepatitis C in 53% (30 of 57 patients), acute or chronic rejection and delayed graft function in 16% (9 of 57 patients), hepatic veno-occlusive disease in 7% (4 of 57 patients), and various miscellaneous or unknown causes in the remainder. Of these patients, 49 of 57 (86%) patients presented with refractory ascites or hepatic hydrothorax, and only 8 of 57 (14%) presented with variceal hemorrhage.[27,30,62–65]

Since 2010, seven publications have presented an additional 121 patients with the largest by Saad et al[24] presenting 38 cases, Feyssa et al[28] presenting 26 cases, and King et al[29] presenting 22 cases. Recurrent hepatitis C was responsible for recurrent PHT in 43% (52 of 121 patients), alcohol use alone or in combination with hepatitis B or C in 8% (10 of 121 patients), and vascular abnormalities or hepatic venous outflow obstruction in 10% (11 of 121 patients). Recurrent hepatitis B, hepatocellular carcinoma, cystic fibrosis, nonalcoholic steatohepatitis, primary biliary cirrhosis, primary sclerosing cholangitis, sarcoidosis, and cholangiopathy were all reported as well but in fewer than 10% of cases. The etiology was not reported or was unknown in 30 patients. Refractory ascites or hepatic hydrothorax continued to be the dominant reported indication for TIPS after transplant with 106 of 121 patients (87%) in this category. A total of 14 of 121 (12%) patients had a TIPS performed after transplant for variceal hemorrhage. A single case was reported for small-for-size syndrome (SFSS).[23,24,28,29,66–68]

There are two aspects for discussion regarding TIPS in liver transplant recipients: technical considerations and the actual clinical outcome of TIPS in this particular population.

Technical Aspects

Early in the clinical practice of TIPS in the United States, there was a debate whether liver transplant anatomy adds to the technical difficulty of the procedure.[22,25,69,70] Intuitively, knowledge of portal and hepatic venous anatomy and surgical anastomoses is paramount as was emphasized by Richard et al[69] and supported by other subsequent authors. As transplant techniques have evolved, surgical anastomoses have changed as well. Traditionally, orthotopic liver transplantation involved caval reconstruction. In most modern centers, the piggyback anastomosis technique has supplanted caval reconstruction, avoiding veno-venous bypass and reducing the warm ischemic time of the graft, ultimately improving outcomes.

Piggyback Anastomosis

Richard and coworkers[69] raised the anatomic concern for piggyback anastomoses posing technical difficulty to the TIPS procedure. Although Saad and coworkers[24] noted that the piggyback anastomosis did not always pose an additional technical challenge, they did support the assertion that this anastomosis could be more difficult, particularly if significantly angulated downward.

Moreover, they noted that the operator must be cognizant of the partly extrahepatic portion of the piggyback anastomosis to avoid extrahepatic punctures.[24] Capacious caval stumps and hepatic venous outflow stenosis were other potential technical challenges to the TIPS procedure in this population.[24,69] The discussions in both studies are not substantiated by data given the small sample sizes.[24,69] In general, multiple studies have consistently demonstrated a technical success rate greater than 80% in placement of TIPS in the posttransplant patient population, but not all studies differentiated which patients had the standard caval interposition or piggyback anastomoses, making it difficult to elucidate the exact technical success rate. However, if conventional TIPS cannot be achieved or there is concern for extrahepatic puncture, an unconventional TIPS approach such as the gun-site technique was performed by Saad et al,[24] increasing the proportion of patients in whom TIPS was technically successful.

Split Grafts, Especially Left Lobe Grafts

Anecdotally, Saad and coworkers[70] added that split grafts, especially undersized grafts such as left lobe grafts in growing children, would pose additional technical difficulty. The orientation of the hepatic and portal veins may be unconventional because the grafts will rotate as they hypertrophy. Moreover, the TIPS procedure is most commonly performed from a right hepatic to right portal vein and to a lesser extent middle hepatic to right portal vein approach. Targeting from the left hepatic vein to the left portal vein is not as commonly performed. To overcome the technical challenges, real-time ultrasound guidance or the gun-site technique were suggested as procedural adjuncts.[70]

Comparative Analysis of Technical Outcomes Between TIPS in Hepatic Grafts and TIPS in Native Livers

A comparative technical analysis between TIPS in transplants and TIPS in native livers was performed by Saad and coworkers.[24] This study compared two different institutions that approached "difficult TIPS" in two different ways. One institution in the study approached an initial technical TIPS failure in a native or transplant liver by reattempting the conventional TIPS procedure another day with a different and usually more experienced operator. The other institution switched from a conventional TIPS approach to an unconventional TIPS approach. The conventional TIPS approach was defined as a single right transjugular approach. Unconventional approaches included unconventional accesses or additional accesses that include femoral access, transhepatic access, gun-site technique, and left paraumbilical vein access.[24] In both institutions, there was no significant difference in technical success between all attempts, including conventional, unconventional, or conversion to unconventional approaches.[24] The overall first attempt technical success and ultimate technical success in both institutions for transplant livers versus native livers was 87% versus 92% for first attempts and 97% versus 97% for ultimate technical success, respectively.[24] The authors did note, however, that the majority of these transplants were whole grafts without angulated piggyback anastomoses and that if there were more split grafts or angulated piggyback anastomoses, the results may not have been equivocal.[24]

Clinical Outcome

In the past decade, with larger case numbers and longer follow-up periods, several studies have evaluated the clinical effectiveness of TIPS in liver transplant recipients. Generally, these studies report that TIPS appears to be less effective clinically in liver transplant recipients than nontransplanted patients[23,24,27,29] with many authors noting poor survival and urging early retransplantation if possible. A review of Model For End-Stage Liver Disease (MELD) score utilization for outcomes predication in posttransplant TIPS patients is discussed. Also, the results of studies using TIPS in the posttransplant patient for refractory ascites, variceal hemorrhage, and evolving indications are presented. Last, special considerations in posttransplant TIPS patients are discussed.

MELD Score and Survival for TIPS After Transplant

Generally, multiple studies have documented a 1-year survival rate nearing 15% for TIPS placement in liver transplant recipients. This compares poorly with the 60% 1-year survival rate for TIPS placement in pretransplant patients.[24,27,30] In the majority of cases, death was attributable to the complications of end-stage liver disease. Feyssa et al[28] and King et al[29] reported that MELD scores above 15 portended a high mortality rate within 3 to 6 months without retransplantation.[24,28,29] Saad and coworkers[24] used a MELD of 17 as a cutoff comparison and demonstrated significant transplant-free survival difference between a pre-TIPS MELD score less than 17 and a pre-TIPS MELD score greater than 17 with 1-year transplant-free survival of 54% versus 8%, respectively. Moreover, they compared the grafts that survived more than 3 months versus those that survived less than 3 months, and the MELD score was statistically significant at 14 ± 4.9 versus 18.6 ± 4.5, respectively ($P = 0.002$).[24]

Posttransplant TIPS for Ascites

In reviewing the literature, nearly 200 patients have had posttransplant TIPS for refractory ascites, hepatic hydrothorax, or both. Generally, although TIPS in liver transplant recipients was safe, it resulted in a poor clinical response. Variations in the literature are noted and are likely attributable to several factors, including an amalgamation of ascitic patients with variceal bleeding patients, varying definitions of clinical success for ascites response, potential for multifactorial etiologies of ascites, and varying degrees of retransplantation thresholds.[24]

Indications Unique to Posttransplant Patients

Given the overall small number of published reports of TIPS in the posttransplant population, it is important to discuss indications that are presented in case reports and small case series, particularly if they are unique to care of post–liver transplant patients. Herein, TIPS for posttransplant portal vein thrombosis, sinusoidal obstruction syndrome (SOS), and SFSS are reviewed.

Just as TIPS accesses can assist in treatment of portal vein thrombosis for patients with native livers, Ciccarelli et al[71] reported the successful treatment of early portal vein thrombosis after transplant through a TIPS augmented with local thrombolysis.

Sinusoidal obstruction syndrome was previously referred to as veno-occlusive disease. Although central vein occlusion is usually present in this entity, progressive outflow obstruction begins in sinusoids. Most often, SOS is seen after stem cell transplantation, but it can also be seen after solid organ transplant with acute allograft dysfunction. In stem cell patients with SOS, TIPS placement did not improve prognosis.[72] However, Campos-Varela et al[66] most recently reported a case of SOS after liver transplant successfully managed with TIPS and recommended consideration of TIPS placement in patients who were refractory to medical treatment for SOS. It is notable that little experience is present in this condition with Lerut et al,[26] Kitajima et al,[73] Sebagh et al,[74] and Senzolo et al,[75] contributing similar cases including seven patients.

Particular to split graft transplants, liver dysfunction may occur because there may not be enough liver mass, which is referred to as SFSS. Typical treatment revolves around control of the portal inflow to the graft or optimizing venous outflow. In a letter, Sampietro et al[76] shared a case in which a temporary TIPS was used to overcome SFSS in a right lobe adult split liver transplant. In a subsequent case report, Xiao et al[77] reported a similar case in which TIPS placement was successful for the treatment of SFSS. Although TIPS placement was feasible and improved the patient's clinical status in both cases, the patients passed away shortly thereafter.

Considerations in Posttransplant Patients

Two studies were case controlled comparing a transplant TIPS group with nontransplant patients undergoing TIPS.[24,27] Kim and coworkers[27] showed a higher infectious complication rate, a high hepatic encephalopathy rate (>80%), and a poor 1-year transplant-free survival rate of 14%. The high encephalopathy rate was suggested by an earlier study by Lerut and coworkers,[20] who documented high levels of calcineurin inhibitors. They postulated that the neurotoxic effect of calcineurin inhibitors was more pronounced because the TIPS functions to bypass their first-pass metabolism in the liver.[20] Conversely, in another case-controlled study, Kim and coworkers[27] showed no difference in hepatic encephalopathy between transplant and nontransplant patients after undergoing TIPS. However, the clinical success rate remained significantly lower for transplanted patients than nontransplant patients (93% vs. 77%, respectively).[27]

Conclusion

In conclusion, TIPS as a prelude to liver transplantation in an attempt to decompress the portal circulation appears to have no effect on blood product and hospital resource utilization. However, using TIPS as an adjunct to preserve a partially thrombosed main portal vein in potential liver transplant recipients has shown promising results in small cohorts. Whole-graft liver transplantation does not pose significant technical difficulty on the TIPS procedure. Anecdotally, split grafts and angulated piggyback anastomoses may increase the technical difficulty of TIPS placement. Liver transplant recipients undergoing TIPS do not survive as well as their counterparts who have not undergone transplantation, and a MELD greater than 15 to 17 is a prognostic indicator of poor graft survival. Liver transplant recipients with ascites may not respond clinically as well as their nontransplant comparisons, although this is subject to graft survival and definitions of clinical success.

Clinical Pearls

- TIPS is routinely performed in the management of patients with portal hypertension and does not preclude liver transplantation.
- TIPS can be placed percutaneously in patients who are nonoperative candidates and can be removed *en bloc* at the time of liver transplantation with the native liver, representing advantages over surgical portosystemic shunts.
- Although TIPS is a successful bridge to liver transplant, studies are contradictory and inconclusive regarding the intentional placement of a TIPS pretransplant for the sole purpose of facilitating surgery.
- Partial portal vein thrombosis can be treated by TIPS placement and may evolve into an accepted indication in pretransplant patients.
- Post–liver transplantation anatomy can be challenging. Knowledge of portal and hepatic venous anatomy and surgical anastomoses is paramount for technically successful TIPS placement.
- Liver transplant recipients fare poorly when undergoing TIPS compared with pretransplant patients with lower survival rates and poorer clinical responses.
- Brief reviews of TIPS for posttransplant portal vein thrombosis, sinusoidal obstruction syndrome, and SFSS have demonstrated success and may warrant additional evaluation.

References

1. Boyer TD, Haskal ZJ. The role of transjugular intrahepatic portosystemic shunt (TIPS) in the management of portal hypertension: update 2009. Hepatology 2010;51:1–16.
2. Saad WE, Saad NE, Davies M, et al. Elective transjugular intrahepatic portosystemic shunt creation for portal decompression in the adult living related liver transplant recipient candidates: preliminary results. J Vasc Interv Radiol 2006;17:995–1002.
3. Organ Procurement Transplant Network. 2012 Annual Data Report. Retrieved June 20, 2014, from http://srtr.transplant.hrsa.gov/annual_reports/2012/Default.aspx.
4. Porte RJ, Hendricks HGD, Slooff MJH. Blood conservation in liver transplantation: the role of aprotinin. J Cardiothorac Vasc Anesthesia 2004;18:S31–S37.
5. Ramos E, Dalmau A, Sabate A, et al. Intraoperative red blood cell transfusion in liver transplantation: influence on patient outcome, predictions of requirements, and measures to reduce them. Liver Transpl 2003;9:1320–1327.
6. Chung SW, Kirkpatrick AW, Kim HLN, et al. Correlation between physiological assessment and outcome after liver transplantation. Am J Surg 2000;179:396–399.
7. Cacciarelli TV, Keefe EB, Moore DH, et al. Effect of intraoperative blood transfusion on patient outcome in hepatic transplantation. Arch Surg 1999;134:25–29.
8. Schroeder RA, Johnson LB, Plotkin JS, et al. Total blood transfusion and mortality after orthotopic liver transplantation. Anesthesiology 1999;91:329–330.
9. Megegaux F, Keeffe EB, Baker E, et al. Comparison of transjugular and surgical portosystemic shunts on the outcome of liver transplantation. Arch Surg 1994;129:1018–1023.
10. Mills JM, Martin P, Gomes A, et al. Transjugular intrahepatic portosystemic shunts: impact on liver transplantation. Liver Transpl Surg 1995;1:229–233.
11. Mor E, Jennings L, Gonwa TA, et al. The impact of operative bleeding on outcome in transplantation of the liver. Surg Gynecol Obstet 1993;176:219–227.
12. Seiders E, Peeters PMJG, TenVergert EM, et al. Prognostic factors for long-term actual patient survival after orthotopic liver transplantation in children. Transplantation 2000;70:1448–1453.

13. Porte RJ, Molenaar IQ, Beglimini B, et al. Aprotinin and transfusion requirements in orthotopic liver transplantation: a multicenter randomized double-blind study. Lancet 2000;355:1303–1309.
14. Findlay JY, Rettke SR. Poor prediction of blood transfusion requirements in adult liver transplantations from preoperative variables. J Clin Anesthesia 2000;12:319–323.
15. Hendriks HG, Van der Meer J, de Wolf JT, et al. Intraoperative blood transfusion requirements in the main determinant of early surgical re-intervention after orthotopic liver transplantation. Transpl Int 2005;17:673–679.
16. Abou Jaoude MM, Almawi WY. Liver transplantation in patients with previous portasystemic shunt. Transpl Proc 2001;33:2723–2725.
17. Langnas AN, Marujo WC, Stratta RJ, et al. Influence of a prior portosystemic shunt on outcome after liver transplantation. Am J Gastroenterol 1992;87:714–718.
18. Brems JJ, Hiatt JR, Klein AS, et al. Effect of prior portosystemic shunt on subsequent liver transplantation. Ann Surg 1989;209:51–56.
19. Rubio Gonzalez EE, Moreno Planas JM, Jimenez Garrido MC, et al. Results of liver transplantation in patients with previous portosystemic shunts. Transpl Proc 2005;37:1491–1492.
20. John TG, Jalan R, Stanley AJ, et al. Transjugular intrahepatic portosystemic stent-shunt insertion as a prelude to orthotopic liver transplantation in patients with severe portal hypertension. Eur J Gastroenterol Hepatol 1996;8:1145–1149.
21. Somberg KA, Lombardero MS, Lawlor SM, et al. A controlled analysis of the transjugular intrahepatic portosystemic shunt in liver transplant recipients. Transplantation 1997;63:1074–1079.
22. Lerut JP, Laterre PF, Goffette P, et al. Transjugular intrahepatic portosystemic shunt and liver transplantation. Transpl Int 1996;9:370–375.
23. Saad WE, Darwish WM, Davies M, et al. Transjugular intrahepatic portosystemic shunts in liver transplant recipients for management of refractory ascites: clinical outcome. J Vasc Interv Radiol 2010;21:218–223.
24. Saad WE, Darwish WM, Davies M, et al. Transjugular intrahepatic portosystemic shunts in liver transplant recipients: technical analysis and clinical outcome. AJR Am J Roetgenol 2013;200:210–218.
25. Amesur NB, Zajko AB, Orons PD, et al. Transjugular intrahepatic portosystemic shunt in patients who have undergone liver transplantation. J Vasc Interv Radiol 1999;10:569–573.
26. Lerut JP, Goffette P, Molle G, et al. Transjugular intrahepatic portosystemic shunt after adult liver transplantation: experience in eight patients. Transplantation 1999;68:379–384.
27. Kim JJ, Dasika NL, Yu E, Fontana RJ. Transjugular intrahepatic portosystemic shunts in liver transplant recipients. Liver Int 2008;28:19:516–520.
28. Feyssa E, Ortiz J, Grewal K, et al. MELD score less that 15 predicts prolonged survival after transjugular intrahepatic portosystemic shunt for refractory ascites after liver transplantation. Transplantation 2011;91:786–792.
29. King A, Masterton G, Gunson B, et al. A case-controlled study of the safety and efficacy of transjugular intrahepatic portosystemic shunts after liver transplantation. Liver Transpl 2011;17:771–778.
30. Choi D, Ashokkumar JB, Orloff MS. Utility of transjugular intrahepatic portosystemic shunts in liver-transplant recipients. J Am Coll Surg 2009;208:539–546.
31. Jabbour N, Gagandeep S, Mateo R, et al. Live donor liver transplantation without blood products: strategies developed for Jehovah's Witnesses offer broad application. Ann Surg 2004;240:350–357.
32. Spanier TB, Klein RD, Naraway SA, et al. Multiple organ failure after liver transplantation. Crit Care Med 1995;23:466–473.
33. Lo CM, Fan ST, Liu CL, et al. Lessons learned from one hundred tight lobe living donor liver transplants. Ann Surg 2004;204:151–158.
34. Wilson MW, Gordon RL, LaBerge JM, et al. Liver transplantation complicated by malpositioned transjugular intrahepatic portosystemic shunts. J Vasc Interv Radiol 1995;6:695–699.
35. Tivener D, Vannucci A, Fagley RE, et al. Atrial laceration caused by removal of a transjugular intrahepatic portosystemic shunt necessitates emergent cardiopulmonary bypass during liver transplant: a case report. Transplant Proc 2011;43:2810–2813.
36. Mazziotti A, Morelli MC, Grazi GL, et al. Beware of TIPS in Liver transplant candidates. Transjugular intrahepatic portosystemic shunt. Hepato-gastroenterology 1996;43:1606–1610.
37. Rumi MN, Schumann R, Freeman RB, et al. Acute transjugular intrahepatic portosystemic shunt migration into pulmonary artery during liver transplantation. Transplantation 1999;67:1492–1494.
38. Hutchins RR, Patch D, Tibballs J, et al. Liver transplantation complicated by embedded transjugular intrahepatic portosystemic shunt: a new method for portal anastomosis—a surgical salvage procedure. Liver Transpl 2000;6:237–238.
39. Jordan Ray M, Savage C, Klintmalm GB, Rees CR. Endovascular caudal retraction of the cranial end of a misplaced Viatorr TIPS Prior to liver transplantation. Proc (Bayl Univ Med Cent) 2012;25:341–343.
40. Clavien PA, Selzner M, Tuttle-Newhall JE, et al. Liver transplantation complicated by misplaced TIPS in the portal vein. Ann Surg 1998;227:440–445.
41. da Silva RF, Arroyo Jr. PC, Duca WJ, et al. Migration of transjugular intrahepatic portosystemic shunt to the right atrium: complications in the intraoperative period of liver transplantation. Transplant Proc 2008;40:3778–3780.
42. Salvalaggio PRO, Koffron AJ, Fryer JP, Abecassis MM. Liver transplantation with simultaneous removal of an intracardiac transjugular intrahepatic portosystemic shunt and a vena cava filter without the utilization of cardiopulmonary bypass. Liver Transpl 2005;11:229–232.
43. Maleux G, Pirenne J, Vaninbroukx J, et al. Are TIPS stent-grafts a contraindication for future liver transplantation? Cardiovasc Interv Radiol 2004;27:140–142.
44. Levi Sandri GB, Lai Q, Lucatelli P, et al. Transjugular Intrahepatic portosystemic shunt for a wait list patient is not a contraindication for orthotopic liver transplant outcomes. Exp Clin Transplant 2013;5:426–428.
45. American College of Radiology (ACR), Society of Interventional Radiology (SIR), Society of Pediatric Radiology (SPR): ACR-SIR-SPR Practice Guideline for the Creation of Transjugular Intrahepatic Portosystemic Shunt (TIPS). [online publication]. Reston, VA: American College of Radiology (ACR);2012.
46. Woodle ES, Darcy M, White HM, et al. Intrahepatic portosystemic vascular stents: a bridge to hepatic transplantation. Surgery 1993;113:344–351.
47. Knechtle SJ. Portal hypertension: A multi-disciplinary approach to current clinical management. New York: Futura 1998;253–263.
48. Freeman RB Jr, FritzMaurice SE, Greenfield AE, et al. Is the transjugular intrahepatic portocaval shunt procedure beneficial for liver transplant recipients? Transplantation 1994;58:297–300.
49. Tripathi D, Therapondos G, Redhead DN, et al. Transjugular intrahepatic portosystemic stent-shunt and its effect on orthotopic liver transplantation. Eur J Gastroenterol Hepatol 2002;827–832.
50. Castellani P, Campan P, Bernardini D, et al. Is transjugular intrahepatic portosystemic shunt really deleterious for liver transplantation issue? A monocentric study on 86 liver transplanted patients. Transplant Proc 2001;33:3468–3469.
51. Valdivieso A, Ventoso A, Gastaca M, et al. Does the transjugular intrahepatic portosystemic influence the outcome of liver transplantation? Transplant Proc 2012;44:1505–1507.
52. Moreno A, Meneu JC, Moreno E, et al. Liver transplantation and transjugular intrahepatic portosystemic shunt. Transplant Proc 2003;35:1869–1870.
53. Dell'Era A, Grande L, Barros-Schelotto P, et al. Impact of prior portosystemic shunt procedures on outcome of liver transplantation. Surgery 2005;137:620–625.
54. Guerrini GP, Pleguezuelo M, Maimone S, et al. Impact of TIPS preliver transplantation for the outcome posttransplantation. Am J Transplant 2009;9:192–200.
55. Bauer J, Johnson S, Durham J, et al. The role of TIPS for portal vein patency in liver transplant patients with portal vein thrombosis. Liver Transpl 2006;12:1544–1551.
56. Ponziani FR, Zocco MA, Senzolo M, et al. Portal vein thrombosis and liver transplantation: implications for waiting list period, surgical approach, early and late follow-up. Transplant Rev (Orlando) 2014;28:92–101.
57. Han G, Qi X, He C, et al. Transjugular intrahepatic portosystemic shunt for portal vein thrombosis with symptomatic portal hypertension in liver cirrhosis. J Hepatol 2011;54:78–88.
58. Qi X, Han G. Transjugular intrahepatic portosystemic shunt in the treatment of portal vein thrombosis: a critical review of the literature. Hepatol Int 2012;6:576–90.
59. D'Avola D, Bilbao JI, Zozaya G, et al. Efficacy of transjugular intrahepatic portosystemic shunt to prevent total portal vein thrombosis in cirrhotic patients awaiting for liver transplantation. Transplant Proc 2012; 44:2603–2605.
60. Gaba RC, Parvinian A. Transjugular intrahepatic portosystemic shunt for maintenance of portal venous patency in liver transplant candidates. J Clin Imaging Sci 2013;3:28.
61. Nolte W, Canelo R, Figulla HR, et al. Transjugular intrahepatic portosystemic stent-shunt after orthotopic liver transplantation in a patient with early recurrence of portal hypertension of unknown origin. Z Gastroenterol 1998;36:159–164.
62. Finkenstedt A, Graziadei IW, Nachbaur K, et al. Transjugular intrahepatic portosystemic shunt in liver transplant recipients. World J Gastroenterol 2009;15:1999–2004.
63. Aboujloud M, Yoshida A, Kim D, et al. Transjugular intrahepatic portosystemic shunts for refractory ascites after liver transplantation. Transplant Proc 2005;37:1248–1250.
64. Van Ha TG, Hodge J, Funaki B, et al. Transjugular intrahepatic portosystemic shunt placement in patients with cirrhosis and concomitant portal vein thrombosis. Cardiovasc Intervent Radiol 2006;29:785–790.
65. Patel NH, Patel J, Behrens G, Savo A. Transjugular intrahepatic portosystemic shunts in liver transplant recipients: technical considerations and review of the literature. Semin Intervent Radiol 2005;22:329–333.

66. Campos-Varela I, Castells L, Dopazo C, et al. Transjugular intrahepatic porto-systemic shunt for the treatment of sinusoidal obstruction syndrome in a liver transplant recipient and review of the literature. Liver Transpl 2012;18:201–205.

67. Ghinolfi D, De Simone P, Catalano G, et al. Transjugular intrahepatic portosystemic shunt for hepatitis C virus-related portal hypertension after liver transplantation. Clin Transplant 2012;26:699–705.

68. El Atrache M, Abouljoud M, Sharma S, et al. Transjugular intrahepatic portosystemic shunt following liver transplantation: can outcomes be predicted? Clin Transplant 2012;26:657–661.

69. Richard HM, III, Cooper JM, Ahn J, et al. Transjugular intrahepatic portosystemic shunts in the management of Budd-Chiari syndrome in the liver transplant patient with intractable ascites: anatomic considerations. J Vasc Interv Radiol 1998;9:137–140.

70. Saad WE, Davies MG, Lee DE, et al. Transjugular intrahepatic portosystemic shunt in liver donor left lateral segment liver transplant recipient: technical considerations. J Vasc Interv Radiol 2005;16:873–877.

71. Ciccarelli O, Goffette P, Laterre PF, et al. Transjugular intrahepatic portosystemic shunt approach and local thrombolysis for treatment of early post-transplant portal vein thrombosis. Transplantation 2001;72:159–161.

72. Senzolo M, Germani G, Cholongitas E, et al. Veno occlusive disease: update on clinical management. World J Gastroenterol 2007;13:3918–3924.

73. Kitajima K, Vaillant JC, Charlotte F, et al. Intractable ascites without mechanical vascular obstruction after orthotopic liver transplantation: etiology and clinical outcome of sinusoidal obstruction syndrome. Clin Transplant 2010;24:139–148.

74. Sebagh M, Debette M, Samuel D, et al. "Silent" presentation of veno-occlusive disease after liver transplantation as part of the process of cellular rejection with endothelial predilection. Hepatology 1999;30:1144–1150.

75. Senzolo M, Patch D, Cholongitas E, et al. Severe venoocclusive disease after liver transplantation treated with transjugular intrahepatic portosystemic shunt. Transplantation 2006;82:132–135.

76. Sampietro R, Ciccarelli O, Wittebolle X, et al. Temporary transjugular intrahepatic portosystemic shunt to overcome small-for-size syndrome after right lobe adult split liver transplantation. Transplant Int 2006;19:1032–1034.

77. Xiao L, Li F, Wei B, et al. Small-for-size syndrome after living donor liver transplantation: Successful treatment with a transjugular intrahepatic portosystemic shunt. Liver Transplant 2012;18:1118–1120.

Chapter 24: Management of Mesenteric and Portal Vein Thrombosis in Nontransplanted Patients

Ron C. Gaba and Wael E.A. Saad

Introduction

The development of mesenteric venous thrombosis (MVT) or portal vein thrombosis (PVT) heralds potentially devastating consequences in patients with liver cirrhosis. Not only are such individuals at risk for intestinal ischemia and portal hypertensive complications,[1] but liver transplant status and surgical outcome may be adversely affected as well[2]; timely and effective management of MVT and PVT is thus of paramount importance. Although standard medical and surgical therapies have constituted the traditional management approaches to MVT and PVT, newer, minimally invasive interventional radiologic (IR) treatment strategies have successfully addressed this condition while affording a targeted approach associated with acceptable safety and efficacy. The purpose of this chapter is to review the current status of IR therapies for MVT and PVT, with a focus on patient selection, procedure technique, and interventional outcomes.

Mesenteric and Portal Vein Thrombosis

Epidemiology and Classification

Partial or complete PVT complicates approximately 5% to 25% of liver cirrhosis cases[3] and is primarily related to stagnant portal venous blood flow in the setting of portal hypertension[4] as well as hemostatic derangement. Although malignancy; inflammatory conditions such as diverticulitis, appendicitis, or pancreatitis; vessel injury from surgery; and hypercoagulable states may also underlie PVT,[1] hepatic cirrhosis is a dominant predisposing condition, present in approximately 30% of PVT cases.[5] Moreover, the incidence of PVT increases with liver disease severity; PVT is uncommon in compensated liver cirrhosis but is more prevalent among decompensated cases requiring transplantation.[6,7]

Portal vein thrombosis may also be a consequence of steal phenomenon caused by end-stage portosystemic shunt syndrome in which there is portal hypertension and a portosystemic collateral "stealing" blood from the portal vein and essentially taking over as the splanchnic venous outflow as PVT sets in.[8]

Acute PVT is new or sudden onset of thrombus and is characterized by a lack of collateral vessel formation. Chronic PVT is defined by venous occlusion with development of mature collateral pathways. In differentiating acute and chronic PVT, specific time frames are not compulsory for classification of disease, although acute thrombus typically refers to a clot 14 or less days old, and chronic thrombus refers to a clot 28 or more days old as per the deep venous thrombosis literature[9]; these time frames are not necessarily directly translatable to PVT, however, because cavernous transformation of the portal vein may occur as early as 6 to 20 days after thrombus development.[10]

Mesenteric venous thrombosis may develop exclusive of or contemporaneously with PVT; whereas primary MVT represents idiopathic thrombus formation, secondary MVT is related to underlying pathology, such as cirrhosis-related slow flow, inflammatory conditions, or prothrombotic states.[11] Interestingly, MVT caused by hypercoagulability typically begins in small peripheral vessels and progresses to involve larger central vessels, but other causes of MVT propagate central to peripheral.[11]

Both MVT and PVT may be defined by anatomic location. One proposed classification scheme designates six thrombosis patterns outlined as follows: type 1, thrombus within intrahepatic portal vein only; type 2, thrombus within main portal vein only; type 3, thrombus within intrahepatic portal vein and main portal vein; type 4, thrombus within superior mesenteric vein; type 5, thrombus within superior mesenteric vein and main portal vein; and type 6, thrombus within superior mesenteric vein, main portal vein, and intrahepatic portal vein.[2] Associated varices (if any) are classified according to the thrombosis or occlusion of the mesenteric or portal venous system and the degree of portal systemic or portoportal collateralization (▶ Fig. 24.1; ▶ Table 24.1).[8]

Clinical Presentation, Diagnosis, and Sequelae

The presentation of acute MVT or PVT may be clinically silent, with a diagnosis made incidentally or upon surveillance imaging (which is commonly performed for hepatocellular carcinoma [HCC] detection in patients with cirrhosis) or may involve symptoms such as vague abdominal pain and diarrhea or fever and chills in the setting of septic thrombus.[1,11] Specific laboratory abnormalities are not routinely present because liver function is preserved by increased hepatic arterial flow; it is known that a decrease in

Table 24.1 Hemodynamic Classification System

		Both Portoportal and Portosystemic Collaterals	
	Purely Portoportal Collateral (Type 1)	Predominantly Portoportal Collaterals with Lesser Portosystemic Branches (Type 2)	Predominantly Portosystemic Collaterals with Lesser Portoportal Branches (Type 3)
Nonocclusive (oncotic) type (type A)	Type 1a	Type 2a	Type 3a
Occlusive type (type b)	Type 1b	Type 2b	Type 3b

Adapted with permission from Saad WE, Lippert A, Saad NE, Caldwell S. Ectopic varices: anatomical classification, hemodynamic classification, and hemodynamic-based management. Tech Vasc Interv Radiol 2013;16:158–175.

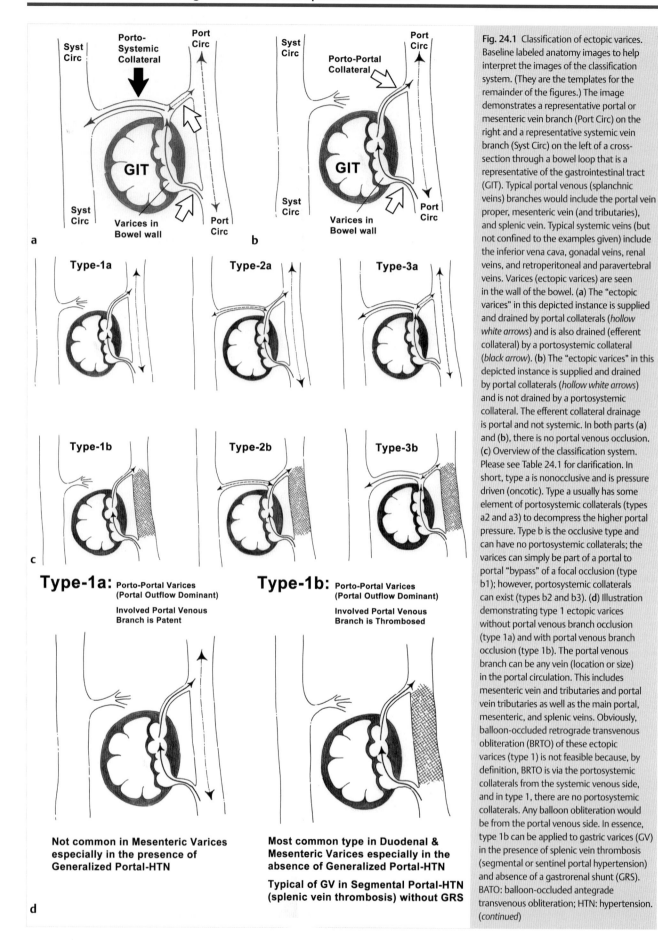

Fig. 24.1 Classification of ectopic varices. Baseline labeled anatomy images to help interpret the images of the classification system. (They are the templates for the remainder of the figures.) The image demonstrates a representative portal or mesenteric vein branch (Port Circ) on the right and a representative systemic vein branch (Syst Circ) on the left of a cross-section through a bowel loop that is a representative of the gastrointestinal tract (GIT). Typical portal venous (splanchnic veins) branches would include the portal vein proper, mesenteric vein (and tributaries), and splenic vein. Typical systemic veins (but not confined to the examples given) include the inferior vena cava, gonadal veins, renal veins, and retroperitoneal and paravertebral veins. Varices (ectopic varices) are seen in the wall of the bowel. (**a**) The "ectopic varices" in this depicted instance is supplied and drained by portal collaterals (*hollow white arrows*) and is also drained (efferent collateral) by a portosystemic collateral (*black arrow*). (**b**) The "ectopic varices" in this depicted instance is supplied and drained by portal collaterals (*hollow white arrows*) and is not drained by a portosystemic collateral. The efferent collateral drainage is portal and not systemic. In both parts (**a**) and (**b**), there is no portal venous occlusion. (**c**) Overview of the classification system. Please see Table 24.1 for clarification. In short, type a is nonocclusive and is pressure driven (oncotic). Type a usually has some element of portosystemic collaterals (types a2 and a3) to decompress the higher portal pressure. Type b is the occlusive type and can have no portosystemic collaterals; the varices can simply be part of a portal to portal "bypass" of a focal occlusion (type b1); however, portosystemic collaterals can exist (types b2 and b3). (**d**) Illustration demonstrating type 1 ectopic varices without portal venous branch occlusion (type 1a) and with portal venous branch occlusion (type 1b). The portal venous branch can be any vein (location or size) in the portal circulation. This includes mesenteric vein and tributaries and portal vein tributaries as well as the main portal, mesenteric, and splenic veins. Obviously, balloon-occluded retrograde transvenous obliteration (BRTO) of these ectopic varices (type 1) is not feasible because, by definition, BRTO is via the portosystemic collaterals from the systemic venous side, and in type 1, there are no portosystemic collaterals. Any balloon obliteration would be from the portal venous side. In essence, type 1b can be applied to gastric varices (GV) in the presence of splenic vein thrombosis (segmental or sentinel portal hypertension) and absence of a gastrorenal shunt (GRS). BATO: balloon-occluded antegrade transvenous obliteration; HTN: hypertension. (*continued*)

Type-2a: Porto-Portal Varices with porto-systemic Collat's (Portal Outflow Dominant)

Involved Portal Venous Branch is Patent

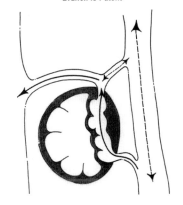

Can be seen in Mesenteric Varices especially in the presence of Generalized Portal-HTN

e

Type-3a: Porto-Systemic Varices (Systemic Outflow Dominant)

Involved Portal Venous Branch is Patent

Most common type of any GIT Varices especially in the presence of Generalized Portal-HTN

Typical of GV in Generalized Portal-HTN with GRS

f

Type-2b: Porto-Systemic Varices (Systemic Outflow Dominant)

Involved Portal Venous Branch is Thrombosed

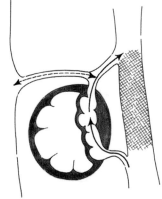

Can be seen in Duodenal & Mesenteric Varices especially in the absence of Generalized Portal-HTN

Type-3b: Porto-Systemic Varices (Systemic Outflow Dominant)

Involved Portal Venous Branch is Thrombosed

Typical of GV in Segmental Portal-HTN (splenic vein thrombosis) with GRS

Fig. 24.1 (*Continued*) (e) Illustration demonstrating type 2 ectopic varices without portal venous branch occlusion (type 2a) and with portal venous branch occlusion (type 2b). The portal venous branch can be any vein (location or size) in the portal circulation. BRTO of these ectopic varices (type 2) is feasible because, by definition, BRTO is via the portosystemic collaterals from the systemic venous side, and in type 2, there are rudimentary portosystemic collaterals. Rudimentary means that it is not the main efferent outflow of the ectopic varices. The main efferent outflow of the ectopic varices in type 2 is portal and not portosystemic. Flow in the existing portosystemic collaterals may be minimal and may even fluctuate. (f) Illustration demonstrating type 3 ectopic varices without portal venous branch occlusion (type 3a) and with portal venous branch occlusion (type 3b). The portal venous branch can be any vein (location or size) in the portal circulation. BRTO of these ectopic varices (type 2) is feasible because, by definition, BRTO is via the portosystemic collaterals from the systemic venous side, and in type 3, there are predominant portosystemic collaterals. Predominant means that it is the main efferent outflow of the ectopic varices. The main efferent outflow of the ectopic varices in type 3 is portosystemic and not portoportal. *Used with permission from Saad WE, Lippert A, Saad NE, Caldwell S. Ectopic varices: anatomical classification, hemodynamic classification, and hemodynamic-based management. Tech Vasc Interv Radiol 2013;16:158–175.*

portal venous blood flow results in an increase in hepatic arterial flow in a mechanism termed the *hepatic arterial buffer response*.[13] Nonetheless, elevation nonspecific liver function test results may be present.[1] Chronic PVT is generally asymptomatic unless complications of portal hypertension or biliary obstruction by enlarged gastric antral, duodenal, or biliary veins—so-called portal cholangiopathy—are present.[14] Preservation of liver function by collateral vessel perfusion averts laboratory abnormalities in chronic PVT.

Both MVT and PVT may be diagnosed with a high sensitivity and specificity using cross-sectional imaging such as contrast enhanced computed tomography (CT) or magnetic resonance (MR) imaging[15]; these studies generally reveal a filling defect in the portal venous system accompanied by atypical or heterogeneous hepatic parenchymal enhancement in acute PVT and show a diminutive or absent portal vein replaced by serpiginous collateral vessels in chronic PVT. Color Doppler ultrasonography may

also be used[16] and demonstrates hyperechoic thrombus within the portal venous system as well as lack of blood flow in acute PVT; chronic PVT findings of hepatic hilar collateral veins are similar to those with CT or MRI. In select instances, mesenteric arteriography can assist in diagnosing small peripheral vein thrombosis that is beyond the imaging resolution of cross-sectional modalities.[17] It is important to distinguish bland MVT or PVT from tumor invasion, which may occur in the setting of HCC; distinguishing features of tumor invasion include vessel distension, casting, filling defect, arterial enhancement or internal color Doppler flow, and contiguity with the intrahepatic tumor.[18] Detection and diagnosis of HCC obviously affect clinical management.

Both MVT and PVT may be associated with several clinically significant consequences, including intestinal ischemia, portal hypertension with variceal hemorrhage, and portal cholangiopathy. Bowel infarction is a particularly devastating occurrence and is suggested by abdominal pain of insidious onset and severity disproportionate to examination findings; overt or occult gastrointestinal (GI) bleeding may also be present.[11] Portal hypertension from chronic PVT may spur variceal hemorrhage, a life-threatening complication associated with immediate mortality rate ranging from 5% to 8% when uncontrolled and up to a 20% overall mortality rate within 6 weeks.[19] Associated varices (if any) are classified according to the thrombosis or occlusion of the mesenteric or portal venous system and the degree of portal systemic or portoportal collateralization (▶ Fig. 24.1; ▶ Table 24.1).[8] Portal cholangiopathy may result in obstructive jaundice or cholangitis requiring biliary drainage.[14] In the long term, PVT also negatively impacts liver transplant patients; not only are auxiliary maneuvers (e.g., intraoperative thrombectomy or jump graft creation) or advanced techniques (e.g., renoportal anastomosis, cavoportal hemitransposition, multivisceral transplantation) required at the time of orthotopic liver transplant (OLT) surgery depending on the extent of clot formation, but posttransplant mortality risk is also increased.[20]

Conventional Medical and Surgical Therapies

Systemic anticoagulation represents the standard first-line therapy for acute MVT and PVT; correction of underlying causal factors should also be pursued. Current treatment recommendations advise for a 3- to 6-month anticoagulation course or long-term anticoagulation in individuals with persistent predisposing risk factors.[1] However, although systemic anticoagulation may result in portal vein recanalization in 40% to 70% of cases,[7,21,22] it does not improve portal hemodynamics, thus contributing to thrombus progression in a small percentage of cases.[4] Moreover, its use may be precluded in individuals with cirrhosis and gastroesophageal variceal bleeding risk. In the setting of chronic PVT, systemic anticoagulation may be used to prevent recurrent thrombosis but should not be initiated before preventive, prophylactic treatment of varices using beta-blockers or endoscopic therapy.[1] Of note, septic MVT or PVT mandates intravenous (IV) antibiotic therapy.

Surgical management of MVT or PVT is not routinely pursued in the absence of profound mesenteric ischemia evidenced by transmural bowel infarction or peritonitis.[23] When clinical signs and imaging features of intestinal necrosis are present, emergent laparotomy and segmental resection are pursued for removal of nonviable bowel segments.[24] As a means of conserving viable intestinal segments, 24-hour delayed follow-up "second look" laparotomy has been proposed to avoid primary resection of bowel that may be viable.[25] Open thrombectomy may also be pursued at the time of surgery,[26,27] although it may be technically difficult to remove all of the thrombus, particularly from small branches of the mesenteric and portal veins. Despite advances in medical and surgical therapy, MVT and PVT remain potentially lethal, particularly in the setting of bowel infarction, with mortality rates up to 30%.[1,28]

Interventional Radiologic Management Approaches and Rationale

Interventional radiologic treatment approaches to MVT and PVT may aim to clear thrombus by several means, including flow-enhanced dispersal, thrombolytic agent–assisted dissolution, direct mechanical disruption, maceration, aspiration, or stent muralization or recanalization. Different interventional approaches allow for these various management strategies and may be used in isolation or combination to optimize therapy.

Transjugular Intrahepatic Portosystemic Shunt Creation

The success of transjugular intrahepatic portosystemic shunt (TIPS) in the management of portal hypertensive complications[29] has prompted translation of this procedure from traditional indications, such as medically refractory gastroesophageal variceal hemorrhage[30] and intractable ascites[31] or hepatic hydrothorax,[32] to newer indications, such as early use in variceal bleeding patients[33] as well as application of TIPS for the treatment of PVT. This developing indication for TIPS may enhance the care of patients with cirrhosis and liver transplant candidates by averting PVT complications and ensuring conventional operative approaches to transplantation, which may be significantly complicated or even precluded in the setting of partial or complete PVT,[4] as well as optimizing posttransplant survival, which is negatively impacted by PVT.[20] TIPS functions to clear clot by providing portal venous access for thrombolytic agent–assisted dissolution, direct mechanical disruption, maceration, or aspiration and by establishing a low-pressure outflow conduit for splanchnic blood volume and concomitantly increasing portal venous flow, which favorably assists the dissolution of PVT in patients with cirrhosis.

When applied for the purpose of direct pharmacomechanical PVT clearance, the TIPS approach into the portal vein confers advantages of theoretically less bleeding risk because of a lower risk of liver capsular transgression, applicability to patients with ascites, larger caliber and more longitudinal access of entry to the portal vein, and a large-bore outflow pathway for clot clearance (e.g., Pullback Fogarty Embolectomy) in cases of PVT compared with transhepatic portal venous access.[34] The main disadvantages of the TIPS approach are poor access to peripheral intrahepatic portal vein branches[34] and potentially greater technical difficulty in obtaining portal venous access compared with ultrasound-guided transhepatic puncture if intrahepatic branches are thrombosed. Another disadvantage of TIPS during pharmacolysis of PVT is that after flow is established, the TIPS may be the predominant outflow and prevent chemical agents from bathing the "end artery" portal vein branches.

Increased portal venous flow velocity after TIPS favorably affects thrombus dissolution. Although the biochemical mechanism of fibrinolysis is well described, the role of hemodynamic factors in this process is often neglected. Originally described by Virchow, flow stasis contributes to vascular thrombosis by reducing laminar clearance of local thrombin and fibrin monomer.[35] Experimental and mathematical models have demonstrated that the shear forces exerted by circulating blood promote mechanical dissolution of nonocclusive thrombi.[36–38] Higher velocity blood flow results in increased rates of mechanical degradation, as well as increased deposition of physiologic fibrinolytic agents.[39] The improved portal venous flow after TIPS creation helps dissolve existing thrombus through flow-enhanced dissolution and may obviate the need for concomitant use of anticoagulation[7,22,40] or mechanical or thrombolytic techniques.[41]

Direct Portal and Mesenteric Vein Thrombolysis and Thrombectomy

A direct transhepatic approach to the portal and mesenteric venous system confers definitive access to clot for potential clearance using thrombolysis or thrombectomy (or both). Catheter-directed thrombolysis (CDT) aims to dissolve thrombus in a targeted fashion through direct intraclot fibrinolytic agent infusion. Contemporary CDT primarily uses recombinant tissue plasminogen activator (TPA), a protein that activates the serine protease enzyme plasmin and initiates fibrinolysis by plasmin-induced degradation of cross-linked fibrin mesh within blood clot, which is consequently more susceptible to further enzymatic proteolysis. The glycoprotein enzyme urokinase and the beta-hemolytic streptococcus glycoprotein streptokinase have also been used in thrombolytic therapy but represent more historical agents; newer fibrinolytic agents that have greater fibrin specificity are also commercially available. CDT has been applied in multiple clinical settings and has a firm basis in systemic arterial and venous recanalization[42-45] as well as hemodialysis graft clot dissolution,[46] among other applications. The efficacy of therapy is greater in acute or soft thrombus compared with chronic, organized clot because of reduced platelet composition and fibrin cross-linking,[47] and thrombolysis may be augmented by concomitant techniques such as ultrasound-accelerated fibrinolytic agent deposition using systems such as the EkoSonic Endovascular System (EKOS Corporation, Bothell, Washington).

Catheter-directed thrombolysis may be supplemented with mechanical thrombectomy, which represents an attractive means to disrupt thrombus caused by more rapid clot clearance compared with enzymatic thrombolysis.[48] Mechanical thrombectomy typically uses clot disruption, maceration, or aspiration using commercially available guidewires, compliant (e.g., Fogarty) or noncompliant (e.g., angioplasty) balloons, rotating devices such as the Arrow-Trerotola percutaneous thrombectomy device (Arrow International, Asheboro, North Carolina) or Trellis Peripheral Infusion System (Covidien, Dublin, Ireland), or rheolytic devices that disrupt the clot through saline injection and aspiration such as the AngioJet Ultra Thrombectomy System (Bayer Healthcare, Leverkusen, Germany), among others. Disadvantages of mechanical devices include risk of vessel injury and cost.[48]

A transhepatic portal venous approach to portal and mesenteric vein thrombolysis and thrombectomy confers benefits of direct access to the portal vein, technically easier access to the peripheral intrahepatic portal vein branches,[34] and more straightforward portal venous access compared with TIPS if intrahepatic branches are thrombosed because direct sonographic guidance may be used instead of solely fluoroscopy. Downsides of transhepatic portal venous access include increased bleeding risk caused by liver capsular traversal, access size limitation, and angulated entry into the main portal vein.[34]

Indirect Mesenteric and Portal Vein Thrombolysis via the Superior Mesenteric Artery

In addition to direct CDT of MVT and PVT, thrombolysis may be undertaken via an indirect approach using the superior mesenteric artery (SMA) as a conduit to deliver thrombolytic agent to the portal and mesenteric venous clot via transcapillary traversal.

Potential benefits of this approach include technical simplicity; theoretically reduced bleeding risk because of avoidance of liver parenchymal puncture; and bathing of small mesenteric capillaries and venules with fibrinolytic agent, allowing restoration of small branch vessel patency.[49] Drawbacks to this procedure include lack of direct fibrinolytic agent infusion into the thrombus, potentially increasing length of thrombolysis,[50] as well as the potential for inducing GI bleeding, especially in the setting of borderline intestinal infarction because of venous engorgement.

Portal Vein Recanalization for Chronic Occlusion

Chronic portal vein occlusion, characterized by fibrotic, shrunken, and cordlike transformation of the portal vein, represents a major therapeutic challenge. Despite cavernous transformation or formation of hepatic hilar collateral vessels in many cases, the splanchnic blood volume may not be adequately drained, rendering patients at risk for portal hypertensive complications. IR recanalization techniques may be used to reestablish patency in chronically occluded venous systems; in the setting of chronic PVT or portal vein occlusion, this may be pursued with the intent of relieving portal hypertension and its complications or reinstating liver transplant candidacy.

Patient Selection
Procedure Indications

Interventional approaches to portal vein clot removal are indicated in patients awaiting liver transplantation to maintain portal vein patency and in the presence of clinical symptoms suggesting intestinal ischemia to prevent progression to intestinal infarction. PVT resulting in portal hypertensive complications, such as variceal hemorrhage, or liver dysfunction, evidenced by findings such as liver enzyme elevation or the development of ascites, may also prompt treatment. Because there has been no objective comparison of the benefits and risks of IR therapies with those of conservative anticoagulation therapy alone,[1] the decision to proceed with IR interventions is best made on a case-by-case basis in collaboration with primary hepatology physicians and transplant surgeons, with the best interest of the patient taken into account and after thorough discussion of the procedure benefits, risks, and alternatives with the patient and family.[1]

Procedure Contraindications

Accepted contraindications to TIPS creation include congestive heart failure, multiple hepatic cysts as in polycystic liver disease, systemic infection or sepsis, unrelieved biliary obstruction, severe pulmonary hypertension, and profound coagulopathy or thrombocytopenia.[51] Similar contraindications—namely, multiple hepatic cysts, unrelieved biliary obstruction, and profound coagulopathy or thrombocytopenia—may preclude direct transhepatic portal venous access. Standard contraindications to thrombolytic agent administration include items such as active internal bleeding or disseminated intravascular coagulation; recent cerebrovascular event, neurosurgery, or intracranial trauma; recent cardiopulmonary resuscitation; major surgery; obstetric delivery;

organ biopsy; major trauma; intracranial tumor; uncontrolled hypertension; and recent major GI bleed.[52]

Procedure Technique and Periprocedure Patient Care

General Considerations

Procedures are performed in the IR suite under IV moderate sedation or general anesthesia with routine hemodynamic, cardiac, and oxygen saturation monitoring and standard sterile site preparation while patients are supine on the angiographic procedure table. Because general anesthesia provides optimal patient comfort and pain relief, airway control, and hemodynamic cardiorespiratory monitoring by an anesthesiologist, leaving the IR physician free to concentrate fully on technical aspects of procedures, it may represent the best option for intraprocedural anesthesia during complex procedures such as TIPS creation.[53]

Regarding preprocedure antibiotic administration, there is no evidence from clinical trials that the use of prophylactic antibiotics is beneficial before TIPS creation; studies comparing transjugular interventions with and without antibiotic treatment have identified no significant differences in infection rates.[54] Nonetheless, routine antibiotic prophylaxis is recommended before TIPS creation by clinical practice guidelines.[55] Although no firm recommendations are available for antibiotic prophylaxis for percutaneous transhepatic portal venous interventions,[55] antibiotic coverage for biliary organisms may be prudent because bile duct traversal is possible. Preprocedure antibiotics are not routinely endorsed before standard venous thrombolysis procedures.[55]

Transjugular Intrahepatic Portosystemic Shunt Creation

The standard technique for TIPS creation is well described[30] but varies slightly in the setting of PVT. Right jugular venous access is routinely gained with dilation to a 10-Fr sheath. The sheath is advanced into the right atrium, and pressure measurements are performed. A 5-Fr catheter is then used to engage a hepatic vein, typically the right. After hepatic venography and pressure measurement, wedged hepatic venography is performed, although the utility of portal venous imaging may be limited in the setting of PVT depending on thrombus extent and degree of portal venous occlusion. Next, a transjugular liver access set is used to access the portal vein. This step represents the most challenging procedure component in the setting of PVT. Unlike patent portal venous targets, occluded portal vein branches may not allow aspiration of blood to confirm portal venous entry, may not normally opacify with contrast during confirmatory venography, and may present a challenge to guidewire cannulation caused by an obstructive clot. In this regard, correlation with cross-sectional imaging for anatomic guidance is valuable, and guidewire passage along the expected course of the portal vein should be observed. After portal vein catheterization is achieved, direct portal, splenic, or mesenteric pressure is measured for portosystemic pressure gradient calculation, and balloon dilation of the hepatic parenchymal tract is performed. Next, direct portography is performed. At this point, thrombolytic agent assisted dissolution, direct mechanical disruption, maceration, or aspiration of clot may be pursued at the discretion of the

primary operating IR physician; the particular technique for each of these interventions is described in later sections.

Subsequently, a metallic stent is deployed across the liver tract; the specialized expanded polytetrafluoroethylene (e-PTFE)–covered VIATORR stent graft (W. L. Gore & Associates, Flagstaff, Arizona) is widely used for TIPS creation because of bile impermeability uniquely suited for hepatic parenchymal tract coverage compared with other stents, and 8- to 12-mm-diameter devices are available. If thrombolysis is pursued via the TIPS approach, it may be prudent to defer stent insertion for 24 to 72 hours until the PVT has been satisfactorily bathed in fibrinolytic agent and some clot clearance has been achieved; this averts systemic loss of thrombolytic agent via the TIPS and avoids large pulmonary embolism. After the stent is deployed, if the distal shunt falls short of the hepatic vein to inferior vena cava (IVC) junction, additional stents may be used to extend the shunt. Balloon angioplasty of the stent is then performed followed by measurement of post-stent portal and right atrial pressures; a final portosystemic pressure gradient measuring 12 mm Hg or less is routinely targeted.[28] Last, completion shunt venography is performed.

Direct Mesenteric and Portal Vein Thrombolysis and Thrombectomy

For direct portal venous access, a peripheral portal vein branch is punctured using a percutaneous transhepatic approach and a 20- to 22-gauge needle using ultrasound or fluoroscopic guidance (or both).[56] Combined use of ultrasound and fluoroscopy for percutaneous portal venous access is associated with a low risk for complications and shorter procedure time compared with fluoroscopy alone.[57–59] Care is taken to avoid excessive liver punctures, which increase bleeding risk. The portal venous puncture may be either right or left sided; whereas right-sided puncture is more in line with the main portal vein, provides more "running room" for central portal vein interventions, and is subject to less radiation to operator hands, left-sided puncture may have a lower bleeding risk, especially in the setting of ascites, and has less risk of pleural complications.[34] As in transjugular puncture of occluded portal vein branches, aspiration of blood or injection of iodinated contrast to confirm portal venous entry may be limited, and guidewire passage may be difficult because of an obstructive clot. After portal venous access is achieved, the percutaneous access is dilated to accept a vascular sheath (typically up to 8 Fr), which is advanced into the main portal vein. Direct portography is then performed followed by baseline portal venous pressure measurement.

Catheter-directed thrombolysis may be initiated with administration of 0.5- to 1.0-mg ("low-dose) TPA or alteplase (Activase; Genentech, South San Francisco, California) per hour through a multi-side-hole catheter embedded within the MVT, PVT, or both. TPA dosing is typically at the discretion of the operating IR physician, but "low-dose" fibrinolytic agent administration is supported by practice guidelines relating to management of acute lower extremity ischemia.[60] Dosing protocols for other thrombolytic agents are readily available.[61] In addition to continuous infusion, fibrinolytic agents may be infused via bolus dose lacing followed by continuous infusion or in a pulse-spray fashion for pharmacomechanical thrombolysis.[48] Systemic IV heparin is concomitantly administered to prevent thrombus propagation and is titrated to achieve a partial thromboplastin time (PTT) of 60 to 80 seconds; subtherapeutic doses of heparin have been deemed acceptable when used in combination with thrombolytic therapy.[60] Patients are continuously monitored in an intensive care unit setting during the entirety of thrombolytic therapy. Laboratory studies, including hematologic parameters such as complete blood count (CBC); coagulation profile, including prothrombin time (PT) and PTT; and fibrinogen levels, are monitored every 4 to 6 hours. Although the clinical progress of CDT may be assessed by evaluating patient clinical symptoms, daily venography is commonly performed in the IR suite to monitor the progress of thrombolytic therapy, ensure catheter positional stability, and allow for catheter repositioning or other interventions as needed. Mechanical thrombectomy using guidewires, balloons, or other devices may be used as an adjunct to CDT to facilitate thrombus removal. Endpoints for CDT include patient symptomatic improvement, complete or near complete clot dissolution, and portal venous pressure reduction.

After completion of percutaneous procedures, vascular sheath removal and liver tract hemostasis are pursued. The vascular access sheath is retracted into the hepatic parenchymal tract using a combination of ultrasound or fluoroscopic guidance (or both). Contrast is injected via the sheath to confirm tip position within the hepatic parenchyma before tract embolization. Embolization of the hepatic parenchymal tract is then performed using Gelfoam torpedoes,[58] metallic coils,[58] or other hemostatic material[62] such as N-butyl cyanoacrylate liquid glue.[34] Care is taken to ensure deployment of the embolic material exclusively within the liver parenchymal tract so as to avert intravascular embolization.

Indirect Mesenteric and Portal Vein Thrombolysis via the Superior Mesenteric Artery

For indirect portal and mesenteric vein thrombolysis via the SMA, routine single-wall puncture arterial access is gained via the right or left common femoral artery using direct sonographic guidance and a 21-gauge needle (e.g., the Micropuncture Introducer Set; Cook Medical, Bloomington, Indiana). Vascular access is dilated to accept a 5-Fr vascular sheath, such as Pinnacle (Terumo, Somerset, New Jersey), for subsequent arteriography. Initial superior mesenteric arteriogram is performed using a 5-Fr catheter such as the Sos Omni Selective (AngioDynamics, Queensbury, New York), SIM 1 (Cook Medical), or C2 (Cook Medical). Arteriography is carried out to include delayed portal venous phase imaging to image the MVT and PVT. Subsequent selective arteriography may be performed after exchange for a 4-Fr angled glide coated catheter such as Glidecath (Terumo) or placement of a coaxial 3-Fr microcatheter such as Renegade Hi-flo (Boston Scientific, Natick, Massachusetts). For treatment, lytic agent may be infused via the SMA trunk or selectively into a segmental distribution if MVT is peripheral and localized. CDT dosing, monitoring, and termination is similar to that described for direct mesenteric and portal vein thrombolysis except that the progress of thrombolytic therapy is monitored using delayed portal venous phase imaging after superior mesenteric arteriogram.

Portal Vein Recanalization for Chronic Occlusion

Portal venous recanalization is usually pursued in an antegrade fashion via a direct transhepatic approach or a TIPS approach. A combined approach via an antegrade approach (e.g., a transsplenic or transmesenteric approach [or both]) can also be performed. The transsplenic approach is percutaneous and is similar to a transhepatic access or approach. The transmesenteric approach is laparotomy and cannulation of a mesenteric venous tributary. Preprocedure assessment of cross-sectional imaging is imperative to delineate the anatomic relationship between patent intrahepatic portal venous channels and a patent hepatic hilar portal venous target. After establishing direct transhepatic portal venous access or TIPS access as previously described, recanalization is initially attempted using a hydrophilic, torqueable guidewire such as the Glidewire (Terumo) or Hi-wire (Cook Medical) and catheter. The guidewire is used to bore into and through the occluded vessel employing techniques such as wire rotation and jabbing. The soft front end of the guidewire is initially used, but traversal into the occluded vein segment may be attempted using the stiff back end of the guidewire if success is not achieved with conventional maneuvers. The catheter is advanced over the guidewire, and injection of iodinated contrast material is used to confirm passage into a patent venous target. If blunt guidewire recanalization is unsuccessful, sharp recanalization using a needle-based system such as the Dextera TLAB Patel Set transjugular liver biopsy system (US Biopsy, Franklin, Indiana) or LABS liver access and biopsy set (Cook Medical) may be attempted. Care should be taken to avoid puncture of a cavernous collateral vessel, which may preclude wire passage into the main portal vein. Of note, if isolated transhepatic or transjugular approaches to portal venous recanalization are unsuccessful, combined methods such as the "gun-sight" approach using intravascular snares and a transhepatic portal venous access[63] or a balloon-targeted approach using transjugular puncture of a transhepatic placed portal venous balloon[64] may be attempted. Other alternative techniques include retrograde recanalization via a transsplenic approach through the splenic venous system[65] or a transmesenteric approach through a mini laparotomy.[66] After traversal of the occluded venous segment is achieved, vessel patency may be reestablished via balloon angioplasty and stent insertion for portal venous reconstruction. The superior mesenteric vein and splenic vein may be reconstructed with stents if occlusion of these vessels results in clinical symptoms.

Procedure Outcomes

Clinical studies of IR procedures for management of MVT and PVT are diverse in terms of investigation types, patient sample sizes, methods applied, and outcomes measured. The following clinical outcomes review comprises a broad and representative, albeit not completely exhaustive, compilation of studies investigating IR treatment of MVT and PVT. Reports of three cases or less are not routinely included.

Transjugular Intrahepatic Portosystemic Shunt Flow-Enhanced Clot Dissolution

Case series and clinical investigations describing TIPS creation for flow-enhanced thrombus dissolution indicate a high level of clinical effectiveness. In 2006, Bauer et al reported nearly 90% improvement in portal venous patency 2 to 45 months post-TIPS for treatment of varying degrees of nonocclusive PVT.[67] In 2006,

Van Ha et al reported 91% (10 of 11) technical success of TIPS recanalization of acute or partial PVT.[68] In 2008, Streitparth et al described successful TIPS in 11 of 13 (85%) patients with PVT.[69] In 2011, Luca et al described 87% patency improvement (complete recanalization in 57%) among 70 patients with nontumoral PVT who underwent TIPS.[70] In 2012, D'Avola et al reported 100% portal vein patency in 15 patients with main trunk or branch vessel partial PVT who underwent TIPS followed by OLT at median 185 days postprocedure.[71] In that study, a control group of 8 patients with similar nonocclusive PVT who did not undergo TIPS showed 50% portal vein patency at OLT performed at median 213 days after PVT diagnosis.[71] In 2012, Senzolo et al described stable PVT (4 of 6, 67%) or complete portal venous repermeation (2 of 6, 33%) in 6 patients who underwent TIPS for PVT.[72] In 2013, Gaba et al reported 100% clot clearance in four cases of PVT and concomitant SMV or splenic vein thrombus within mean 79 days of TIPS creation.[73] In that series, portal venous flow was increased more than fivefold after TIPS to a mean of greater than 80 cm/s—normal portal venous flow velocity approximates 16-40 cm/s[74]—and no recurrence of PVT was identified after mean 460 days of imaging follow-up.[73] The findings of these studies are further supported by report of at least one individual case describing use of TIPS to keep the portal vein open for liver transplantation.[75] These data all suggest clinical effectiveness of TIPS for PVT clearance. Once a contraindication to TIPS creation, PVT may now represent an unequivocal procedural indication for TIPS given the efficacy demonstrated in such investigations.

Transjugular Intrahepatic Portosystemic Shunt Thrombolysis and Thrombectomy

For more extensive PVT, TIPS with CDT or thrombectomy (or both) has shown satisfactory success rates. In 1995, Blum et al described 100% technically successful portal venous flow restoration in 7 patients who underwent TIPS, balloon thrombectomy, and CDT (using urokinase or TPA for mean 7 hours) for treatment of noncavernomatous PVT.[76] In 1998, Walser reported on 15 patients with noncavernomatous PVT who were treated with TIPS[77]; shunt creation was successful in 12 of 15 (80%) cases, and PVT was cleared using some combination of adjunctive angioplasty, CDT, mechanical thrombectomy, and stent placement.[76] In 1999, Ganger et al reported the results of 11 patients with PVT who were treated with TIPS and mechanical thrombectomy.[78] TIPS was successful in 9 of 11 (82%) cases, with restoration of portal venous patency; complications occurred in 2 of 9 (22%) technically successful cases.[78] In 2006, Senzolo et al described technically successful portal venous recanalization in 19 of 28 (73%) patients with PVT using TIPS and concomitant catheter or balloon thrombectomy (or both).[79] In 2009, Liu et al reported the outcomes of 26 PVT patients treated with TIPS and urokinase CDT.[80] Outcomes were reported cumulatively with 6 patients undergoing direct transhepatic CDT, and were significant for complete recanalization in 26 of 32 (81%) cases.[80] In 2010, Liu et al described successful TIPS with adjunctive thrombus clearing interventions in 26 patients.[81] In 2011, Wang et al reported the outcomes of 12 patients who underwent TIPS and urokinase CDT for treatment of acute MVT.[82] After a mean 4 days of CDT, mesenteric venous patency was reestablished in 100% of patients with attendant substantial clinical improvement

and no MVT recurrence over mean 3-year follow-up.[82] Four puncture site complications were minor.[82] In 2011, Luo et al described 13 patients who underwent successful TIPS, balloon maceration, sheath aspiration thrombectomy, and urokinase CDT for PVT recanalization.[83] Portal venous patency was achieved in all cases with clinical improvement in more than 90% of patients; one patient developed intraperitoneal hemorrhage and died.[83] In all, adjunctive CDT or thrombectomy can enhance the effectiveness of TIPS in clot clearance for MVT and PVT.

Direct Mesenteric and Portal Vein Thrombolysis and Thrombectomy

Prior investigations have demonstrated the utility of direct transhepatic manipulation of PVT. In 2002, Lopera et al described technically successful transhepatic clearance of MVT and PVT in 3 patients using CDT or mechanical disruption.[84] In 2005, Kim et al reported the outcomes of 11 patients with MVT who underwent transhepatic CDT and thrombectomy.[85] Seven of 11 patients (64%) underwent mechanical thrombectomy using either the AngioJet thrombectomy device (Bayer Healthcare) or the Helix Clot Buster thrombectomy device (ev3 Inc., Plymouth, Minnesota), and 10 of 11 (91%) patients underwent TPA or urokinase CDT for up to 45 hours.[85] Mesenteric venous patency was restored in 10 of 11 (91%) cases, and no recurrent MVT or death was documented over mean 42 months of clinical follow-up.[85] Complications included one case of hemothorax and one death caused by preexisting sepsis.[85] In 2009, Di Minno et al described 18 patients who underwent direct transhepatic urokinase CDT for MVT management.[86] Restoration of mesenteric venous patency was achieved in 16 of 18 (89%) cases, and three 30-day mortality cases (secondary to sepsis, pneumonia, and myocardial infarction) were unrelated to treatment.[86] In 2010, Liu et al described successful direct transhepatic PVT recanalization with adjunctive clot clearing interventions in 18 patients.[81]

Indirect Portal and Mesenteric Vein Thrombolysis via the Superior Mesenteric Artery

Case series and clinical investigations describing indirect MVT and PVT thrombolysis via the SMA have shown variable degrees of clinical effectiveness and safety. In 2005, Hollingshead et al. described the results of indirect SMA thrombolysis as a sole therapy for MVT and PVT in six patients.[12] After administration of urokinase or TPA for a mean 42 hours, 3 of 6 (50%) patients showed partial (less than 90%) clot clearance, and 3 of 6 (50%) patients demonstrated no (0%) clot clearance.[12] Three of six (50%) patients experienced a major complication (two bleeding events, one death).[12] Of note, the investigation also described the outcomes of concomitant indirect SMA thrombolysis and direct portal venous thrombolysis in 4 patients; results included complete and partial clot clearance in 1 of 4 (25%) and 3 of 4 (75%) cases, respectively, but were also notable for bleeding complications in 3 of 4 (75%) cases.[12] In 2009, Liu et al reported the outcomes of 14 patients treated with indirect MVT and PVT thrombolysis in whom urokinase was administered via an SMA placed catheter.[80] After treatment, 2 of 14 (14%) patients showed partial recovery of portal venous and superior mesenteric venous flow, partial thrombolysis, and complete symptomatic relief, and 11 of 14 (79%) had intact MVT and PVT but dramatically improved clinical symptoms; 1 of 14 (7%) patients had no improvement and subsequently required bowel resection to treat intestinal infarction.[80] The authors concluded that indirect MVT and PVT thrombolysis is inferior to direct thrombolytic approaches.[80] In 2012, Wang et al described 47 patients with acute extensive MVT and PVT who were treated with urokinase thrombolysis via an SMA catheter for a mean 7.1 days[87]; a portion of this cohort was initially reported in 2010.[49] Technical success was achieved in all cases, 45 of 47 (96%) patients showed clinical improvement, and imaging follow-up revealed near complete disappearance and partial recanalization of MVT and PVT in 29 of 47 (64%) and 16 of 47 (36%) patients. Two of 47 (4%) patients required laparotomy and resection of necrotic bowel, and 2 of 47 (4%) patients had recurrent MVT or PVT within 5 years.

Portal Vein Recanalization for Chronic Occlusion with Combined Therapeutic Approaches

Variable outcomes for chronic portal vein recanalization are reflective of the technical difficulty of this procedure. In 1993, Radosevich et al reported 60% (6 of 10) technical success in portal vein recanalization via a TIPS approach with or without adjunctive transhepatic portal venous recanalization.[88] In 1999, Stein et al described portal vein reconstruction attempted in 21 patients using a TIPS (5 patients) or TIPS plus transhepatic approach (16 patients).[89] Technically successful recanalization was achieved in 18 of 21 (86%) cases, and the primary patency rate was 64% at 43 months of follow-up.[89] In 2004, Bilbao et al described successful TIPS recanalization of chronic PVT in 6 patients using auxiliary methods such as ultrasound guidance and "gunshot" technique.[90] In 2006, Van Ha et al reported 75% (3 of 4) technical success of TIPS recanalization of chronic PVT with cavernous transformation.[68] In 2009, Han et al described 65 patients who underwent TIPS for PVT treatment with or without adjunctive transhepatic or transsplenic portal vein recanalization.[91] TIPS were successfully created in 54 of 65 (83%) patients, with 36 undergoing TIPS alone, 15 undergoing concomitant transhepatic recanalization, and 3 undergoing simultaneous transsplenic recanalization.[91] In 2011, Han et al reported on 57 patients with chronic PVT who underwent TIPS, which were successfully created in 43 of 57 (75%) cases; one procedure-related death was encountered.[92] In 2012, Qi et al described 20 patients with cavernous portal vein transformation who underwent attempted TIPS recanalization; the technical success rate was 35% (7 of 20).[93] In 2013, Salem described portal vein recanalization in 30 patients using portal vein thromboembolectomy–TIPS (PVTE-TIPS) to reestablish portal vein patency before OLT.[94] All cases were technically successful using a combination of percutaneous and transjugular access (with snaring), and none required main portal vein stenting; 15 of 30 (50%) patients were successfully transplanted after portal vein recanalization.[94]

Procedure-Related Complications

The benefits of TIPS, transhepatic portal venous access, and CDT for clearance of PVT must be weighed against possible risks. When performed by experienced operators in properly selected candidates,[95,96] TIPS may be created with a reasonable safety profile; some adverse effects include hepatic encephalopathy, liver failure with deterioration of liver function, bleeding, and infection.[97] TIPS complications that particularly affect subsequent transplantation are uncommon, and the presence of TIPS does not typically impact operative technique or result in detrimental effects on posttransplant patient clinical outcomes.[98,99] As a matter of caution, IR operators should take great care in proper stent length selection as well as device deployment because shunt extension into the portal vein or hepatic level IVC and right atrium, either caused by device misplacement or migration, may leave inadequate room for vascular cross-clamping at the time of surgery.

Bleeding, either intraperitoneal or liver subcapsular, is the most common procedure-related complication after transhepatic portal venous access in patients with portal hypertension, occurring with an incidence approximating 16%.[100] Anticoagulation contributes to bleeding frequency, as seen in the islet cell transplant literature in which hemorrhage occurs in up to 13% of cases,[58] and independent risk factors for hemorrhagic complications include systemic anticoagulation with a heparin dose of 45 units/kg or more.[58] Fortunately, effective hepatic parenchymal tract embolization significantly reduces bleeding,[58,62] but extreme care should be taken in vascular access management after PVT interventions, particularly if CDT and anticoagulation are involved. Because hemorrhagic events may be heightened during CDT, close clinical and laboratory monitoring are also recommended.

Conclusion

Minimally invasive IR treatment strategies constitute an emerging means to manage MVT and PVT. Although techniques such as TIPS and transhepatic portal venous recanalization have demonstrated many successes to date, more clinical investigation is necessary to further define the safety and efficacy of these procedures, and conception, design, and execution of prospective comparative studies assessing IR therapies against conventional medical and surgical treatments will help delineate their role in the treatment algorithm for MVT and PVT in the future.

References

1. DeLeve LD, Valla DC, Garcia-Tsao G. Vascular disorders of the liver. Hepatology 2009;49:1729–1764.
2. Englesbe MJ, Kubus J, Muhammad W, et al. Portal vein thrombosis and survival in patients with cirrhosis. Liver Transpl 2010;16:83–90.
3. Fimognari FL, Violi F. Portal vein thrombosis in liver cirrhosis. Intern Emerg Med 2008;3:213–218.
4. Francoz C, Valla D, Durand F. Portal vein thrombosis, cirrhosis, and liver transplantation. J Hepatol 2012;57:203–212.
5. Ogren M, Bergqvist D, Bjorck M, et al. Portal vein thrombosis: prevalence, patient characteristics and lifetime risk: a population study based on 23,796 consecutive autopsies. World J Gastroenterol 2006;12:2115–2119.
6. Okuda K, Ohnishi K, Kimura K, et al. Incidence of portal vein thrombosis in liver cirrhosis. An angiographic study in 708 patients. Gastroenterology 1985;89: 279–286.
7. Francoz C, Belghiti J, Vilgrain V, et al. Splanchnic vein thrombosis in candidates for liver transplantation: usefulness of screening and anticoagulation. Gut 2005;54:691–697.
8. Saad WE, Lippert A, Saad NE, Caldwell S. Etopic varices: anatomical classification, hemodynamic classification, and hemodynamic-based management. Tech Vasc Interv Radiol 2013;16:158–175.
9. Vedantham S, Grassi CJ, Ferral H, et al. Reporting standards for endovascular treatment of lower extremity deep vein thrombosis. J Vasc Interv Radiol 2009; 20:S391–S408.

10. De Gaetano AM, Lafortune M, Patriquin H, et al. Cavernous transformation of the portal vein: patterns of intrahepatic and splanchnic collateral circulation detected with Doppler sonography. AJR Am J Roentgenol 1995;165:1151–1155.

11. Kumar S, Sarr MG, Kamath PS. Mesenteric venous thrombosis. N Engl J Med 2001;345:1683–1688.

12. Hollingshead M, Burke CT, Mauro MA, et al. Transcatheter thrombolytic therapy for acute mesenteric and portal vein thrombosis. J Vasc Interv Radiol 2005;16:651–661.

13. Zipprich A. Hemodynamics in the isolated cirrhotic liver. J Clin Gastroenterol 2007;41(suppl 3):S254–S258.

14. Khan MR, Tariq J, Raza R, Effendi MS. Portal hypertensive biliopathy: review of pathophysiology and management. Trop Gastroenterol 2012;33:173–178.

15. Kreft B, Strunk H, Flacke S, et al. Detection of thrombosis in the portal venous system: comparison of contrast-enhanced MR angiography with intraarterial digital subtraction angiography. Radiology 2000;216:86–92.

16. Tessler FN, Gehring BJ, Gomes AS, et al. Diagnosis of portal vein thrombosis: value of color Doppler imaging. AJR Am J Roentgenol 1991;157:293–296.

17. Bradbury MS, Kavanagh PV, Bechtold RE, et al. Mesenteric venous thrombosis: diagnosis and noninvasive imaging. Radiographics 2002;22:527–541.

18. Demirjian A, Peng P, Geschwind JF, et al. Infiltrating hepatocellular carcinoma: seeing the tree through the forest. J Gastrointest Surg 2011;15:2089–2097.

19. Bosch J, Abraldes JG, Groszmann R. Current management of portal hypertension. J Hepatol 2003;38(suppl 1):S54–S68.

20. Englesbe MJ, Schaubel DE, Cai S, et al. Portal vein thrombosis and liver transplant survival benefit. Liver Transpl 2010;16:999–1005.

21. Senzolo M, Sartori MT, Lisman T. Should we give thromboprophylaxis to patients with liver cirrhosis and coagulopathy? HPB (Oxford) 2009;11:459–464.

22. Amitrano L, Guardascione MA, Menchise A, et al. Safety and efficacy of anticoagulation therapy with low molecular weight heparin for portal vein thrombosis in patients with liver cirrhosis. J Clin Gastroenterol 2010;44:448–451.

23. Brunaud L, Antunes L, Collinet-Adler S, et al. Acute mesenteric venous thrombosis: case for nonoperative management. J Vasc Surg 2001;34:673–679.

24. Clavien PA. Diagnosis and management of mesenteric infarction. Br J Surg 1990;77:601–603.

25. Levy PJ, Krausz MM, Manny J. The role of second-look procedure in improving survival time for patients with mesenteric venous thrombosis. Surg Gynecol Obstet 1990;170:287–291.

26. Klempnauer J, Grothues F, Bektas H, Pichlmayr R. Results of portal thrombectomy and splanchnic thrombolysis for the surgical management of acute mesentericoportal thrombosis. Br J Surg 1997;84:129–132.

27. Inahara T. Acute superior mesenteric venous thrombosis: treatment by thrombectomy. Ann Surg 1971;174:956–961.

28. Rhee RY, Gloviczki P, Mendonca CT, et al. Mesenteric venous thrombosis: still a lethal disease in the 1990s. J Vasc Surg 1994;20:688–697.

29. Boyer TD, Haskal ZJ. American Association for the Study of Liver Diseases Practice Guidelines: the role of transjugular intrahepatic portosystemic shunt creation in the management of portal hypertension. J Vasc Interv Radiol 2005;16:615–629.

30. Gaba RC, Omene BO, Podczerwinski ES, et al. TIPS for treatment of variceal hemorrhage: clinical outcomes in 128 patients at a single institution over a 12-year period. J Vasc Interv Radiol 2012;23:227–235.

31. Salerno F, Camma C, Enea M, et al. Transjugular intrahepatic portosystemic shunt for refractory ascites: a meta-analysis of individual patient data. Gastroenterology 2007;133:825–834.

32. Dhanasekaran R, West JK, Gonzales PC, et al. Transjugular intrahepatic portosystemic shunt for symptomatic refractory hepatic hydrothorax in patients with cirrhosis. Am J Gastroenterol 2010;105:635–641.

33. Garcia-Pagan JC, Caca K, Bureau C, et al. Early use of TIPS in patients with cirrhosis and variceal bleeding. N Engl J Med 2010;362:2370–2379.

34. Saad WE, Madoff DC. Percutaneous portal vein access and transhepatic tract hemostasis. Semin Intervent Radiol 2012;29:71–80.

35. Lowe GD. Virchow's triad revisited: abnormal flow. Pathophysiol Haemost Thromb 2003;33:455–457.

36. Sersa I, Tratar G, Blinc A. Blood clot dissolution dynamics simulation during thrombolytic therapy. J Chem Inf Model 2005;45:1686–1690.

37. Sersa I, Vidmar J, Grobelnik B, et al. Modelling the effect of laminar axially directed blood flow on the dissolution of non-occlusive blood clots. Phys Med Biol 2007;52:2969–2985.

38. Sersa I, Tratar G, Mikac U, Blinc A. A mathematical model for the dissolution of non-occlusive blood clots in fast tangential blood flow. Biorheology 2007;44:1–16.

39. Bajd F, Sersa I. A concept of thrombolysis as a corrosion-erosion process verified by optical microscopy. Microcirculation 2012;19:632–641.

40. Delgado MG, Seijo S, Yepes I, et al. Efficacy and safety of anticoagulation on patients with cirrhosis and portal vein thrombosis. Clin Gastroenterol Hepatol 2012;10:776–783.

41. Lodhia N, Salem R, Levitsky J. Transjugular intrahepatic portosystemic shunt with thrombectomy for the treatment of portal vein thrombosis after liver transplantation. Dig Dis Sci 2010;55:529–534.

42. Results of a prospective randomized trial evaluating surgery versus thrombolysis for ischemia of the lower extremity. The STILE trial. Ann Surg 1994; 220:251–266;discussion 266–258.

43. Ouriel K, Shortell CK, DeWeese JA, et al. A comparison of thrombolytic therapy with operative revascularization in the initial treatment of acute peripheral arterial ischemia. J Vasc Surg 1994;19:1021–1030.

44. Ouriel K, Veith FJ, Sasahara AA. A comparison of recombinant urokinase with vascular surgery as initial treatment for acute arterial occlusion of the legs. Thrombolysis or Peripheral Arterial Surgery (TOPAS) Investigators. N Engl J Med 1998;338:1105–1111.

45. Watson LI, Armon MP. Thrombolysis for acute deep vein thrombosis. Cochrane Database Syst Rev 2004:CD002783.

46. Cynamon J, Pierpont CE. Thrombolysis for the treatment of thrombosed hemodialysis access grafts. Rev Cardiovasc Med 2002;3(suppl 2):S84–S91.

47. Roberts AC. Principles of selective thrombolysis. In: Baum S, Pentecost MJ, editors. Abrams' Angiography Interventional Radiology, 2nd ed. Philadelphia: Lippincott Williams & Wilkins; 2006, pp 220–232.

48. Valji K. Standard angiographic and interventional techniques. In: Valji K, editor. Vascular and Interventional Radiology, 2nd ed. Philadelphia: Elsevier; 2006, pp 15–48.

49. Wang MQ, Guo LP, Lin HY, et al. Transradial approach for transcatheter selective superior mesenteric artery urokinase infusion therapy in patients with acute extensive portal and superior mesenteric vein thrombosis. Cardiovasc Intervent Radiol 2010;33:80–89.

50. Rosen MP, Sheiman R. Transhepatic mechanical thrombectomy followed by infusion of TPA into the superior mesenteric artery to treat acute mesenteric vein thrombosis. J Vasc Interv Radiol 2000;11:195–198.

51. Boyer TD, Haskal ZJ. The role of transjugular intrahepatic portosystemic shunt in the management of portal hypertension. Hepatology 2005;41:386–400.

52. Thrombolytic therapy in thrombosis: a National Institutes of Health consensus development conference. Ann Intern Med 1980;93:141–144.

53. DeGasperi A, Corti A, Corso R, et al. Transjugular intrahepatic portosystemic shunt (TIPS): the anesthesiological point of view after 150 procedures managed under total intravenous anesthesia. J Clin Monit Comput 2009;23: 341–346.

54. Deibert P, Schwarz S, Olschewski M, et al. Factors and prevention of early infection after implantation or revision of transjugular intrahepatic portosystemic shunts: results of a randomized study. Dig Dis Sci 1998;43:1708–1713.

55. Venkatesan AM, Kundu S, Sacks D, et al. Practice guidelines for adult antibiotic prophylaxis during vascular and interventional radiology procedures. Written by the Standards of Practice Committee for the Society of Interventional Radiology and Endorsed by the Cardiovascular Interventional Radiological Society of Europe and Canadian Interventional Radiology Association [corrected]. J Vasc Interv Radiol 2010;21:1611–1630;quiz 1631.

56. Owen RJ, Ryan EA, O'Kelly K, et al. Percutaneous transhepatic pancreatic islet cell transplantation in type 1 diabetes mellitus: radiologic aspects. Radiology 2003;229:165–170.

57. Goss JA, Soltes G, Goodpastor SE, et al. Pancreatic islet transplantation: the radiographic approach. Transplantation 2003;76:199–203.

58. Villiger P, Ryan EA, Owen R, et al. Prevention of bleeding after islet transplantation: lessons learned from a multivariate analysis of 132 cases at a single institution. Am J Transplant 2005;5:2992–2998.

59. Venturini M, Angeli E, Maffi P, et al. Technique, complications, and therapeutic efficacy of percutaneous transplantation of human pancreatic islet cells in type 1 diabetes: the role of US. Radiology 2005;234:617–624.

60. Patel NH, Krishnamurthy VN, Kim S, et al. Quality improvement guidelines for percutaneous management of acute lower-extremity ischemia. J Vasc Interv Radiol 2013;24:3–15.

61. Kandarpa K. Commonly used medications. In: Kandarpa K, Aruny JE, editors. Handbook of Interventional Radiologic Procedures, 3rd ed. Philadelphia: Lippincott Williams & Wilkins; 2002. p. 653–685.

62. Froud T, Yrizarry JM, Alejandro R, Ricordi C. Use of D-STAT to prevent bleeding following percutaneous transhepatic intraportal islet transplantation. Cell Transplant 2004;13:55–59.

63. Haskal ZJ, Duszak R, Jr., Furth EE. Transjugular intrahepatic transcaval portosystemic shunt: the gun-sight approach. J Vasc Interv Radiol 1996;7:139–142.

64. Jourabchi N, McWilliams JP, Lee EW, et al. TIPS placement via combined transjugular and transhepatic approach for cavernous portal vein occlusion: targeted approach. Case Rep Radiol 2013;2013:635391.

65. Rasinska G, Wermenski K, Rajszys P. Percutaneous transsplenic embolization of esophageal varices in a 5-year-old child. Acta Radiol 1987;28:299–301.

66. Matsui O, Yoshikawa J, Kadoya M, et al. Transjugular intrahepatic portosystemic shunt after previous recanalization of a chronically thrombosed portal vein via a transmesenteric approach. Cardiovasc Intervent Radiol 1996;19:352–355.

67. Bauer J, Johnson S, Durham J, et al. The role of TIPS for portal vein patency in liver transplant patients with portal vein thrombosis. Liver Transpl 2006;12: 1544–1551.

68. Van Ha TG, Hodge J, Funaki B, et al. Transjugular intrahepatic portosystemic shunt placement in patients with cirrhosis and concomitant portal vein thrombosis. Cardiovasc Intervent Radiol 2006;29:785–790.

69. Streitparth F, Santosa F, Milz J, et al. [Transjugular intrahepatic portosystemic shunt in patients with portal vein thrombosis]. Rofo 2008;180:899–905.

70. Luca A, Miraglia R, Caruso S, et al. Short- and long-term effects of the transjugular intrahepatic portosystemic shunt on portal vein thrombosis in patients with cirrhosis. Gut 2011;60:846–852.

71. D'Avola D, Bilbao JI, Zozaya G, et al. Efficacy of transjugular intrahepatic portosystemic shunt to prevent total portal vein thrombosis in cirrhotic patients awaiting for liver transplantation. Transplant Proc 2012;44:2603–2605.

72. Senzolo M, Sartori TM, Rossetto V, et al. Prospective evaluation of anticoagulation and transjugular intrahepatic portosystemic shunt for the management of portal vein thrombosis in cirrhosis. Liver Int 2012;32:919–927.

73. Gaba RC, Parvinian A. TIPS for maintenance of portal venous patency in liver transplant candidates. J Clin Imaging Sci 2013;3:29.

74. McNaughton DA, Abu-Yousef MM. Doppler US of the liver made simple. Radiographics 2011;31:161–188.

75. McHugh PP, Bietz GJ, Jeon H, et al. Transjugular intrahepatic portosystemic shunt to keep vein open. Liver Transpl 2009;15:558–560.

76. Blum U, Haag K, Rossle M, et al. Noncavernomatous portal vein thrombosis in hepatic cirrhosis: treatment with transjugular intrahepatic portosystemic shunt and local thrombolysis. Radiology 1995;195:153–157.

77. Walser EM, NcNees SW, DeLa Pena O, et al. Portal venous thrombosis: percutaneous therapy and outcome. J Vasc Interv Radiol 1998;9:119–127.

78. Ganger DR, Klapman JB, McDonald V, et al. Transjugular intrahepatic portosystemic shunt (TIPS) for Budd-Chiari syndrome or portal vein thrombosis: review of indications and problems. Am J Gastroenterol 1999;94:603–608.

79. Senzolo M, Tibbals J, Cholongitas E, et al. Transjugular intrahepatic portosystemic shunt for portal vein thrombosis with and without cavernous transformation. Aliment Pharmacol Ther 2006;23:767–775.

80. Liu FY, Wang MQ, Fan QS, et al. Interventional treatment for symptomatic acute-subacute portal and superior mesenteric vein thrombosis. World J Gastroenterol 2009;15:5028–5034.

81. Liu FY, Wang MQ, Duan F, et al. Interventional therapy for symptomatic-benign portal vein occlusion. Hepatogastroenterology 2010;57:1367–1374.

82. Wang MQ, Liu FY, Duan F, et al. Acute symptomatic mesenteric venous thrombosis: treatment by catheter-directed thrombolysis with transjugular intrahepatic route. Abdom Imaging 2011;36:390–398.

83. Luo J, Yan Z, Wang J, et al. Endovascular treatment for nonacute symptomatic portal venous thrombosis through intrahepatic portosystemic shunt approach. J Vasc Interv Radiol 2011;22:61–69.

84. Lopera JE, Correa G, Brazzini A, et al. Percutaneous transhepatic treatment of symptomatic mesenteric venous thrombosis. J Vasc Surg 2002;36:1058–1061.

85. Kim HS, Patra A, Khan J, et al. Transhepatic catheter-directed thrombectomy and thrombolysis of acute superior mesenteric venous thrombosis. J Vasc Interv Radiol 2005;16:1685–1691.

86. Di Minno MN, Milone F, Milone M, et al. Endovascular thrombolysis in acute mesenteric vein thrombosis: a 3-year follow-up with the rate of short and long-term sequaelae in 32 patients. Thromb Res 2010;126:295–298.

87. Wang Y, Wang MQ, Liu FY, et al. [Transradial approach for transcatheter selective superior mesenteric artery urokinase infusion therapy in patients with acute extensive portal and superior mesenteric vein thrombosis]. Zhonghua Yi Xue Za Zhi 2012;92:1448–1452.

88. Radosevich PM, Ring EJ, LaBerge JM, et al. Transjugular intrahepatic portosystemic shunts in patients with portal vein occlusion. Radiology 1993;186: 523–527.

89. Stein M, Link DP. Symptomatic spleno-mesenteric-portal venous thrombosis: recanalization and reconstruction with endovascular stents. J Vasc Interv Radiol 1999;10:363–371.

90. Bilbao JI, Elorz M, Vivas I, et al. Transjugular intrahepatic portosystemic shunt (TIPS) in the treatment of venous symptomatic chronic portal thrombosis in non-cirrhotic patients. Cardiovasc Intervent Radiol 2004;27:474–480.

91. Han GH, Meng XJ, Yin ZX, et al. [Transjugular intrahepatic portosystemic shunt and combination with percutaneous transhepatic or transsplenic approach for the treatment of portal vein thrombosis with or without cavernomatous transformation]. Zhonghua Yi Xue Za Zhi 2009;89:1549–1552.

92. Han G, Qi X, He C, et al. Transjugular intrahepatic portosystemic shunt for portal vein thrombosis with symptomatic portal hypertension in liver cirrhosis. J Hepatol 2011;54:78–88.

93. Qi X, Han G, Yin Z, et al. Transjugular intrahepatic portosystemic shunt for portal cavernoma with symptomatic portal hypertension in non-cirrhotic patients. Dig Dis Sci 2012;57:1072–1082.

94. Salem R. Portal vein thromboembolectomy/TIPS: a novel preliver transplant interventional approach to rendering the untransplantable patient transplant-ready. J Vasc Interv Radiol 2013;24(suppl):S61.

95. Gaba RC, Khiatani VL, Knuttinen MG, et al. Comprehensive review of TIPS technical complications and how to avoid them. AJR Am J Roentgenol 2011; 196:675–685.

96. Gaba RC, Couture PM, Bui JT, et al. Prognostic capability of different liver disease scoring systems for prediction of early mortality after transjugular intrahepatic portosystemic shunt creation. J Vasc Interv Radiol 2013; 24(3): 411–420.

97. Freedman AM, Sanyal AJ, Tisnado J, et al. Complications of transjugular intrahepatic portosystemic shunt: a comprehensive review. Radiographics 1993;13:1185–1210.

98. Tripathi D, Therapondos G, Redhead DN, et al. Transjugular intrahepatic portosystemic stent-shunt and its effects on orthotopic liver transplantation. Eur J Gastroenterol Hepatol 2002;14:827–832.

99. Moreno A, Meneu JC, Moreno E, et al. Liver transplantation and transjugular intrahepatic portosystemic shunt. Transplant Proc 2003;35:1869–1870.

100. Ohta M, Hashizume M, Kawanaka H, et al. Complications of percutaneous transhepatic catheterization of the portal venous system in patients with portal hypertension. J Gastroenterol Hepatol 1996;11:630–634.

Chapter 25: Percutaneous Mesocaval Shunts

Robert K. Kerlan Jr., Sue J. Rhee, and Jeanne M. LaBerge

Introduction

Transjugular intrahepatic portosystemic shunts (TIPS) have replaced surgical shunting as the preferred method to manage symptomatic complications related to portal hypertension that fail conservative treatment. Unfortunately, not all patients are candidates for conventional TIPS creation.

One situation that makes the creation of TIPS difficult is the presence of chronic portal vein (PV) thrombosis (▸ Fig. 25.1). Although recanalization of the PV can be achieved in up to 80% of individuals, in some cases it is not possible. In patients in whom it is not possible, a surgical shunt may be used as an alternative. Unfortunately, patients with advanced liver disease have significant operative morbidity and mortality related to the operation.

An innovative alternative to the open surgical shunt, the percutaneous mesocaval shunt, was originally described by Nyman et al.[1] In this procedure, a direct communication is created between the superior mesenteric vein (SMV) and the inferior vena cava (IVC). This chapter will describe the technique of creating a percutaneous mesocaval shunt.

Indications and Contraindications

- Bleeding in patients with chronic PV occlusion

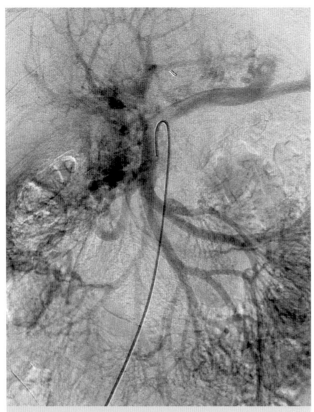

Fig. 25.1 Venous phase of superior mesenteric arteriogram reveals occlusion of the extrahepatic portal vein and numerous varices.

- Intractable ascites in patients with chronic PV occlusion
  - Failed percutaneous transhepatic PV reconstruction
  - Poor surgical candidate
  - Failed surgical shunt

Technique

There are two methods to perform a percutaneous mesocaval shunt: (1) a combined transabdominal and transvenous approach and (2) an exclusively transvenous approach.

Combined Transabdominal and Transvenous Approach

The first method uses a combined percutaneous and transvenous approach.[1] The procedure is reasonably entailed and should be performed under general anesthesia. Prophylactic antibiotics should be administered.

The patient is placed supine on the computed tomography (CT) table. Survey images are obtained to delineate a safe route that extends through the SMV into the IVC. As a 22-gauge needle will be used to puncture, transgression through liver and bowel is acceptable. Routes extending through the pancreatic parenchyma or duodenum insinuated between the IVC and SVC are not acceptable and should be avoided.

A skin site is selected, and the area is sterilely prepped and draped. A 22-gauge 15- or 20-cm-length needle is then advanced with CT guidance from the anterior abdominal wall through the SMV and into the IVC (▸ Fig. 25.2). Blood is aspirated through the needle to confirm an intravascular position. Subsequently, a 260–cm, 0.014-in diameter guidewire is advanced through the needle into the IVC. Wire position is confirmed with CT scanning.

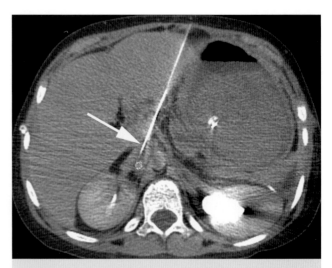

Fig. 25.2 A 22-gauge needle (*arrow*) is advanced from the anterior abdominal wall through the superior mesenteric vein into the inferior vena cava.

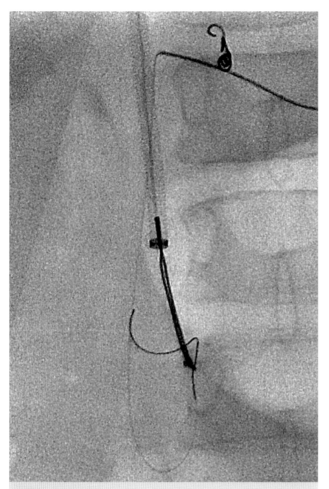

Fig. 25.3 A 0.018-in guidewire is snared in the inferior vena cava from a jugular approach.

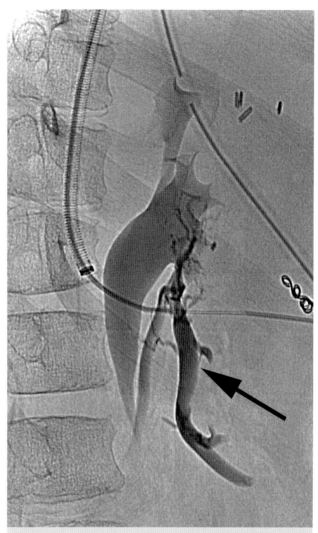

Fig. 25.4 A small amount of contrast is ejected through the transjugular 4-Fr catheter confirming the distal tip is within the superior mesenteric vein (*arrow*).

The patient is subsequently transferred under general anesthesia to the fluoroscopic suite, where the skin overlying the right internal jugular vein is sterilely prepped and draped. Ultrasound-guided access to the right internal jugular vein is established, and a 10-Fr sheath is placed. An Amplatz goose-neck or other snare is used to capture the free end of the 0.014-in guidewire (▶ Fig. 25.3) and pull it externally through the 10-Fr angled sheath and out the neck. Of note, the 0.014-in guidewire needs to be advanced through the indwelling 22-gauge needle while the free end of the wire is being pulled.

Next, a low-profile 3.5- or 4-Fr, 5-mm-diameter, 2-cm-length angioplasty balloon catheter is advanced over the 0.014-in guidewire. The transabdominal 22-gauge needle is retracted to a position proximal to its ventral entry into the SMV. The angioplasty balloon is inflated across the tract extending from the IVC to the SMV. As the SMV cannot be seen, its position must be estimated.

The balloon catheter is then removed and replaced with a 4-Fr angled catheter. A side-arm adaptor is placed on the 4-Fr catheter allowing injection of contrast through the catheter to assess the position of the catheter tip. This catheter is advanced over the 0.014-in wire through the 10-Fr sheath across the IVC wall into the anticipated position of the SMV. A small amount of contrast is injected accompanied by gentle manipulation until the catheter tip is securely within the SMV (▶ Fig. 25.4).

A second guidewire is then advanced through the 4-Fr catheter whose internal diameter will easily accommodate an additional 0.014- or 0.018-in guidewire. This wire is advanced securely within a branch of the SMV. When a secure position has been achieved, the original 0.014-in guidewire is removed through the 22-gauge needle, and the needle is removed. The 4-Fr catheter can then be advanced well into the SMV and the 0.014- or 0.018-in wire removed. A 0.035- or 0.038-in stiff exchange wire is then advanced through the 4-Fr catheter into a stable position within the SMV vascular bed.

The 4-Fr catheter is then removed. The tapered dilator is then reinserted through the 10-Fr sheath, and the sheath–dilator combination is advanced through the IVC wall across the retroperitoneal tract securely into the SMV. The dilator is removed, and contrast is injected through the sheath to confirm the position of the tip and established landmarks for stent graft deployment.

A stent graft is selected with a length adequate to line the tract from the SMV to the IVC and a diameter sufficient to decompress the portal venous system (usually 8 or 10 mm in diameter). A VIATORR (W.L. Gore, Flagstaff, AZ) stent graft is well suited for this purpose because the uncovered distal end stent graft may

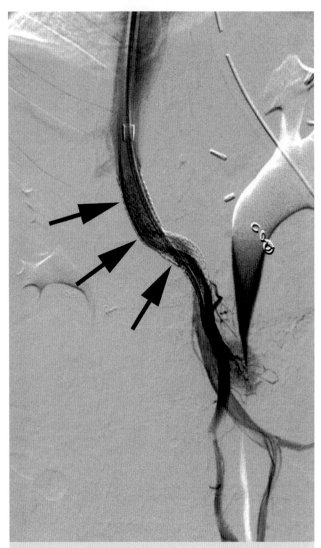

Fig. 25.5 A stent graft (*arrows*) is deployed connecting the superior mesenteric vein to the inferior vena cava.

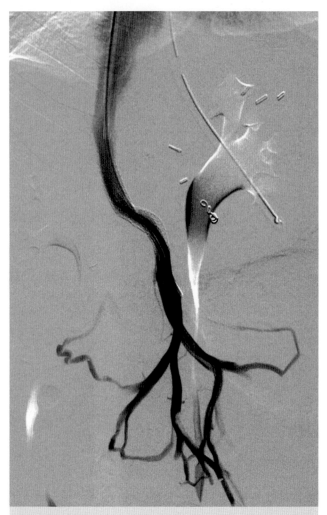

Fig. 25.6 A completion venogram is performed confirming the stent graft is widely patent and well positioned.

allow additional flow into the shunt from the splenic vein. However, in the setting of splenic vein thrombosis, a fully covered stent graft can be used because additional inflow from the splenic vein would not be expected.

The selected stent graft is then advanced through the 10-Fr sheath and is deployed into the appropriate position extending from the SMV into the IVC (▶ Fig. 25.5). The stent deployment platform is then removed and an 8- or 10-mm-diameter angioplasty balloon is inserted over the wire. The stent graft is then dilated to its full diameter. The angioplasty balloon is then removed and replaced with a diagnostic catheter over the indwelling wire. Venography can then be performed to assess the stent position (▶ Fig. 25.6). Extension and further stent dilatation are performed as necessary. Subsequently, the sheath is removed, and hemostasis is achieved by manual compression.

Exclusively Transvenous Approach

The exclusively transvenous approach does not rely on the presence of a transabdominal wire extending through the SMV into the IVC. This technique was described by Hong et al[2] and builds on a technique for creation of a direct intrahepatic portosystemic shunt described by Petersen and Binkert.[3]

Using general anesthesia, access is obtained from both the right common femoral and right internal jugular approach. A 12-Fr, 80-cm-length sheath with a 6-cm slit cut 10 cm from the tip is used. A 10-Fr by 30-cm-length sheath is inserted from the jugular approach. A through-and-through guidewire extends into the jugular sheath and exits the femoral sheath using standard snare techniques, and the sheaths are advanced until a coaxial configuration is achieved. A side-firing 8-Fr intravascular ultrasound probe (AcuNav; Acuson/Siemens, Mountain View, CA) is inserted through the femoral sheath, and an 8-Fr transjugular access set (AngioDynamics, Latham, NY) is inserted through the jugular The metal cannula from the Rösch–Uchida transjugular access set (Coo, Inc., Bloomington, IN) is advanced through the jugular sheath and out the precut slit. When the cannula is oriented properly, the 22-gauge needle is advanced out the cannula through the inferior vena caval wall into the SMV inferior to the uncinate process of the pancreas into the SMV. After confirming appropriate position with contrast injection, the 0.018-in guidewire is advanced through the needle well into the superior mesenteric venous system. The 5-Fr catheter is then advanced over the needle–wire system into the superior mesenteric venous system, and a 0.035-in Amplatz wire is placed securely into the vein. This guidewire supports the passage of the 10-Fr sheath through the 12-Fr sheath into the SMV. A VIATORR stent graft with a diameter of 8 or 10 mm is then positioned through the sheath and deployed with its distal end in the SMV and proximal end within the IVC bridging the entire retroperitoneal tract. Venography and pressure measurement are then performed with balloon dilatation of the stent as necessary.

Outcomes

Because this procedure has only been rarely reported, reliable outcome data reporting significant numbers of patients are not yet available. However, on the basis of the limited number of case reports, an acceptable safety and therapeutic profile has been suggested.

Technical and Hemodynamic Results

The technical success rate is difficult to know with certainty because the number of these procedures that have been attempted and were unsuccessful is unknown. Moreover, the patient must have anatomy suitable for a percutaneous approach including an SMV of sufficient size coupled with a route from the SMV to the IVC devoid of transverse duodenum and, ideally, pancreas.

When a successful shunt is established, the hemodynamic results should parallel that of a successful TIPS with a final portosystemic gradient falling to below 10 mm Hg. The only issue in establishing this parallel is that whereas TIPS is a shunt to the suprahepatic cava (in essence, a mesoatrial shunt), the percutaneous mesocaval shunt is to the infrahepatic IVC. Therefore, if there is an obstruction of the IVC more centrally (potentially caused by an enlarged caudate lobe of the liver), the shunt may not be as effective.

Follow-up imaging with ultrasonography or CT (► Fig. 25.7) has shown prolonged patency of percutaneous mesocaval shunts. Routine imaging follow-up should be obtained at the same intervals performed for patients undergoing TIPS or if bleeding recurs. Shunt revision may be necessary when shunt dysfunction is detected.

Clinical Outcomes

Resolution of bleeding has been reported in all cases of successful mesocaval shunt creation; however, because fewer than 10 of these procedures have been reported to date, the true efficacy of percutaneous mesocaval shunt creation remains unknown.

Likewise, serious complications have not been reported, although the potential for procedure-related bleeding, intestinal

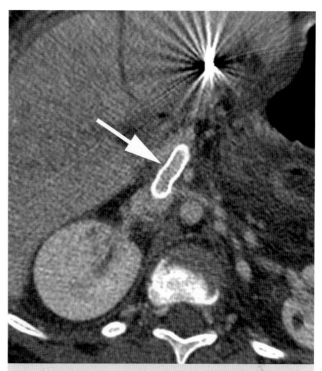

Fig. 25.7 An axial contrast enhanced computed tomographic image confirms the stent graft extending from the superior mesenteric vein to the inferior mesenteric vein to be patent.

injury, pancreatitis, infection, and vascular occlusion must be recognized. A significant complication in the patients undergoing this procedure has the potential to be life threatening.

Conclusion

Percutaneous mesocaval shunt creation is an unusual procedure in which portal decompression can be achieved in patients with unsuitable anatomy for TIPS creation. To be successful, the superior mesenteric venous system must allow decompression of the bleeding varices. The safety and efficacy profile are unknown because of the small number of patients in whom this procedure has been performed.

References

1. Nyman U, Semba CP, Chang H, et al. Percutaneous creation of a mesocaval shunt. J Vasc Interv Radiol 1996;7:769–773.
2. Hong R, Dhanani RS, Louie JD, Sze DY. Intravascular ultrasound-guided mesocaval shunt creation in patients with portal or mesenteric venous occlusion. J Vasc Interv Radiol 2012;23:136–141.
3. Petersen B, Binkert C. Intravascular ultrasound-guided direct intrahepatic portacaval shunt: midterm follow-up. J Vasc Interv Radiol 2004;15:927–938.

Chapter 26: Splenic Artery Embolization for Management of Hypersplenism and Portal Hypertension

Raj A. Jain and Charles E. Ray Jr.

Introduction

Partial splenic embolization (PSE) is a technique that provides many benefits in the setting of hypersplenism and portal hypertension (PHT); these include decreasing the incidence of variceal bleeding and hepatic encephalopathy while increasing liver protein production, platelet counts, and white blood cell (WBC) counts. A recent review article by Koconis et al nicely documents the history, efficacy, and safety of PSE.[1]

Splenic embolization using autologous clot was first described in 1973 by Maddison for treatment of hemorrhage from gastrointestinal varices.[2] Early in the experience with splenic embolization, there were unacceptably high rates of splenic abscess, pneumonia, sepsis, splenic rupture, and death. This was predominately because of very aggressive embolization techniques and the lack of antibiotic prophylaxis. These severe complications limited the popularity of the procedure. Improved clinical results were obtained with the addition of decreased embolization volume, antibiotic prophylaxis, and adequate pain control as initially described by Spigos et al.[3]

The clinical utility of PSE was slow to develop because of the concurrent development and popularity of both transjugular intrahepatic portosystemic shunts (TIPS) and the subsequent development of balloon-occluded retrograde transvenous obliteration (BRTO) in the management of PHT and varices. However, in the correct clinical context, PSE is a safe and effective procedure that should be considered for the management of patients with hypersplenism and PHT.

Results and Outcomes

Hemodynamic Results

Chikamori et al evaluated 37 patients who underwent PSE for hypersplenism.[4] The authors found that the wedged hepatic venous pressure before PSE averaged 39 ± 10 cm H_2O, which was reduced to 33 ± 8 cm H_2O after PSE. Additionally, the flow volumes in the splenic vein decreased from 477 ± 200 mL/min before PSE to 319 ± 187 mL/min after PSE. However, in this study, there was no significant change in the flow volume within the portal vein (PV).[4] This last finding is likely due to the increase in mesenteric arterial flow after PSE, which results in increased mesenteric venous flow, offsetting the decreased splenic venous flow and thus maintaining portal venous flows.[5]

Clinical Outcome

The reported ideal degree of splenic devascularization from PSE is widely variable throughout the literature, ranging from 20% to 70%. Sangro et al recommend a goal of 60% to 70% devascularization to maintain a good response without adverse outcomes. In their experience, there was a relapse of hypersplenism in patients with less than 50% devascularization.[6]

Other investigators have had success with 30% to 40% embolization, with the plan to repeat PSE as needed to control the underlying sequelae.[7]

Similar to patients undergoing splenectomy, it may be worthwhile to administer *Haemophilus influenzae*, pneumococcal, and meningococcal vaccination before PSE in case there is an inadvertent high percentage of splenic embolization. In a review of patients with splenic trauma, Nakae et al compared 24 patients who underwent splenectomy with 34 patients who underwent splenic preservation treatment (embolization, partial splenectomy, or splenorrhaphy). They found that there was no significant difference in the levels of IgM or specific IgG antibodies against 14 types of *Streptococcus pneumoniae* capsular polysaccharide between the two groups. This suggests that embolization is as detrimental to immune function as splenectomy and that vaccination should be performed.[8]

In terms of embolic agent choice, Gelfoam (Upjohn, Kalamazoo, Michigan) is the embolic agent most frequently described in the literature.[1] Coils, medium to large polyvinyl alcohol (PVA) particles, *N*-butyl cyanoacrylate (NBCA), or absolute alcohol can also be used depending on operator preference and goals of the embolization. One advantage of NBCA and absolute alcohol as embolic agents is that they do not rely on the patient's coagulation status. There is considerable variability in the literature with regard to how distal the embolization should be; more distal embolizations (i.e., distal to the splenic hilum) may result in higher complication rates[9] but may also prevent development of collaterals that can lead to a recurrence of hypersplenism.[10] In a recent meta-analysis, Schnüriger et al found that the main minor complication from more distal embolization was a higher rate of segmental splenic infarction.[11] In a separate small series of children with hypersplenism from thalassemia, the lower pole splenic artery was selectively embolized, which was thought to help reduce the development of left-sided pleural effusions.[12]

Partial splenic embolization is effective in decreasing the rate of variceal bleeding in patients with PHT, regardless of the etiology. Pålsson et al followed a cohort of 26 severely ill patients with bleeding esophageal varices and thrombocytopenia.[13] These patients were treated a total of 52 times over the course of 20 plus years with PSE, using Gelfoam as the embolic agent with a splenic devascularization goal of 30% to 40%. The average number of esophageal variceal bleeding episodes per patient decreased from 4.3 ± 2.9 before PSE to 1.1 ± 1.7 after PSE ($P < 0.001$).[13] In the aforementioned review article by Koconis et al, there were four studies that had a combined 50 patients with an average of 2.4 variceal bleeding episodes per year that decreased to an average of 0.48 bleeding episodes per year, a reduction of 80%.[1]

In a study by Ohmagari et al, 17 patients with portal hypertensive gastropathy were treated with PSE and compared with 13 control participants. When compared with control participants, PSE resulted in an 11% reduction in gastric mucosal hemoglobin content ($P < 0.01$). There was also a 71% rate of improvement in portal hypertensive gastropathy in the PSE group compared with 8% in the control group at follow-up endoscopy ($P < 0.05$).[14]

Partial splenic embolization has been found to be effective at improving synthetic liver function. In the review article by Koconis et al, there were two studies that had a combined 40 patients who had improved total cholesterol levels, total protein levels, albumin levels, and prothrombin time that persisted for more than 1 year after PSE.[1] The etiology for this improvement remains unclear but may be related to increased mesenteric arterial flow, with subsequent improvement in the nutritional levels in the PV.

Platelet and WBC counts also improve after PSE in patients with hypersplenism. Alzen et al described their experience with 17 patients ranging in age from 1 to 31 years in which hypersplenism was defined as an enlarged spleen in a patient with pancytopenia.[15] The main etiologies for splenomegaly in this patient population were PV thrombosis (five patients) and cystic fibrosis with concomitant cirrhosis (three patients). All patients were embolized with 150- to 355-micron PVA particles with a goal devascularization of 30% to 60%. Ten of the 17 (59%) patients developed a temporary left-sided effusion or ascites. The mean platelet count increased from 51,000/µL to 275,000/µL two weeks after the procedure; this increase was likely due to decreased splenic sequestration. Additionally, the mean WBC count increased from 2800 to 8200/µL two weeks after the procedure, potentially because of decreased leukocyte pooling in the spleen.[15]

Nagata et al treated 15 patients with hypersplenism, with NBCA diluted 3 to 1 or 4 to 1 with ethiodized oil. Goal devascularization in this study was 60 to 80%. These authors reported that the mean platelet count increased from 45,600 to 174,000/µL two weeks after the procedure and remained elevated at 88,100/µL 2 months after the procedure and 97,600/µL 2 years after the procedure.[16] This overall improvement in platelet count likely helps control variceal bleeding.

Similarly, in a series of 32 patients, N'Kontchou et al demonstrated that platelet counts increased by an average of 185% at 1 month after PSE, with 31 of 32 (97%) patients achieving platelet counts greater than 80,000/µL (only one patient was above that threshold before the procedure).[17] At 6 months, there was still an average increase of 95% compared with baseline counts, with 20 of 32 patients (63%) above 80,000/µL. Additionally, average leukocyte counts increased by an average of 51% at 1 month and remained elevated by 30% at 6 months. Finally, this study demonstrated usefulness in alleviating pain, which can arise from splenomegaly; all four of the patients in this series with painful splenomegaly treated with PSE experienced resolution of their pain.[17]

Combination Therapy

In a prospective study by Ohmoto and Yamamoto, 52 patients with cirrhosis, esophageal varices, and thrombocytopenia were assigned to one of two groups: one treated with endoscopic variceal band ligation (EVL) combined with PSE and the other one treated with EVL alone.[18] PSE was carried out to a 60% to 80% devascularization. The combination group had lower relative risks of new varices (RR = 0.390; $P = 0.024$), variceal bleeding (RR = 0.191; $P = 0.021$), and death (RR = 0.193; $P = 0.012$). The long-term cumulative variceal bleeding rate in the combination group was nearly 50% less than in the EVL alone group, with follow-up performed out to 7 years ($P = 0.029$).[18]

In a prospective study by Tania et al, 33 patients with esophageal varices were treated with a combination of EVL with PSE and compared with 25 patients who underwent EVL alone.[19] The combination therapy group had statistically significantly lower rates of recurrent esophageal varices at 6, 12, and 24 months of 21.1%, 37%, and 58.1%, respectively, compared with the EVL alone group of 58.1%, 70.7%, and 80.4%, respectively.[19]

BRTO is a method of treating gastric varices through a gastrorenal shunt and can be performed via a transjugular or transfemoral route. The transjugular approach has been associated with a high rate of esophageal variceal development after the procedure (51%–56% at 3 years after the procedure).[20] Given that PSE decreases portal venous pressure, it was hypothesized that combining PSE with BRTO might reduce the development of esophageal varices. In a recent study by Chikamori et al, 14 patients were treated with PSE in combination with BRTO to treat gastric varices in patients with a gastrorenal shunt.[21] This combination treatment group was compared with 19 patients treated only with BRTO. In the combination therapy group, PSE was performed 7 to 14 days before the obliteration procedure. Gastric varices resolved in 100% of patients in both groups, and there was no significant difference in the 3-year survival rate between the two groups. However, the 3-year cumulative occurrence rate of esophageal varices was only 9% in the combination group but was 45% in the group undergoing BRTO alone ($P < 0.05$).[21] This report demonstrates that PSE added to BRTO may be more effective for the long-term prevention of esophageal varices.

Partial splenic embolization added to the obliteration of portosystemic shunts (PSS) may reduce the degree of hepatic encephalopathy. In a study by Yoshida et al, 25 patients with hepatic encephalopathy were divided into two groups; 14 patients underwent obliteration of PSS followed by PSE, and 11 control patients underwent only obliteration of PSS.[22] Serum ammonia levels were lower in the combination group at 6 months, 9 months, 1 year, and 2 years after treatment. Grades of encephalopathy were also lower in the PSE group at 3 months, 6 months, 9 months, and 1 year after treatment.[22]

Transplant Population

Partial splenic embolization has been described as a safe and effective technique to decompress the portal system before live donor liver transplantation, resulting in improved outcomes. Severe PHT increases the risk of intraoperative bleeding and graft hyperperfusion, especially in small-for-size grafts that are often seen in the live donor setting. Additionally, well-developed portal venous collaterals lead to difficulty with perihepatic dissection. In a study by Umeda et al, 60 patients with liver failure from viral or alcoholic etiologies with severe PHT were randomized to two groups: one group underwent proximal splenic artery embolization 12 to 18 hours before live donor liver transplantation, and the other group served as a control.[23] Splenic embolization was carried out with coils delivered proximal to the origin of the main pancreatic artery (dorsal pancreatic). There was a statistically significant decrease in portal venous flow and a concurrent increase in hepatic arterial flow in the proximal splenic embolization population. This procedure led to statistically significant decreased operating room time, blood loss, need for transfusion, ascites, posttransplant portal venous velocities, and mortality. Additionally, two patients in the control group developed splenic arterial steal syndrome after transplant and required subsequent proximal splenic embolization.[23]

Partial splenic embolization is a useful technique in the post–liver transplant population in which either the splenic artery or the gastroduodenal artery steals flow from the transplant hepatic artery. The majority of these cases involve increased flow via the splenic artery as a result of hypersplenism, although steal from the gastroduodenal artery may occur in the setting of superior mesenteric artery stenosis.[24] Steal syndrome is a rare complication, occurring in fewer than 6% of transplants, but it results in graft ischemia, particularly of the bile ducts.[9] It is often a diagnosis of exclusion after rejection, infection, and vascular thrombosis have been ruled out as a cause of elevated liver enzymes, decreased liver function, and cholestasis. The diagnosis requires careful attention to the dynamic celiac artery angiogram and should be suspected when there is persistent flow in the hepatic arterial branches at the same time that there is portal venous flow from the spleen.[24] Other diagnostic criteria for splenic artery steal syndrome include a splenic arterial diameter of 4 mm or larger or 150% larger in diameter than the hepatic artery. The diagnosis can be made as early as 3 weeks or as late as 5.5 years after transplant; however, the majority are diagnosed within 3 months.[9]

Given the higher risk of infection in the transplant population caused by the administration of immunosuppressive medications, PSE should be performed cautiously with the goal of less than 30% devascularization even if this necessitates repeat intervention.[24] In a study by Nussler et al, 29 post-liver transplant patients who were diagnosed with splenic arterial steal syndrome underwent coil embolization of the splenic artery.[9] There were rather high rates of adverse outcomes, including PV thrombosis (10.3%), sepsis (46.2%), need for splenectomy (27.6%), and death (17.2%). These complications, however, occurred in the first 15 patients in whom the endovascular technique used distal rather than proximal splenic artery coil embolization. In the latter 14 patients, coil embolization was carried out in the more proximal splenic artery, thus maintaining distal collateral splenic flow, and resulted in no complications and rapid normalization of liver function.[9] These results demonstrate the importance of performing the coil embolization in a proximal location for this particular patient population.

Complications

As with other embolization procedures, patients often develop postembolization syndrome, which consists of fever, nausea, decreased appetite, and abdominal pain that begins 1 to 2 days after the procedure and lasts for up to 2 weeks. Fevers most likely arise from the release of pyrogens by inflammatory cells within the infarcted region and can be reduced by administration of steroids. Abdominal pain can typically be controlled with nonsteroidal antiinflammatory drugs.[25]

A wide range of minor complications may occur after PSE, including left pleural effusion, ascites, leukocytosis, ileus, and prolonged pain. Depending on the size and symptoms, the pleural effusion and ascites may require drainage. Major complications from PSE more often occur in the setting of a higher percentage of devascularization and include splenic abscess, PV thrombosis, pancreatitis, severe pneumonia, sepsis, bacterial peritonitis, and death. Splenic abscesses often respond to antibiotic management; however, some patients require percutaneous or surgical drainage.[25] Finally, the combination of decreased portal flow and increased platelet number after PSE is thought to contribute to the risk of developing PV thrombosis, which is initially managed with anticoagulation.[26]

In the reported literature, 15 patients with serious complications have been reported; in only 11 of these patients was the degree of embolization reported.[1] In eight of these 11 cases, there was 70% or greater devascularization of the spleen. Taking the overall number of patients treated with PSE from published series of at least 10 patients, Koconis et al were able to identify four deaths out of 401 patients, resulting in a 1% mortality rate for the procedure.[1] This compares with a 2.8% mortality rate reported for TIPS patients.[27]

Procedural Aspects

A typical step-by-step procedure, as performed at the authors' institution, is as follows:

1. Administer antibiotics and consider vaccinations before the procedure.
2. Access the common femoral artery using a micropuncture technique.
3. Exchange the micropuncture system for a 5-Fr vascular sheath.
4. Select the celiac axis with a 5-Fr C2 catheter and perform a celiac artery angiogram.
5. Advance either the C2 catheter or a microcatheter and microwire through the C2 catheter to selectively catheterize the splenic artery and perform a splenic artery angiogram (▶ Fig. 26.1).
6. Deliver embolic agent of choice to achieve 30% to 60% embolization. The authors' institution typically uses larger (700–900 micron) particles.
7. Perform a postembolization splenic angiogram (▶ Fig. 26.2).
8. Remove catheters and perform a common femoral angiogram through the sheath to evaluate for closure device.
9. Remove the femoral sheath and obtain hemostasis with a closure device or manual pressure.
10. Admit the patient overnight for monitoring and pain control.
11. Continue antibiotics for 7 to 14 days after the procedure and a steroid dose pack for 7 days after the procedure; monitor for signs of infection, and maintain adequate pain control.

Conclusion

Partial splenic embolization is a safe and effective method for treating patients with hypersplenism and PHT and shows particular promise when used in combination with other therapies. PSE has been shown to be effective in the transplant population as well. See ▶ Table 26.1 for a summary of indications and contraindications.

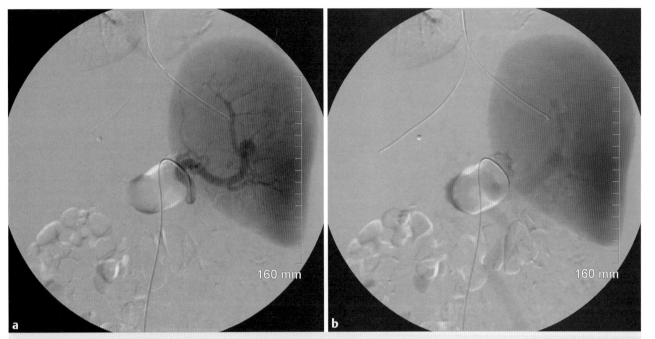

Fig. 26.1 Selective distal embolization procedure used in the treatment of portal hypertension. Preembolization angiography. (a) Selective splenic angiography, arterial phase, demonstrating a normal branching pattern and intraparenchymal appearance of the splenic arterial distribution. (b) Selective splenic angiography, venous phase, demonstrating homogeneous splenic parenchymal blush and normal splenic venous flow.

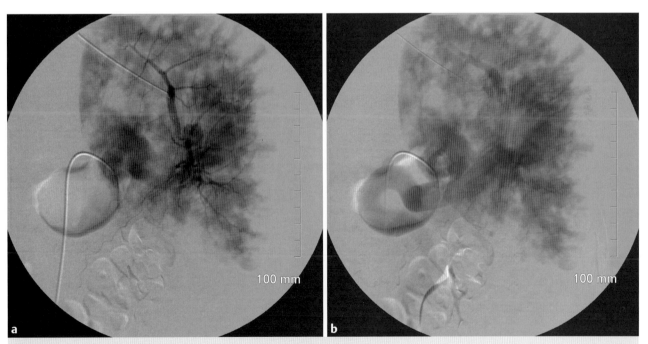

Fig. 26.2 Selective distal embolization procedure used in the treatment of portal hypertension. Postembolization angiography. (a) Selective splenic angiography, arterial phase, post–Gelfoam embolization demonstrating truncated arterial supply and a patchy heterogenous appearance to the splenic parenchyma. Devascularization here would be estimated at 60% to 70%. (b) Selective splenic angiography, venous phase, post–Gelfoam embolization redemonstrating patchy parenchymal enhancement.

Table 26.1 Indications and Contraindications for Splenic Artery Embolization in the Setting of Portal Hypertension

Indications
Hypersplenism (treat both thrombocytopenia and leukopenia)
Variceal bleeding (gastric or esophageal)
Prevention of esophageal varices in combination with BRTO or endoscopic techniques
Before liver transplant to reduce PHT
After liver transplant with splenic artery steal syndrome
Contraindications
Infection
Pyrexia
Sepsis

BRTO: balloon-occluded retrograde transvenous obliteration; PHT: portal hypertension.

Clinical Pearls

Technical Pearls

- Embolic agent used for PSE include Gelfoam, particles, coils, and NBCA.
- The goal (procedural endpoint) is 30% to 60% embolization.
- Antibiotics should be administered before and after the procedure.
- PSE is useful in combination therapy.

Outcomes Pearls

- Postembolization syndrome commonly occurs.
- Minor complications include ascites, hydrothorax, leukocytosis, and pain.
- The procedural endpoint is 30% to 60% embolization with major complications occurring at higher percentage embolizations.
- PSE can increase the risk of PV thrombosis (reduced inflow to the PV).

References

1. Koconis KG, Singh H, Soares G. Partial splenic embolization in the treatment of patients with portal hypertension: a review of the English language literature. J Vasc Interv Radiol 2007;18:463–481.
2. Maddison FE. Embolic therapy of hypersplenism. Invest Radiol 1973;8:280–281.
3. Spigos DG, Jonasson O, Mozes M, Capek V. Partial splenic embolization in the treatment of hypersplenism. AJR Am J Roentgenol 1979;132:777–782.
4. Chikamori F, Kuniyoshi N, Kawashima T, Takasae Y. Short-term portal hemodynamic effects of partial splenic embolization for hypersplenism. Hepatogastroenterology 2007;54(78):1847–1849.
5. Porter BA, Frey CF, Link DP, et al. Splenic embolization monitored by the video dilution technique. AJR Am J Roentgenol 1983;141(5):1063–1065.
6. Sangro B, Bilbao I, Herrero I, et al. Partial splenic embolization for the treatment of hypersplenism in cirrhosis. Hepatology 1993;18(2):309–314
7. Harned RK 2nd, Thompson HR, Kumpe DA, et al. Partial splenic embolization in five children with hypersplenism: effects of reduced-volume embolization on efficacy and morbidity. Radiology 1998;209:803–806.
8. Nakae H, Shimazu T, Miyauchi H, et al. Does splenic preservation treatment (embolization, splenorrhaphy, and partial splenectomy) improve immunologic function and long-term prognosis after splenic injury? J Trauma 2009;67(3): 557–563.
9. Nussler NC, Settmacher U, Haase R, et al. Diagnosis and treatment of arterial steal syndromes in liver transplant recipients. Liver Transpl 2003;9:596–602.
10. Shah R, Mahour GH, Ford EG, Stanley P. Partial splenic embolization. An effective alternative to splenectomy for hypersplenism. Am Surg 1990;56(12):774–777.
11. Schnüriger B, Inaba K, Konstantinidis A, et al. outcomes of proximal versus distal splenic artery embolization after trauma: a systematic review and meta-analysis. J Trauma 2011;70(1):252–260.
12. Stanley P, Shen TC. Partial embolization of the spleen in patients with thalassemia. J Vasc Interv Radiol 1995;6:137–142.
13. Pålsson, B, Hallén M, Forsberg AM, Alwmark A. Partial splenic embolization: long-term outcome. Langenbecks Arch Surg 2003;387:421–426.
14. Ohmagari K, Toyonaga A, Tanikawa K. Effects of transcatheter splenic arterial embolization on portal hypertensive gastric mucosa. Am J Gastroenterol 1993; 88(11):1837–1841.
15. Alzen G, Basedow J, Luedemann M, et al. Partial splenic embolization as an alternative to splenectomy in hypersplenism—single center experience in 16 years. Klin Padiatr 2010;222:368–373.
16. Nagata Y, Wray R, Tsugi T, et al. Midterm results of partial splenic embolization using N-butyl cyanoacrylate. J Vasc Interv Radiol 2010;21(2):S113.
17. N'Kontchou G, Serror O, Bourcier V, et al. Partial splenic embolization in patients with cirrhosis: efficacy, tolerance and long-term outcome in 32 patients. Eur J Gastroenterol Hepatol 2005;17(2):179–184.
18. Ohmoto K, Yamamoto S. Prevention of variceal recurrence, bleeding, and death in cirrhosis patients with hypersplenism, especially those with severe thrombocytopenia. Hepatogastroenterology 2003;50(54):1766–1769.
19. Taniai N, Onda M, Tajiri T. Endoscopic variceal ligation (EVL) combined with partial splenic embolization (PSE). Hepatogastroenterology 1999;46(29):2849–2853.
20. Chikamori F, Kuniyoshi N, Shibuya S, Takase Y. Eight years of experience with transjugular retrograde obliteration for gastric varices with gastrorenal shunts. Surgery 2001;129(4):414–420.
21. Chikamori F, Kuniyoshi N, Kawashima T, Takase Y. Gastric varices with gastrorenal shunt: combined therapy using transjugular retrograde obliteration and partial splenic embolization. AJR Am J Roentgenol 2008;191:555–559.
22. Yoshida H, Mamada Y, Taniai N, et al. Long-term results of partial splenic artery embolization as supplemental treatment for portal-systemic encephalopathy. Am J Gastroenterol 2005;100(1):43–47.
23. Umeda Y, Yagi T, Sadamori H, et al. Preoperative proximal splenic artery embolization: a safe and efficacious portal decompression technique that improves the outcome of live donor liver transplantation. Transplant Int 2007;20:947–955.
24. Saad WEA. Management of nonocclusive hepatic artery complications after liver transplantation. Tech Vasc Interv Radiol 2007;10(3):221–232.
25. Yoshida H, Mamada Y, Taniai N, Tajiri T. Partial splenic embolization. Hepatol Res 2008;38:225–233.
26. Noula J, Sourge I, Deckert F, et al. Acute portal vein thrombosis after splenic embolization and splenectomy for autoimmune pancytopenia. Eur J Pediatr Surg 2005;15:358–360.
27. Papatheodoridis GV, Goulis J, Leandro G, et al. Transjugular intrahepatic portosystemic shunt compared with endoscopic treatment for prevention of variceal rebleeding: a meta-analysis. Hepatology 1999;30(3):612–622.

Chapter 27: Pediatric Portal Interventions

Ravi N. Srinivasa, Narasimham L. Dasika, Alexandria Jo, and Wael E.A. Saad

Introduction

While portal interventions on adults have become commonplace, as most interventionalists are comfortable with the variety of different approaches, portal interventions in children are perhaps more daunting due to their relative infrequency and operator trepidation around performing complex interventions on children. While it is easy to say kids are just small adults, and one can tailor the procedure to a small adult, this is only partially true given certain considerations in children (including preoperative, intraoperative, and postoperative management) that one should be aware of when treating children. Furthermore, certain conditions may present in the pediatric population that may be best managed according to a different algorithm than an adult counterpart. Additionally, these complex portal interventions likely get triaged to larger academic institutions with pediatric liver transplant programs and dedicated children's hospitals; therefore, these interventions may not be a routine practice. With children, interventional radiologists can provide a great service by offering a minimally invasive approach in managing a life-threatening disease process. In lieu of creating a surgical splenorenal or mesocaval shunt, creating a transjugular portosystemic shunt (TIPS) can be life-saving in a child with variceal bleeding. Congenital abnormalities, such as direct portosystemic shunts and Abernethy malformations, may be discovered early in the pediatric population and be managed with minimally invasive interventional techniques.

Children commonly present in ways similar to adults including with variceal bleeding, ascites, or hepatic hydrothorax. However, the etiology of portal hypertension in children is certainly different than in adults. In adults, portal hypertension is often the result of alcohol consumption or underlying liver cirrhosis secondary to hepatitis or non-alcoholic steatohepatosis (NASH); in children, the causes may be congenital or acquired. Post–chemotherapy-related liver disease after leukemia treatment is one situation where a child may present with portal hypertension. Long-term jejunal tube feeding in the setting of chronic liver disease may result in stomal variceal formation, which may be prone to bleeding. Children with biliary atresia may undergo liver transplantation and be susceptible to the complications that go along with it, including hepatic artery occlusion or portal vein anastomotic narrowing. Another etiology in senestral (left-sided) portal hypertension due to splenic thrombosis is dehydration in infants and small children. These are all complications that can be managed from a minimally invasive interventional approach, and, in children, this is generally preferable compared to larger open-surgical operations.

The remainder of this chapter is divided along technical (procedural) lines.

Transjugular Intrahepatic Portosystemic Shunts (TIPS)

Due to the longer life expectancy of children relative to their adult counterparts with portal hypertension, TIPS creation

may be a bridge to liver transplantation in the setting of portal hypertension. Although the techniques for placement of a TIPS are similar among adults and children, factors to consider include the smaller size of the liver and consequently the smaller size of the hepatic veins and portal branches. Shunts may also need to be tailored and may eventually be modified as the child grows.[1] Depending on the degree of portal hypertension and the specific circumstances, direct transhepatic portal access or transjugular transhepatic portal sclerotherapy without placement of a TIPS may be options to consider to avoid potential complications associated with creation of a TIPS, such as hepatic encephalopathy, liver failure and right heart failure.[1,2] Children are much more susceptible to these potential risks if appropriate pre-procedural screening or planning is not undertaken.

In the setting of a variceal hemorrhage, often the first line of management may be endoscopic with banding, vasoconstricting medication injection, or glue directly into the varices. In the setting of a life-threatening hemorrhage, a Sengstaken-Blakemore occlusion balloon may also be placed. Medical management may include beta-blockers, vasopressin, pressor support, and/or octreotide with supportive therapy with blood and fluid resuscitation.

Technique

Creation of a TIPS in a child is similar to that in an adult. Internal jugular vein access is obtained and, depending on the size of the child, ideally a 10-F, 40-cm sheath is placed. A catheter such as an MPA or C2 Cobra catheter (with tip cut off) is utilized to select a hepatic vein branch (right or middle). Venography is performed with contrast and then with CO_2 while the catheter is wedged, in order to obtain a map of the portal venous system. A Rosch Uchida set or a Colapinto needle is used to make a puncture into a portal venous branch from the hepatic vein. Once needle positioning is confirmed with contrast, a wire is placed into the portal venous system. A catheter is then passed into the portal venous system and a stiff wire such as an Amplatz wire is placed. Pressures are measured, the tract is measured, the balloon dilated, and a stent is placed. Eight- to 10-mm diameter Viatorr stentgrafts (Gore & Associates, Flagstaff, AZ) can be placed to establish TIPS in larger children and adolescents as shown in ► Fig. 27.1. However, in smaller prepubertal children, balloon-expandable stents are preferred to provide adequate—but not excessive—portal decompression but at the same time allow subsequent expansion of the shunt to 8 to 10 mm as the child grows. As a general rule, 8- to 10-mm TIPS can take a child into adolescence and adulthood.

Variceal sclerotherapy using sotradecol, alcohol, and/or coils should also be performed. Patients should be admitted postoperatively to assess for complications, which, similar to adults, include bleeding, hepatic encephalopathy and liver failure.

TIPS in pediatric transplant recipients can be particularly challenging because the recipients commonly have split grafts. Left hepatic lobe split grafts are particularly challenging because of

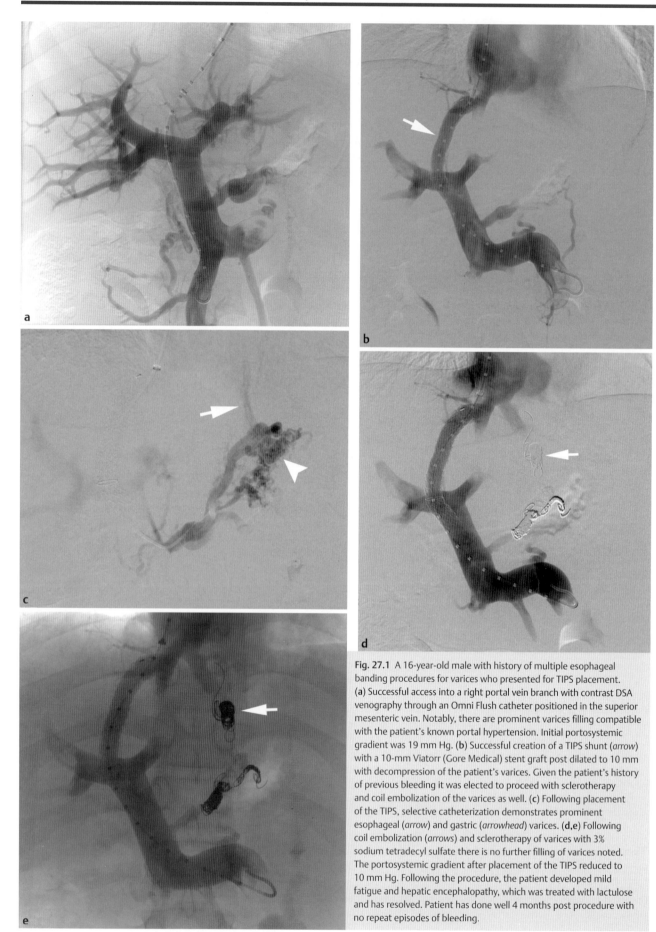

Fig. 27.1 A 16-year-old male with history of multiple esophageal banding procedures for varices who presented for TIPS placement. (a) Successful access into a right portal vein branch with contrast DSA venography through an Omni Flush catheter positioned in the superior mesenteric vein. Notably, there are prominent varices filling compatible with the patient's known portal hypertension. Initial portosystemic gradient was 19 mm Hg. (b) Successful creation of a TIPS shunt (*arrow*) with a 10-mm Viatorr (Gore Medical) stent graft post dilated to 10 mm with decompression of the patient's varices. Given the patient's history of previous bleeding it was elected to proceed with sclerotherapy and coil embolization of the varices as well. (c) Following placement of the TIPS, selective catheterization demonstrates prominent esophageal (*arrow*) and gastric (*arrowhead*) varices. (d,e) Following coil embolization (*arrows*) and sclerotherapy of varices with 3% sodium tetradecyl sulfate there is no further filling of varices noted. The portosystemic gradient after placement of the TIPS reduced to 10 mm Hg. Following the procedure, the patient developed mild fatigue and hepatic encephalopathy, which was treated with lactulose and has resolved. Patient has done well 4 months post procedure with no repeat episodes of bleeding.

the size of the liver and vessels as well as the unfamiliar orientation of the vessels because most operators are used to right-sided TIPS (from right or middle hepatic to right portal trajectories). Moreover, split left lobe grafts (especially segment 2/3 grafts) grow, rotate, and may have rotated vessels conventionally oriented.[3-5]

Portal Vein Recanalization

Portal vein thrombosis (PVT) occurs at a rate of approximately 12% in pediatric patients after liver transplantation. Patients with late PVT, defined as detection 30 or more days after transplant, often present with variceal bleeding, which can cause significant morbidity. Pediatric liver transplant patients pose unique challenges to successful portal vein recanalization due to altered anatomy, postoperative fibrosis, and smaller caliber vessels. However, essentially the same techniques that are utilized in adults can be similarly employed in children to recanalize an occluded portal vein. In children, generally portal vein occlusion/stenosis is most likely in the setting of a liver transplant. Young children most commonly receive liver transplants in the setting of biliary atresia. Splenic vein thrombosis, which may propagate to PVT, may be due to infection and/or dehydration in small children, especially in warm/tropical environments.

Recanalization of the portal vein can be performed from either a transhepatic or trans-splenic approach (▶ Fig. 27.2). The trans-splenic approach may be preferable in some situations due to the straight-line approach provided the splenic vein is patent. A transhepatic portal vein approach using ultrasound or fluoroscopic guidance can also be performed. Generally stenting should be performed with balloon expandable covered stents such as the iCast stent (Atrium Medical) (▶ Fig. 27.2). This allows for the stent to be dilated as needed in the future as the child grows. Again, similar to TIPS, 8- to 10-mm portal vein stents can take a child into adolescence/adulthood.

Depending on the degree, length, and chronicity of occlusion, recanalization may be difficult and may require multiple approaches and potentially sharp recanalization. Follow-up ultrasound and/or MRI of these patients is advisable both initially for diagnosis as well as in follow-up to ensure no restenosis. It is easier to remedy any problems if they are discovered early. A pure subacute/acute stenosis may potentially respond to angioplasty alone; however, more chronic long-standing occlusions that have progressed over time likely require support with a stent.

The tract, whether trans-splenic or transhepatic, should be embolized with either coils, gelfoam pledgets, or glue (N-butyl cyanoacrylate). Particularly with the trans-splenic (especially in the setting of splenomegaly) approach, there is a definite concern for post-procedural bleeding, and therefore the patient should be admitted to the hospital postoperatively to assess for signs of bleeding. As these pediatric cases are commonly performed with general anesthesia, one has to ensure that when the patient awakens from anesthesia there is not a sudden increase in intra-abdominal pressure, which results in bleeding. It may be wise to hold pressure at the puncture site while the patient is waking up from anesthesia, particularly with the trans-splenic approach in children. A follow-up ultrasound should also be performed the subsequent day to ensure that no acute complications develop from the access and to ensure stent patency.

Variceal Sclerotherapy

Children with portal hypertension, similar to their adult counterparts, can develop spontaneous splenorenal shunts, esophageal and gastric varices, and enteric varices. Enteric varices are an uncommon manifestation of portal hypertension and occur in about 5% of patients with portal hypertension. Treatment may include surgery, TIPS, enteroscopic sclerotherapy, percutaneous embolization, and occasionally the stenting of a stenosed portal vein. Treatment planning should begin with MRI/MRV of the portal venous system to minimize radiation dose in the pediatric population. MRI/MRV provides for treatment planning prior to performing a procedure. Approaches to treating varices are similar to that in adults, though—if possible in smaller children—avoiding a TIPS at least initially is preferable until they reach full-grown size. Transhepatic access to the portal venous system is preferred in children with a balloon antegrade transvenous obliteration approach (BATO) with coils and sodium tetradecyl sulfate (STS) (▶ Fig. 27.3). Depending how superficial the varices are, 1% STS may be preferred over 3% STS. Following sclerotherapy of the varices, embolization of the transhepatic portal tract can be performed with coil/gelfoam pledgets or glue (N-butyl cyanoacrylate). Direct percutaneous access into the varices using ultrasound guidance with direct sclerotherapy could also be performed in this setting.

Gastrorenal shunts (a prerequisite for conventional balloon-occluded retrograde transvenous obliteration–BRTO) in the setting of gastroesophageal varices or isolated gastric varices have recently been described in children.[2,6] Prior to this recent report, gastrorenal shunts (GRS), and thus conventional BRTO, were only described in adults.[2] According to the report, conventional BRTO for children with bleeding gastric varices is technically feasible along similar lines with BRTO in adults albeit with smaller balloon sizes and less foam sclerosant volumes.[2] Partial splenic embolization has also been described as an adjunct to variceal sclerosis in the setting of partial or complete portal vein thrombosis and/or complete splenic vein thrombosis (see below).[2]

Splenic Embolization

Partial splenic embolization is usually performed for either (1) symptomatic portal hypertension or (2) hypersplenism (not synonymous with symptomatic portal hypertension) for the management of thrombocytopenia or pancytopenia. In the treatment of symptomatic portal hypertension, the authors resort to partial splenic embolization either to augment other management approaches (BRTO, for example) or as the only/least-invasive option for managing portal hypertension (managing gastroesophageal varices without a shunt, for example). Recently recanalized portal vein and/or splenic vein is a relative contraindication to splenic embolization because it reduces the inflow to the splenic/portal vein and thus may predispose to premature rethrombosis after the recanalization.

Complications from splenic embolization are post-embolization syndrome, liquefactive infarction with superadded infection (abscess formation), and severe flank pain. Unlike in adults, the flank pain after splenic embolization in children can be a source of considerable morbidity requiring hospital admission for hydration and pain management. In order to reduce the risk of liquefactive infarction and make the post-procedural pain manageable, the authors prefer to do multiple[2] embolization sessions with 25% to 35% of the splenic parenchymal infarcted per session.

(Text continued on page 230)

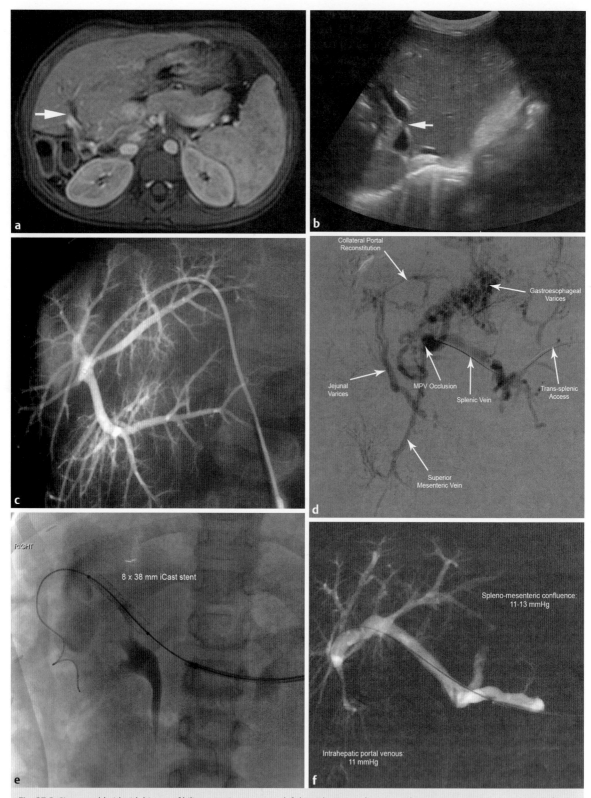

Fig. 27.2 Six-year-old girl with history of biliary atresia status post left lateral segment liver transplant 6 years prior. Severe stenosis of the portal vein is demonstrated at the anastomosis (*arrows*) on (**a**) MRI and (**b**) ultrasound. (**c**) Percutaneous access from a left and right (not pictured) transhepatic approach was initially attempted but was unsuccessful. (**d**) A trans-splenic approach was then performed as it was felt that this would provide an easier straight-line approach to recanalization. CO_2 splenic venography demonstrated main portal vein occlusion at the splenomesenteric confluence, large gastroesophageal varices, and jejunal varices from the superior mesenteric vein at the hepaticojejunal anastomosis site. The patient notably presented with jejunal variceal bleeding and these varices were treated with gelfoam slurry embolization. (**e**) After initial conservative approaches, recanalization of the portal vein was performed with the backend of a V18 wire with successful placement of an 8- × 38-mm iCast covered stent over an Amplatz wire. (**f**) Post stenting portography demonstrated a widely patent portal vein with no significant pressure gradient between the splenic vein and intrahepatic portal vein.

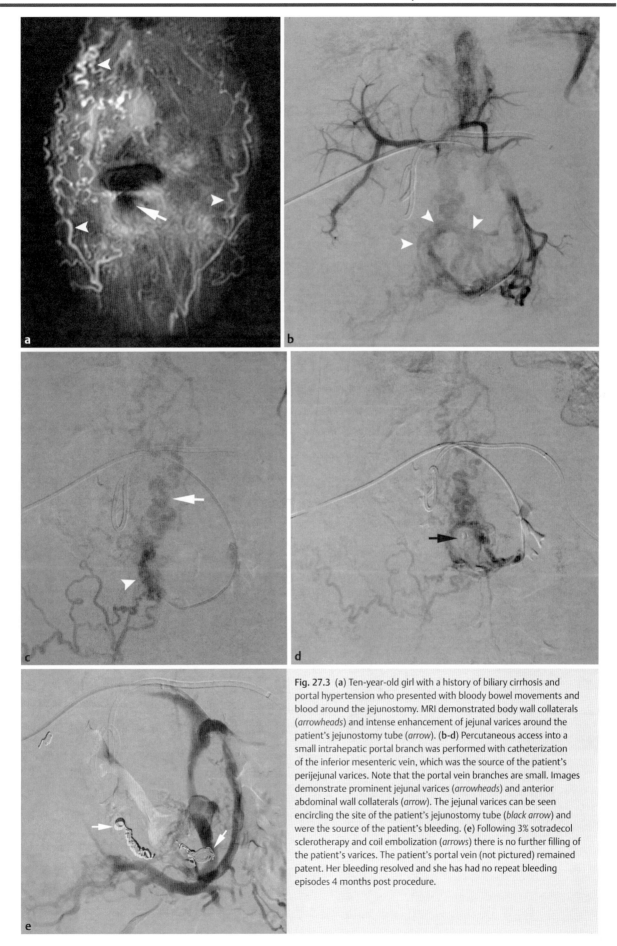

Fig. 27.3 (a) Ten-year-old girl with a history of biliary cirrhosis and portal hypertension who presented with bloody bowel movements and blood around the jejunostomy. MRI demonstrated body wall collaterals (*arrowheads*) and intense enhancement of jejunal varices around the patient's jejunostomy tube (*arrow*). (b-d) Percutaneous access into a small intrahepatic portal branch was performed with catheterization of the inferior mesenteric vein, which was the source of the patient's perijejunal varices. Note that the portal vein branches are small. Images demonstrate prominent jejunal varices (*arrowheads*) and anterior abdominal wall collaterals (*arrow*). The jejunal varices can be seen encircling the site of the patient's jejunostomy tube (*black arrow*) and were the source of the patient's bleeding. (e) Following 3% sotradecol sclerotherapy and coil embolization (*arrows*) there is no further filling of the patient's varices. The patient's portal vein (not pictured) remained patent. Her bleeding resolved and she has had no repeat bleeding episodes 4 months post procedure.

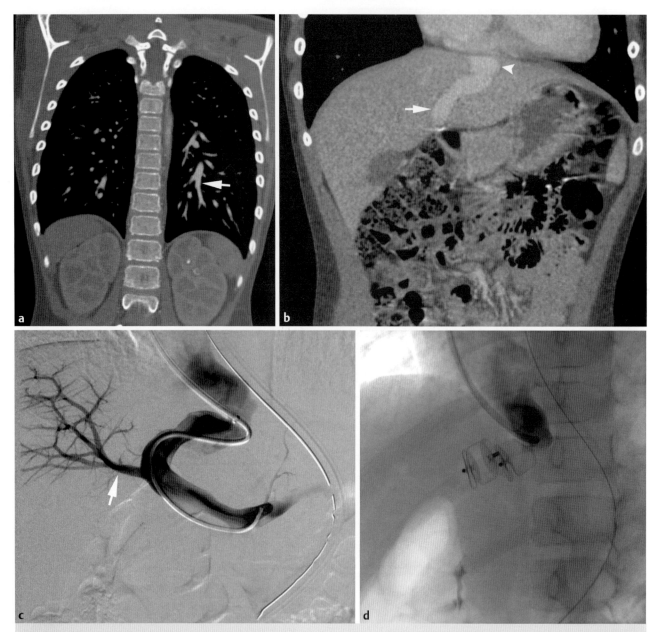

Fig. 27.4 (a) Prominent left lower lobe pulmonary arteries (*arrow*) are noted in this 7-year-old boy. Cardiomegaly was also noted (not pictured). (b) There is direct congenital portosystemic shunt between the left portal vein (*arrow*) and the left hepatic vein (*arrowhead*). Hepatic vein is isodense to the portal vein, also compatible with shunt physiology. Also the right heart chambers are dilated (not fully pictured) from the significant shunting. (c) Cannulation of an intrahepatic congenital portosystemic shunt from the left hepatic vein to the left portal vein. A relative small right portal vein (*arrow*) is noted which is well developed. The hepatic veins were also noted to be well developed (not pictured). Occlusion balloon was then placed in the shunt for 20 minutes with repeat contrast portography demonstrating satisfactory portal flow into the liver with only 7 mm Hg increase in portosystemic gradient. Therefore, it was determined to be safe to occlude the shunt. (d) Two 16-mm Amplatzer Vascular Plug generation 2 (AVP2) plugs placed into the shunt. Follow-up ultrasound 2 years later demonstrated complete occlusion of the shunt and the patient was doing symptomatically well with no shortness of breath.

The interval between sessions would be at least 6 to 8 weeks, and the schedule of the sessions can be tailored to the child's schedule (school and summer activity schedule). If large areas of the spleen are embolized (intentionally or inadvertently), careful surveillance of the platelet count may be warranted to make sure the platelet count does not become excessively high. Excessively high platelet counts may lead to thrombogenic states and thrombose the splenic and portal veins, particularly when coupled with the reduced inflow effect of embolizing a large portion of the spleen.

Congenital Portosystemic Shunts

Congenital intrahepatic portosystemic shunts (IPSVS) can cause significant changes in flow dynamics in the portal circulation and result in elevated right heart pressures as well as potentially high-output cardiac failure.[7-17] Congenital IPSVS represents an abnormal intrahepatic connection between branches of the portal vein and the hepatic vein and is due to a persistent communication between the vitelline veins of the omphalomesenteric system and the sinus venosus due to a focal absence of sinusoid formation (► Fig. 27.4). Abernethy malformations are another entity of portosystemic shunts where there is an extrahepatic portosystemic shunt as a result of persistent embryonic vessels.[7–17] There are two main types/categories of Abernathy malformation: Type-I is complete diversion of portal blood flow away from the liver with resultant no-flow to the liver, and Type-II is partial diversion of portal flow away from the liver with residual inline portal flow into the liver. Partial diversion (Type-II) is subclassified into: Type-IIa, where the fistula arises from the portal vein branches (left or right, and including patent ductus venosus); Type-IIb, where the fistula arises from the main portal vein (including its bifurcation or the confluence of its tributaries: the splenic and mesenteric veins), and Type-IIc, where the fistula arises from the tributaries of the portal vein (splenic and/or mesenteric veins).[4–6]

Patients with hepatopulmonary shunts can develop hepatopulmonary syndrome as a result of efflux of venous effluents from the liver into the lungs. The exact mechanism is unknown but is likely due to a combination of upregulation of nitric oxide production and inability of the liver to metabolize vasoactive mediators, resulting in V/Q mismatch, diffusion limitation, and shunting through pulmonary AVMs. These patients may present with cyanosis, clubbing, polycythemia, and impaired exercise tolerance from hypoxemia. Serious complications may include systemic embolization, pulmonary hemorrhage, or cerebral abscesses.[7,8]

The most common presenting symptom of congenital portosystemic shunts, however, is hepatic encephalopathy secondary to hyperammonemia. Often closure of congenital intrahepatic portosystemic shunts is clinically indicated. Alternately, if closure is neither possible nor feasible due to poorly developed hepatic or portal veins, then liver transplantation could be considered. Prior to closure, thorough hepatic and portal venography with pressure measurements should be performed, and test balloon occlusion of the shunt should be performed with repeat venography and pressure measurements prior to definitive embolization of the shunt. The easiest method for occlusion of these large shunts is to utilize the Amplatzer Vascular Plug (AVP2). The key is treating these earlier rather than later because as the shunt becomes larger over time it becomes more difficult to embolize.

Pearls/Take-Home Points

- Portal hypertension presents in children similarly to adults; however, the etiologies of portal hypertension are different.
- A higher prevalence of portal hypertension cases in children is associated with splenic/portal vein thrombosis and splenomegaly-associated hyperdynamic portal circulation, compared to adults.
- Infections and dehydration cause of portal vein thrombosis in children, unlike adults.
- Left-lobe split transplant grafts pose technical challenges to TIPS creation compared to whole-graft transplants or native (non-transplant) livers.
- An 8-mm diameter stent for TIPS or a portal vein stent usually is large enough to take the patient to adulthood.
- In small children unable to tolerate stents for TIPS or portal vein stent diameters greater than 6 mm, it is best to place balloon-expandable stents and not self-expanding stents. Balloon-expandable stents allow subsequent sequential

dilations to reach the 8 to 10 mm diameters that can take children to adulthood.
- Gastric varices can be associated with gastrorenal shunts in prepubertal children, and thus conventional-BRTO is technically feasible in these children.
- Pain after partial splenic embolization appears to have a greater impact on morbidity in children than in adults, and this may be due to the medical community's and society's limited tolerance of children in pain.
- The authors prefer to perform 2 to 3 sessions of smaller portion (25%–35%) partial splenic embolizations instead of a one-time 60% to 80% embolization of the spleen to reduce pain-associated morbidity and liquefactive necrosis of the spleen in children.
- It is best to occlude symptomatic congenital intrahepatic porto-systemic shunts earlier than in late stages when the embolization procedure is technically more challenging and clinical response is less common.

References

1. Heyman MB, Laberge JM, Somberg KA, et al. Transjugular intrahepatic portosystemic shunts (TIPS) in children. J Pediatr 1997;131(6):914–919.
2. Saad WE, Anderson CL, Patel RS, et al. Management of gastric varices in the pediatric population with balloon-occluded retrograde transvenous obliteration (BRTO) utilizing sodium tetradecyl sulfate foam sclerosis with or without partial splenic artery embolization. Cardiovasc Intervent Radiol 2015;38(1):236–41.
3. Saad WE, Davies MG, Lee DE, et al. Transjugular intrahepatic portosystemic shunt in a living donor left lateral segment liver transplant recipient: technical considerations. J Vasc Interv Radiol 2005;16(6):873–877.
4. Saad WE, Darwish WM, Davies MG, Waldman DL. Transjugular intrahepatic portosystemic shunts in liver transplant recipients for management of refractory ascites: clinical outcome. J Vasc Interv Radiol 2010;21(2):218–223.
5. Saad WE, Darwish WM, Davies MG, et al. Transjugular intrahepatic portosystemic shunts in liver transplant recipients: technical analysis and clinical outcome. AJR Am J Roentgenol 2013;200(1):210–218.
6. Saad WE, Kitanosono T, Koizumi J, Hirota S. The conventional balloon-occluded retrograde transvenous obliteration procedure: indications, contraindications, and technical applications. Tech Vasc Interv Radiol, 2013;16(2):101–151.
7. Alonso J, Sierre S, Lipsich J, et al. Endovascular treatment of congenital portal vein fistulas with the Amplatzer occlusion device. J Vasc Interv Radiol 2004;15:989–993.
8. Florio F, Nardella M, Balzano S, Giacobbe A, Perri F. Congenital intrahepatic portosystemic shunt. Cardiovasc Intervent Radiol 1998;21:421–424.
9. Gallego C, Miralles M, Marin C, et al. Congenital hepatic shunts. Radiographics 2004;24(3):755–772.
10. Konstas AA, Digumarthy SR, Avery LL, et al. Congenital portosystemic shunts: imaging findings and clinical presentations in 11 patients. Eur J Radiol 2010; 80(2):175–181.
11. Lautz TB, Tantemsapya N, Rowell E, Superina RA. Management and classification of type II congenital portosystemic shunts. J Pediatr Surg 2011;46:308–314
12. Lee SA, Lee YS, Lee KS, Jeon GS. Congenital intrahepatic portosystemic venous shunt and liver mass in a child patient: successful endovascular treatment with an Amplatzer vascular plug (AVP). Korean J Radiol 2010;11(5):583–586.
13. Morikawa N, et al. Resolution of hepatopulmonary syndrome after ligation of a portosystemic shunt in a pediatric patient with an abernethy malformation. J Pediatr Surg 2008;43:e35–e38.
14. Park JH, Cha SH, Han JK, Han MC. Intrahepatic portosystemic venous shunt. AJR Am J Roentgenol 1990;155(3):527–528.
15. Scalabre A, Gorincour G, Hery G, et al. Evolution of congenital malformations of the umbilical-portal-hepatic venous system. J Pediatr Surg 2012;147:1490–1495.
16. Stringer MD. The clinical anatomy of congenital portosystemic venous shunts. Clin Anat 2008;21:147–157.
17. Nacif LS, Paranagua-Vezozzo DC, Galvao FHF, et al. Significance of CT scan and color Doppler duplex ultrasound in the assessment of Abernethy malformation. BMC Medical Imaging 2015;15:37.

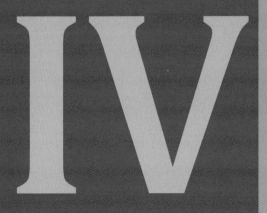

Chapter 28: Vascular Anatomy and Classification Schema of Gastric Varices Relevant to Balloon-Occluded Retrograde Transvenous Obliteration

Minhaj S. Khaja, Shozo Hirota, Kaoru Kobayashi, Satoshi Yamamoto, and Wael E.A. Saad

Introduction

The complex, highly variable anatomy and hemodynamics of the portal circulation associated with gastric varices (GVs) are challenging. However, it is essential for interventional radiologists to understand the pathological anatomy and hemodynamics of GVs in these patients when making clinical management decisions. Additionally, a thorough understanding is necessary for describing the technical details of the balloon-occluded retrograde transvenous obliteration (BRTO) and balloon-occluded antegrade transvenous obliteration (BATO) procedures. Given the considerable variability in anatomy, pathology, and hemodynamics, numerous descriptive and categorical classifications have been described in the past two decades by Japanese physicians. This chapter reviews the descriptive anatomy as well as the classification schema that have been described that are relevant to the BRTO procedure.

Descriptive Anatomy

The anatomy of the gastric variceal system (GVS), the entity that is sclerosed by the BRTO procedure, is summarized in ▶ Table 28.1. This section delineates the descriptive and radiographic anatomy of the GVS relevant to GVs and the BRTO procedure. Additional multimodality detailed radiographic anatomy has previously been published by one of the authors.

The GVS can be divided into three main components: (1) an afferent (portal venous inflow) part, (2) a central variceal part, and (3) an efferent (systemic venous outflow) part (▶ Fig. 28.1a-28.1d).

Afferent (Portal Venous Inflow) Feeder(s)

The afferent feeders of the GVS are portal venous branches that arise from the splenic vein and supply the GVs (▶ Fig. 28.1a). These portal venous inflow vessels do not communicate directly with the true (intragastric, submucosal) GVs but rather communicate with the GVS, outside of the stomach, usually in the extragastric or false GVs (described later) (▶ Fig. 28.2; ▶ Fig. 28.3; ▶ Fig. 28.4; ▶ Fig. 28.5). The portal venous (afferent) feeders include the left gastric vein (LGV), also known as the coronary vein, the posterior gastric vein (PGV), and the short gastric vein(s) (SGV or SGVs). The PGV is usually singular but can be duplicated or have an early bifurcation. There are usually multiple SGVs, but one may predominate amid the other SGVs. On occasion, it may be difficult to differentiate between a lateral-lying PGV or a medial-lying SGV, although neither has any technical implications.

The LGV (coronary vein) travels to the left from its origin in the very distal splenic vein or proximal main portal vein. Commonly, the LGV heads cephalad as it travels leftward as if targeting the gastroesophageal junction just below the medial aspect of the left

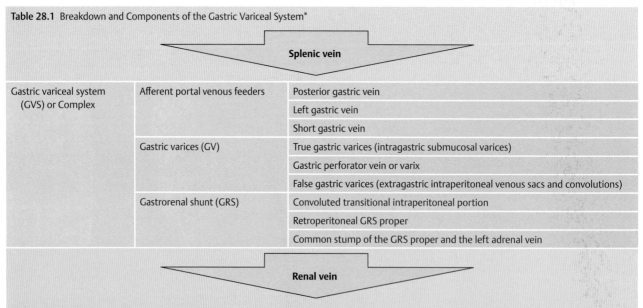

Table 28.1 Breakdown and Components of the Gastric Variceal System*

		Splenic vein
Gastric variceal system (GVS) or Complex	Afferent portal venous feeders	Posterior gastric vein
		Left gastric vein
		Short gastric vein
	Gastric varices (GV)	True gastric varices (intragastric submucosal varices)
		Gastric perforator vein or varix
		False gastric varices (extragastric intraperitoneal venous sacs and convolutions)
	Gastrorenal shunt (GRS)	Convoluted transitional intraperitoneal portion
		Retroperitoneal GRS proper
		Common stump of the GRS proper and the left adrenal vein
		Renal vein

*The gastric variceal system is hemodynamically a splenorenal shunt (portosystemic shunt, respectively). This tabulation breaks down the gastric variceal system or complex from the portal (splenic) side at the very top to the systemic (renal) side at the very bottom. In other words, the tabulation (relative to flow) moves from proximal to distal.[1]
Adapted from Saad WE. Vascular anatomy and the morphologic and hemodynamic classifications of gastric varices and spontaneous portosystemic shunts relevant to the BRTO procedure. Tech Vasc Interv Radiol 2013;16:60–100. With permission from the author and Elsevier.

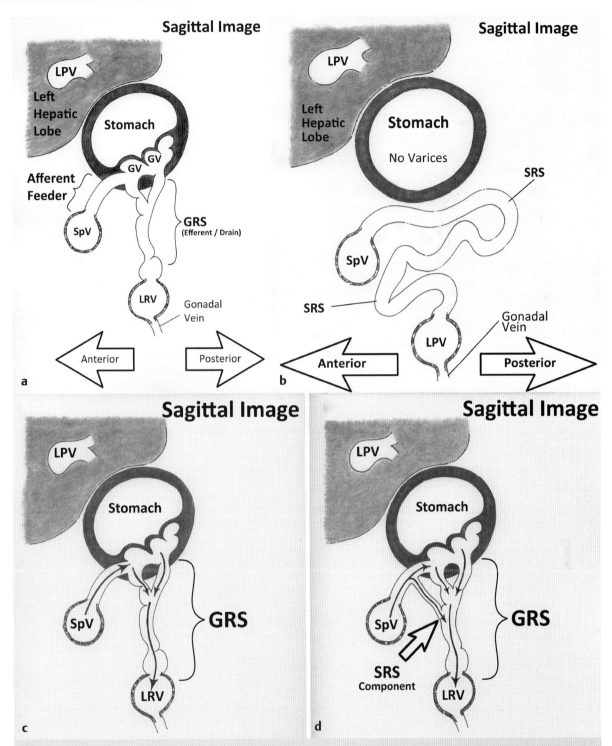

Fig. 28.1 Sagittal illustrations depicting gastrorenal shunt (GRS) and splenorenal shunt (SRS) anatomic features and hemodynamics.
(a) The key labeled sagittal drawing of the basic anatomy of gastric varices (GVs) and their draining GRS. The afferent portal venous feeders originate from the splenic vein (SpV) or portosplenic venous axis. This supplies the GVs, which in turn are drained by the efferent systemic venous system. The most common efferent drainage is the GRS, which commonly empties into the left renal vein (LRV). LPV: intrahepatic left portal vein. (b) Sagittal drawing of the basic anatomy of morphologic or anatomic SRS. The afferent portal venous feeders come off the SpV or portosplenic venous axis. The SRS does not supply any varices and does not run through the wall of the gastrointestinal tract (GIT). The most common efferent drainage is the left renal vein (LRV). The SRS, as depicted, commonly meanders (long and tortuous) and is not a straight, short portosystemic shunt. Sagittal drawing of the basic anatomy and hemodynamics of a GRS without (c) and with (d) a direct SRS component. Please see part A for labeling purposes. Basic GRSs are actually SRSs (or more accurately, spleno-gastro-renal shunts) (c). Occasionally, a direct SRS or connection is seen (d, *hollow arrow*, SRS component). *From Saad WE. Vascular anatomy and the morphologic and hemodynamic classifications of gastric varices and spontaneous portosystemic shunts relevant to the BRTO procedure. Tech Vasc Interv Radiol 2013;16:60–100. With permission from the author and Elsevier.*

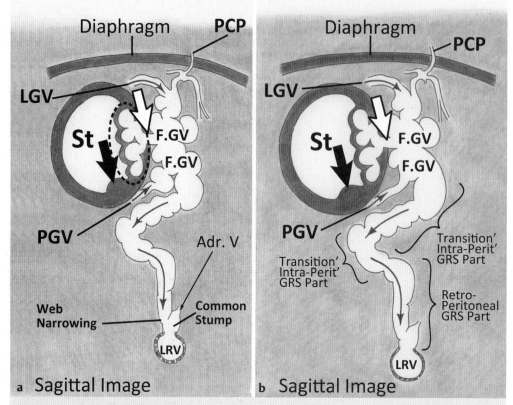

Fig. 28.2 Sagittal illustrations depicting the detailed anatomy of the gastric variceal system (GVS). (**a**) Labeled sagittal drawing of the detailed anatomy of gastric varices (GVs) and their draining gastrorenal shunt (GRS). For simplified and basic anatomy, see Fig. 28.1a. The GVS is composed of the afferent portal venous feeders, the central variceal part, and the GRS (systemic venous drainer or drainers). The central variceal part has the extragastric or false GVs (F.GV), the intragastric submucosal or true GVs (T.GV) (*dashed ellipse*) and a perforator vein or varix communicating between the false and true GVs (*hollow arrow*). The cluster of false GVs is the central part of the GVS where the true GVs, the afferent feeders, and the GRS all communicate. Please see the simplified illustration in Fig. 28.5. The degree of convolutions of the false GVs varies considerably from one GVS system to the other. Notice the difference in convolutions and sacculations between (**a**) and (**b**). The GRS is composed of an intraperitoneal convoluted or transitional part and a retroperitoneal part. The transitional or intraperitoneal part is usually more tortuous and drains the false GVs as it transitions from intraperitoneal to retroperitoneal. The retroperitoneal part is usually more straight and is composed of two subparts: the GRS proper and the common venous stump (common stump), which is the common drain of the GRS proper and the left adrenal vein (Adr. V). LGV: left gastric vein; LRV: left renal vein; PCP: pericardiophrenic vein; PGV: posterior gastric vein; St: stomach. *From Saad WE. Vascular anatomy and the morphologic and hemodynamic classifications of gastric varices and spontaneous portosystemic shunts relevant to the BRTO procedure. Tech Vasc Interv Radiol 2013;16:60–100. With permission from the author and Elsevier.*

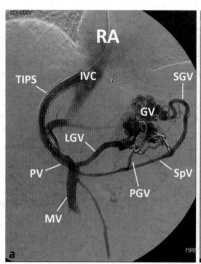 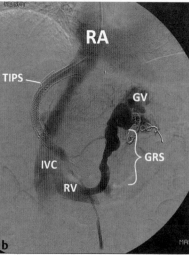

Fig. 28.3 Portal venogram through a transjugular intrahepatic shunt (TIPS). showing the gastric varices (GVs) and the gastrorenal shunt (GRS) and its parts. (**a,b**) Two digitally subtracted angiogram images (portograms) in sequence performed through a TIPS. The TIPS is patent. There is a small diminutive splenic vein (SpV), which most likely represents a recanalized, previously thrombosed splenic vein. There is also reversal of flow in the splenic vein. The GVs (**a,b**) are supplied by the short gastric vein (SGV); the posterior gastric vein (PGV); and, most dominantly, the left gastric vein (LGV). The GVs empty into the GRS, which then empties into the left renal vein (LRV), which anatomically empties into the inferior vena cava (IVC) and right atrium (RA). MV: mesenteric vein; PV: main portal vein. *From Saad WE. Vascular anatomy and the morphologic and hemodynamic classifications of gastric varices and spontaneous portosystemic shunts relevant to the BRTO procedure. Tech Vasc Interv Radiol 2013;16:60–100. With permission from the author and Elsevier.*

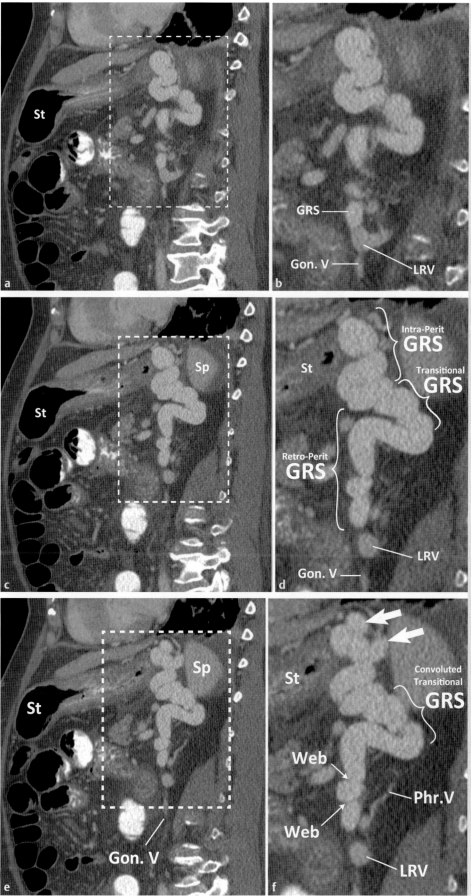

Fig. 28.4 Detailed anatomy of the gastric varices (GVs) and gastrorenal shunt (GRS) on sagittal and coronal reformats with fluoroscopic correlation. This aids in the preprocedural imaging planning. (a–l) Contrast-enhanced sagittal reformats of a CT image with magnified insets (b,d,f,h). The proximal to distal description is flow based. The proximal GRS is caudal and nearest to the GVs. The distal GRS is retroperitoneal as the GRS merges with the left renal vein (LRV). The proximal GRS is the convoluted portion, which starts intraperitoneal (intraperitoneal convoluted portion) and passes retroperitoneally to merge with the vertically oriented (relatively straight) retroperitoneal distal portion of the GRS. The convoluted portion that passes intra- to retroperitoneally is referred to by the current authors as the "transitional portion" of the GRS (d). (continued)

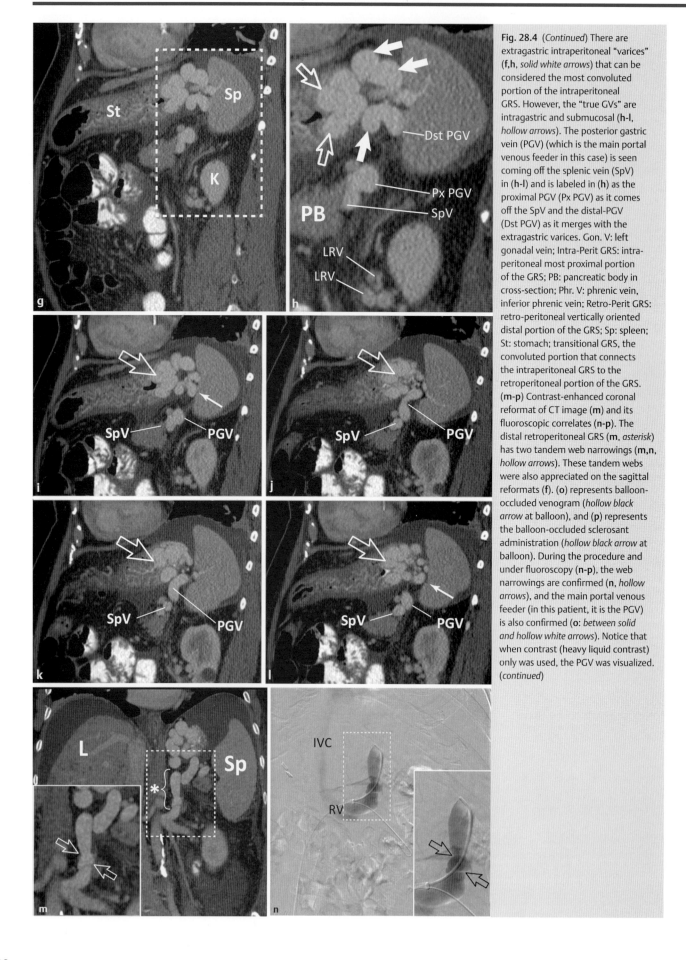

Fig. 28.4 (*Continued*) There are extragastric intraperitoneal "varices" (**f,h**, *solid white arrows*) that can be considered the most convoluted portion of the intraperitoneal GRS. However, the "true GVs" are intragastric and submucosal (**h-l**, *hollow arrows*). The posterior gastric vein (PGV) (which is the main portal venous feeder in this case) is seen coming off the splenic vein (SpV) in (**h-l**) and is labeled in (**h**) as the proximal PGV (Px PGV) as it comes off the SpV and the distal-PGV (Dst PGV) as it merges with the extragastric varices. Gon. V: left gonadal vein; Intra-Perit GRS: intra-peritoneal most proximal portion of the GRS; PB: pancreatic body in cross-section; Phr. V: phrenic vein, inferior phrenic vein; Retro-Perit GRS: retro-peritoneal vertically oriented distal portion of the GRS; Sp: spleen; St: stomach; transitional GRS, the convoluted portion that connects the intraperitoneal GRS to the retroperitoneal portion of the GRS. (**m-p**) Contrast-enhanced coronal reformat of CT image (**m**) and its fluoroscopic correlates (**n-p**). The distal retroperitoneal GRS (**m**, *asterisk*) has two tandem web narrowings (**m,n**, *hollow arrows*). These tandem webs were also appreciated on the sagittal reformats (**f**). (**o**) represents balloon-occluded venogram (*hollow black arrow* at balloon), and (**p**) represents the balloon-occluded sclerosant administration (*hollow black arrow* at balloon). During the procedure and under fluoroscopy (**n-p**), the web narrowings are confirmed (**n**, *hollow arrows*), and the main portal venous feeder (in this patient, it is the PGV) is also confirmed (**o**: *between solid and hollow white arrows*). Notice that when contrast (heavy liquid contrast) only was used, the PGV was visualized. (*continued*)

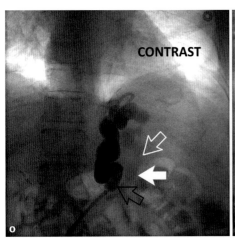
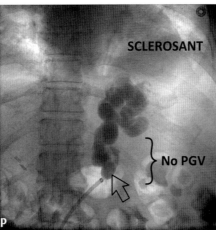

Fig. 28.4 (*Continued*) (**o**, *between solid and hollow white arrows*); however, when the foam sclerosant (lighter foam) is used (**p**) the PGV is not visualized. The take-home point is that the foam sclerosant acts differently from the heavier liquid nonionic contrast. Occasionally, the opposite may occur. The portal feeder may be seen on the GRS contrast venogram but will be seen during sclerosant administration. *From Saad WE. Vascular anatomy and the morphologic and hemodynamic classifications of gastric varices and spontaneous portosystemic shunts relevant to the BRTO procedure. Tech Vasc Interv Radiol 2013;16:60–100. With permission from the author and Elsevier.*

hemidiaphragm. It terminates near the midline and almost always in the cephalad portion of the GVS. The LGV, strictly speaking, should be a right-sided component of the spontaneous portosystemic shunt because it arises from the portal vein at or near the midline. However, the PGV and SGVs are left-sided components of the greater portosystemic shunt effect of the GVS.[1] This is important to the later discussions of laterality, afferent dominance, and classification systems that determine GVs management.

The posterior gastric vein travels straight up or slightly to the left of the GVS, arising from the middle or near middle splenic vein. The PGV can be singular or duplicated, and its course may be straight, meandering, or spiral. The SGV arises from the splenic hilum or very proximal splenic vein just beyond the hilum. The SGV then travels medially toward the GVS and enters the GVS, commonly higher than the PGV. It usually enters the GVS slightly higher than the PGV (ventral to the GVS). As previously

mentioned, it may be difficult to differentiate a PGV from SGV; however, SGVs are shorter and smaller than the PGV and usually arise from the splenic hilum or just outside of it.[1] From a hemodynamic standpoint, however, differentiation of these two veins is not important because they both arise from the proximal half of the splenic vein and are clearly left-sided components of the portosystemic shunt effect of the GVS.

The portal venous feeders of the GVS vary in dominance. Whereas the LGV is the dominant inflow vessel in some patients, the PGV/SGVs are dominant in others. In some patients, all three vessels (LGV, PGV, and SGVs) are codominant. This combination of codominant afferent feeders signifies a complex GVS. The SGV is rarely, if ever, the sole dominant portal venous feeder in a patient with a patent splenic vein in the authors' experience. However, in the setting of splenic and/or portal venous thrombosis, the SGV becomes the main and only portal venous feeder because the

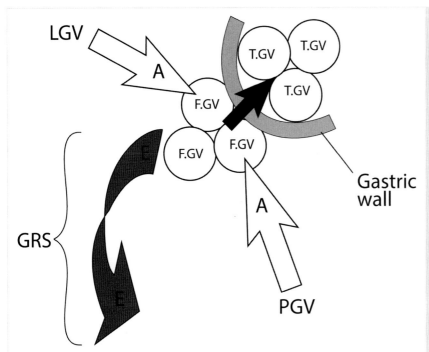

Fig. 28.5 Illustrations depicting the anatomic relationships of the different components of the gastric variceal system (GVS). The GVS is composed of the afferent portal venous feeders (*hollow arrows*), the central variceal part, and the gastrorenal shunt (GRS; systemic venous drainer or drainers). The central variceal part has the extragastric or false gastric varices (F.GV), the intragastric submucosal or true gastric varices (T.GV), and a perforator vein or varix communicating between the false and true GVs (*black arrow*). The GRS is the efferent (*curved arrow*) systemic venous drainage. The cluster of false GVs is the central part of the GVS where the true GVs, the afferent feeders (A), and the GRS all communicate. *From Saad WE. Vascular anatomy and the morphologic and hemodynamic classifications of gastric varices and spontaneous portosystemic shunts relevant to the BRTO procedure. Tech Vasc Interv Radiol 2013;16:60–100. With permission from the author and Elsevier.*

only splenic outflow is through the SGVs and gastric wall varices. In this specific situation, the gastric wall varices are not only confined to the proximal stomach (fundus and cardia) but also involve the distal stomach (body, antrum, and gastric outlet).[1]

Patients with bleeding GVs (13% to 53%) have been shown to have higher rebleeding rates than patients with esophageal varices (11% to 22%) after transjugular intrahepatic portosystemic shunts (TIPS).[2] Moreover, TIPS has shown variable results with GVs (wide range of rebleeding, 13% to 53%) and has shown more consistent results with esophageal varices (narrower range of rebleeding, 11% to 20%).[2] Based on these reported outcomes, there are two theories, based on hemodynamics, as to why TIPS have poorer and less consistent results with GVs than esophageal varices. The first theory is that portosystemic shunting through the gastrorenal shunt (GRS) varies significantly in volume, and therefore large GRSs may not be affected by the TIPS and may even compete with the TIPS. As such, a low portosystemic pressure gradient may reflect a large GRS with high flow. It is commonly believed that TIPS is not effective in managing GVs in the setting of a low (<12 mm Hg) portosystemic gradient presumably because of a large shunt.[2] The second theory is that the portal venous feeders (PGV or SGV) of GVs are farther away from the TIPS compared with the LGV in patients with EVs. As a result, the TIPS may be effective in decompressing GVs with a dominant LGV and less effective in decompressing GVs with a dominant PGV or SGV.[2] The Saad GVs management classification is based on the latter theory in which LGV-dominant GVs would likely respond to TIPS and PGV- or SGV-dominant GVs would respond less to TIPS and that BRTO may have a greater and more effective role in managing these patients (see later discussion).

Central Variceal Part of the Gastric Variceal System

The central elements of the GVS are composed of the true submucosal intragastric and false extragastric varices (▶ Table 28.1; ▶ Fig. 28.2; ▶ Fig. 28.4; ▶ Fig. 28.5). The submucosal intragastric varices are the ones that bleed. There may be thickened folds in the stomach that do not have varices beneath them. These folds may represent mere thickened rugae (gastric folds) or autothrombosed GVs. Between the intra- and extragastric varices is a perforator vein/varix (▶ Fig. 28.2; ▶ Fig. 28.5).

The extragastric varices are saccules or convolutions located outside the gastric wall (▶ Fig. 28.2; ▶ Fig. 28.4; ▶ Fig. 28.5). The extragastric varices play a key role in the GVS because the afferent portal feeders empty into them, the perforator vein arises from them and penetrates the gastric wall to the true intragastric varices, and the GRS (efferent venous drainer) arises from them and empties into the left renal vein (LRV). Whereas some patients have elaborate false varices and convolutions, others have a simple network composed of one simple varix or chamber. As such, the degree of extragastric variceal complexity varies considerably among patients.

Efferent Systemic Venous Drainage

The efferent systemic venous drainage of the GVS can vary widely in complexity. Simple efferent drainage may only have a GRS present, but more complex systems may have multiple draining systemic veins such as the inferior phrenic or pericardiophrenic vein, whose hemodynamic significance also varies (see the later discussion of the Kiyosue and Hirota classifications).[3–5] For the purpose of this section, the detailed anatomical description is focused on the GRS and the pericardiophrenic or inferior phrenic vein (IPV).

The Gastrorenal Shunt

The GRS arises from the intraperitoneal extragastric varices or convolutions in the lesser sac. The intraperitoneal portion of the GRS is usually convoluted and transitions from an intra- to a retroperitoneal location as it travels caudally and posteriorly (▶ Fig. 28.4).

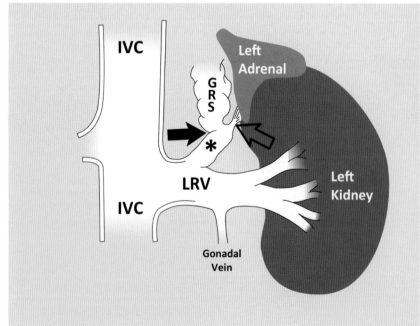

Fig. 28.6 Anatomy of the distal gastrorenal shunt (GRS). This is a drawing illustrating the detailed anatomy of the distal GRS where it anastomoses with the left renal vein (LRV). The anatomy is not as simple. The gastrorenal shunt proper (GRS) actually does not fuse with the LRV directly but actually merges with the venous outflow (adrenal vein, *hollow black arrow*) of the left adrenal gland (left adrenal) to form a common stump (*asterisk*), which acts as the outflow of both the gastric varices (not shown) and the left adrenal vein. This common trunk (*asterisk*) then merges (anastomoses) with the LRV, which in turn empties in the inferior vena cava (IVC). A weblike narrowing is commonly encountered at the GRS-to-common stump junction (*solid black arrow*). From Saad WE. Vascular anatomy and the morphologic and hemodynamic classifications of gastric varices and spontaneous portosystemic shunts relevant to the BRTO procedure. Tech Vasc Interv Radiol 2013;16:60–100. With permission from the author and Elsevier.

As such, the name of this portion of the GRS is the "intraperitoneal transitional (convoluted) portion of the GRS" After the GRS transitions into the retroperitoneum, it usually becomes less convoluted and travels inferiorly in the retroperitoneum, where it reaches the confluence of the common stump of the left adrenal vein and itself (GRS) (▶ Fig. 28.2; ▶ Fig. 28.3; ▶ Fig. 28.4).

Commonly, the retroperitoneal portion has one or more web-like narrowings, which most commonly occurs at the junction of the GRS proper (the retroperitoneal portion of the GRS) and the common stump (▶ Fig. 28.2; ▶ Fig. 28.3; ▶ Fig. 28.4; ▶ Fig. 28.6; ▶ Fig. 28.7). The various angles at which the GRS proper dumps into the common stump are shown in ▶ Fig. 28.7. Rarely (<2% of GVs cases with GRS), the GRS has a common anastomosis with the left gonadal vein rather than the left adrenal vein. When this occurs, the GRS passes posterior to the LRV and ends in a common insertion with the gonadal vein at the inferior aspect of the LRV. In addition, the GRS may be duplicated. Duplicated GRS have been encountered in fewer than 2% of patients with GRS and GVs.[1]

Pericardiophrenic Vein

The pericardiophrenic vein, IPV, and phrenic vein are more or less synonymous. The pericardial vein and IPV are collectively referred to as the pericardiophrenic vein. The IPV is composed of two parts: the transverse portion (infradiaphragmatic, horizontally oriented portion) and a vertically oriented portion (▶ Fig. 28.8). The vertically oriented portion is further separated into ascending and descending components. The ascending part usually siphons around the transverse portion and anastomoses with it. The GVS is usually located inferior to the ascending part of the IPV. The descending part of the IPV contributes to the GRS proper by anastomosing with the left adrenal vein. When the IPV is large (>3 mm in diameter), the ascending and medial parts of the transverse portion are usually disproportionately dilated or ectatic.[1] Additionally, the IPV can be duplicated or be part of a complex phrenic venous plexus. When rudimentary, the IPV can be interrupted with various isolated veins that interconnect with one another via collaterals.

The pericardial vein usually runs along the edge of the left heart descending from the left subclavian or brachiocephalic vein (▶ Fig. 28.8). It travels caudally and pierces the left hemidiaphragm after which it anastomoses with the transverse portion of the IPV just lateral to the anastomosis of the ascending part of the IPV with the transverse part of the IPV. The current authors previously published data regarding the visualization of the IPV and pericardiophrenic veins. In 130 patients with balloon-occluded retrograde venography (BORV), an IPV was seen in 75% of cases and a pericardiophrenic vein in an additional 40%.[6]

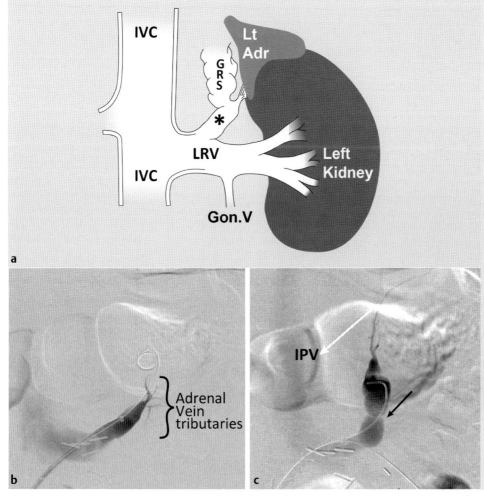

Fig. 28.7 Variations in the anatomy of the distal gastrorenal shunt (GRS). (a) Drawing illustrating the detailed anatomy of the distal GRS. Please see Fig. 28.6 for anatomic and labeling detail. Lt Adr: left adrenal gland; Gon. V: left gonadal vein. (b,c) Retrograde venograms of the same patient opacifying the common stump of the GRS outflow. They may look very different venograms, but they are actually from the same patient. After the GRS proper is selected (c), the stump of adrenal venous tributaries is only seen (solid black arrows). Injection of contrast in the distal GRS opacifies an inferior phrenic vein (IPV). (continued)

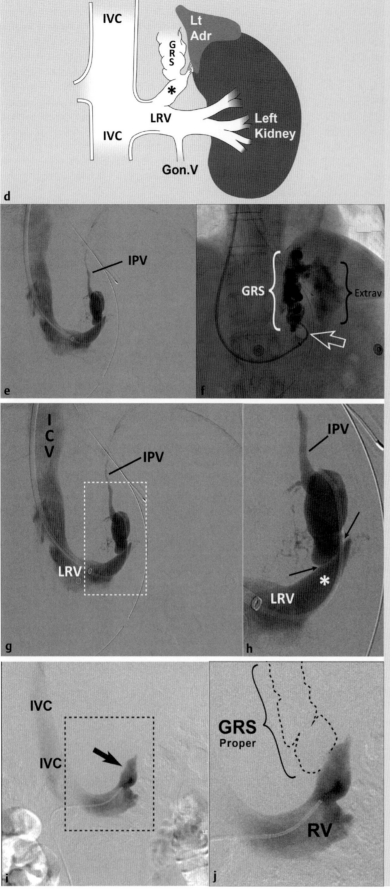

Fig. 28.7 (*Continued*) Compare with two different patients in (**d-f**) and (**g,h**). (**d**) Drawing illustrating the detailed anatomy of the distal GRS. (**e-f**) Retrograde venograms of the same patient opacifying the common stump of the GRS outflow. After the GRS proper is selected (**e**) a typical weblike narrowing is seen between the GRS proper and the common stump (see **g,h** for detail). Please compare with two different patients in **a-c**. (**f**) Balloon occlusion with a balloon-occlusion catheter inflated with air (**f**, *hollow white arrow*). With balloon occlusion, the entire GRS (**f**) is visualized. Incidentally noted is active extravasation (**f**, *Extrav*) of contrast from the submucosal gastric varices into the gastric fundus. (**g,h**) Images of the retrograde venograms of the same patient as in (**d-f**) detailing the anatomy of the distal GRS. The typical weblike narrowing (**h**, *between solid black arrows*) is seen between the GRS proper and the common stump (**h**, *asterisk*). The common stump empties into the left renal vein (LRV) and then into the inferior vena cava (IVC). These venograms are relatively forceful injections where only the IPV is opacified or visualized. Only balloon occlusion that causes stasis of flow and contrast opacification allows full visualization of the GRS proper (see **f**). (**i-n**) Retrograde venograms of a different patient of the common stump of the GRS outflow with a line drawing beneath each venographic image. The purpose of these images is to show the anatomic variations of the "take-off" (or rather, the confluence) of the GRS (**i-n**) with the common stump (**k-n**, *asterisk*) of the GRS with the left adrenal vein. (**i,j**) Shows the more common relationship between the GRS proper and the common stump, where the GRS proper merges at an angle between 10 and less than 12 o'clock. It is common to not visualize the GRS proper without balloon-occlusion venography as seen in (**i**). Only the inflow effect (a vacating effect or wash-in on venography) is seen (**i**, *solid black arrow*). (*continued*)

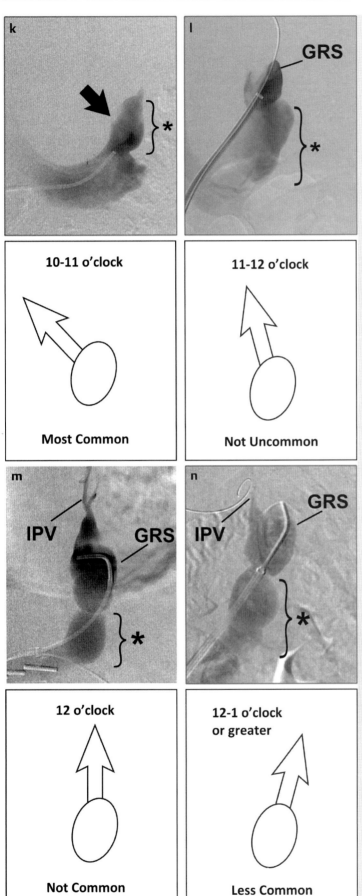

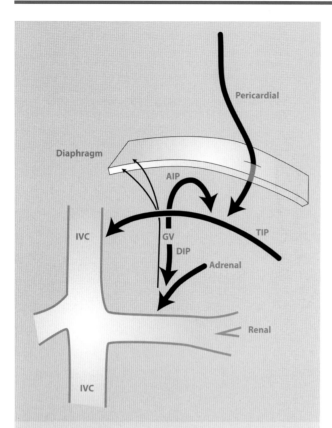

Fig. 28.8 Venous anatomy of the pericardiophrenic and left adrenal vein and their anastomoses. The percardiophrenic vein complex is composed of a pericardial vein (pericardial) that anastomoses with the left subclavian vein near the left subclavian–left brachiocephalic vein junction (near the anastomosis of the left internal jugular and the left subclavian). The pericardial vein courses inferiorly along the left heart border, transgresses the left hemidiaphragm, and anastomoses with the transverse subdiaphragmatic portion of the inferior phrenic vein (TIP). The TIP courses below the diaphragm and anastomoses with the lateral (usually anterolateral aspect) of the immediate infracardiac inferior vena cava (IVC). Occasionally, the TIP anastomosis close to or into the left hepatic vein as it empties in the IVC. The vertical portion of the inferior phrenic vein (IPV) is divided into the ascending part (AIP) and the descending part (DIP). The AIP ascends toward the diaphragm and typically, but not necessarily, arcs posterior and superiorly to the TIP and descends to anastomoses with the TIP usually close to the midclavicular line. The arcing of the AIP around the TIP, and then its anastomosis with the TIPS forms a loop, especially when the AIP and TIPS are hypertrophic. The distance between the pericardial vein anastomosis with the TIP and the DIP anastomosis with the TIPS varies in length but is usually within 2 cm in distance. The DIP courses inferiorly and usually anastomoses with the left adrenal venous outflow (left adrenal vein) to form a common trunk (see Fig. 28.6, *asterisk*) that in turn anastomoses with the superior aspect of the left renal vein (renal). The DIP is presumed to be the anatomical origin of the gastrorenal shunt when gastric varices (GVs) develop. The DIP and the AIP may not be contiguous and may be replaced by a series of relaying retroperitoneal venous segments that connect (relay) via retroperitoneal collaterals. The IPV may also be duplicated (contiguous or interrupted). In addition, other innominate retroperitoneal veins can anastomose with the left-sided intercostal, subcostal, or lumbar veins. The IPV complex is a collective of the AIP, the DIP, and the TIP. *From Saad WE. Vascular anatomy and the morphologic and hemodynamic classifications of gastric varices and spontaneous portosystemic shunts relevant to the BRTO procedure. Tech Vasc Interv Radiol 2013;16:60–100. With permission from the author and Elsevier.*

Retroperitoneal Veins

There are numerous other systemic venous draining veins, which are collectively referred to as retroperitoneal veins. These are commonly seen on BORV.[6]

Variations in Systemic Venous Drainage

In more than 93% of the first 60 consecutive BRTO cases performed by one of the authors (WES), the GRS was singular and emptied on the superior aspect of the LRV via a common trunk with the left adrenal vein.[1] This drainage pathway was also seen on 88.3% of 130 patients during BORV performed by the authors.[6] This is the conventional or most common systemic venous drainage.

From the same group of 60 consecutive BRTO procedures, fewer than 2% of patients had a singular GRS that emptied on the ventral or inferior aspect of the LRV via a common trunk with the venous outflow of the left gonadal vein. The significance of this anatomy is that it poses difficulty in catheterization and balloon occlusion, particularly from a femoral approach (a jugular approach is slightly favorable but still difficult in this setting).[1] Also reported is a drainage configuration in which in addition to the conventional drainage pathway described earlier is a large (>3 mm in diameter) IPV (seen in 3% to 5% of patients [WES]).[1] The significance of this anatomy is that it may pose considerable decompression (escape) of contrast and subsequently sclerosant to fill the GVs completely. This size IPV (>3 mm in diameter) usually requires coil embolization from either the GVS side or from the systemic venous side (from the inferior vena cava side). Moreover, IPVs that have diameter larger than 5 mm may even make it feasible to place an additional balloon occlusion catheter (BRTO approach).

Classifications

The following are classifications that have been described over the past 2 decades. In addition, there are new classifications of gastric, duodenal, and mesenteric varices. The new classifications (the Saad gastroduodenal and mesenteric variceal classification and Saad classifications for GVs [inflow and outflow]) may be helpful in planning the management of small bowel (duodenal and mesenteric) varices and GVs, respectively. These two new classifications have a management component that discusses the options for decompression (TIPS or recanalization of thrombosed portal vessels) and not just obliterative options, as has commonly been described in the literature.

Saad Gastroduodenal and Mesenteric Variceal Classification and Classification-Based Management

This is a global classification system that applies to all splanchnic (gastric, duodenal, and mesenteric) varices. However, its application is primarily for duodenal and mesenteric varices (▶ Fig. 28.9). The management strategies for the treatment of the above types within this classification are primarily based on whether the varices have portal or systemic outflow dominance and the presence and absence of generalized portal hypertension.[1]

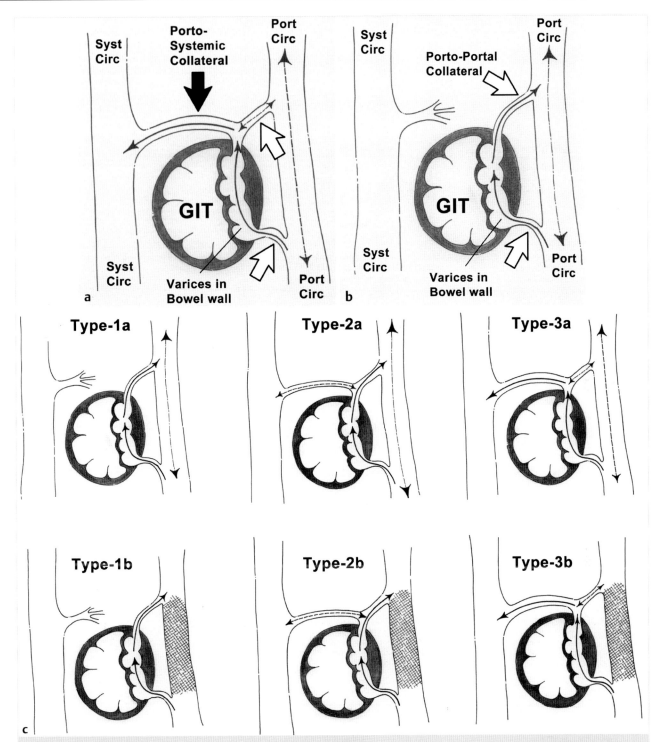

Fig. 28.9 Classification of ectopic varices (gastric, duodenal, mesenteric, and stomal varices). (**a,b**) Baseline labeled anatomy images to help interpret the images of the classification system. (They are the templates for the remainder of the figures.) The image demonstrates a representative portal or mesenteric vein branch (Port Circ) on the right and a representative systemic vein branch (Syst Circ) on the left of a cross-section through a bowel loop, which is a representative of the gastrointestinal tract (GIT). Typical portal venous (splanchnic veins) branches include the portal vein proper, the mesenteric vein (and tributaries), and the splenic vein. Typical systemic veins (but not confined to the examples given) include the inferior vena cava, gonadal veins, renal veins, and retroperitoneal and paravertebral veins. Varices (ectopic varices) are seen in the wall of the bowel. (**a**) The "ectopic varices" in this depicted instance is supplied and drained by portal collaterals (*hollow black arrows*) and is also drained (efferent collateral) by a portosystemic collateral (*black arrow*). (**b**) The "ectopic varices" in this depicted instance is supplied and drained by portal collaterals (*hollow black arrows*) and is not drained by a portosystemic collateral. The efferent collateral drainage is portal and not systemic. (**c**) Overview of the classification system. In short, type a is nonocclusive and is pressure driven (oncotic). Type a is usually with some element of portosystemic collaterals (types a2 and a3) to decompress the higher portal pressure. Type b is the occlusive type and can have no portosystemic collaterals; the varices can simply be part of a portal-to-portal "bypass" of a focal occlusion (type b1); however, portosystemic collaterals can exist (types b2 and b3). (*continued*)

Type-1a: Porto-Portal Varices (Portal Outflow Dominant)

Involved Portal Venous Branch is Patent

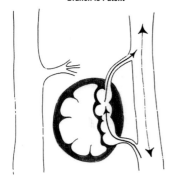

Not common in Mesenteric Varices especially in the presence of Generalized Portal-HTN

d

Type-1b: Porto-Portal Varices (Portal Outflow Dominant)

Involved Portal Venous Branch is Thrombosed

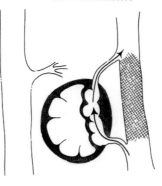

Most common type in Duodenal & Mesenteric Varices especially in the absence of Generalized Portal-HTN

Typical of GV in Segmental Portal-HTN (splenic vein thrombosis) without GRS

Type-2a: Porto-Portal Varices with porto-systemic Collat's (Portal Outflow Dominant)

Involved Portal Venous Branch is Patent

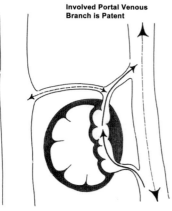

Can be seen in Mesenteric Varices especially in the presence of Generalized Portal-HTN

e

Type-2b: Porto-Systemic Varices (Systemic Outflow Dominant)

Involved Portal Venous Branch is Thrombosed

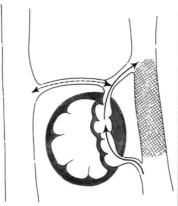

Can be seen in Duodenal & Mesenteric Varices especially in the absence of Generalized Portal-HTN

Type-3a: Porto-Systemic Varices (Systemic Outflow Dominant)

Involved Portal Venous Branch is Patent

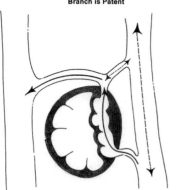

Most common type of any GIT Varices especially in the presence of Generalized Portal-HTN

f **Typical of GV in Generalized Portal-HTN with GRS**

Type-3b: Porto-Systemic Varices (Systemic Outflow Dominant)

Involved Portal Venous Branch is Thrombosed

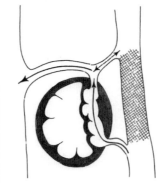

Typical of GV in Segmental Portal-HTN (splenic vein thrombosis) with GRS

Fig. 28.9 (*Continued*) (**d**) Illustration demonstrating type 1 ectopic varices without portal venous branch occlusion (type 1a) and with portal venous branch occlusion (type 1b). The portal venous branch can be any vein (location or size) in the portal circulation. This includes mesenteric vein and tributaries and portal vein tributaries as well as the main portal, mesenteric, and splenic veins. Obviously, balloon-occluded retrograde transvenous obliteration (BRTO) of these ectopic varices (type 1) is not feasible because, by definition, BRTO is via the portosystemic collaterals from the systemic venous side, and in type 1, there are no portosystemic collaterals. Any balloon obliteration would be from the portal venous side (balloon-occluded antegrade transvenous obliteration [BATO]). In essence, type 1b can be applied to gastric varices (GVs) in the presence of splenic vein thrombosis (segmental or sentinel portal hypertension) and absence of a gastrorenal shunt (GRS). HTN: hypertension. (**e**) Illustration demonstrating type 2 ectopic varices without portal venous branch occlusion (type 2a) and with portal venous branch occlusion (type 2b). The portal venous branch can be any vein (location or size) in the portal circulation. BRTO of these ectopic varices (type 2) is feasible because, by definition, BRTO is via the portosystemic collaterals from the systemic venous side, and in type 2, there are rudimentary portosystemic collaterals. Rudimentary means that it is not the main efferent outflow of the ectopic varices. The main efferent outflow of the ectopic varices in type 2 is portal and not portosystemic. Flow in the existing portosystemic collaterals may be minimal and may even fluctuate. (**f**) Illustration demonstrating type 3 ectopic varices without portal venous branch occlusion (type 3a) and with portal venous branch occlusion (type 3b). The portal venous branch can be any vein (location or size) in the portal circulation. BRTO of these ectopic varices (type 2) is feasible because, by definition, BRTO is via the portosystemic collaterals from the systemic venous side, and in type 3, there are predominant portosystemic collaterals. Predominant means that it is the main efferent outflow of the ectopic varices. The main efferent outflow of the ectopic varices in type 3 is portosystemic and not portoportal. *From Saad WE. Vascular anatomy and the morphologic and hemodynamic classifications of gastric varices and spontaneous portosystemic shunts relevant to the BRTO procedure. Tech Vasc Interv Radiol 2013;16:60–100. With permission from the author and Elsevier.*

Hirota Balloon-Occluded Retrograde Venography Classifications and Kiyosue Classification for Efferent Outflow: Management Based on Drainage (Efferent) Veins as seen on Presclerosant Balloon-Occluded Retrograde Venography

As described by the title, this is a classification system based on findings of BORV (▶ Fig. 28.10).

Kiyosue Classification for Afferent Inflow and Classification-Based Management: Management Based on Portal Venous (Afferent) Feeders

This is not only a morphologic or anatomic classification but is also a hemodynamic classification (▶ Fig. 28.11).

Saad Classification for Afferent Inflow and Efferent Outflow of Gastroesophageal Varices and Classification-Based Management

This is a classification system based on the dominance of the portal venous afferent feeders in the presence or absence of a GRS and the presence or absence of splenic vein thrombosis (▶ Fig. 28.12). The unique matter of this classification is the presence or absence of splenic vein thrombosis and the option of decompression (TIPS creation, splenic embolization, or both) instead of the only option of variceal obliteration. Moreover, this classification partly stems from the Sarin classification-based management system presented by Al-Osaimi and Caldwell.[3]

Fukuda-Hirota Hemodynamic Classification for Gastric Varices

This is different from the Hirota BORV classification described earlier. The Hirota BORV classification is based on BRTO.

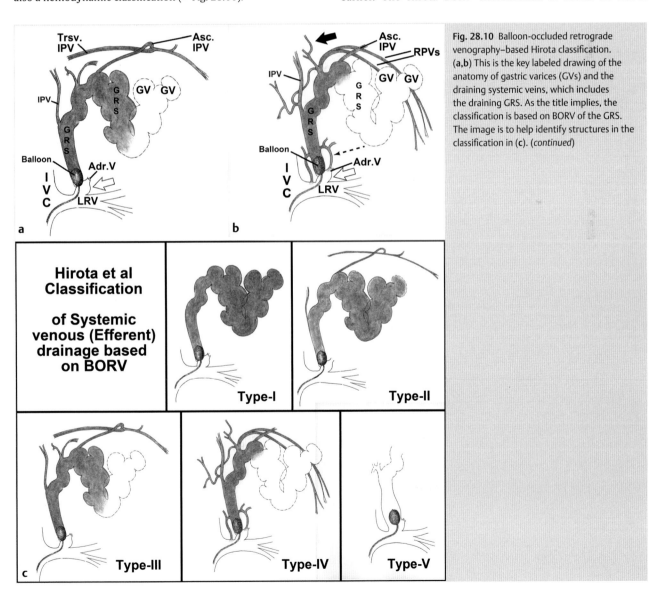

Fig. 28.10 Balloon-occluded retrograde venography–based Hirota classification. (a,b) This is the key labeled drawing of the anatomy of gastric varices (GVs) and the draining systemic veins, which includes the draining GRS. As the title implies, the classification is based on BORV of the GRS. The image is to help identify structures in the classification in (c). *(continued)*

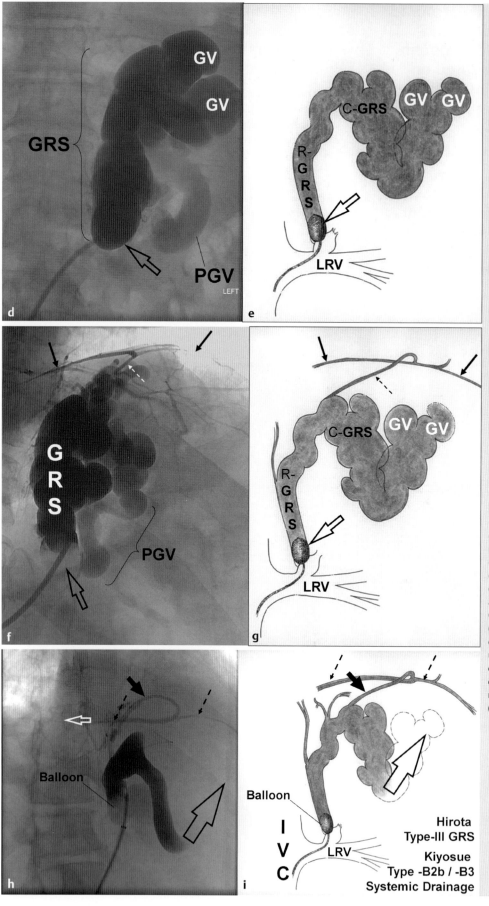

Fig. 28.10 (*Continued*) The inferior phrenic vein (IPV) has a vertical part and a horizontally oriented subdiaphragmatic transverse part (Trsv. IPV). The vertical part is composed of an ascending portion (Asc. IPV) and a descending portion. When the descending portion anastomoses with the adrenal vein or the common trunk of the adrenal vein and the GRS proper (*hollow arrows*), it forms the GRS. Occasionally, there are retroperitoneal veins or adrenal venous collaterals (*dashed arrow*) that communicate between the distal GRS (distal relative to blood flow) and the left adrenal vein(s). Additional venous collaterals (*solid black arrow*) can communicate between the gastric variceal system (GVS) and the azygous–hemiazygos axis or esophageal varices. Adr. V: adrenal vein; Asc. IPV: ascending portion of the vertical part of the inferior phrenic vein; IVC: inferior vena cava; LRV: left renal vein; RPVs: innominate retroperitoneal veins; Trsv. IPV: transverse portion of the inferior phrenic vein. (c) Schematic classification based on the anatomical BORV classification by Hirota. Type I (**d,e**) is the simplest GVS by BORV drained by the GRS and without other systemic venous draining veins (significant or insignificant). Because of the lack of decompression of contrast by venous collaterals, the entire GVS is opacified by contrast. The *hollow black arrow* points to the occlusive balloon. Type II (**f,g**) is a simple GVS drained by the GRS and with insignificant (nondecompressive) systemic venous draining veins, which are typically inferior phrenic veins. Because of the negligible decompression of contrast by the small collaterals and IPV, the entire GVS is opacified by contrast. Type III (**h,i**) is a more complex GVS drained by the GRS and with an additional significant (decompressive) systemic venous draining vein (typically IPV, which is usually >3 mm in diameter). Because of the significant decompression of contrast by the large IPV, the GVS is not completely opacified by contrast. (*continued*)

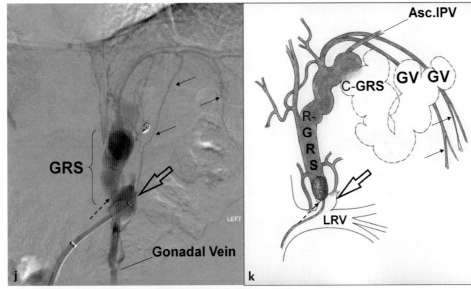

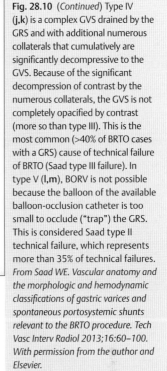

Fig. 28.10 (*Continued*) Type IV (j,k) is a complex GVS drained by the GRS and with additional numerous collaterals that cumulatively are significantly decompressive to the GVS. Because of the significant decompression of contrast by the numerous collaterals, the GVS is not completely opacified by contrast (more so than type III). This is the most common (>40% of BRTO cases with a GRS) cause of technical failure of BRTO (Saad type III failure). In type V (l,m), BORV is not possible because the balloon of the available balloon-occlusion catheter is too small to occlude ("trap") the GRS. This is considered Saad type II technical failure, which represents more than 35% of technical failures. *From Saad WE. Vascular anatomy and the morphologic and hemodynamic classifications of gastric varices and spontaneous portosystemic shunts relevant to the BRTO procedure. Tech Vasc Interv Radiol 2013;16:60–100. With permission from the author and Elsevier.*

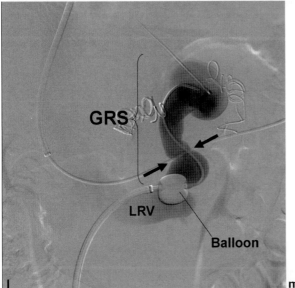

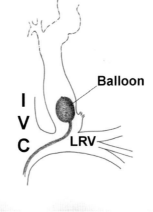

This is a hemodynamic classification system (based on celiac and superior mesenteric angiography) that has not shown a particular management value (▶ Fig. 28.13).[7]

based on left gastric artery angiography. The classification is simple: whereas type 1 has portosystemic flow in the GRS, type 2 has no portosystemic flow in the GRS on left gastric artery angiography.

Matsumoto Hemodynamic Classification of Gastric Varices for Predicting the Aggravation of Esophageal Varices After Balloon-Occluded Retrograde Venography Classifications

This is a hemodynamic classification system that has not shown a particular management value but has shown to be a predictor for the aggravation of esophageal varices after BRTO.[8] It is

Conclusion

There is considerable anatomic variation and complexity in the GVS. The GVS is composed of the afferent portal venous feeders, the central GVs, and the GRS (outflow). The GRS is part of the greater GVS, which, from a hemodynamic standpoint, is a spleno-renal shunt (spleno-gastric-renal shunt). The morphologic splenorenal shunt, however, is not associated with varices. Numerous anatomic and hemodynamic classification systems exist and have been described. They commonly have particular management or outcome applications or implications, respectively.

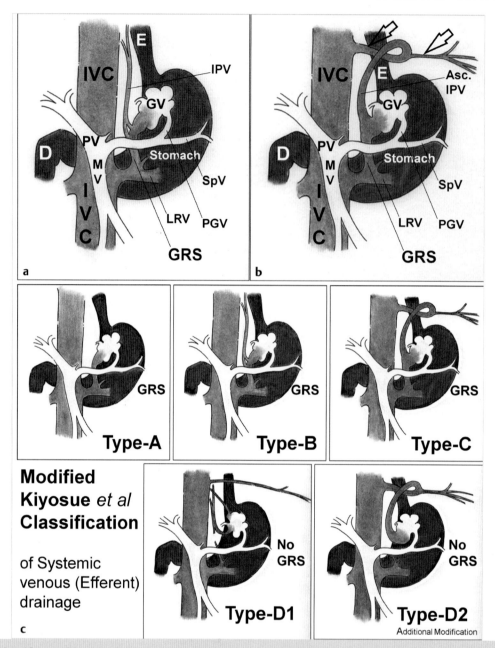

Fig. 28.11 Saad modification of the Kiyosue classification of the systemic venous drainage of gastric varices (GVs). **(a,b)** The key labeled drawing of the anatomy of GVs and the draining systemic veins, which includes the draining gastrorenal shunt (GRS), if present. The image is to help identify structures in the classification in **(c)**. The primary difference between **(a)** and **(b)** is the size and morphology of the inferior phrenic vein (IPV). The IPV has a vertical part and a horizontally oriented subdiaphragmatic transverse part (*hollow black arrows*). The vertical part is composed of an ascending portion (Asc. IPV) and a descending portion. When the descending portion anastomoses with the adrenal vein, it forms the GRS. Asc. IPV: ascending portion of the vertical part of the inferior phrenic vein; D: duodenum; E: esophagus; IVC: inferior vena cava; LRV: left renal vein; MV: mesenteric vein; PGV: posterior gastric vein; PV: main portal vein; SpV: splenic vein. **(c)** Schematic classification based on the anatomical classification of Kiyosue et al.[5,6] Type A is the simplest gastric variceal system (GVS) drained by the GRS and without other systemic venous draining veins (significant or insignificant). Type B is a simple GVS drained by the GRS and with insignificant (nondecompressive) systemic venous draining veins, which are typically IPVs but can also be other retroperitoneal veins (innominate veins, hemiazygos tributaries, intercostal veins, and adrenal veins). Type C is a more complex GVS drained by the GRS and with an additional significant (decompressive) systemic venous draining vein (IPV, usually >3 mm in diameter, Saad interpretation of diameter estimate). Type D is a GVS that is not drained by the GRS. In other words, no GRS exists. However, there is significant systemic venous drainage by other retroperitoneal or phrenic vein(s). In type D1, the decompressive systemic venous draining veins have no particular predominance and include IPVs but can also be other retroperitoneal veins such as innominate retroperitoneal veins, hemiazygos tributaries, intercostal veins, and adrenal veins. Type D GVs represent more than 40% of technical failures (Saad type III failure). Type D2 is the same as type D1, but there is a predominant systemic venous draining vein (usually >3 mm in diameter) that can be accessible and is amenable to balloon-occluded retrograde transvenous obliteration (BRTO) via unconventional systemic veins. These predominant draining routes include (1) hemiazygos–azygos axis, (2) IPV (usually the ascending portion leading to the transverse portion as drawn), and (3) pericardial vein (or pericardiophrenic vein). *From Saad WE. Vascular anatomy and the morphologic and hemodynamic classifications of gastric varices and spontaneous portosystemic shunts relevant to the BRTO procedure. Tech Vasc Interv Radiol 2013;16:60–100. With permission from the author and Elsevier.*

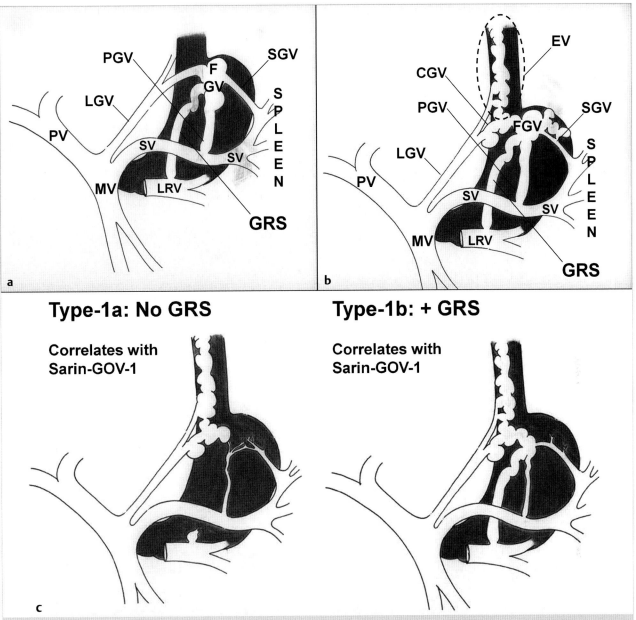

Type-1a: No GRS

Correlates with
Sarin-GOV-1

Type-1b: + GRS

Correlates with
Sarin-GOV-1

Fig. 28.12 Anatomic and hemodynamic classification of isolated gastric varices (GVs) and gastroesophageal varices. This is similar (with added complexity) to the Fukuda-Hirota classification. **(a,b)** The key labeled drawing of the basic anatomy of esophageal and GVs and their draining gastrorenal shunt (GRS). The drawings are the key for the structure identification and labeling of the classification system illustrated and described in **(c,d,e,f)**. The afferent portal venous feeders of the GVs comes off the splenic vein (SV) or portosplenic venous axis. These include the left (LGV), posterior (PGV), and short (SGV) gastric veins. The GVs are in turn drained by the efferent systemic venous system, which as drawn here is the GRS, which empties into the left renal vein (LRV). The gastroesophageal varices can be classified into esophageal varices (EVs) and GVs. The GVs can be subclassified into fundic (F.GV) and cardia (C.GV). MV: mesenteric vein; PV: portal vein (main portal vein). **(c)** Saad type 1 GVs are isolated cardia GVs without fundic varices that probably correlate with the endoscopic Sarin classification. The dominant portal venous feeder in these cases is the LGV, which comes off the distal SV, proximal main PV, or splenoportal junction. The posterior and short gastric portal venous feeders are diminutive. Variations to Saad type 1 are the presence or absence of associated esophageal varices or the presence (type 1b) or absence (type 1a) of a draining GRS. Because of that the main portal venous feeder (LGV) is central or close to the main PV, the hemodynamics of this type 1 varices are very similar to those of esophageal varices, especially in the absence of a GRS (type 1a). As a result, type 1 GVs would probably respond favorably to a transjugular intrahepatic portosystemic shunt (TIPS), especially in the absence of a GRS (type 1a). If a GRS is present (type 1b), the GVs may respond to TIPS with LGV embolization. Obviously, a balloon-occluded retrograde transvenous obliteration (BRTO) can be performed; however, if EV exist without endoscopic control, a TIPS is preferred. (*continued*)

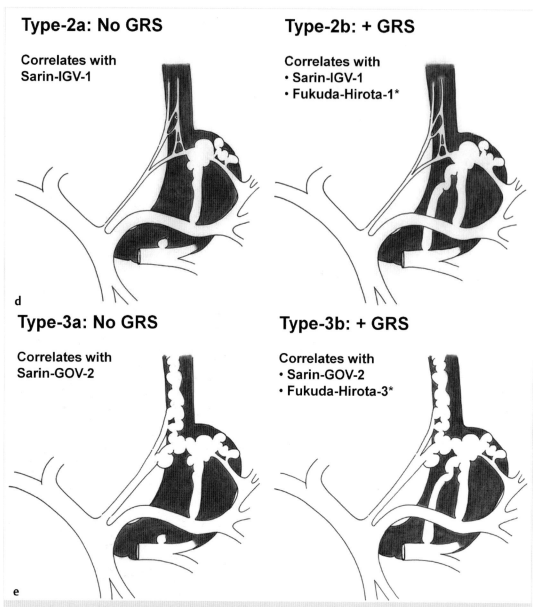

Type-2a: No GRS

Correlates with
Sarin-IGV-1

Type-2b: + GRS

Correlates with
• Sarin-IGV-1
• Fukuda-Hirota-1*

d

Type-3a: No GRS

Correlates with
Sarin-GOV-2

Type-3b: + GRS

Correlates with
• Sarin-GOV-2
• Fukuda-Hirota-3*

e

Fig. 28.12 (*Continued*) (**d**) Saad type 2 GVs are isolated fundic GVs without cardia GVs that probably correlate with endoscopic Sarin classification (IGV-1) and the Fukuda-Hirota type 1 (please see Fig. 28.13). The dominant portal venous feeder in these cases is the posterior (PGV) and short (SGV) gastric vein, which come off the proximal SV near the splenic hilum and distant from the liver and main PV. The left gastric portal venous feeder is diminutive. Variations to Saad type 2 is the presence (type 2b) or absence (type 2a) of a draining GRS. Because of that the main portal venous feeders (PGV, SGV, or both) is at a distance from the main PV and liver, a TIPS may be less effective, especially in the presence of a large (high-flow) GRS. In the presence of a GRS (type 2b), especially a large one, a BRTO is preferred. If there is no GRS (type 2a), a TIPS with portal venous feeder embolization would be effective. (**e**) Saad type III GVs are complex cardiofundic GVs with a high association with esophageal varices and probably correlate with endoscopic Sarin classification (GOV-2) and the Fukuda-Hirota type 3. All three portal venous feeders are involved and have variable dominance. These are usually complex and large variceal systems. Variations to Saad type 3 are the presence (type 3b) or absence (type 3a) of a draining GRS. When the GRS is present (type 3b), the GRS is usually large and has significant flow acting as an outflow to the three enlarged portal venous feeders (PGV, SGV, and LGV). In the absence of a GRS (type 3a), a TIPS is recommended with multiple portal venous feeder embolizations or trans-TIPS on-occluded antegrade transvenous obliteration (BATO) approach sclerosis. In the presence of a large GRS (type 3b), a BRTO with or without a TIPS is recommended. (*continued*)

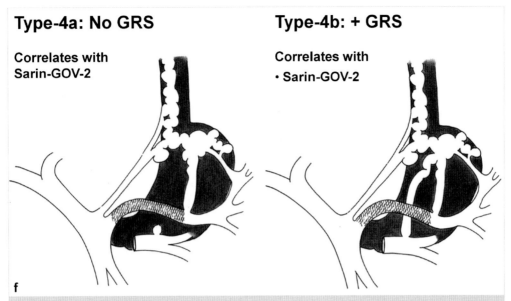

Type-4a: No GRS

Correlates with
Sarin-GOV-2

Type-4b: + GRS

Correlates with
• Sarin-GOV-2

Fig. 28.12 (*Continued*) (**f**) Saad type 4 GVs are similar to type 2 or type 3 (and are more likely to be similar to type 3), but is the presence of splenic with or without portal venous thrombosis. In these cases, the decisive factor is whether the PV is patent. If there are a patent PV and a GRS, a BRTO procedure would be reasonable. If the PV is occluded in the presence of a GRS, then the GRS most likely will be the outflow of the mesenteric and SVs, and BRTO is ill advised unless the PV is recannulated (with or without a TIPS) or there is significant cavernous transformation of the PV that can replace the PV as a hepatic inflow and a mesenteric outflow. In the absence of a GRS and in the presence of SV thrombosis with or without PV thrombosis, splenic artery embolization would be recommended. *From Saad WE. Vascular anatomy and the morphologic and hemodynamic classifications of gastric varices and spontaneous portosystemic shunts relevant to the BRTO procedure. Tech Vasc Interv Radiol 2013;16:60–100. With permission from the author and Elsevier.*

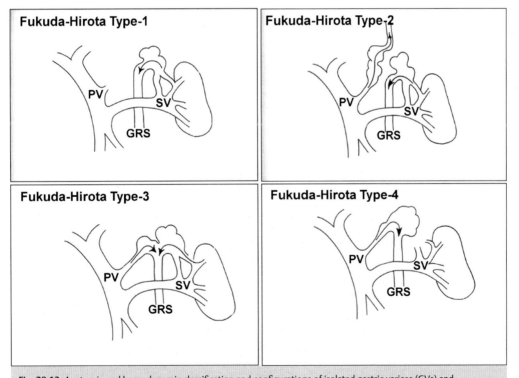

Fig. 28.13 Anatomic and hemodynamic classification and configurations of isolated gastric varices (GVs) and gastroesophageal varices in the experience of Fukuda and Hirota and coworkers. Type 1 (Saad type 2b) has fundic varices with predominant short and posterior gastric veins without esophageal varices. Type 2 is similar to type-1 but has additional esophageal varices that are not hemodynamically connected with the GVs and do not contribute to the gastrorenal shunt (GRS) outflow. Type 3 (Saad type 3b) has the complex gastroesophageal varices with all having the GRS as the primary outflow. Type 4 (Saad type 1b) has GVs that are supplied solely or predominantly by the left gastric vein (LGV). PV: portal vein; SV: splenic vein. *From Saad WE. Vascular anatomy and the morphologic and hemodynamic classifications of gastric varices and spontaneous portosystemic shunts relevant to the BRTO procedure. Tech Vasc Interv Radiol 2013;16:60–100. With permission from the author and Elsevier.*

References

1. Saad WE. Vascular anatomy and the morphologic and hemodynamic classifications of gastric varices and spontaneous portosystemic shunts relevant to the BRTO procedure. Tech Vasc Interv Radiol 2013;16:60–100.

2. Saad WEA, Darcy MD. Transjugular intrahepatic portosystemic shunt (TIPS) versus balloon-occluded retrograde transvenous obliteration (BRTO) for the management of gastric varices. Semin Intervent Radiol 2011;28:339–349.

3. Al-Osaimi AMS, Caldwell SH. Medical and endoscopic management of gastric varices. Semin Intervent Radiol 2011;28:273–282.

4. Saad WEA. The history and evolution of balloon-occluded retrograde transvenous obliteration (BRTO): from the United States to Japan and back. Semin Intervent Radiol 2011;28:283–287.

5. Kiyosue H, Mori H, Matsumoto S, et al. Transcatheter obliteration of gastric varices: part 1: anatomic classification. Radiographics 2003;23 911–920.

6. Maeda H, Hirtoa S, Yamamoto S, et al. Radiologic variations in gastrorenal shunts and collateral veins from gastric varices in images obtained before balloon-occluded retrograde transvenous obliteration. Cardiovasc Intervent Radiol 2007;30:410–414.

7. Fukuda T, Hirota S, Sugimoto K, et al. "Downgrading" of gastric varices with multiple collateral veins in balloon-occluded retrograde transvenous obliteration. JVIR J Vasc Intervent Radiol 2005;16:1379–1383.

8. Matsumoto A, Hamamoto N, Nomura T, et al. Balloon-occluded retrograde transvenous obliteration of high risk gastric fundal varices. Am J Gastroenterol 1999;94:643–649.

Chapter 29: The Conventional Balloon-Occluded Retrograde Transvenous Obliteration Procedure

Minhaj S. Khaja and Wael E.A. Saad

Introduction

Transvenous obliteration of gastric varices can be performed from the systemic-venous side (draining veins/shunts) or from the portal-venous side (portal afferent feeders). When balloon-occluded transvenous obliteration is performed from the systemic veins, it is referred to as balloon-occluded retrograde transvenous obliteration (BRTO) (▶ Fig. 29.1; ▶ Fig. 29.2). However, when balloon-occluded transvenous obliteration is performed from the portal vein and its afferent feeders, it is referred to as balloon-occluded antegrade transvenous obliteration (BATO) (▶ Fig. 29.3).[1] BRTO is the conventional obliterative procedure because it is the least invasive choice of access or approach via a transfemoral, transrenal route[2–5] (▶ Fig. 29.1; ▶ Fig. 29.2). However, BATO is considered an alternative or adjunctive approach.[1,6] The objective of BRTO and BATO is complete obliteration of the gastric varices while preserving anatomical hepatopetal flow of the splenoportal circulation.

This chapter discusses the indications, contraindications, and technical considerations of the conventional BRTO procedure. The indications of concomitant portal venous modulators such as splenic embolization or the creation of a transjugular intrahepatic portosystemic shunt (TIPS) are briefly mentioned.

Indications and Contraindications

The two clinical indications for BRTO are gastric variceal bleeding (impending, prior or current or active) and, to a lesser extent, refractory debilitating hepatic encephalopathy.[7]

The contraindications to BRTO are only relative contraindications at best. The contraindications include (i) severe uncorrected coagulopathy (which in this clinical setting is likely caused by liver failure), (ii) splenic vein thrombosis (segmental portal hypertension), (iii) portal vein thrombosis, and (iv) uncontrolled esophageal variceal bleeding. In patients with severe, uncorrected coagulopathy, commonly associated with liver failure, BRTO is probably being performed as an emergent, heroic measure to stop life-threatening gastric variceal bleeding. This is particularly true when the alternative (TIPS) has a high mortality rate in the setting of severe hepatic failure. The most serious contraindication, although not an absolute contraindication, is chronic portal vein thrombosis in which the gastrorenal shunt (GRS) is the only splenomesenteric (splanchnic) outflow.

Uncontrolled esophageal variceal bleeding can be considered a contraindication to BRTO when performed solely. To clarify, a combined TIPS with BRTO or TIPS with trans-TIPS BATO can be performed as necessary. Hypothetically, if the gastric varices are primarily supplied by the left gastric vein (which usually supplies uncontrolled esophageal varices), they usually respond to a TIPS equally as effectively as esophageal varices.[8]

Performing BRTO in the presence of portal vein thrombosis may have potentially grave consequences and is a serious dilemma for the team managing the patient. Because the entire splenic and

mesenteric outflow may be through the GRS, closure of the shunt could cause splenic engorgement and more thrombosis and, potentially, venous mesenteric ischemia. In this scenario, BRTO, if performed at all, is performed as part of a greater portal procedure (beyond the scope of this chapter). Similar to portal vein thrombosis, performing BRTO in a patient with isolated splenic vein thrombosis is a dilemma. In the opinion of the current authors, the primary endovascular management, especially in the presence of splenomegaly, is partial splenic (arterial) embolization with or without BRTO.[9]

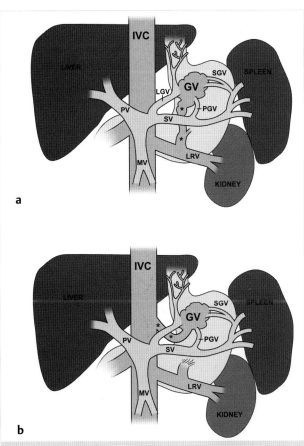

Fig. 29.1 Illustrations of common anatomy for the conventional balloon-occluded retrograde transvenous obliteration (BRTO) procedure. (**a**) The basic portosystemic venous anatomy of gastric varices (GVs) pertinent to the conventional BRTO procedure with the classic gastrorenal shunt (*asterisk*), which is more common than a direct gastrocaval shunt. (**b**) The basic portosystemic venous anatomy of GVs pertinent to the conventional BRTO procedure but with the less common direct gastrocaval shunt (*asterisk*). IVC: inferior vena cava; LGV: left gastric vein; LRV: left renal vein; MV: mesenteric vein; PGV: posterior gastric vein; PV: portal vein; SGV: short gastric vein; SV: splenic vein. (*Reproduced with permission from Saad WE, Kitanosono T, Koizumi J, Hirota S. The conventional balloon-occluded retrograde transvenous obliteration procedure: indications, contraindications and technical applications. Tech Vasc Intervent Radiol 2013;16:101–151.*)

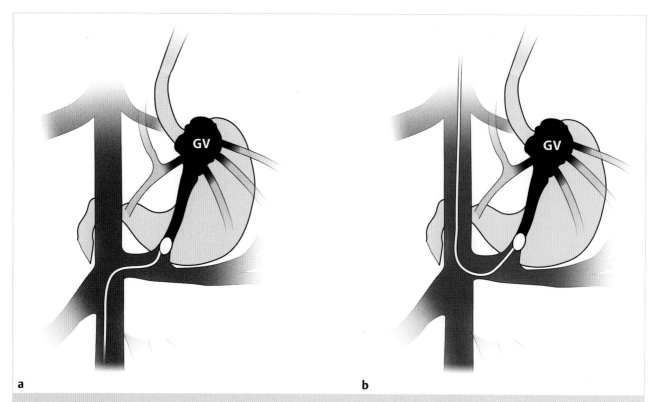

Fig. 29.2 Illustration of the basic approach of the conventional balloon-occluded retrograde transvenous obliteration (BRTO) procedure. (**a**) BRTO through a transfemoral approach with the balloon in the gastrorenal shunt (GRS). BRTO is obliteration from the systemic vein side, and balloon-occluded antegrade transvenous obliteration is obliteration from the portal venous side. (**b**) BRTO through a transfemoral approach with the balloon in the GRS. GV: gastric varices. (*Reproduced with permission from Saad WE, Kitanosono T, Koizumi J, Hirota S. The conventional balloon-occluded retrograde transvenous obliteration procedure: indications, contraindications and technical applications. Tech Vasc Intervent Radiol 2013;16:101–151.*)

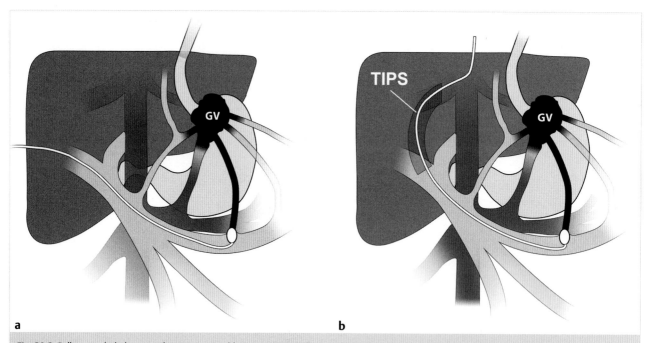

Fig. 29.3 Balloon-occluded antegrade transvenous obliteration (BATO). Illustration demonstrating BATO (balloon occlusion from the portal venous side) and its subclassification into percutaneous transhepatic obliteration (PTO; **a**) and trans-TIPS (transjugular intrahepatic portosystemic shunt; **b**) obliteration. GV: gastric varices. (*Reproduced with permission from Saad WE, Kitanosono T, Koizumi J, Hirota S. The conventional balloon-occluded retrograde transvenous obliteration procedure: indications, contraindications and technical applications. Tech Vasc Intervent Radiol 2013;16:101–151.*)

Table 29.1 Procedural Steps of the Conventional Balloon-Occluded Retrograde Transvenous Obliteration Procedure

	Broad Procedural Steps	Specific Procedural Steps
1.	Access and approach (see ▸ Fig. 29.5)	• Venous access (femoral vs. jugular) • Approach from infrarenal IVC or suprarenal IVC
2.	Selective catheterization (see ▸ Figs. 29.6, 29.7, 29.8, 29.9, 29.10, 29.11, 29.12, 29.13)	• Catheterization of the left renal vein • Catheterization of the common stump of the adrenal vein and GRS • Selective catheterization of the GRS proper
3.	"Trapping" of the gastric variceal system (see ▸ Figs. 29.14, 29.15, 29.16, 29.17, 29.18, 29.19, 29.20, 29.21)	• Balloon occlusion of the GRS (with balloon manipulation) • Collateral vein embolization or sclerosis • BATO debranching
4.	Balloon-occluded retrograde venography	
5.	Sclerosant administration (see ▸ Figs. 29.22, 29.23)	• Preferably microcatheter catheterization of the gastric variceal system • Preferably even distribution of the sclerosant mixture
6.	Additional intraprocedural imaging (if any) (see ▸ Fig. 29.19c-e)	• Cone-beam dynamic computed tomography • Hemodynamic analysis and imaging
7.	Indwelling sclerosant with indwelling temporary balloon or balloon-occlusion catheter	
8.	Deflation of balloon (deflation of balloon-occlusion catheter)	

BATO: balloon-occluded antegrade transvenous obliteration; GRS: gastrorenal shunt; IVC; inferior vena cava.
Reproduced with permission from Saad WE, Kitanosono T, Koizumi J, Hirota S. The conventional balloon-occluded retrograde transvenous obliteration procedure: indications, contraindications and technical applications. Tech Vasc Intervent Radiol 2013;16:101–151.

Technique of the Balloon-Occluded Retrograde Transvenous Obliteration Procedure

The hemodynamic endpoint of BRTO is the complete obliteration of the gastric varices while preserving the anatomical hepatopetal flow through the splenoportal veins. The concept of BRTO (▸ Fig. 29.1; ▸ Fig. 29.2) is to access and occlude the GRS with subsequent reflux of sclerosant throughout the gastric variceal system without spillage into the portal circulation.[2–4] The basic steps of the BRTO procedure are listed and summarized in ▸ Table 29.1. The following is a detailed description of the procedural steps of BRTO of gastric varices. For the inventory used, particularly balloon-occlusion catheters and sclerosants, see Saad et al.[10]

The operator should note that in the setting of active gastric variceal bleeding, transoral gastric tamponade insufflation balloons (e.g., the Blakemore tube) should be used. However, if the gastric Blakemore tube is placed and inflated, it is of utmost importance that the gastric balloon be deflated (intraprocedurally) during the catheterization stage of the BRTO procedure; if inflated, the balloon compresses and distorts the varices and creates additional difficult anatomy for the BRTO procedure (▸ Fig. 29.4). Additionally, the compression of the gastric varices by the Blakemore balloon will not allow for adequate filling of the varices by the sclerosant, even with appropriate balloon occlusion of the gastrorenal shunt, and complete obliteration or sclerosis of the gastric varices will be virtually impossible. As a result of incomplete obliteration, if bleeding continues after the BRTO, then a balloon-occluded antegrade transvenous obliteration, TIPS, or both is required because the draining GRS at that point will be sclerosed or thrombosed.

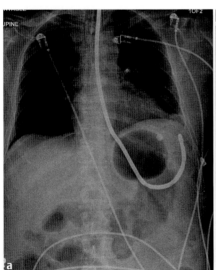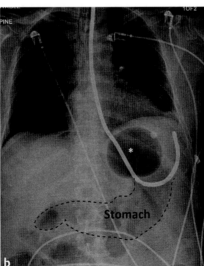

Fig. 29.4 Balloon-occluded retrograde transvenous obliteration (BRTO) attempt in the presence of an inflated Blakemore (gastric or fundic) balloon. (The balloon must be deflated.) Chest radiography with the upper abdomen with a Blakemore tube inflated (**a,b**) and pulled back in the stomach fundus (*asterisk*). (*continued*)

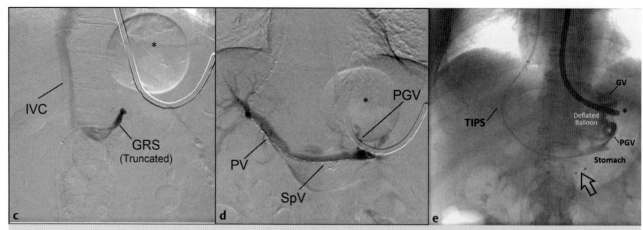

Fig. 29.4 *(Continued)* **(c,d)** Digital subtraction venograms, one from the gastrorenal shunt **(c**, GRS) and a splenoportogram **(d)**. In both venograms the portal feeders in the splenoportogram **(d)**, which is the posterior gastric vein (PGV) or the gastric varices (GVs) drainer, which is the GRS, are truncated because of the significant compressive nature of the fundic balloon *(asterisk)*. The gastric varices themselves (not visualized) are completely compressed (which is the purpose of the balloon). It is paramount that the gastric balloon be deflated (intraprocedurally) during the early part (catheterization stage) of the BRTO procedure. An inflated gastric balloon compresses the gastric varices and distorts, or even compresses, the GRS anatomy, making the BRTO procedure difficult or impossible. In addition, even in the advent of balloon occluding the GRS, inadequate filling of the GVs by the sclerosant will occur because the GVs are compressed. As a result, complete obliteration or sclerosis of the GVs is virtually impossible in the presence of an inflated balloon. IVC: inferior vena cava; PV: main portal vein; SpV: splenic vein. **(e)** Selective venogram of the PGV leading to the GVs, which are in the gastric fundus *(asterisk)*. The fundic balloon has been deflated to allow visualization of the GVs. The PGV is selected from a balloon-occluded antegrade transvenous obliteration (BATO) approach via a newly established transjugular intrahepatic portosystemic shunt (trans-TIPS BATO). In addition, note the BRTO balloon *(open arrow)*. *(Reproduced with permission from Saad WE, Kitanosono T, Koizumi J, Hirota S. The conventional balloon-occluded retrograde transvenous obliteration procedure: indications, contraindications and technical applications. Tech Vasc Intervent Radiol 2013;16:101–151.)*

Access and Approach

For conventional BRTO (via the GRS), the approach is invariably transrenal to the GRS.[2-5] However, the access and approach to the left renal vein can be transfemoral or transjugular[2-4,6,11-16] (▶ Fig. 29.1; ▶ Fig. 29.2). The transjugular approach is advantageous in that it is less likely to introduce infection compared with the transfemoral approach and is likely better tolerated by the patient. Bacteremia suspected from the indwelling balloon has been described in 2.4% of cases.[11] However, the transjugular approach requires longer reinforced sheaths to reach the GRS (at least 50- to 55-cm length), which may not be easily available to all operators. Conversely, the transfemoral approach requires shorter reinforced sheaths (40- to 45-cm length) and frees the right internal jugular vein for additional access, particularly when adjunctive transcaval phrenic vein embolization is required or for additional TIPS creation. The primary advantage of the transfemoral approach is the "pushability" of the coaxial wire and catheter system. Selection of the left renal vein and GRS from a jugular approach usually requires Cobra-shaped selective catheters and balloon-occlusion catheters. Alternatively, a Simmons-shaped catheter is usually required to select the GRS from a femoral approach, although Cobra-shaped catheters may also be used.

The distance between the common stump (of the left adrenal vein and GRS) and the inferior vena cava (IVC) can vary. Additionally, the origin of the common stump may vary in angulation as it arises from the superior aspect of the left renal vein (▶ Fig. 29.5; ▶ Fig. 29.6). The GRS is easier to select from a femoral approach when it is situated closer to the IVC and has a steeper (more perpendicular) angle with relation to the renal vein. Conversely, selection of the GRS is easier from the jugular approach when it originates farther from the IVC and has a shallower (more

parallel) angle with the left renal vein (▶ Fig. 29.6). However, this anatomical and technical divide may be moot when using the transfemoral pullback straight-sheath selection approach described later.

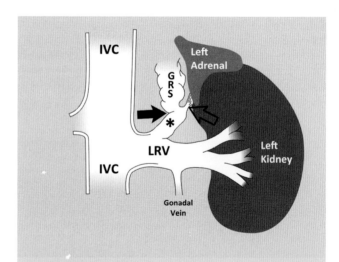

Fig. 29.5 Anatomy of the distal gastrorenal shunt (GRS) and its venous outflow. The GRS commonly does not empty directly into the left renal vein (LRV) but actually empties in the LRV via a common stump *(asterisk)* with the left adrenal vein *(open arrow)*. Commonly, there is a weblike narrowing *(solid black arrow)* at the junction of the GRS (the GRS proper) with the common trunk *(asterisk)*. IVC: inferior vena cava. *(Reproduced with permission from Saad WE, Kitanosono T, Koizumi J, Hirota S. The conventional balloon-occluded retrograde transvenous obliteration procedure: indications, contraindications and technical applications. Tech Vasc Intervent Radiol 2013;16:101–151.)*

Catheter Selection of the Gastrorenal Shunt

The selection of the GRS is actually a three-step process, and any one of the steps can pose a significant technical challenge to the catheter selection process. The three-in-one selection includes (i) from the IVC to the left renal vein, (ii) from the left renal vein to the common stump of the left adrenal vein and the GRS, and (iii) from the common stump to the GRS proper (▶ Fig. 29.7). The complexity of the selection is because the GRS is commonly a

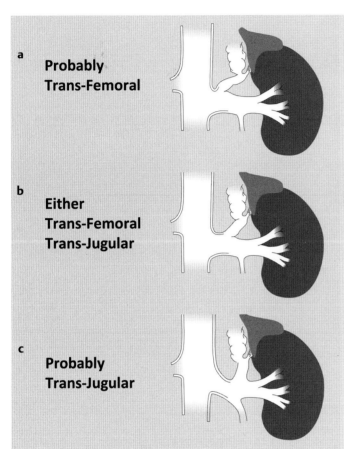

Fig. 29.6 Choice of approach (transjugular or transfemoral) based on the varying anatomy of the distal gastrorenal shunt (GRS) and its venous outflow. The GRS commonly does not empty directly into the left renal vein (LRV) but actually empties in the LRV via a common stump with the left adrenal vein. For labeling of anatomical structure, see ▶ Fig. 29.5. (a) The takeoff of the common stump of the GRS is close to the junction of the LRV with the inferior vena cava (IVC) and makes a shallower angle (more parallel to the LRV) with the LRV. Catheterization in this setting is more favorable via a transfemoral approach. The primary factor for a transfemoral approach here is the short distance between the GRS (common stump) and the IVC. (b) The takeoff of the common stump of the GRS is more or less midway between the LRV–IVC junction and the left renal hilum. In addition, the GRS makes a shallower angle (more parallel to the LRV) with the LRV. This anatomical setting is between ▶ Fig. 29.6a and Fig. 29.6c, and catheterization in this setting can be via a transfemoral or transjugular approach (depending on operator preference and availability of inventory). (c) The takeoff of the common stump of the GRS is a distance from the junction of the LRV with the IVC and makes a steep angle (more perpendicular to the LRV) with the LRV. Catheterization in this setting is more favorable via a transjugular approach. (*Reproduced with permission from Saad WE, Kitanosono T, Koizumi J, Hirota S. The conventional balloon-occluded retrograde transvenous obliteration procedure: indications, contraindications and technical applications. Tech Vasc Intervent Radiol 2013;16:101–151.*)

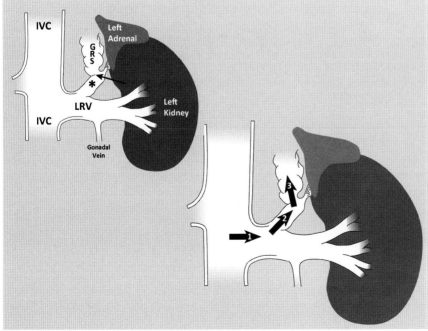

Fig. 29.7 Catheter selection steps of the gastrorenal shunt (GRS) from the inferior vena cava (IVC). The GRS commonly does not empty directly into the left renal vein (LRV) but actually empties in the LRV via a common stump (*asterisk*) with the left adrenal vein. Commonly, there is a weblike narrowing (*solid black arrow*) at the junction of the GRS (the GRS proper) with the common trunk (*asterisk*). From the IVC, the operator should select three catheter selections from the IVC to the LRV (*arrow in step 1*), from the LRV to the common trunk of the adrenal vein and the GRS (*arrow in step 2*), and from the common stump to the GRS proper (*arrow in step 3*). (*Reproduced with permission from Saad WE, Kitanosono T, Koizumi J, Hirota S. The conventional balloon-occluded retrograde transvenous obliteration procedure: indications, contraindications and technical applications. Tech Vasc Intervent Radiol 2013;16:101–151.*)

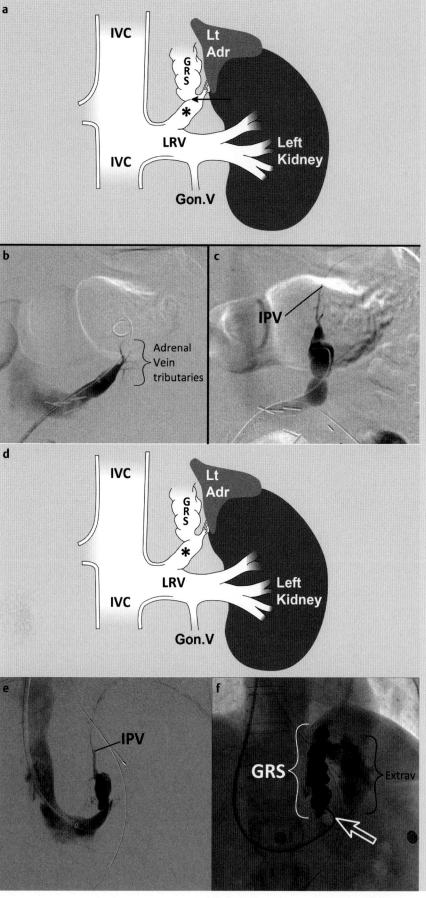

Fig. 29.8 Varying anatomy of the distal gastrorenal shunt (GRS) and its venous outflow in different patients. (**a**) The GRS commonly does not empty directly into the left renal vein (LRV) but actually empties in the LRV via a common stump (*asterisk*) with the left adrenal vein. Commonly, there is a weblike narrowing (*solid black arrow*) at the junction of the GRS (the GRS proper) with the common trunk (*asterisk*). IVC: inferior vena cava. (**b**) Venogram of the common stump refluxing contrast into the smaller adrenal veins (tributaries). Neither the GRS proper nor its effect (inflow or wash-in) is visualized in this venogram. (**c**) Venogram in a completely different patient from (**b**) of the common stump and distal GRS refluxing contrast into inferior phrenic vein (IPV). The common stump is seen inferiorly with the adrenal vein stump barely visualized (*arrow*). (**d**) See (**a**) for labeling. (**e**) Venogram in a completely different patient from (**a-c**) of the common stump and distal GRS refluxing contrast into the IPV. The common stump is seen inferior to the GRS proper with a web-narrowing in between *arrows* (**g,h**). (**f**) Balloon-occluded retrograde venogram (BORV) of the gastric variceal system in the same patient as in (**e,g,h**). The occlusive balloon (*open arrow*) of the balloon-occlusion catheter is filled with air. Contrast is seen filling the GRS and is also seen extravasating (Extrav) from the gastric varices into the fundus of the stomach. (*continued*)

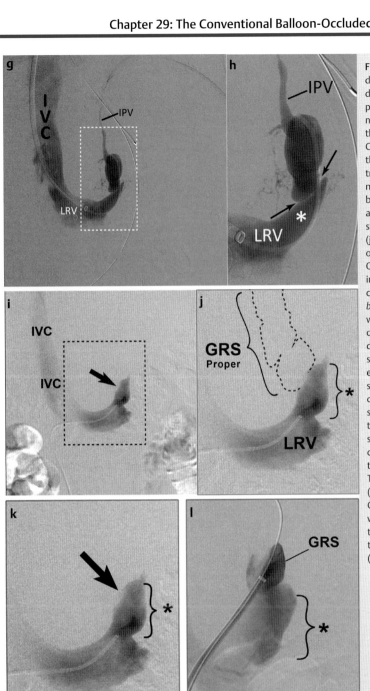

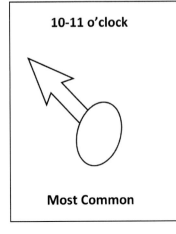

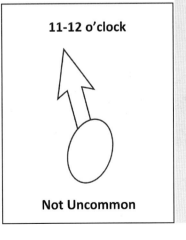

Fig. 29.8 (*Continued*) (**g**) Venogram in the same patient as (**d-f**) detailing the venographic anatomy of the common stump and distal GRS (**h** is a magnified inset). The catheter is in the distal GRS proper and has reached there by being advanced through a web narrowing (*between solid arrows*, **h**). Contrast is seen refluxing into the IPV and emptying into the common stump (*asterisk*) of the GRS and the adrenal vein(s). The common stump empties into the LRV and subsequently the IVC. Web narrowings are difficult to traverse with catheters and wires. However, when traversed, they make very effective "choke points" that do not necessarily require balloon sizes greater than 10 mm to occlude (**f**). (**i**) Venogram in a completely different patient from parts **b** and **c** of the common stump and distal GRS and the adrenal vein with a magnified inset (**j**) via a Simmons II catheter. Contrast is seen in the common outflow stump (*asterisk*) of the adrenal vein and the GRS proper. Occasionally, the GRS is not seen, but its effect (wash-in) is seen in the venogram of the common stump. Operators must be cognizant of this and identify it. Identifying the wash-in (**i**, *solid black arrow*) of the GRS is important because it tells the operator where to direct the selection catheter and wire to selectively catheterize the GRS proper. The GRS proper is not seen but is drawn out in (**j**). The GRS proper merges with the common stump at different angles and approaches (see **k-n** for detailed examples). (**k-n**) The GRS proper merges with the common stump at different angles and approaches. These are different common stump venograms with accompanying simplified schematic demonstrating the different angles and approaches for the merging of the GRS proper with the common venous outflow stump of the GRS proper and the left adrenal vein. (**k**) The most common relationship in which the GRS proper anastomoses at the 10 to 11 o'clock position with the common stump (*asterisk*). The *solid black arrow* denotes the inflow of the GRS proper (**i,j**). (**l**) Demonstrates another very common relationship where the GRS proper (GRS) anastomosis at the 11 to 12 o'clock position with the common stump (*asterisk*). The GRS is right on top of the common stump but because the adrenal vein comes from the lateral aspect of the stump the GRS is inclined medially. (*continued*)

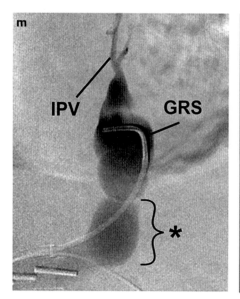

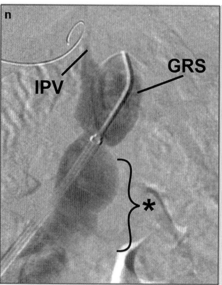

Fig. 29.8 (*Continued*) (**m**) A frequent relationship in which the GRS proper (GRS) anastomoses at the 12 o'clock position with the common stump (*asterisk*). Incidentally noted is contrast reflux into the IPV. (**n**) The least frequent relationship in which the GRS proper (GRS) anastomoses at the 12 to 1 o'clock position with the common stump (*asterisk*). (*Reproduced with permission from Saad WE, Kitanosono T, Koizumi J, Hirota S. The conventional balloon-occluded retrograde transvenous obliteration procedure: indications, contraindications and technical applications. Tech Vasc Intervent Radiol 2013;16:101–151.*)

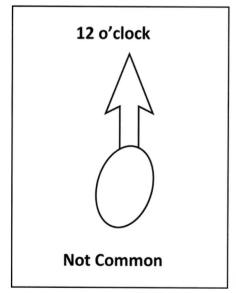

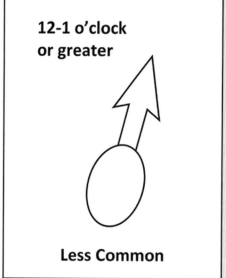

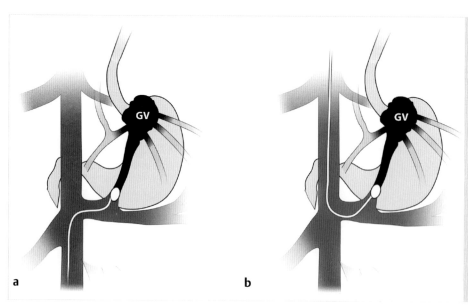

Fig. 29.9 Catheter shape and selection of the gastrorenal shunt (GRS). (**a**) Illustration of a femoral approach balloon-occluded retrograde transvenous obliteration (BRTO) for obliteration of gastric varices (GVs). (**b**) Illustration of a jugular approach BRTO for obliteration of GVs.

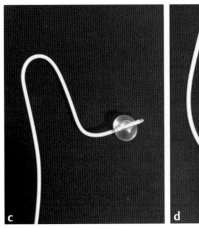
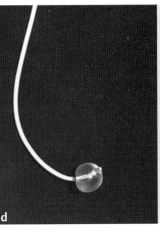

Fig. 29.9 (*Continued*) (**c**) Photograph of a Simmons II-shaped balloon occlusion catheter (Terumo, Tokyo, Japan), which is typically used in Japan for a femoral approach BRTO. (**d**) Photograph of a Cobra-shaped balloon occlusion catheter (Terumo, Tokyo, Japan), which is typically used in Japan for a jugular approach BRTO. (*Reproduced with permission from Saad WE, Kitanosono T, Koizumi J, Hirota S. The conventional balloon-occluded retrograde transvenous obliteration procedure: indications, contraindications and technical applications. Tech Vasc Intervent Radiol 2013;16:101–151.*)

gastroadrenorenal shunt (▶ Fig. 29.8) where the gastric variceal drainage (the shunt) merges with the left adrenal vein to form a common stump (*asterisks* in ▶ Fig. 29.5 and ▶ Fig. 29.8).

For the purpose of the anatomical description below, the portosystemic shunt draining the gastric varices into the "common gastroadrenal stump/common stump" is referred to as the GRS proper. Occasionally, there is little discernible difference between the common stump and the GRS proper. However, not infrequently, a web is found across the junction of the GRS proper with the adrenal vein stump (▶ Fig. 29.8), which is difficult to catheterize, especially when there is very little wire and catheter "purchase" into the common stump. For further details of this anatomy, please see Chapter 28.

When no discernible difference between the adrenal vein stump and the GRS proper (and no web narrowing) is found, it is easy to make this three-stage selection using a Cobra- or

Simmons-shaped balloon-occlusion catheter from a transjugular or transfemoral approach, respectively (▶ Fig. 29.9). However, because these balloon-occlusion catheters are not currently available in the United States, American interventionalists have to selectively catheterize the GRS proper with a selective catheter and then perform an over-wire exchange for one of the commercially available straight balloon-occlusion catheters. This exchange requires adequate stiff wire "purchase" in an area of anatomy that may not allow a lot of wire purchase. Certain techniques described later can be used to selectively catheterize the GRS proper and advance a reinforced sheath and balloon-occlusion catheter in the setting of difficult anatomy.

As discussed, Cobra-shaped catheters are typically used to select the GRS from the transjugular approach (▶ Fig. 29.10). However, the Cobra catheter may also be helpful in selecting the GRS proper from the common stump in the presence of a web

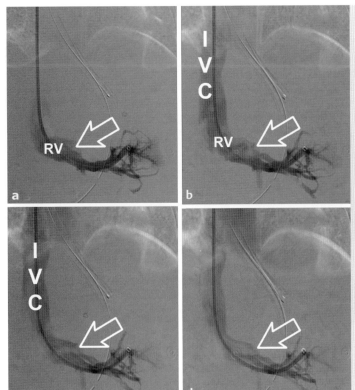

Fig. 29.10 Cobra-shaped catheter for selection of the gastrorenal shunt (GRS) from the jugular approach. (**a-d**) Four images in sequence of a digital subtraction venogram through a reinforced sheath (Cook Corp, Bloomington, IN), which is advanced in the left renal hilum from a jugular approach. Noted in these images is an inflow wash-in effect (*open white arrow*) of the GRS as it empties in the left renal vein (RV) and subsequently into the inferior vena cava (IVC). (*continued*)

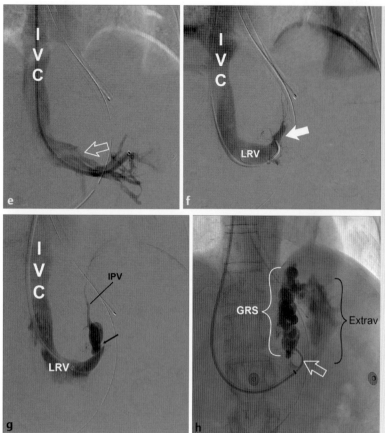

Fig. 29.10 *(Continued)* **(e,f)** Selective venograms during catheterization of the GRS. The operator identifies the GRS site from the inflow (wash-in) that was seen initially (**a-e**, *open white arrow*). The stump of the common trunk of the GRS proper and the adrenal vein is noted (**f**, *solid white arrow*). **(g,h)** Selective venograms during catheterization of the GRS beyond a web-narrowing (**g**, *solid black arrow*). Contrast is seen opacifying the inferior phrenic vein (IPV). Contrast is seen emptying into the left renal vein (LRV) and subsequently the inferior vena cava (IVC). The web narrowing is a hindrance to catheterization; however, after it is transgressed, it is a perfect choke point for balloon occlusion as seen in (**h**). **(h)** The balloon is inflated with air and contrast is seen opacifying the GRS. In addition, there is extravasation (Extrav) of contrast from the GRS (from the gastric varices specifically) and into the gastric lumen. *(Reproduced with permission from Saad WE, Kitanosono T, Koizumi J, Hirota S. The conventional balloon-occluded retrograde transvenous obliteration procedure: indications, contraindications and technical applications. Tech Vasc Intervent Radiol 2013;16:101–151.)*

narrowing at the GRS proper to common stump junction from a femoral approach. The Cobra shape helps catheterize the left renal vein. Next, the Cobra catheter is then flipped upward so that it "scrapes" the superior aspect of the left renal vein as it is pulled back until it selects the upward-pointing common stump. A JB-2 catheter may also be used without the need to flip the catheter upward. If the left renal vein has been successfully selected and there is room to form a reverse-shaped catheter, it can be used to select the common stump. A reverse-shaped catheter is especially helpful in selection if the common stump or the GRS proper points

medially in the 9 to 11 o'clock position (▶ Fig. 29.8d; ▶ Fig. 29.8e). Reverse-shaped catheters that can be formed in the left renal vein include a Simmons I or an SOS-shaped catheter. A reverse-shaped Simmons II catheter is ideal for selecting the GRS in a picturesque manner (▶ Fig. 29.11).

However, in the author's opinion (WES), selection of the GRS with a Simmons II catheter provides little wire purchase for an exchange, especially in the setting of a web narrowing that is difficult to transgress. ▶ Fig. 29.11 demonstrates an infrequently achieved selection while highlighting how difficult it is to

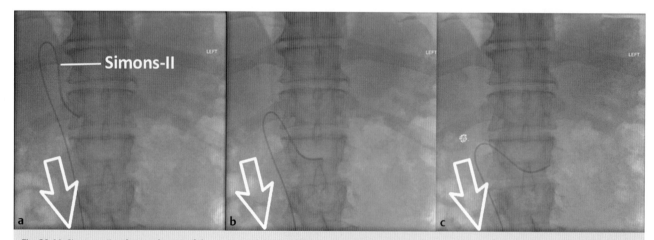

Fig. 29.11 Simmons II catheter selection of the gastrorenal shunt (GRS) from the inferior vena cava (IVC) via a femoral approach. **(a-f)** A series of fluoroscopic images obtained during GRS selection using a 5-Fr Simmons II–shaped catheter. Because of the shape of the Simmons II catheter, it selects the left renal vein (LRV) and the GRS. *(continued)*

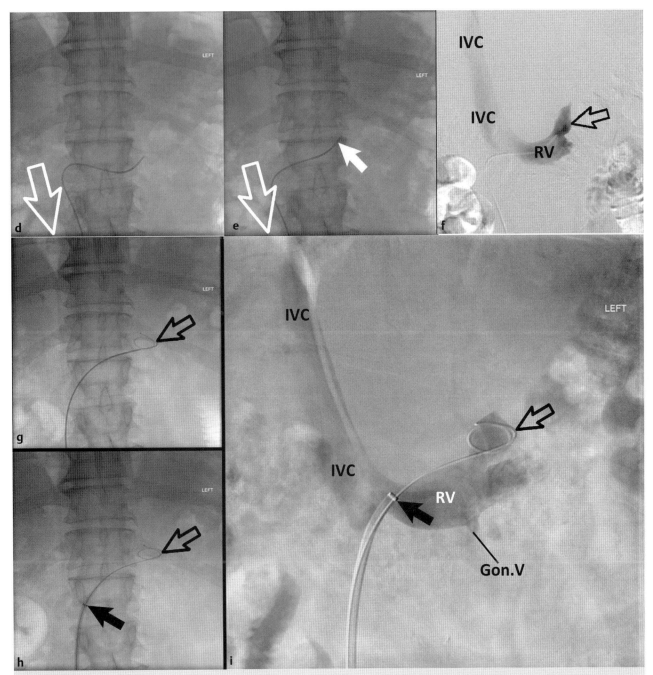

Fig. 29.11 (*Continued*) The Simmons II catheter is formed easily within the suprarenal IVC (because the IVC is usually wide and patulous) and is then pulled down (**a-e**, *open white directional arrow*) with it pointing toward the left (toward the LRV). As the catheter engages the left renal vein (**b,c**), it is pulled down farther (**d,e**, *open white directional arrow*) so that it points upward (**e**, *solid white arrow*) and selects the common stump (**f**, *open black arrow*) of the GRS and the left adrenal vein. The digitally subtracted venogram (**f**) demonstrates the commons stump (*open black arrow*) with contrast emptying into the left renal vein (RV) and IVC. The GRS proper is not visualized. The advantage of utilizing a Simmons II reverse curve catheter from the IVC is that it is more stable and selects the LRV and GRS in one step (by forming it in the IVC and pulling down). (**g-i**) After the Simmons II catheter has selected the common stump of the GRS proper and left adrenal vein, a superstiff Amplatz wire (*open black arrow*) is advanced to achieve wire purchase so that the Simmons II catheter can be exchanged for the straight balloon-occlusion catheter. The advancement of a reinforced sheath (**h,i**, *solid black arrow*) also helps with the exchange of the Simmons II catheter for the balloon-occlusion catheter. This needs to be done in the United States because we do not have Simmons II–shaped balloon-occlusion catheters as the one photographed in (**b**). The digitally subtracted venogram (**i**) through the reinforced sheath (*solid black arrow*) shows how tenuous the wire purchase can be. Rarely does the operator catch a break when the Amplatz wire actually glides into the GRS proper or a phrenic vein and provides adequate wire purchase for an exchange as seen in ▶ Fig. 29.12. (**i**) Contrast is seen filling the common stump of the GRS proper and the left adrenal vein with the Amplatz wire within it (*open black arrow*), the left RV, and the IVC. Incidentally noted is a small part of the left gonadal vein (Gon.V). (*Reproduced with permission from Saad WE, Kitanosono T, Koizumi J, Hirota S. The conventional balloon-occluded retrograde transvenous obliteration procedure: indications, contraindications and technical applications. Tech Vasc Intervent Radiol 2013;16:101–151.*)

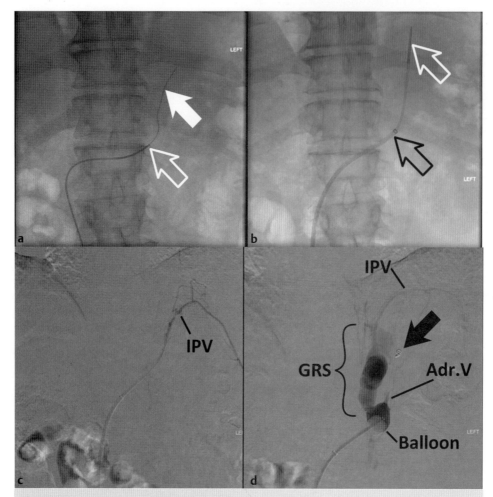

Fig. 29.12 Simmons II catheter selection of the gastrorenal shunt (GRS) from the inferior vena cava (IVC) via a femoral approach with fortuitous wire purchase in one of the phrenic veins. (**a-d**) A series of images obtained during GRS selection using a 5-Fr Simmons II–shaped catheter. Because of the shape of the Simmons II catheter, it selects the left renal vein (LRV) and the GRS. The Simmons II catheter is formed easily within the suprarenal IVC (because the IVC is usually wide and patulous) and is then pulled down with it pointing toward the left (toward the LRV). As the catheter engages the left renal vein, it is pulled down farther so that it points upward (**a**, *open white arrow*) and selects the common stump. Fortuitously, the Amplatz wire (**a**, *solid white arrow*) has passed into a phrenic vein instead of coiling in the common stump as is the case in (**b**). This allows the catheter (**a,b**, *open white arrow*) and reinforced sheath (**b**, *open black arrow*) to be advanced over the Amplatz wire. The other advantage to getting immediate inferior phrenic vein (**c**, IPV) access besides wire purchase is that coil embolization (**d**, *solid black arrow*) can be performed as a final step before the exchange of the catheter for the balloon occlusion catheter. (**d**) Demonstrates a balloon-occlusion retrograde venogram (BORV) of the GRS. The balloon is inflated in the common stump of the GRS proper (GRS) and the left adrenal vein (Adr.V). Contrast is still seen filling another IPV in addition to the IPV that was embolized (*solid black arrow*). For continuation of this case, see ▶ Fig. 29.17. (*Reproduced with permission from Saad WE, Kitanosono T, Koizumi J, Hirota S. The conventional balloon-occluded retrograde transvenous obliteration procedure: indications, contraindications and technical applications. Tech Vasc Intervent Radiol 2013;16:101–151.*)

acquire wire purchase for a sheath or balloon-occlusion catheter exchange. The operator may catch a lucky break where an Amplatz wire can be advanced through the selection catheter (usually a Simmons II catheter via a femoral approach) and passes straight into a phrenic vein. Access to the phenic vein should provide adequate wire purchase for catheter exchange, sheath advancement, and subsequent balloon-occlusion catheter advancement (▶ Fig. 29.12).

One of the current authors (WES) uses another technique for the selection of the GRS from a femoral approach, called the pull-back reinforced straight-sheath (PRESS) technique (▶ Fig. 29.13).

The first step of the technique involves selective catheterization of the left renal vein using, for example, a Cobra-shaped catheter. Next, a Rosen wire (Cook Corp., Bloomington, Indiana) is placed deep in the renal hilum. However, if possible, it would be best if the Rosen wire were placed in a left gonadal vein or a left-sided IVC. A 9- or 10-Fr, 38- to 45-cm reinforced sheath (9-Fr or 10-Fr TIPS Sheath, Cook Corp.) is advanced over the Rosen wire (▶ Fig. 29.13a). Next, the sheath dilator is removed. The sheath is then pulled back as the operator injects contrast through the sheath. As the sheath is retracted, its tip scrapes the superior aspect of the left renal vein and selects the common stump of the GRS. The position of the sheath with the GRS is confirmed with contrast injection (▶ Fig. 29.13b; ▶ Fig. 29.13c). Even if the sheath does not pop directly into the GRS, its tip is usually in near-enough proximity to allow visualization of the GRS by angiography. At this point, the operator advances a 5-Fr angled tip vertebral catheter (▶ Fig. 29.13d; ▶ Fig. 29.13e) or an SOS-shaped catheter beyond the web narrowing into the GRS (▶ Fig. 29.13f; ▶ Fig. 29.13g).

Together, the Rosen wire and reinforced sheath provide a stable platform that supports the selective catheterization of the GRS and maintains transfemoral access into the left renal vein. Sheath access into the left femoral vein can be easily lost if the GRS is near the IVC. The presence of the safety Rosen wire allows for easy reestablishment of left renal vein catheterization, if necessary. After the GRS proper has been selected and

adequate catheter purchase has been achieved, a coiled-tip Amplatz or super-stiff Amplatz wire (Cook, Corp.) is advanced into the GRS proper (▶ Fig. 29.13g). A Rosen or any J-tipped wire is not preferred because anecdotally, they may cause extravasation and spasm; therefore, a straight-tip stiff wire is preferred. When wire access into the GRS is stabilized with a stiff guidewire, the safety Rosen wire can be removed to allow advancement of the reinforced sheath into the GRS with its dilator. Together, the stiff wire and reinforced sheath provide support for the advancement of most balloon-occlusion catheters. Alternatively, if the sheath is sufficiently sized (usually at least 10 Fr), a low-profile balloon-occlusion catheter (maximum of 7-Fr, 8- to 10-mm balloon) can be advanced without removal of the safety Rosen wire (▶ Fig. 29.13g).

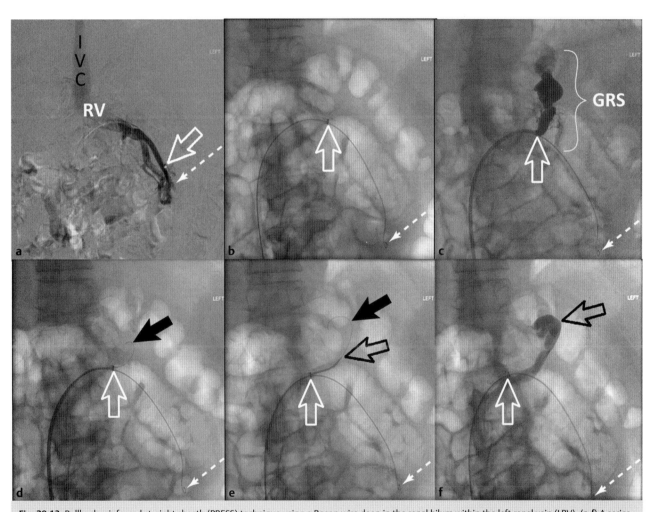

Fig. 29.13 Pullback reinforced straight sheath (PRESS) technique using a Rosen wire deep in the renal hilum within the left renal vein (LRV). (**a-f**) A series of images obtained during gastrorenal shunt (GRS) selection using a 10-Fr reinforced (braided) sheath passed over a Rosen wire that is placed in the LRV. The operator advances the reinforced sheath (9- or 10-Fr braided 38- to 45-cm-long sheath, Cook Corp. Bloomington, Indiana) (*open white arrow*) over the 0.035-inch Rosen wire (*dashed white arrow*), which has been placed in the left renal vein by a 5-Fr Cobra catheter selection earlier. A gonadal or left-sided IVC is preferable, but a deep purchase of the LRV (lower renal poll) works as well. This is because the straight reinforced sheath needs to be bowed so that it "scrapes" the ceiling of the left renal vein as it is pulled back (**b,c**). As the sheath is pulled back, contrast is injected until the GRS is visualized. Occasionally, the sheath pops in the GRS and "autoselects" the GRS as seen in (**c**). However, even if the sheath does not select the GRS, the GRS is frequently visualized with contrast and allows planning for catheterization. After the GRS is catheterized and visualized, a selection catheter can be used to obtain wire and catheter access of the GRS. Usually, the catheter (usually a 5-Fr angled tip as in **d-f**, *open black arrow*, but can be a reverse-curve catheter such as an SOS omni selective catheter) is advanced through the reinforced sheath and adjacent to the safety or anchoring Rosen wire (*dashed white arrow*) as seen in (**d-f**). When catheterizing using the selection catheter, a 0.035-inch hydrophilic guidewire (**d,e**, *solid black arrow*) is usually used carefully as to not cause perforations in the GRS. The Rosen wire acts as a safety to maintain access to the LRV but also acts as an anchoring stabilizer throughout the catheterization and is removed just before the advancement of the sheath into the GRS. (*continued*)

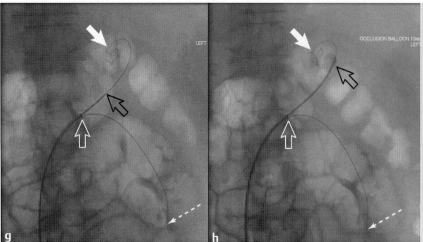

Fig. 29.13 (*Continued*) (**g,h**) After the catheter is advanced into the GRS (**g**, *open black arrow*) and venography has confirmed that the catheter is truly in the GRS and not an adjacent venous system, an Amplatz wire is advanced in the GRS (*solid white arrow*). If the balloon occlusion catheter (**h**, *open black arrow*) is small enough (low profile), it can also be advanced adjacent to the anchoring Rosen wire (**h**, *dashed white arrows*). (*Reproduced with permission from Saad WE, Kitanosono T, Koizumi J, Hirota S. The conventional balloon-occluded retrograde transvenous obliteration procedure: indications, contraindications and technical applications. Tech Vasc Intervent Radiol 2013;16:101–151.*)

Rarely, the GRS merges (anastomoses) with the inferior aspect of the left renal vein via a common trunk with the left gonadal vein, rather than along the superior aspect of the renal vein via a common trunk with the left renal vein. This poses a particularly difficult catheterization, especially from the femoral approach. A transjugular approach is probably easier to catheterize these GRSs.

Gastric Variceal System Occlusion "Trapping"

"Trapping" refers to the cessation of flow within the gastric variceal system. This part of the BRTO procedure includes numerous technical categories of which only one or possibly all may need to be used to achieve adequate gastric variceal system obliteration, particularly based on the size and complexity of the gastric variceal system (▶ Fig. 29.14). These technical categories include (i) balloon positioning and manipulation, (ii) venous collateral embolization or obliteration, (iii) adjunctive balloon inflation (BRTO or BATO), and (iv) confirmation balloon-occluded retrograde venography (BORV). As previously mentioned, the patient may have a gastric Blakemore tube in place; if so, it should be deflated during the trapping stage of the BRTO procedure (▶ Fig. 29.4). An inflated gastric balloon compresses the gastric varices and distorts, or even compresses, the GRS, making the BRTO procedure difficult or impossible (see earlier).

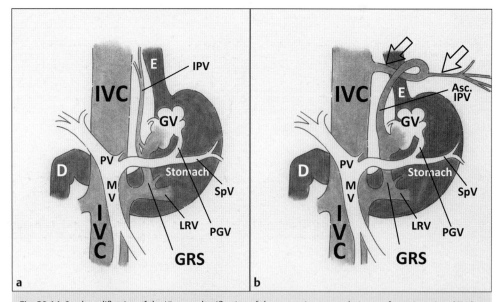

Fig. 29.14 Saad modification of the Kiyosue classification of the systemic venous drainage of gastric varices (GVs). (**a**) The anatomy of GVs and the draining systemic veins, which includes the draining gastrorenal shunt (GRS), if present. The image is to help identify structures in the classification in (**c**). The primary difference between (**a**) and (**b**) is the size and morphology of the inferior phrenic vein (IPV). The IPV has a vertical part and a horizontally oriented subdiaphragmatic transverse part (*open black arrows*). The vertical part is composed of an ascending portion (Asc. IPV) and a descending portion. When the descending portion anastomoses with the adrenal vein, it forms the GRS. Asc. IPV: ascending portion of the vertical part of the inferior phrenic vein; D: duodenum; E: esophagus; IVC: inferior vena cava; LRV: left renal vein; MV: mesenteric vein; PGV: posterior gastric vein; PV: main portal vein; SpV, splenic vein. (*continued*)

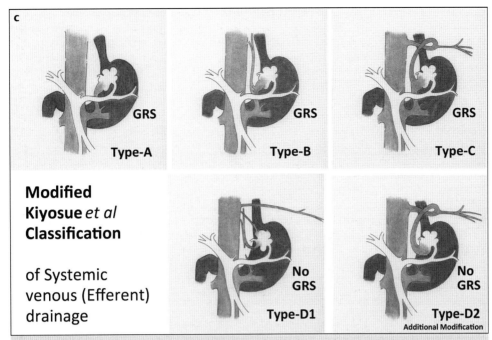

Fig. 29.14 (*Continued*) (**c**) Schematic classification based on the anatomical classification of Kiyosue et al.[4] Type A is the simplest gastric variceal system drained by the GRS and without other systemic venous draining veins (significant or insignificant). Type B is a simple gastric variceal system drained by the GRS and with insignificant (nondecompressive) systemic venous draining veins, which are typically inferior phrenic veins but can also be other retroperitoneal veins (innominate veins, hemiazygous tributaries, intercostal veins, and adrenal veins) (see **a** for detailed labeling). Type C is a more complex gastric variceal system drained by the GRS and with an additional significant (decompressive) systemic venous draining vein (inferior phrenic vein, usually >3 mm in diameter, Saad interpretation of diameter estimate) (see **b** for detailed labeling). Type D is a gastric variceal system that is not drained by the GRS. In other words, no GRS exists. However, there is significant systemic venous drainage by other retroperitoneal or phrenic vein(s). In type D1, the decompressive systemic venous draining veins have no particular predominance and include inferior phrenic veins but can also be other retroperitoneal veins such as innominate reroperitoneal veins, hemiazygous tributaries, intercostal veins, and adrenal veins. Type D GVs represent more than 40% of technical failures (Saad type III failure). Type D2 is the same as type D1, but there is a predominant systemic venous draining vein (usually >3 mm in diameter) that can be accessible, and it is amenable to balloon-occluded retrograde transvenous obliteration via unconventional systemic veins. These predominant draining routes include (i) the hemiazygous–azygous axis, (ii) inferior phrenic vein (usually the ascending portion leading to the transverse portion as drawn), and (iii) pericardial vein (or pericardiophrenic vein). (*Reproduced with permission from Saad WE, Kitanosono T, Koizumi J, Hirota S. The conventional balloon-occluded retrograde transvenous obliteration procedure: indications, contraindications and technical applications. Tech Vasc Intervent Radiol 2013;16:101–151.*)

In some patients, trapping of complex gastrosystemic variceal systems may require elaborate accesses and technical approaches. For example, some patients may require the placement of additional balloon occlusions in a second GRS if the system has two, or in a large phrenic or retroperitoneal vein (usually ≥3 mm in size).

Balloon Positioning, Manipulation, and Occlusion

The primary component of the "trapping" step is the use of a balloon-occlusion catheter to occlude the GRS outflow. Knowledge of the commercially available balloon-occlusion catheter inventory is paramount for the planning of the BRTO procedure. The available inventory in the United States and Japan are available for reference.[10] The point of balloon occlusion is cessation of blood flow through the gastric variceal system with minimal escape of sclerosant (as seen with contrast). Simple gastric variceal systems

(particularly from a drainage standpoint) are simply occluded by an adequately sized balloon without the need for adjunctive collateral pathway venous embolization. After the balloon catheter is inflated and occlusion is achieved, previously visualized collaterals may not serve as significant drainage pathways, either because of changed hemodynamics or occlusion of the collaterals by the balloon-occlusion catheter itself.

During "trapping," the balloon-occlusion catheters should be positioned at or just above certain "choke points" in the GRS. These "choke points" are key areas of narrowing (particularly web narrowings) in the GRS. The most common site of weblike narrowing is at the junction between the common trunk of the GRS and the left adrenal vein (▶ Fig. 29.8); however, other areas of narrowing may be found closer to the gastric variceal complex. The balloons can and should be oversized to target the "choke points" because the balloons are compliant and will conform rather than rupture.

Commonly, operators early in their experience with BRTO may believe that occlusion of the variceal system should occur very near to the left renal vein. However, occlusion at the renal vein is not necessarily the best option as long as higher choke points are feasible and can be reached by catheter and wire manipulation. In addition, higher balloon occlusion would be feasible as long as the occlusion does not exclude the gastric varices proper (intragastric submucosal gastric varices). See ▶ Fig. 29.19 for additional details of a high-balloon occlusion, which serves as an example.

If the inflated balloon is too small to occlude high in the GRS, then the balloon should be pulled down to "cork" a lower "choke point" as depicted in the case presented in ▶ Fig. 29.15. Conversely, if the balloon inflated down low (near the left renal vein) is too small to occlude the GRS at that level, then the balloon should be advanced upward beyond a higher choke point and pulled down to "cork" the GRS shown in the case presented in ▶ Fig. 29.16. High balloon occlusion may also be used in an attempt to occlude the outflow higher than the take-off of systemic venous

collaterals, which may act as escape routes for contrast and sclerosant and thus prevent an adequate diagnostic BORV and a completely obliterating (adequate) BRTO, respectively (▶ Fig. 29.17). Occasionally, occluding the GRS outflow high, but not higher than the collateral, may be beneficial. For example, the most cephalad aspect of the balloon may occlude the orifice of the venous collateral, or the altered hemodynamics may be significant enough to have preferential contrast and subsequent sclerosant flow to the GRS instead of the collateral (▶ Fig. 29.18). Balloon inflation at a higher "choke point" has been described to be necessary in 5% of BRTO procedures and has been successful in avoiding collateral embolization.[13]

Another advantage of a higher than usual balloon inflation is reduction of the sclerosant–reagent dose.[16] This was described by Fukuda and coworkers and was referred to as the "downgrade technique."[16] The move toward sclerosant dose reduction stemmed from the use of ethanolamine oleate, which potentially caused hemoglobinuria and renal failure, particularly at dosages

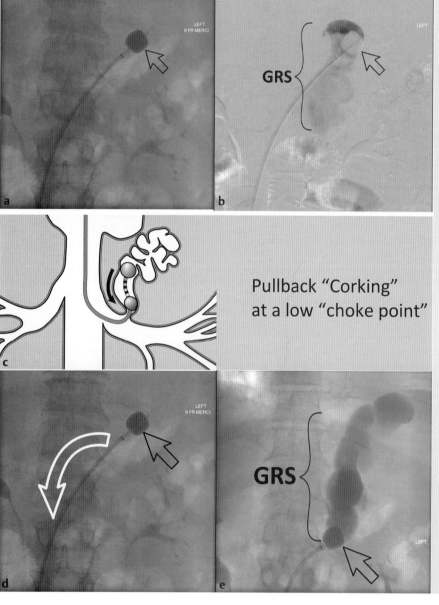

Fig. 29.15 Manipulation of the balloon-occlusion catheter by pulling it down to "cork" a gastric variceal system at a lower "choke point." Fluoroscopic image (a) and digitally subtracted venogram (b) with an inflated high balloon occlusion catheter (*open black arrow*) that is "floating" in a spatial gastrorenal shunt (GRS). (c-e) A depiction of pulling down the balloon to "cork" the GRS to a lower "choke point" instead of having it float up higher in a particular GRS, where it is wider (c). (d) Demonstrates the high balloon (*open black arrow*), and the *curved directional arrow* depicts the action of pulling the balloon occlusion catheter so that it "corks" the GRS as seen in (d). After the balloon (*open arrow*) is brought down to occlude (cork) the GRS where it is narrowed, a complete balloon-occluded retrograde venogram (BORV) is performed, and the entire GRS is visualized. (*continued*)

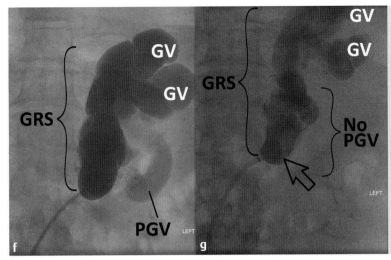

Fig. 29.15 (*Continued*) (**f,g**) Fluoroscopic images during BORV (continued contrast injection from **d**) demonstrating an occlusive balloon (*open arrow*) and resultant opacification of the entire gastric variceal system which is composed of the GRS and the gastric varices (GVs). In addition, the posterior gastric vein (PGV) is visualized descending down to the splenic vein, which is not opacified with contrast. (**g**) Fluoroscopic image after the sclerosant mixture (lipiodol, Sotradecol, air) has been instilled. The balloon is still inflated (*open arrow*). Notice that the posterior gastric vein (PGV) is not visualized. Only the gastric variceal system is filled with the sclerosant. (*Reproduced with permission from Saad WE, Kitanosono T, Koizumi J, Hirota S. The conventional balloon-occluded retrograde transvenous obliteration procedure: indications, contraindications and technical applications. Tech Vasc Intervent Radiol 2013;16:101–151.*)

exceeding 30 to 40 cm.[3–6,16] This has become less of a problem with the advent of foam sclerosants, particularly with detergent agents such as 3% sodium tetradecyl sulfate. In fact, creating a sclerosant mixture in a foam or froth state is in itself another strategy to reduce the sclerosant dosage. ▶ Table 29.2 briefly summarizes the strategies and methods to reduce sclerosant dosages. Details regarding foam sclerosants and their advantages can be found in Saad et al.[10]

Venous Collateral Embolization or Obliteration

Decompressive venous collaterals can vary in number, size, and location, and their presence is the most common cause of technical failure, representing more than 40% of BRTO failures (Saad type III failure).[7] These veins can include adrenal veins (▶ Fig. 29.21), phrenic veins (inferior phrenic or pericardiophrenic) (▶ Fig. 29.17; ▶ Fig. 29.21), or innominate retroperitoneal veins (▶ Fig. 29.18; ▶ Fig. 29.20). These veins do not need to be occluded for ideal gastric variceal system trapping before balloon occlusion. However, in up to 39% of BRTO procedures, these veins are encountered and require embolization, balloon manipulation, or additional balloon occlusion.[11] Balloon occlusion may change the hemodynamics and decompressive nature of the veins, where a previously decompressive vein now serves as an escape route for contrast and sclerosant after the balloon-occlusion catheter is inflated. If there continues to be significant venous collaterals that create preferential flow into them and not into the GRS, then

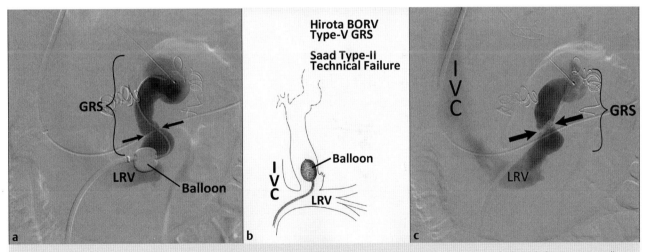

Fig. 29.16 Manipulation of the balloon-occlusion catheter by advancing it higher to "cork" a gastric variceal system at a higher "choke point." Digitally subtracted image (**a**) and a drawing (**b**) depicting the findings in (**a**). The inflated low-lying balloon occlusion catheter is not occlusive and is "floating" in a spatial gastrorenal shunt (GRS). In essence, this is a Hirota balloon-occluded retrograde venography (BORV) type V in which the BORV is not possible because the balloon of the available balloon-occlusion catheter is too small to occlude ("trap") the GRS. This is considered a Saad type II technical failure if occlusion of the GRS is not achieved at a higher point. Proof of poor occlusion of the GRS is contrast emptying in the left renal vein (LRV). Notice that there is a narrowing higher up the GRS (*between the solid black arrows*). (**c**) Subtracted image venogram as the deflated balloon occlusion catheter as it is advanced higher up the GRS and through and above the narrowing described earlier (*between the solid black arrows*). The GRS is not yet occluded (balloon deflated) and thus contrast empties in the LRV and subsequently the inferior vena cava (IVC). (*Reproduced with permission from Saad WE, Kitanosono T, Koizumi J, Hirota S. The conventional balloon-occluded retrograde transvenous obliteration procedure: indications, contraindications and technical applications. Tech Vasc Intervent Radiol 2013;16:101–151.*)

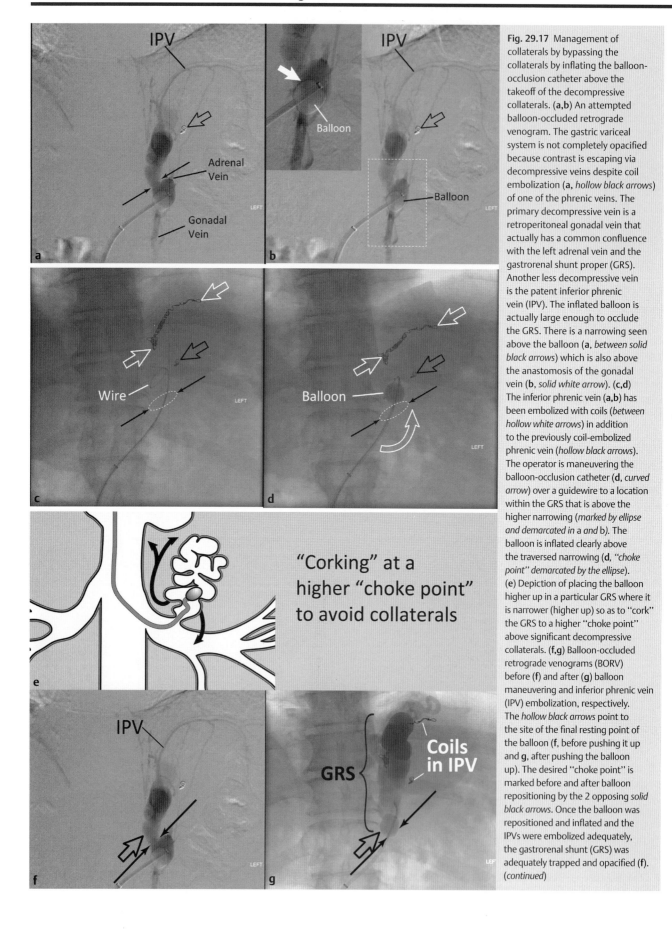

Fig. 29.17 Management of collaterals by bypassing the collaterals by inflating the balloon-occlusion catheter above the takeoff of the decompressive collaterals. (a,b) An attempted balloon-occluded retrograde venogram. The gastric variceal system is not completely opacified because contrast is escaping via decompressive veins despite coil embolization (a, *hollow black arrows*) of one of the phrenic veins. The primary decompressive vein is a retroperitoneal gonadal vein that actually has a common confluence with the left adrenal vein and the gastrorenal shunt proper (GRS). Another less decompressive vein is the patent inferior phrenic vein (IPV). The inflated balloon is actually large enough to occlude the GRS. There is a narrowing seen above the balloon (a, *between solid black arrows*) which is also above the anastomosis of the gonadal vein (b, *solid white arrow*). (c,d) The inferior phrenic vein (a,b) has been embolized with coils (*between hollow white arrows*) in addition to the previously coil-embolized phrenic vein (*hollow black arrows*). The operator is maneuvering the balloon-occlusion catheter (d, *curved arrow*) over a guidewire to a location within the GRS that is above the higher narrowing (*marked by ellipse and demarcated in* a *and* b*).* The balloon is inflated clearly above the traversed narrowing (d, *"choke point" demarcated by the ellipse*). (e) Depiction of placing the balloon higher up in a particular GRS where it is narrower (higher up) so as to "cork" the GRS to a higher "choke point" above significant decompressive collaterals. (f,g) Balloon-occluded retrograde venograms (BORV) before (f) and after (g) balloon maneuvering and inferior phrenic vein (IPV) embolization, respectively. The *hollow black arrows* point to the site of the final resting point of the balloon (f, before pushing it up and g, after pushing the balloon up). The desired "choke point" is marked before and after balloon repositioning by the 2 opposing *solid black arrows*. Once the balloon was repositioned and inflated and the IPVs were embolized adequately, the gastrorenal shunt (GRS) was adequately trapped and opacified (f). (*continued*)

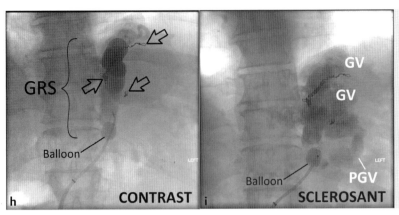

Fig. 29.17 (*Continued*) (**h**) BORV obtained once the gastric variceal system was adequately "trapped" by repositioning the balloon and inflating it and coil embolizing the inferior phrenic veins (*hollow black arrows*). Once adequate "trapping" has been achieved, sclerosant is administered to displace the residual contrast within the gastric variceal system. (**i**) The completion image with the foam sclerosant fully administered in the entire gastric variceal system including the gastric varices (GV) and the afferent posterior gastric vein (PGV). (*Reproduced with permission from Saad WE, Kitanosono T, Koizumi J, Hirota S. The conventional balloon-occluded retrograde transvenous obliteration procedure: indications, contraindications and technical applications. Tech Vasc Intervent Radiol 2013;16:101–151.*)

Table 29.2 Strategies and Methods for Reducing Sclerosant–Reagent in Balloon-Occluded Retrograde Transvenous Obliteration of Gastric Varices

Strategy	Technical Details	Comments
Multiple-session "lavage technique"	Performing the BRTO as need be with a 30- to 40-cc limit per session	• Requires multiple sessions (increased morbidity) • Effective in > 95% of cases within 2 to 3 sessions
Adjunct sclerosant	Using two sclerosants: primary sclerosants and either D50% or ETOH	• May sustain the complications (disadvantages) of both sclerosants • One-session treatment
"Downgrading technique"	Occluding the GRS higher and closer to the GVs and thus "trapping" less of the gastric variceal system and focusing on the GVs themselves	• Not commonly feasible • One-session treatment
Foam or froth sclerosant	Adding a gas (CO_2 or air) to the sclerosant to form a foam (33%–50% gas) or froth (< 33% gas)	• Reduces the sclerosant–reagent dose : volume ratio • May have more even distribution than liquid-state sclerosant mixtures • One-session treatment

BRTO: Balloon-occluded retrograde transvenous obliteration; D50%: 50% dextrose solution; ETOH: absolute (98%–99%) alcohol or ethanol; GRS: gastrorenal shunt; GVs: gastric varices.
Reproduced with permission from Saad WE, Kitanosono T, Koizumi J, Hirota S. The conventional balloon-occluded retrograde transvenous obliteration procedure: indications, contraindications and technical applications. Tech Vasc Intervent Radiol 2013;16:101–151.

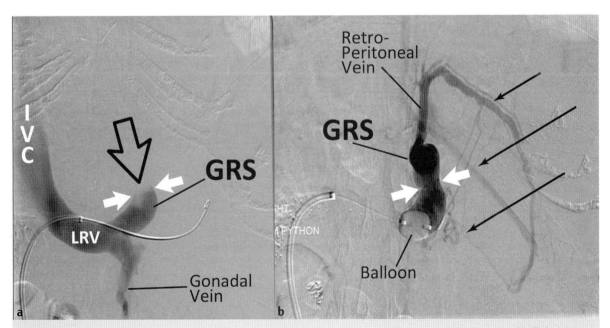

Fig. 29.18 Management of collaterals by simply inflating the balloon-occlusion catheter higher, but not necessarily above, the takeoff of decompressive collaterals. (**a**) An initial venogram before catheter selection of the gastrorenal shunt (GRS). The entire GRS is not visualized and only is inflow effect (*directional open arrow*) in the form of wash-in. A "choke point" is identified (*between solid white arrows*) (please correlate with the same choke point *between solid white arrows* in **b**). Contrast is seen opacifying the left renal vein (LRV), gonadal vein, and inferior vena cava (IVC). (**b**) An attempted balloon-occluded retrograde venography (BORV) in which the balloon has been inflated at the junction of the GRS and the LRV. It is not placed at the higher choke point (*between solid white arrows* in **a** and **b**). Contrast is seen leaving ("escaping") from the GRS into a prominent vertically oriented paraumbilical retroperitoneal vein, which is further decompressed by posterior intercostal veins (*solid black arrows*). (*continued*)

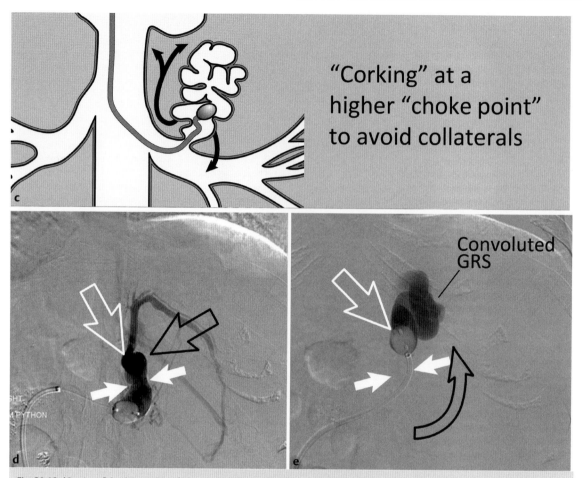

Fig. 29.18 (*Continued*) (**c-e**) Depiction of placing the balloon up higher in a particular GRS, where it is narrower (up higher) so as to "cork" the GRS to a higher "choke point" above significant decompressive collaterals. However, the case shows (**a,b,d,e**) the balloon not to be above the decompressive vein but positioning and inflation of the balloon just below or at (juxta) to the takeoff of the decompressive collateral. In some instances, this is enough to change the hemodynamics and be enough to create preferential flow of contrast (and subsequently sclerosant) into the GRS and not the decompressive collaterals. (**d** demonstrates the low position of the balloon below a higher "choke point" (*between the solid white arrows*). The *open white arrows* points to the takeoff of the retroperitoneal vein described in (**b**). The *open black arrow* points to the proposed new balloon position above the higher "choke point" (*between the solid white arrows*). (**e**) Depicts the pushing up of the deflated balloon (*curved open white arrow*) so that the balloon can be inflated higher and occlude the takeoff of the retroperitoneal vein (**d,e**, *straight open white arrow*). The retroperitoneal vein is no longer visualized, and the GRS is now adequately "trapped." (*Reproduced with permission from Saad WE, Kitanosono T, Koizumi J, Hirota S. The conventional balloon-occluded retrograde transvenous obliteration procedure: indications, contraindications and technical applications. Tech Vasc Intervent Radiol 2013;16:101–151.*)

embolization of these collaterals is warranted. Up to 32% of BRTO procedures require adjuvant coil embolization of venous collaterals (7% retroperitoneal/adrenal and 25% inferior phrenic).[11]

When embolization of collateral veins is necessary, the primary embolic agent is metallic coils (usually 0.035- or 0.018-in microcoils).[11] Coils range from 2 to 6 mm in coil diameter, although anecdotally, coils up to 7 to 8 mm have been used.[11] Almost all coiling occurs of collaterals that are catheterized from the gastric variceal system (► Fig. 29.17; ► Fig. 29.20; ► Fig. 29.21). Other embolic agents can be used such as Gelfoam (Pfizer, New York, New York) and liquid embolic agents (*N*-butyl cyanoacrylate (Cordis Neurovascular, Warrenton, New Jersey) or ethylene vinyl alcohol copolymer (Onyx, ev3 Neurovascular, Irvine, California). Gelfoam or liquid embolic agents have been used in up to 2% to 3% of BRTO cases and are usually required when there are numerous

small collaterals present.[11] The necessity of liquid embolic agents is demonstrated in ► Fig. 29.21 in which an inferior phrenic vein was coil embolized; however, the contrast continued to escape via small, enumerable adrenal and retroperitoneal venules (► Fig. 29.21c). The venules were embolized or obliterated with both Gelfoam and *N*-butyl cyanoacrylate.

If the use of Gelfoam or liquid embolic agents is contemplated, another alternative can be used. This is the sclerosant mixture itself that is used for the BRTO (whether this sclerosant mixture is ethanolamine oleate or 3% sodium teradecyl sulfate). This technique is referred to as "staged sclerosis" and is a way to manage Kiosue type B1, B2, B3, and potentially, type D gastric variceal systems.[4,5] Staged sclerosis is performed by initially injecting the sclerosant into the decompressing veins preferentially while avoiding overspill into the larger systemic circulation (IVC, left

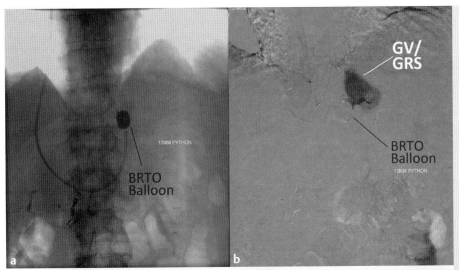

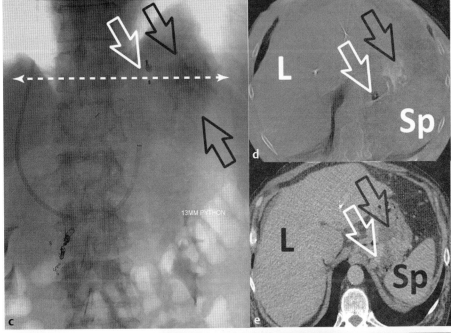

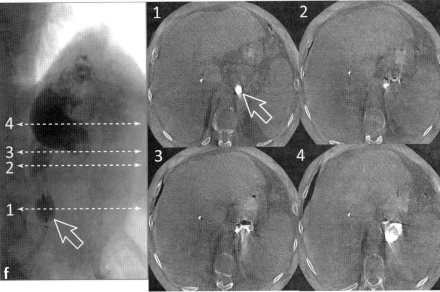

Fig. 29.19 Pulling down the balloon-occlusion catheter to include the entirety of the gastric variceal system unless a desired higher occlusion is required. Fluoroscopic image (a) and digitally subtracted venogram (b) demonstrating a very high balloon occlusion where the balloon is adjacent to the gastric varices (GV). A balloon occlusion of this size is quite rare to be as high as it is achieved here. It is usually achieved in simple (nonconvoluted) gastric variceal systems or gastrorenal shunts (GRS). If balloon-occluded retrograde transvenous obliteration (BRTO) is to be technically successful, all the GVs should be above the balloon. If so, then BRTO can proceed with sclerosant administration. However, if not all the GVs are above the balloon, then the balloon must be pulled down to "cork" a lower "choke point" if any are available. The only reasons why part of the GVs are obliterated and not all with additional sparing of the GRS would be (i) to reduce the sclerosant dose (particularly ethanolamine oleate reaching a dose of 30–40 cc), which is described and called "downgrade BRTO," and (ii) to try to spare the GRS (the splenorenal hemodynamic component of the greater GV system) to preserve the outflow of the splanchnic circulation in case the portal vein is thrombosed. (c-e) Fluoroscopic image of the inflated balloon (now inflated with air; *open white arrow*) in the same position, if not higher, than in (b). There is extravasation of contrast into the gastric fundus (*open black arrow*). The horizontal interrupted bidirectional arrow is the level at which the cone-beam computed tomography (CBCT) image (d) and preprocedural CT image (e) are obtained. In both the CBCT and preprocedural CT images the location of the occlusive balloon (*white open arrow*) and the gastric fundus (*black open arrow*) are noted, respectively (this applies to all three images of c-e). L: liver; Sp: spleen. The key issue with evaluating the gastric varices and the greater gastric variceal system by intraprocedural CBCT is to compare the CBCT images with the preprocedural CT or magnetic resonance (MR) images. Identifying the extent and distribution of the sclerosant should be made by the CBCT by correlating the structures' sizes, locations, and shapes between the CBCT images and the preprocedural CT or MR images. (*continued*)

275

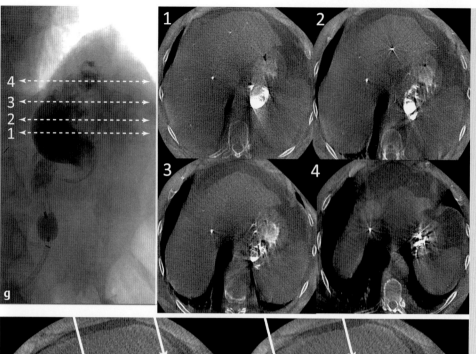

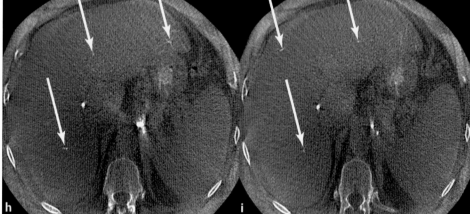

Fig. 29.19 (*Continued*) (f) and (g) Fluoroscopic image after sclerosant injection in the same patient as in (a-e) with *numbered bidirectional arrows*, which are the axial levels of the CBCT images to help the reader identify the level of the axial CBCT images. The *open arrows* correlate and point to the occlusion balloon of the BRTO. (h,i) Two axial CBCT images in the same patient as in a-e, demonstrating the very small quantities of lipiodol laden sclerosant in the intrahepatic portal venous branches (*solid white arrows*). (*Reproduced with permission from Saad WE, Kitanosono T, Koizumi J, Hirota S. The conventional balloon-occluded retrograde transvenous obliteration procedure: indications, contraindications and technical applications. Tech Vasc Intervent Radiol 2013;16:101–151.*)

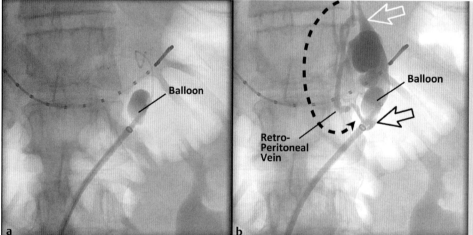

Fig. 29.20 Occlusion balloon being bypassed by a collateral vein. Fluoroscopic image (a) of a contrast inflated balloon in the gastrorenal shunt (GRS). Balloon-occluded retrograde venography (BORV) (b) demonstrates a retroperitoneal venous collateral that takes off (*white open arrow*) above the balloon and heads caudad, circumventing (in the direction of the *curved dashed arrow*) the balloon by anastomosing with the GRS inferior to the balloon (*black open arrow*). (*continued*)

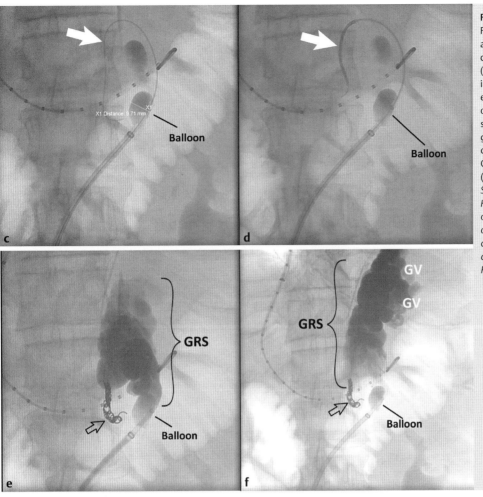

Fig. 29.20 (*Continued*) (c,d) Fluoroscopic images during wire and catheter catheterization of the collateral from above the balloon (*solid white arrow*). (e,f) Fluoroscopic images during BORV after coil embolization (*open black arrow*) of the decompressive collateral showing adequate "trapping" of the gastric variceal system. As a result, contrast is seen opacifying the GRS and the gastric varices (GVs). (*Reproduced with permission from Saad WE, Kitanosono T, Koizumi J, Hirota S. The conventional balloon-occluded retrograde transvenous obliteration procedure: indications, contraindications and technical applications. Tech Vasc Intervent Radiol 2013;16:101–151.*)

renal vein or azygous–hemiazygous system). The operator waits for the sclerosant to take its maximal sclerotic and thrombotic effect and then resumes sclerosant injection, which now goes into the gastric variceal system.

Occasionally, the venous collateral is large (arbitrarily, equal to or larger than 3 mm in diameter; 2% to 3% of BRTO procedures), and its catheterization is technically not feasible. In these cases, a second systemic venous access may be performed, and catheterization of this collateral can be performed retrograde from the IVC or left renal vein.[11] If these collaterals connect to the IVC in a nontortuous manner and are large enough (see next section), an additional BRTO balloon can be introduced and inflated (see later discussion).

Balloon-Occluded Retrograde Venography

BORV actually is not limited to use after "trapping" but actually goes hand in hand with "trapping" because it is the venogram that makes the finding of a well-trapped gastric variceal system (the ultimate technical endpoint) (▶ Figs. 29.15f; 29.17a; 29.17e-g; 29.18b; 29.18c-e; 29.20; 29.21; 29.22). The purpose of BORV is to (i) confirm the technical endpoint of adequate "trapping" of the gastric variceal system, (ii) look for systemic venous escape routes, (iii) identify portal venous afferent feeders (left gastric veins, posterior gastric veins, and short gastric veins), and 4) identify the "overspill" point where cessation of subsequent sclerosant

instilment should occur (▶ Fig. 29.23). Points 3 and 4 are actually the same because sclerosant instilment should be stopped on identifying the portal venous feeder(s) of the gastric variceal system. Notice that the purpose of the BORV is not to assess subsequent sclerosant volumes. This is because the consistency, specific gravity, and fluid dynamics of the contrast (a heavy liquid) are different than those of the 50% air foam sclerosant (or even the 25% to 30% froth sclerosant), which is commonly used in the United States. One can argue that because both contrast and foam act differently, the visualization of portal feeders may vary in the timing of the injection (contrast or sclerosant) and may even show different portal venous feeders. To clarify, dependent feeders such as posterior gastric veins may be visualized more readily with contrast compared with sclerosant, and less dependent feeders (more ventral and anterior) such as the left gastric vein may be visualized more readily with the foam sclerosant and less likely with the contrast (please see the later discussion of sclerosant injection and accompanying images).

Occasionally, the BORV correlates well with the final sclerosis fluoroscopic image. However, on occasion, the portal venous feeders are seen on BORV, but serendipitously are not seen on the final sclerosis fluoroscopic image. Rarely, the portal venous feeders are not seen on BORV (rare because the operator must push to see them) and are seen on the final sclerosis fluoroscopic image.

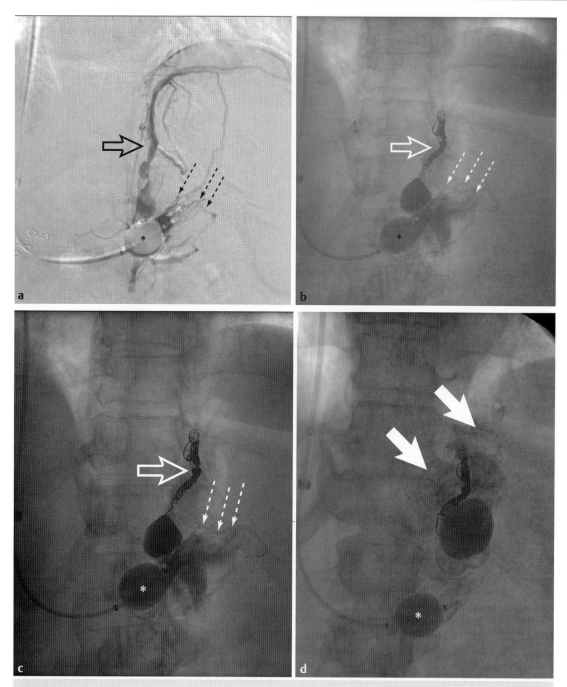

Fig. 29.21 Coil embolization of a phrenic vein (inferior phrenic vein) and gelfoam embolization of numerous adrenal and retroperitoneal veins. Digital subtraction venogram (**a**) with the balloon (*asterisk*) inflated in the gastrorenal shunt (GRS). The GRS is not visualized because contrast is escaping via a phrenic vein (*open arrow*) and possibly numerous small adrenal and retroperitoneal veins (*dashed arrows*). (**b**) Fluoroscopy during venography after coil embolization of the phrenic vein (*open white arrow*). However, the GRS is still not seen because the cumulative effect of the small enumerable adrenal and retroperitoneal veins (*dashed arrows*) is still considerably decompressive to the contrast. The *asterisk* demonstrates a contrast-filled balloon. (**c,d**) Fluoroscopy during balloon-occluded retrograde venography (BORV) (*asterisk*, balloon) after coil embolization of the phrenic vein (*open white arrow*). However, the GRS is still not seen because the cumulative effect of the small enumerable adrenal and retroperitoneal veins (*dashed arrows*) is still considerably decompressive to the contrast. It is not feasible to embolize these veins because they are enumerable and too small. At this point, the operator used a Gelfoam slurry to embolize the small veins, relying on the preferential flow into these veins. Other liquid embolic agents may also be used such as dextrose 50% and absolute alcohol. *N*-butyl cyanoacrylate may also be used, although the risk of glue sticking to the balloon may be a problem. A third, and possibly the most reasonable, option is to use the sclerosant mixture (to be used for the BRTO) itself. The sclerosant is injected in small volumes, relying on the preferential flow to the veins. The operator then waits for the occlusive sclerosant to take effect. The operator then tests with contrast, and if the decompressive veins are occluded, the operator proceeds with the main dose of sclerosant administration with the intent to fill or sclerose the entire gastric variceal system (**d**). (**d**) The sclerosant (*solid white arrows*) in the gastric varices (*asterisk*, balloon). (*Reproduced with permission from Saad WE, Kitanosono T, Koizumi J, Hirota S. The conventional balloon-occluded retrograde transvenous obliteration procedure: indications, contraindications and technical applications. Tech Vasc Intervent Radiol 2013;16:101–151.*)

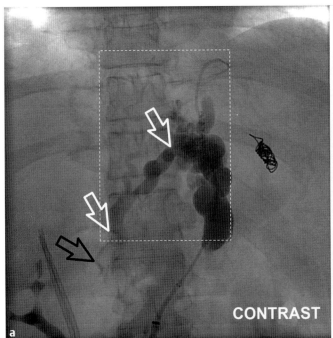
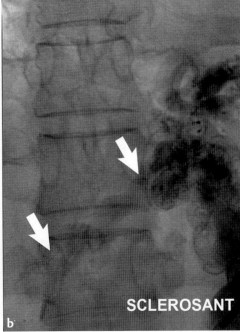

Fig. 29.22 Balloon-occluded retrograde venography (BORV) and sclerosant filling of the gastric variceal system. (a) BORV showing the left gastric vein (LGV) (*open white arrow*) meandering down medial to the gastric variceal system. At the lower end of the LGV where it communicates with the portal vein, contrast is seen flowing out and away from the LGV and into the portal vein (*open black arrow*). The *dashed box* is the outline of the postsclerosant image in (b). (b) Final fluoroscopic image after sclerosant administration correlating well with the BORV image in (a). The sclerosant is seen filling the entire length of the left gastric vein (*between solid white arrows*). (*Reproduced with permission from Saad WE, Kitanosono T, Koizumi J, Hirota S. The conventional balloon-occluded retrograde transvenous obliteration procedure: indications, contraindications and technical applications. Tech Vasc Intervent Radiol 2013;16:101–151.*)

Cone-Beam Computed Tomography Imaging (if Used)

Cone-beam computed tomography (CBCT) helps operators gain confidence with the BRTO procedure by helping correlate the fluoroscopic findings with the preprocedural cross-sectional imaging (▶ Fig. 29.19c-e). CBCT is not necessary for the BRTO procedure, although for the reasons mentioned earlier, the authors recommend that CBCT be used in the early experience of operators and institutions. CBCT can be performed during the BORV stage or after sclerosant mixture instilment, particularly when there is a question of identifying portal venous collaterals. In the authors' opinion, the best time (highest yield of findings) to perform CBCT is after the foam contrast instilment (▶ Fig. 29.19). Regardless of the timing or stage of the procedure when CBCT is performed, when using multiple balloons to trap the gastric varices, it is best to fill one with air and the other with one-third strength contrast, which aids in differentiating them on CBCT.

Cone-beam CT has high spatial resolution and lower contrast resolution than conventional diagnostic CT. As such, performing CBCT during the BORV stage of the BRTO procedure will cause beam-hardening artifact and reduced diagnostic yield. Conversely, rotational angiography may help identify portal venous feeders if they cannot be clearly identified by conventional venography. Additionally, CBCT is very sensitive in detecting lipiodol in the portal circulation or lung bases if it is included in the sclerosant mixture (▶ Fig. 29.19h,i).

Indwelling Balloon Inflation (Sclerosant Dwell Time)

The classic description of balloon inflation and sclerosant dwell time is 12 to 24 hours (overnight inflation).[3–7,12–16] This range of time was described in the Japanese literature using ethanolamine oleate in its liquid form or state. However, with 3% sodium tetradecyl sulfate in the foam state, the average balloon inflation time has been described to be approximately 6 hours.[11] Experienced operators may reduce the inflation dwell time (to less than 6 hours) in small gastric variceal systems. In other words, the inflation time is proportional to the size of the gastric variceal system (sclerosant volumes) and the GRS (blood flow within the GRS).

BRTO or BATO balloons can be inflated with one-third contrast (and two-thirds saline), or they can be filled with air. Some balloon-occlusion catheters and their stopcocks are water tight and not air tight. If air is used with these balloons, premature deflation may occur and result in nontarget embolization. The advantages of using air in a balloon is that air makes the balloon softer and more compliant and that air-filled balloons can be well differentiated from surrounding contrast of sclerosant. Moreover, contrast-filled balloons may cause beam-hardening artifact on CBCT, as discussed previously.

Premature balloon rupture has been described in nearly 9% of BRTO procedures using ethanolamine oleate and up to 15% of BRTO procedures using 3% sodium tetradecyl sulfate.[11,17]

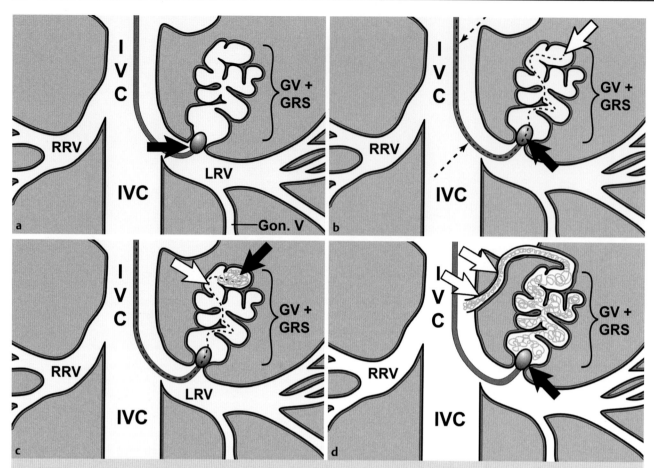

Fig. 29.23 Steps in sclerosant administration using a coaxial microcatheter. (**a**) Simplified drawings of the anatomy of gastric varices (GVs) and the gastric variceal system (GV+GRS). The balloon (*solid black arrow*) is depicted in the distal gastrorenal shunt (GRS). *Gastric variceal system* is the collective term of the GVs and the GRS. Gon. V: left gonadal vein; IVC: inferior vena cava; LRV: left renal vein; RRV: right renal vein. (**b**) A microcatheter (*dashed meandering black line*) is depicted to be placed coaxially through the balloon occlusion catheter shaft (*between straight dashed arrows*) and through the balloon (*solid black arrow*) and into the gastric variceal system. The microcatheter is place as cephalad as possible (*black outlined white arrow*). If the microcatheter is too large for the inner diameter of the available balloon-occlusion catheter, the microcatheter can be placed adjacent to the balloon. IVC: inferior vena cava; RRV: right renal vein. (**c,d**) The role of the microcatheter is to improve the equal distribution of the sclerosant throughout the gastric variceal system and not rely on mere displacement of the sclerosant cephalad from the balloon (*solid black arrow*) of the balloon-occlusion occlusion catheter. The sclerosant is administered as the microcatheter is pulled back toward the balloon. Thus, sclerosant administration usually starts cephalad and ventral, which is closest to the GVs. The sclerosant administration at the end can be just from the balloon-occlusion catheter. The sclerosant administration is stopped when the portal venous feeders are visualized; as in this depiction it is the left gastric vein (*between white arrows*) as seen in ▶ Fig. 29.22. (*Reproduced with permission from Saad WE, Kitanosono T, Koizumi J, Hirota S. The conventional balloon-occluded retrograde transvenous obliteration procedure: indications, contraindications and technical applications. Tech Vasc Intervent Radiol 2013;16:101–151.*)

However, despite the relatively frequent occurrence of balloon rupture, it usually has little effect on the hemodynamic and clinical success rate and is usually a mere technical nuisance.[11,17] Early rupture (within 1 to 1.5 hours from initial inflation and sclerosant administration) may have a higher negative impact on the clinical success because the sclerosant has a higher likelihood to not have caused complete thrombosis of the gastric variceal system.

Balloon Deflation and Removal

The balloon-occlusion catheter can be deflated and removed at bedside, but the current authors recommend that it be removed under fluoroscopy, particularly when the balloon is left inflated for less than 6 hours. When deflating under fluoroscopy, the balloon can be quickly be reinflated if the sclerosant mixture appears loose or mobile. Moreover, it is important to document that the balloon is still intact and inflated (to document the true inflation dwell time of the balloon) and that the radiopaque contrast is in place and has not mobilized.

Conclusion

In conclusion, the conventional BRTO procedure for the management of gastric varices is a technically complex procedure with potentially many adjuvant techniques and complementary procedures. The BRTO procedure has several important steps (▶ Table 29.1), which actually starts with the preprocedural planning based on patient presentation and imaging and terminates with removal of the occlusion catheters.

References

1. Saad WE, Kitanosono T, Koizumi J. Balloon-occluded antegrade transvenous obliteration with or without balloon-occluded retrograde transvenous obliteration for the management of gastric varices: concept and technical applications. Tech Vasc Interventional Radiol 2012;15:203–225.

2. Olson E, Yune HY, Klatte EC. Transrenal-vein reflux ethanol sclerosis of gastroesophageal varices. AJR Am J Roentgenol 1984;143:627–628.

3. Kanagawa H, Mima S, Kouyama H, et al. Treatment of gastric fundal varices by balloon-occluded retrograde transvenous obliteration. J Gastroenterol Hepatol 1996;11:51–58.

4. Kiyosue H, Mori H, Matsumoto S, et al. Transcatheter obliteration of gastric varices: part 1: anatomic classification. Radiographics 2003;23:911–920.

5. Kiyosue H, Mori H, Matsumoto S, et al. Transcatheter obliteration of gastric varices: part-2: strategy and techniques based on hemodynamic features. Radiographics 2003;23:921–937.

6. Saad WE. The history and evolution of balloon-occluded retrograde transvenous obliteration (BRTO): from the United States to Japan and back. Semin Interv Radiol Sep 2011;28(3):283–287.

7. Saad WE, Sabri SS. Balloon-occluded transvenous obliteration (BRTO): technical results and outcomes. Management of gastric varices: endoscopic, BRTO, & TIPS. Semin Intervent Radiol 2011;28(3):333–338.

8. Saad WE. Vascular anatomy and the morphologic and hemodynamic classifications of gastric varices and spontaneous portosystemic shunts relevant to the BRTO procedure. Tech Vasc Interv Radiol 2013;16:60–100.

9. Saad WE, Kitanosono T, Koizumi J, Hirota S. The conventional balloon-occluded retrograde transvenous obliteration procedure: indications, contraindications, and technical applications. Tech Vasc Interv Radiol 2013;15:101–151.

10. Saad WE, Nicholson D, Koizumi J. Inventory used for balloon-occluded retrograde (BRTO) and antegrade (BATO) transvenous obliteration: sclerosants and balloon occlusion device. Tech Vasc Interv Radiol 2012;15:226–240.

11. Saad WE, Nicholson D, Lippert A, et al. Balloon rupture during balloon-occluded retrograde transvenous obliteration (BRTO) of gastric varices utilizing sodium tetradecyl sulfate: Incidence and consequences. Vasc Endovasc Surg 2012;46:664–670.

12. Chikamori F, Kuniyoshi N, Shibuya S, Takase Y. Transjugular retrograde obliteration for chronic portosystemic encephalopathy. Abdom Imaging 2000;25:567–571.

13. Chikamori F, Kuniyoshi N, Shibuya S, Takase Y. Combination treatment of transjugular retrograde obliteration and endoscopic embolization for portosystemic encephalopathy with esophageal varices. Hepatogastroenterology 2004;51: 1379–1381.

14. Hirota S, Matsumoto S, Tomita S, et al. Retrograde transvenous obliteration of gastric varices. Radiology 1999;211:349–356.

15. Fukuda T, Hirota S, Sugimura K. Long-term results of balloon-occluded retrograde transvenous obliteration for the treatment of gastric varices and hepatic encephalopathy. JVIR J Vasc Interv Radiol 2001;12:327–336.

16. Fukuda T, Hirota S, Sugimoto K, et al. "Downgrading" of gastric varices with multiple collateral veins in balloon-occluded retrograde transvenous obliteration. JVIR J Vasc Interv Radiol 2005;16:1379–1383.

17. Park SJ, Chung JW, Kim H-C, et al. The prevalence, risk factors, and clinical outcome of balloon rupture in balloon-occluded retrograde transvenous obliteration of gastric varices. JVIR J Vasc Intervent Radiol 2010;21:503–507.

Chapter 30: Balloon-Occluded Antegrade Transvenous Obliteration and Variations of Balloon-Occluded Retrograde Transvenous Obliteration in the Treatment of Gastric Varices

Minhaj S. Khaja and Wael E.A. Saad

Introduction

Devastating hemorrhage from portosystemic varices remains a major cause of morbidity and mortality in patients with portal hypertension (PHT).[1] Endovascular and surgical portosystemic shunting procedures are effective at reducing the portal pressure but may result in serious complications such as encephalopathy or hepatic insufficiency.[2] Additionally, even with a lowered portosystemic gradient, high-risk varices, such as those found in the gastric antrum, may still be at risk of hemorrhage.[3] Embolization of varices using macroscopic coils or glue is commonly recommended but also fails to eliminate this risk entirely.[4] Chemical-based sclerosis of varices, although frequently resulting in worsened PHT, have proven to be very effective in eradicating the varices at risk.[5]

Because many variceal systems have multiple feeding and multiple draining pathways, combinations of antegrade and retrograde techniques are frequently useful. Balloon-occluded transvenous obliteration from the systemic veins is referred to as balloon-occluded retrograde transvenous obliteration (BRTO), and balloon-occluded transvenous obliteration from the portal veins is referred to as balloon-occluded antegrade transvenous obliteration (BATO) (▶ Fig. 30.1; ▶ Fig. 30.2).[6]

BATO is a collective term referring to three technical approaches: percutaneous transhepatic obliteration (PTO), obliteration via transjugular portosystemic shunt (TIPS) access (▶ Fig. 30.2a), and other unconventional accesses, including transiliocolic vein obliteration (TIO).[6] This chapter reviews variations of conventional BRTO, including BATO, combined BATO and BRTO, and use of vessels other than the conventional left renal vein.

Technique

The first choice of access for endovascular obliteration of gastric varices is via the traditional transrenal route (▶ Fig. 30.1).[7-10] Alternative routes are used for gastric varices when there is no gastrorenal shunt[11-14] or as additional access to the transrenal BRTO route.[15,16] Further alternative routes for transvenous obliteration are used in the management of nongastric varices (ectopic varices) such as duodenal, mesenteric, and stomal varices.[17-28]

Alternative or adjunctive routes can be classified into portal venous access routes and systemic venous access routes. The

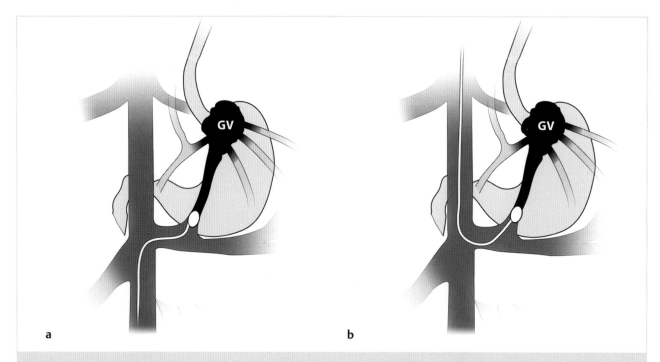

Fig. 30.1 The basic approach of the conventional balloon-occluded retrograde transvenous obliteration (BRTO) procedure. (a) BRTO through a transfemoral approach with the balloon in the gastrorenal shunt. BRTO is obliteration from the systemic vein side, and balloon-occluded antegrade transvenous obliteration is obliteration from the portal venous side. (b) BRTO through a transfemoral approach with the balloon in the gastrorenal shunt. GV: gastric varices. (*With permission from Saad WE, Kitanosono T, Koizumi J, Hirota S. The conventional balloon-occluded retrograde transvenous obliteration procedure: indications, contraindications and technical applications. Tech Vasc Intervent Radiol 2013;16:101–151.*)

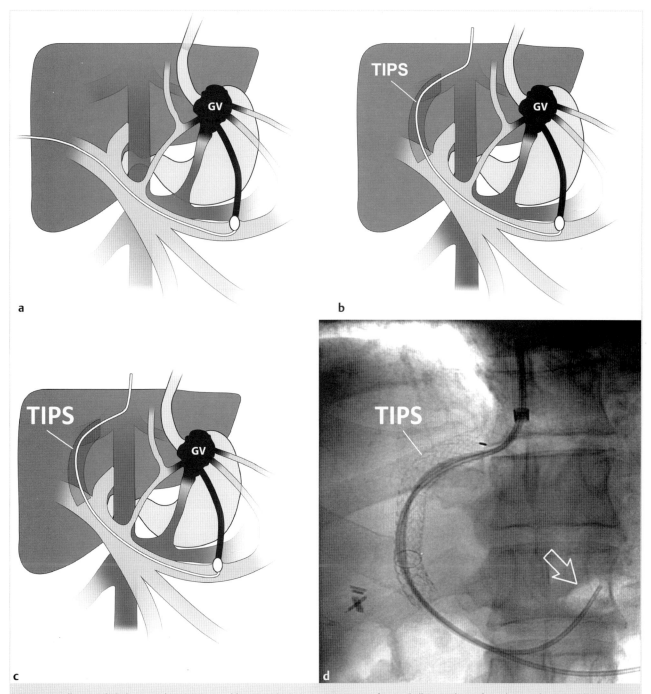

Fig. 30.2 Balloon-occluded antegrade transvenous obliteration (BATO). Demonstration of BATO (balloon occlusion from the portal venous side) and its subclassification into percutaneous transhepatic obliteration (PTO: **a**) and trans-TIPS (transjugular intrahepatic portosystemic shunt: **b**) obliteration. GV: gastric varices. (**c,d**) Illustration demonstrating trans-TIPS BATO (**c**) and a fluoroscopic image of a trans-TIPS BATO (**d**). The illustration depicts the BATO balloon in the posterior gastric vein, and the fluoroscopic image demonstrates an air-filled BATO balloon (*hollow arrow*) occluding the left gastric vein (coronary vein). (*With permission from Saad WE, Kitanosono T, Koizumi J, Hirota S. The conventional balloon-occluded retrograde transvenous obliteration procedure: indications, contraindications and technical applications. Tech Vasc Intervent Radiol 2013;16:101–151.*)

most common alternative route described is the percutaneous transhepatic route, which is commonly referred to in the Japanese literature as PTO.[15,16] Less commonly used alternative access methods include but are not confined to transcaval, transphrenic, transileocolic, trans-TIPS, transgonadal, transazygous, and transrenal capsular vein approaches.[17–28]

Balloon-Occluded Antegrade Transvenous Obliteration

Balloon-occluded antegrade transvenous obliteration is balloon-assisted sclerosant obliteration of varices from a portal venous approach and not from the traditional retrograde approach (BRTO)

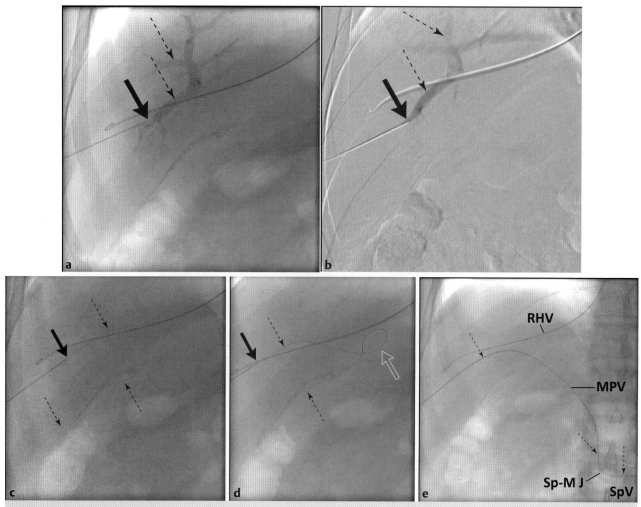

Fig. 30.3 Percutaneous transhepatic access for the purpose of a percutaneous transhepatic obliteration procedure. Fluoroscopic image (**a**) and a digitally subtracted portogram (**b**) alternative during a limited portogram on access of the right-sided portal vein branches with a 21-gauge needle. The operator passes the 21-gauge needle into the right hepatic lobe. Contrast is injected through the needle (*solid black arrow* at needle tip) as it is retracted. The needle retraction is stopped when a small portal vein branch is visualized (*dashed arrows*). This technique is identical to that of percutaneous transhepatic cholangiography. (**c**) Fluoroscopic image with a 0.018-inch guidewire (*dashed arrows*) (Terumo, Corp, Tokyo, Japan) being advanced through the 21-gauge needle (*solid arrow* at needle tip). The 0.018-inch guidewire arcs into a lower portal vein branch, where the wire tip rests in this image. (**d**) Fluoroscopic image obtained as the 0.018-inch guidewire (*dashed arrows*) is being advanced farther through the 21-gauge needle (*solid arrow* at needle tip) and into the more central (and larger) right-sided portal vein branches. The 0.018-inch guidewire is now buckled (*hollow arrow*), which allows the wire to pass, in an atraumatic manner, more centrally into larger portal vein branches. (**e**) Fluoroscopic image obtained after the 0.018-inch guidewire has been exchanged for a 0.035-inch guidewire (*dashed arrows*) using a transitional sheath (usually 4 to 6 French). The operator watches the 0.035-inch wire and whether it follows the expected morphology of the portal circulation. In this instance, the guidewire appears to pass down the main portal vein (MPV) and takes a left turn probably at the splenomesenteric confluence or junction (Sp-M-J) and into the splenic vein (SpV). This is a probability and cannot be a certainty without venography. Incidentally noted is a Rosen wire in the right hepatic vein (RHV). (*With permission from Saad WE, Kitanosono T, Koizumi J. Balloon-occluded antegrade transvenous obliteration with or without balloon-occluded retrograde transvenous obliteration for the management of gastric varices: concept & technical applications. Tech Vasc Intervent Radiol 2012;15:203–225.*)

from the systemic veins. It includes the percutaneous transhepatic approach, trans-TIPS approach, and (percutaneous or open surgical cutdown) approaches via ileocolic veins or mesenteric tributaries (TIO).

Portal Venous Routes

Percutaneous transhepatic obliteration is actually the first described route used solely for the obliteration (embolization) of gastric and esophageal varices. PTO, commonly used in the 1970s, predates the TIPS era.[29-33] With the advent of BRTO in the early 1990s, it has been used as a second choice approach or an adjunct to the traditional BRTO approach.[15,16] PTO is the most commonly described alternative or adjunctive access.[15,16] The portal access is obtained similarly to a right-sided percutaneous transhepatic cholangiography (PTC) and can be performed under moderate sedation (▶ Fig. 30.3; ▶ Fig. 30.4). General anesthesia may be helpful in patients who cannot tolerate the procedure under moderate sedation or if the operator predicts a prolonged intervention involving a PTO and BRTO.

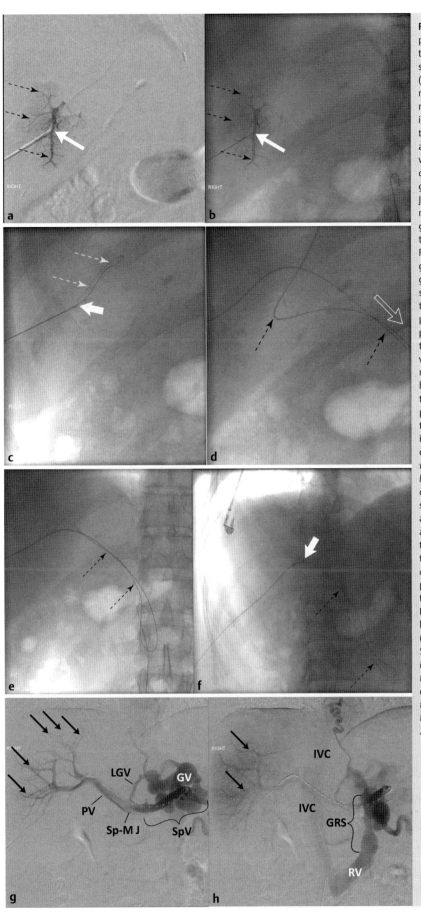

Fig. 30.4 Percutaneous transhepatic access and portography for the purpose of a percutaneous transhepatic obliteration procedure. Digitally subtracted portogram (**a**) and fluoroscopic image (**b**) during a limited portogram on access of the right-sided portal vein branches with a 21-gauge needle. The operator passes the 21-gauge needle into the right hepatic lobe. Contrast is injected through the needle (*solid white arrow* at needle tip) as it is retracted. The needle retraction is stopped when a small portal vein branch is visualized (*dashed arrows*). (**c**) Fluoroscopic image with a 0.018-inch guidewire (*dashed arrows*) (Terumo, Corp, Tokyo, Japan) being advanced through the 21-gauge needle (*solid arrow* at needle tip). The 0.018-inch guidewire (*dashed arrows*) buckles and conforms to the accessed portal vein branch (**a,b**). (**d**) Fluoroscopic image obtained after the 0.018-inch guidewire has been exchanged for a 0.035-inch guidewire (*white dashed arrows*) using a transitional sheath (usually 4 to 6 French). The operator watches the 0.035-inch wire (*black dashed arrows*) as it is pushed (*hollow arrow* depicting directional central push) centrally. The 0.035-inch wire is a soft floppy-tipped Benston wire (Cook Corp, Bloomington, IN), which has a propensity to buckle in an atraumatic manner into the more central larger portal vein branches. (**e**) Fluoroscopic image obtained after the 0.035-inch guidewire (*dashed arrows*) was passed more centrally. The 0.035-inch wire follows the expected morphology of the portal circulation in the main portal vein. (**f**) Fluoroscopic image obtained after a short (11-cm) 7-Fr sheath (*solid white arrow*) over the 0.035-inch guidewire (*dashed black arrows*). (**g,h**) Two digitally subtracted images of a diagnostic portal angiogram/portogram in sequence. The images demonstrate the pathologic anatomy (morphology) of the gastric varices (GV) and its draining gastrorenal shunt (GRS). Despite the relatively large GRS, contrast is observed in the intrahepatic portal vein branches (*solid black arrows*). The dominant portal venous feeder is the posterior gastric vein (not marked or labeled), and the left gastric vein (LGV) is relatively rudimentary. IVC: inferior vena cava; PV: main portal vein; RV: left renal vein; Sp-M-J: splenomesenteric junction (confluence of the splenic and mesenteric veins); SpV: splenic vein. (*With permission from Saad WE, Kitanosono T, Koizumi J. Balloon-occluded antegrade transvenous obliteration with or without balloon-occluded retrograde transvenous obliteration for the management of gastric varices: concept and technical applications. Tech Vasc Interventional Rad 2012;15:203–225.*)

The patient is placed supine with his or her arm at mid-abduction. The right upper quadrant is prepared and draped in the standard surgical manner. Some operators use real-time ultrasound to access a right-sided portal vein radical. However, the current authors use real-time fluoroscopy in an attempt to access smaller, more peripheral portal vein branches that may not be visualized clearly by ultrasound. A 21- or 22-gauge needle is passed into the right hepatic lobe (▶ Fig. 30.3; ▶ Fig. 30.4). Contrast is injected as the needle is retracted until a portal vein radical is visualized. After confirming location within a portal vein radical, a 0.018-inch guidewire is advanced into the more central portal vein branches. A transitional graduated dilator (Accustick, Boston Scientific, Natick, Massachusetts; or Neph-set, Cook, Inc., Bloomington, Indiana) with a metal stiffener is advanced over the wire (▶ Fig. 30.3; ▶ Fig. 30.4). This set is used to upsize the wire to a 0.035-inch wire. The transitional dilator is then exchanged for a vascular sheath that is appropriately sized for the occlusion catheter to be used. Planning for what type and size of occlusion catheter is based on prior imaging, which is usually computed tomography (CT) venography or magnetic resonance (MR) venography. Ideally, coronal projections or reformats would be available for planning the intervention. A 7-Fr sheath is required to accommodate most 10- to 11-mm occlusion catheters, which are usually the maximum required to occlude afferent (portal-venous side) feeders to gastric varices and ectopic varices (duodenal and mesenteric varices; see later discussion). After the adequately-sized

vascular sheath is placed, a splenic, mesenteric, or portal venogram is performed that is pertinent to the varix that needs obliteration (▶ Fig. 30.4).

The **TIPS approach** is the least described alternative or adjunctive access to the portal venous system (▶ Fig. 30.2c,d).[26,34–36] It is usually a preexisting TIPS, and the access is rarely created for the sole purpose of the varices obliteration procedure.[34,36] In a study by Park et al,[37] 6.7% of BRTO cases (n = 5 of 75) were performed with a combined preexisting trans-TIPS approach and a traditional transrenal BRTO approach.[30] After the 9- or 10-Fr TIPS sheath is placed via standard approach, a splenic, mesenteric, or portal venogram is performed that is pertinent to the varix that needs obliteration (▶ Fig. 30.5).

The advantages of this approach is that it is commonly performed through a preexisting TIPS, and no additional access risk is taken.[34–36] However, the largest disadvantage of this access is that it is an invasive route and takes time and resources to establish. In addition, it is a long and indirect access route (especially compared with the percutaneous transhepatic route), particularly when the target vessel is a distance from the liver such as gastric varices and distal colonic.

After the portal venous branches leading to the varices in question are identified, the operator must plan occlusion of these branches. The smaller veins are embolized with coils or vascular plugs. After the "debranching" of the gastric varix is performed, the major (largest) portal venous branch is occluded using the

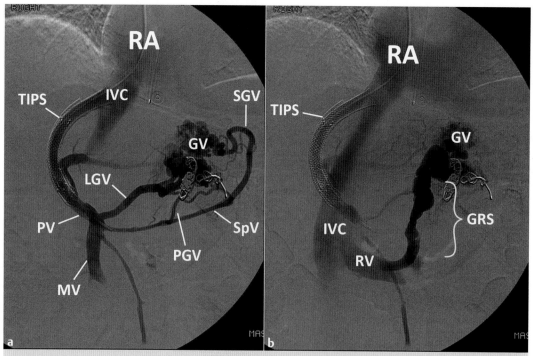

Fig. 30.5 Portal venogram through a transjugular intrahepatic shunt (TIPS) showing gastric varices (GV) and the gastrorenal shunt (GRS) and its parts. **(a,b)** Two digitally subtracted angiogram (portograms) in sequence performed through a TIPS. The TIPS is patent. There is a small diminutive splenic vein **(a,** SpV) that most likely represents a recannulated previously thrombosed splenic vein. There is also reversal of flow in the splenic vein **(a,** SpV). The gastric varices **(a,b,** GV) are supplied by the short gastric vein (SGV), the posterior gastric vein (PGV), and most dominantly the left gastric vein (LGV). The GVs empty into the gastrorenal shunt (GRS) that then empties into the left renal vein (LRV), which anatomically empties into the inferior vena cava (IVC) and right atrium (RA). MPV: main portal vein; MV: mesenteric vein. (*With permission from Saad WE. Vascular anatomy and the morphologic and hemodynamic classifications of gastric varices and spontaneous portosystemic shunts relevant to the BRTO-procedure. Tech Vasc Intervent Radiol 2013;16:60–100.*)

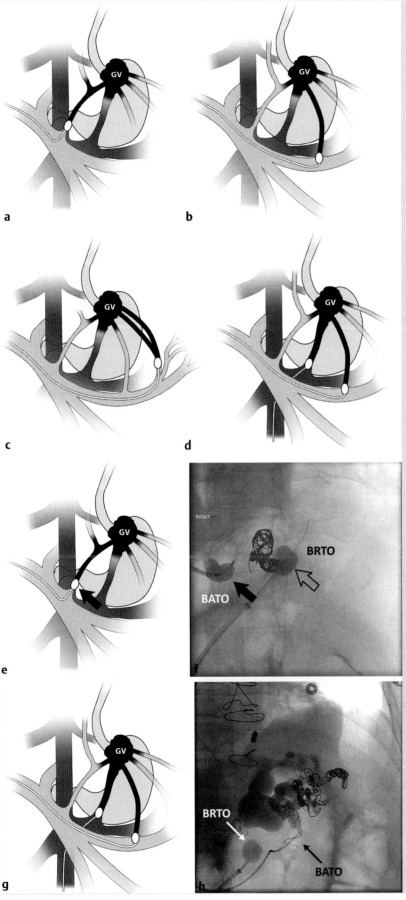

Fig. 30.6 Variations of balloon-occluded antegrade transvenous obliteration (BATO), including combining with conventional balloon-occluded retrograde transvenous obliteration (BRTO). (a-d) Four illustrations demonstrating the various BATO approaches ending with a balloon inflated in the portal venous feeders of the gastric varices (GV), from right to left in the body and in the illustration, in the left gastric vein (a), the posterior gastric vein (b), and the short gastric vein (c). (d) Illustrates a combined BATO (in the posterior gastric vein [PGV]) and BRTO. An illustration (e) and a fluoroscopic spot image (f) demonstrating the BATO approaches ending with a balloon inflated in the left gastric vein (LGV) leading to the GV and the short gastric vein (c). In the illustration, there is no BRTO balloon, but the fluoroscopic image demonstrates a combined BATO (in the LGV) and BRTO. An illustration (g) and a fluoroscopic spot image (h) demonstrating a combined BATO and BRTO. The BATO balloon is inflated in the PGV, leading to the GV, and the BRTO balloon is in the GRS. (*With permission from Saad WE, Kitanosono T, Koizumi J. Balloon-occluded antegrade transvenous obliteration with or without balloon-occluded retrograde transvenous obliteration for the management of gastric varices: concept and technical applications. Tech Vasc Interventional Radiol 2012;15:203–225.*)

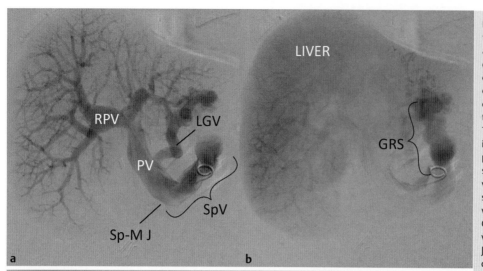

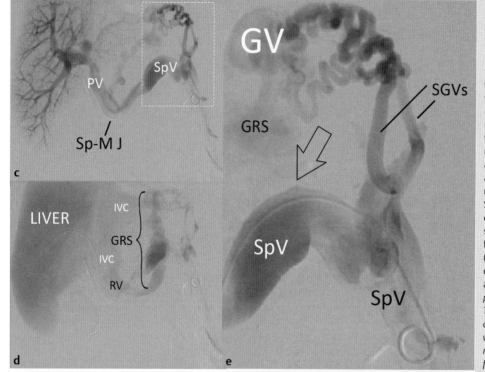

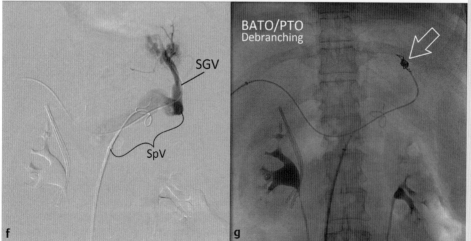

Fig. 30.7 Simple percutaneous transhepatic obliteration (PTO) and gastric variceal debranching combined with conventional balloon-occluded retrograde transvenous obliteration (BRTO). PTO is a form of balloon-occluded antegrade transvenous approach (BATO). (a,b) Two digitally subtracted portograms in sequence performed with a pigtail catheter in the mid-to-distal splenic vein (SpV). There are gastric varices associated with a gastrorenal shunt (GRS). The dominant portal venous feeder to the varices and GRS is the LGV. RPV: right portal vein; PV: main portal vein; Sp-M J: splenomesenteric junction/confluence. Two digitally subtracted portograms in sequence (c,d) performed with a pigtail catheter in the proximal (close to splenic hilum) splenic vein (SpV) with a magnified inset (e). Again seen are the gastric varices (GV), which are associated with a GRS. The dominant portal venous feeder to the varices and GRS is the left gastric vein (a,b); however, relatively small SGV do contribute to the GV and GRS. A small venous nipple (*hollow arrow*) is where the absent posterior gastric vein usually arises. IVC: inferior vena cava; PV: main portal vein; RV: left renal vein; Sp-M J: splenomesenteric junction/confluence. Digitally subtracted short gastric venogram (f) and fluoroscopic spot image (g) before (f) and during (g) the embolization of the SGV. The approach is via a PTO approach. SpV: splenic vein. (*With permission from Saad WE, Kitanosono T, Koizumi J. Balloon-occluded antegrade transvenous obliteration with or without balloon-occluded retrograde transvenous obliteration for the management of gastric varices: concept and technical applications. Tech Vasc Interventional Radiol 2012;15:203–225.*)

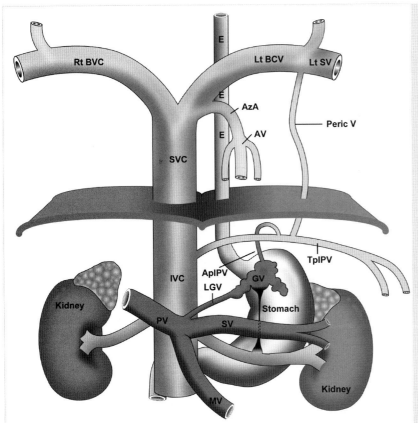

Fig. 30.8 An illustration of the venous anatomy around gastric varices without a gastrorenal shunt. The descending part of the vertical portion of the inferior phrenic vein is believed to form the gastrorenal shunt by anastomosing with the adrenal vein. ApIPV: ascending part of the vertical portion of the inferior phrenic vein; AV: azygous vein; AzA: azygous arch; E: esophagus; GV: gastric varices/varix; IVC: inferior vena cava; LGV: left gastric vein (coronary vein); Lt BCV: left brachiocephalic vein; Lt SV: left subclavian vein; MV: mesenteric vein(s); Peric V: pericardial vein; PV: portal vein; Rt BCV: right brachiocephalic vein; SV: splenic vein; SVC: superior vena cava; TpIPV: transverse portion of the inferior phrenic vein. (*With permission from Araki T, Saad WE. Balloon-occluded retrograde transvenous obliteration of gastric varices from unconventional systemic veins in the absence of gastrorenal shunts. Tech Vasc Intervent Radiol 2012;15:241–253.*)

balloon-occlusion catheter (▶ Fig. 30.6; ▶ Fig. 30.7). If the access to the portal circulation is via an established TIPS, two balloon-occlusion catheters can be passed through the TIPS and occlude the two major portal venous branches (if any).

After the varix has been "trapped" by embolizing smaller portal venous branches (debranching) and balloon occlusion of the main portal venous branch with or without balloon occlusion of the shunt from the renal vein (traditional BRTO), the sclerosant is instilled (▶ Fig. 30.7). If the varix is adequately "trapped" from the portal venous side (BATO) and from the systemic venous side (BRTO) with occlusion balloons, sclerosant distribution without the need for additional microcatheter extensions is usually sufficient.

Systemic Venous Routes

Routes for Gastric Varices

The use of systemic access veins in an obliterative intervention is a backup choice to the gastrorenal shunt. The identifiable systemic veins are (i) the left inferior phrenic vein, which empties into the inferior vena cava (IVC); (ii) the pericardial vein, which anastomoses with the inferior phrenic vein and empties into the left subclavian/left brachiocephalic vein; and (iii) paraesophageal veins, which empty into the azygous and hemiazygos system and then empty to the superior vena cava (SVC) via the azygous arch (▶ Fig. 30.8). These veins are commonly used for access when 1) there is no other alternative (no gastrorenal shunt) or 2) in addition to the gastrorenal shunt if they provide "escape routes" for the sclerosant to travel into the systemic circulation from the gastric varices.[9-19] In a study by Araki et al,[15] 14.5% (n = 11 of 76)

of patients presenting with gastric varices did not have the typical gastrorenal shunt, and alternative systemic venous access routes were used in an attempt to perform a BRTO via them[14]; 82% (n = 9 of 11) had identifiable systemic venous access routes; and the remaining patients (18%, n = 2 of 11) had numerous innominate collaterals (more similar to a retroperitoneal plexus of veins).[14]

These alternative veins are difficult to access from the major systemic venous access veins (the IVC, left brachiocephalic vein, and SVC, respectively) (▶ Fig. 30.8). They also require smaller balloons to occlude them. Intuitively, if these veins are small and difficult to cannulate, the risk of extravasation is higher. The BRTO procedure performed solely from these veins (no additional BRTO from the gastrorenal shunt) require smaller volumes of sclerosants compared with traditional BRTO via a gastrorenal shunt: 12 mL (usually <20 mL) versus an average of 20 to 30 mL (usually <40 mL), respectively.[14,16,37-40] Additional technical details regarding these pathways can be found in the literature.[41]

Routes for Duodenal Varices

These systemic veins are commonly quite difficult to access. The gastrorenal shunt is not an option in duodenal varices. These systemic veins include the renal capsular veins (right, left, or both), gonadal veins (right, left, or both), and right renal vein.[23,24,28] More than 50% of duodenal variceal transvenous obliteration cases in the literature are performed using the BRTO technique from the systemic venous side of the portosystemic varices.[21-28] The remaining cases have been approached from the antegrade portal venous side (BATO technique) via a TIPS approach or more commonly by a percutaneous transhepatic approach (PTO).

Conclusion

When necessary, modifications and alternatives to the traditional BRTO are valuable techniques that can potentially improve the technical and clinical results of transvenous obliteration of gastric, duodenal, and other ectopic varices. These methods include BATO from the portovenous side (trans-TIPS or PTO) and a BRTO from unconventional systemic veins such as the left inferior phrenic, pericardiac, and azygous-hemiazygos veins. Use of these techniques requires in-depth knowledge of the variceal venous anatomy; careful preprocedural planning; and high-level technical skills with microcatheters, occlusion balloons, and embolization.

Clinical Pearls

- Balloon-occluded retrograde transvenous obliteration (BRTO) and balloon-occluded antegrade transvenous obliteration (BATO) are two technical approaches that can be performed solely or in combination on different types of ectopic varices (duodenal or mesenteric varices, for example) and are not specific to gastric varices.
- BRTO is retrograde variceal obliteration from the systemic veins, and there are variations of this approach depending on the feasible anatomy.
- BATO is antegrade variceal obliteration from the portal venous circulation, and there are variations of this approach depending on the feasible anatomy.
- BATO approaches include:
  - Percutaneous transhepatic obliteration (PTO)
  - Trans-TIPS obliteration
  - Transiliocolic obliteration (TIO)
- BRTO is the more conventional approach because the access is usually readily available (systemic veins) and is less invasive than BATO approaches (see immediate points above).
- BRTO approaches are basically through the portosystemic shunts that are commonly associated with ectopic varices.

References

1. Garcia-Tsao G, Bosch J. Management of varices and variceal hemorrhage in cirrhosis. N Engl J Med 2010;362:823–832.
2. Boyer TD, Haskal ZJ. American Association for the Study of Liver Diseases: The role of transjugular intrahepatic portosystemic shunt (TIPS) in the management of portal hypertension: update 2009. Hepatology 2010;51:306.
3. Jalan R, Redhead DN, Forrest EH, Hayes PC. Relationship between directly measured portal pressure gradient and variceal hemorrhage. Am J Gastroenterol 1995;90:1994–1996.
4. Vangeli M, Patch D, Terreni N, et al. Bleeding ectopic varices—treatment with transjugular intrahepatic portosystemic shunt (TIPS) and embolisation. J Hepatol 2004;41:560–566.
5. Tesdal IK, Filser T, Weiss C, et al. Transjugular intrahepatic portosystemic shunts: adjunctive embolotherapy of gastroesophageal collateral vessels in the prevention of variceal rebleeding. Radiology 2005;236:360–367.
6. Saad WE, Kitanosono T, Koizumi J. Balloon-occluded antegrade transvenous obliteration with or without balloon-occluded retrograde transvenous obliteration for the management of gastric varices: concept and technical applications. Tech Vasc Interventional Rad 2012;15:203–225.
7. Olson E, Yune HY, Klatte EC. Transrenal-vein reflux ethanol sclerosis of gastroesophageal varices. AJR Am J Roentgenol 1984;143:627–628.
8. Kanagawa H, Mima S, Kouyama H, et al. Treatment of gastric fundal varices by balloon-occluded retrograde transvenous obliteration. J Gastroenterol Hepatol 1996;11:51–58.
9. Kiyosue H, Mori H, Matsumoto S, et al. Transcatheter obliteration of gastric varices. Part 1. Anatomic classification. Radiographics 2003;23:911–920.
10. Kiyosue H, Mori H, Matsumoto S, et al. Transcatheter obliteration of gastric varices: part 2. Strategy and techniques based on hemodynamic features. Radiographics 2003;23:921–937.
11. Ibukuro K, Sugihara T, Tanaka R, et al. Balloon-occluded retrograde transvenous obliteration (BRTO) for a direct shunt between the inferior mesenteric vein and the inferior vena cava in a patient with hepatic encephalopathy. J Vasc Interv Radiol 2007;18:121–125.
12. Tajiri T, Onda M, Yamashita K, et al. Interventional radiology for portal hypertension. PTO.TIO. Nippon Geka Gakkai Zasshi 1996;97:70–77.
13. Chikamori F, Kuniyoshi N, Kagiyama S, et al. Role of percutaneous transhepatic obliteration for special types of varices with portal hypertension. Abdom Imaging 2007;32:92–95.
14. Fukatsu H, Kawamoto H, Harada R, et al. Gastric fundal varices with an exposed microcoil after the combined BRTO and PTO therapy. Endoscopy 2007;39:E247–E248.
15. Araki T, Hori M, Motosugi U, et al. Can balloon-occluded retrograde transvenous obliteration be performed for gastric varices without gastrorenal shunts? J Vasc Interv Radiol 2010;21:663–670.
16. Arai H, Abe T, Takagi H, Mori M. Efficacy of balloon- occluded retrograde transvenous obliteration, percutaneous transhepatic obliteration and combined techniques for the management of gastric fundal varices. World J Gastroenterol 2006;12:3866–3873.
17. Ninoi T, Nakamura K, Kaminou T, et al. TIPS versus transcatheter sclerotherapy for gastric varices. AJR Am J Roentgenol 2004;183:369–376.
18. Ota K, Okazaki M, Higashihara H, et al. Combination of transileocolic vein obliteration and balloon-occluded retro-grade transvenous obliteration is effective for ruptured duodenal varices. J Gastroenterol 1999;34:694–699.
19. Ono S, Irie T, Kuramochi M, et al. Successful treatment of mesenteric varices with balloon-occluded retrograde transvenous obliteration via an abdominal wall vein. J Vasc Interv Radiol 2007;18:1033–1035.
20. Ibukuro K, Sugihara T, Tanaka R, et al. Balloon-occluded retrograde transvenous obliteration (BRTO) for a direct shunt between the inferior mesenteric vein and the inferior vena cava in a patient with hepatic encephalopathy. J Vasc Interv Radiol 2007;18:121–125.
21. Kimura T, Haruta I, Isobe Y, et al. A novel therapeutic approach for rectal varices: a case report of rectal varices treated with double balloon-occluded embolotherapy. Am J Gastroenterol 1997;92:883–886.
22. Akazawa Y, Murata I, Yamao T, et al. Successful management of bleeding duodenal varices by endoscopic variceal ligation and balloon-occluded retrograde transvenous obliteration. Gastrointest Endosc 2003;58:794–797.
23. Tominaga K, Montani A, Kuga T, et al. Combined balloon- occluded embolization for treatment of concurrent duodenal, gastric, and esophageal varices: a case report. Gastrointest Endosc 2001;53:665–668.
24. Onozato Y, Kakizaki S, Iizuka H, et al. Ectopic varices rupture in the gastroduodenal anastomosis successfully treated with N-butyl-2-cyanoacrylate injection. Acta Med Okayama 2007;61:361–365.
25. Zamora CA, Sugimoto K, Tsurusaki M, et al. Endovascular obliteration of bleeding duodenal varices in patients with liver cirrhosis. Eur Radiol 2006;16:73–79.
26. Haruta I, Isobe Y, Ueno E, et al. Balloon-occluded retrograde transvenous obliteration (BRTO), a promising nonsurgical therapy for ectopic varices: a case report of successful treatment of duodenal varices by BRTO. Am J Gastroenterol 1996;91:2594–2597.
27. Ohta M, Yasumori K, Saku M, et al. Successful treatment of bleeding duodenal varices by balloon-occluded retrograde transvenous obliteration: a transjugular venous approach. Surgery 1999;126:581–583.
28. Sonomura T, Horihata K, Yamahara K, et al. Ruptured duodenal varices successfully treated with balloon-occluded retrograde transvenous obliteration: usefulness of micro- catheters. AJR Am J Roentgenol 2003;181:725–727.
29. Tsurusaki M, Sugimoto K, Matsumoto S, et al. Bleeding duodenal varices successfully treated with balloon-occluded retrograde transvenous obliteration (B-RTO) assisted by CT during arterial portography. Cardiovasc Intervent Radiol 2006;29:1148–1151.
30. Funaro AH, Ring EJ, Freiman DB, et al. Transhepatic obliteration of esophageal varices using the stainless steel coil. AJR Am J Roentgenol 1979;133:1123–1125.
31. Scott J, Dick R, Long RG, Sherlock S. Percutaneous transhepatic obliteration of gastro-oesophageal varices. Lancet 1976;2:53–55.
32. Lunderquist A, Simert G, Tyle NU, Vang J. Follow-up of patients with portal hypertension and esophageal varices treated with percutaneous obliteration of gastric coronary vein. Radiology 1977;122:59–63.
33. Lunderquist A, Vang J. Transhepatic catheterization and obliteration of the coronary vein in patients with portal hypertension and esophageal varices. N Engl J Med 1974;291:646–649.

34. Lunderquist A, Vang J. Sclerosing injection of esophageal varices through transhepatic selective catheterization of the gastric coronary vein. A preliminary report. Acta Radiol Diagn (Stockh) 1974;15:546–550.

35. Chikamori F, Kuniyoshi N, Shibuya S, Takase Y. Transjugular retrograde obliteration for chronic portosystemic encephalopathy. Abdom Imaging 2000;25: 567–571.

36. Chikamori F, Kuniyoshi N, Shibuya S, Takase Y. Combination treatment of transjugular retrograde obliteration and endoscopic embolization for portosystemic encephalopathy with esophageal varices. Hepatogastroenterology 2005;51: 1379–1381.

37. Park SJ, Chung JW, Kim H-C, et al. The prevalence, risk factors, and clinical outcome of balloon rupture in balloon-occluded retrograde transvenous obliteration of gastric varices. J Vasc Interv Radiol 2010;21:503–507.

38. Hong CH, Kim HJ, Park JH, et al. Treatment of patients with gastric variceal hemorrhage: endoscopic N-butyl-2-cyanoacry: late injection versus balloon-occluded retrograde transvenous obliteration. J Gastroenterol Hepatol 2009;24: 372–378.

39. Yamagami T, Kato T, Hirota T, et al. Infusion of 50% glucose solution before injection of ethanolamine oleate during balloon-occluded retrograde transvenous obliteration. Australas Radiol 2007;51:334–338.

40. Kitamoto M, Imamura M, Kamada K, et al. Balloon-occluded retrograde transvenous obliteration of gastric fundal varices with hemorrhage. AJR Am J Roentgenol 2002;178(5):1167–1174

41. Araki T, Saad WE. Balloon-occluded retrograde transvenous obliteration of gastric varices from unconventional systemic veins in the absence of gastrorenal shunts. Tech Vasc Interventional Radiol 2012;15:241–253.

Chapter 31: Clinical Outcomes of Balloon-Occluded Retrograde Transvenous Obliteration and Balloon-Occluded Antegrade Transvenous Obliteration

Paula M. Novelli and Wael E.A. Saad

Introduction

Gastric variceal bleeding is a major complication of portal hypertension (PHT). Although less common than bleeding associated with esophageal varices, gastric variceal bleeding is associated with a higher mortality rate[1,2] and less effective endoscopic treatment options. Despite decades of varying endoscopic, percutaneous, and surgical treatment strategies, the literature is relatively less established, and treatment consequently is more empiric.[3] From an interventional radiology perspective, transjugular intrahepatic portosystemic shunts (TIPS) to decompress the portal circulation and balloon-occluded retrograde transvenous obliteration (BRTO) are both used to address bleeding gastric varices.[4–6] The primary indications for BRTO are gastric variceal bleeding and hepatic encephalopathy refractory to medical management in the presence of gastrorenal shunt.[4,7–37] The bleeding control rate of gastric varices after BRTO is reported as high as 91% to 100%,[7,8] and gastric varices occluded by BRTO have recurrence rates of 0 to 10%.[38–44] Because BRTO diverts blood into the portal circulation and potentially into the liver, there is a favorable significant reduction in encephalopathy in most, if not all, patients treated with BRTO. Although transient and long-term preservation of hepatic function[45] can occur after BRTO, the obliteration of a low-pressure portal diversion pathway can lead to changes in portal hemodynamics that aggravate PHT and result in bleeding from esophageal varices. The 1-, 2-, and 3-year esophageal variceal bleeding rates after BRTO are 27% to 35%, 45% to 66%, and 45% to 91%, respectively.[45]

The classic BRTO procedure is performed from a femoral or jugular venous access site with cannulation of the gastrorenal shunt through the left renal vein. Occlusion of the shunt using balloon-occlusion catheters is followed by placement of a coaxial microcatheter for retrograde injection of a sclerosing agent. The balloon is deflated and removed after confirmation of shunt thrombosis after a dwell period. A detailed description of the BRTO procedure is described in Chapter 29 of this book.

Candidates for the BRTO Procedure

Spontaneous gastrorenal shunts develop in up to 85% of patients with gastric varices.[4,46,47] These patients with shunts that can be occluded by available balloon occlusion catheters are candidates for the classic BRTO procedure.[48] Despite having treatable shunts, patients with a large (>5 cm) hepatocellular carcinoma (HCC) or large-volume intractable ascites are not candidates for BRTO.[13] HCC itself significantly reduces survival in patients undergoing BRTO.

Technical Success

Using patient selection criteria discussed and when performed as described earlier, technical success for BRTO ranges from 79% to 100%.[4,7,9–13,19–23,29,30,31,34,35,46,48] This success does not rely on additional adjunctive obliterative procedures such as balloon-occluded antegrade transvenous obliteration (BATO) and endoscopic sclerotherapy.

Technical success (defined as sclerosant completely filling the gastric varices and gastrorenal shunt) can also be achieved in patients with incomplete variceal obliteration using staged procedures with treatment goals completed over additional sessions. This alternate approach can be used to limit the volume of sclerosant per session. Dose-related hemolysis and hemoglobinuria-induced renal dysfunction can occur with ethanolamine oleate (EO) and sodium tetradecyl sulfate (STS) sclerosant agents.[49]

Five centers studying 210 patients undergoing staged or sequential BRTO have reported progressive and complete obliteration of the gastric varices.[5,13,31,33,48] Cumulatively, these studies show technical success in 71% after one treatment, 88% after the second, and 91% after three treatment sessions.

BATO as an adjunct or rescue technique along with the classic BRTO is a useful modification for control of gastric varices to increase technical success. BATO alone is successful in 44% to 100% of cases.[32,50] Approaching the varices from the portal venous side is most easily achieved through an existing TIPS. Transhepatic and transiliocolic routes are also used. BATO in conjunction with BRTO can reduce sclerosant overspill from the gastric varices into the portal vein (PV). Despite a relatively straightforward procedure, technical failure may occur for a variety of reasons. We have previously classified these technical factors into categories I to IV shown in ▶ Table 31.1.[45]

The actual incidence of each of these type I to IV technical failures is difficult to determine from analyzing the existing literature as scant details of technical failures are reported in most of the large-scale reviews and studies.[12] Three studies evaluated 14 technical failures in 160 BRTO procedures. The studies reported type I failures in 2 of the 14; type II failures accounted for 5 of the 14 failures. Type III failures were to blame for 6 of the 14 technical failures. Type IV failure occurred in 1 of 14.[10,11,19] Type I and II technical failures are often related to operator inexperience and lack of appropriate catheters and occlusion balloons. A retrospective study on 41 BRTO procedures using a variety of occlusion balloon catheters available in the United States showed that a balloon occlusion catheter greater than 20 mm is rarely required. In that study, 75% of the gastrorenal shunts could be occluded using 13-mm balloons, but 30% could be occluded using 10-mm size balloons. Balloon catheters between 14 and 20 mm were necessary in 25%. In Asia, vascular sheaths, diagnostic catheters, and occlusion balloons are designed for BRTO. These specifically designed catheters can facilitate cannulation and occlusion of the shunts.[7,38,46]

Type IV technical complications involve rupture of the balloon occlusion catheter early in the procedure. This early rupture requires instillation of added sclerosant through another occlusion balloon catheter. The reported incidence of type IV failure in

Table 31.1 Causes of Balloon-Occluded Retrograde Transvenous Obliteration Technical Failures

Type	Description
I	Failure to cannulate the gastrorenal shunt with or without contrast or sclerosant extravasation
II	Failure to occlude a large shunt with available occlusion balloons
IIIa	Failure to opacify the shunt in the setting of a complex multi-collateral gastrorenal or gastric variceal system
IIIb	Failure to opacify the shunt and extravasation of contrast or sclerosant into the retroperitoneum
IV	Occlusion balloon rupture occurring before effective variceal obliteration

the literature from Japan ranges from 2.8% to 8.7% of BRTO procedures.[30,51] BRTO in Japan uses EO as the sclerosant. EO is not available in the United States; therefore, 3% STS is used as the sclerosant. Typically, in the United States, a mixture of Lipiodol (Guerbet LLC, Bloomington, Indiana)–STS–air/CO_2 is used to created a fluoroscopically visible foam. A study by Saad et al[52] specifically looked at the incidence of balloon rupture using STS as the sclerosing agent through balloon occlusion catheters available in the United States. In this retrospective study of 41 consecutive BRTO procedures on 40 patients, a balloon rupture rate of 15% was reported (double the 2.3%–8.7% incidence reported rates in the Japanese and Korean literature).[51] The study concluded that dwell time (described as either greater than 6 hours or less than 6 hours) did not influence balloon rupture. Furthermore, the

study revealed a trend for latex balloon occlusion catheters to be more prone to rupture during BRTO despite being inflated to industry specifications.

Rarely does balloon catheter rupture pose a serious harm to patient or impact procedure clinical success. The more likely scenario is operator frustration with the need to exchange the catheter system.

In the immediate post-BRTO period, transient fever, hematuria, and abdominal pain have been observed in a large percentage of patients.[49] More serious procedure-related complications are rarely reported and include asymptomatic and symptomatic pulmonary embolus, anaphylactic reactions to EO, and pulmonary edema.

Portal vein thrombosis and renal vein thrombosis are also potential complications of BRTO. Interestingly, when postprocedural imaging (cone-beam computed tomography [CT] or fluoroscopy) demonstrates small overspill of sclerosant into the intrahepatic PVs this is usually without clinical consequence.[12] See ▶ Table 31.2 for procedure-related complications.

Follow-up endoscopic examinations reveal localized mucosal changes in the region of treated gastric varices in a majority of patients. A typical gastric ulceration pattern with or without associated bleeding has also been reported.[30] These endoscopically visible changes usually respond to short-term conservative therapy.

Postprocedure Imaging Evaluation

Imaging success is usually fluoroscopically apparent at the completion of the procedure; therefore, strict time frames for cross-sectional imaging or ultrasound follow-up are not strictly

Table 31.2 Procedure-Related Complications of Balloon-Occluded Retrograde Transvenous Obliteration

Study	Patients (n)	Complication	Rate
Cho et al[12]	49	Death	2/4 (4.3%)
		Pulmonary embolus	2/49 (4.3%)
		Left renal vein thrombus	1/49 (2.2%)
		Hemoglobinuria	26/49 (53.1%)
Saad et al[55]	39	Spontaneous bacterial peritonitis	4/49 (8.2%)
		Partial portal vein thrombosis	1/39 (2.5%)
		Partial left renal vein thrombosis	1/39 (2.5%)
		Cardiac arrhythmia	1/39 (2.5 %)
		Pulmonary embolus	1/39 (2.5%)
Jang et al[53]	183	Pulmonary embolus	5/183 (2.7%)
		Left renal infarct	1/183 (0.5%)
		Gastrorenal shunt rupture	1/183 (0.5%)
Watanabe et al[58]	77	Portal vein thrombosis	3/77 (3.9%)
		Renal vein thrombosis	2/77 (2.6%)
		Splenic vein thrombosis	2/77 (2.6%)

Based on data from Cho SK, Shin SW, Lee IH, et al. Balloon-occluded retrograde transvenous obliteration of gastric varices: outcomes and complications in 49 patients. AJR Am J Roentgenol 2007;189(6):W365–W372.[12]; Jang SY, Kim GH, Park SY, et al. Clinical outcomes of balloon-occluded retrograde transvenous obliteration for the treatment of gastric variceal hemorrhage in Korean patients with liver cirrhosis: a retrospective multicenter study. Clin Mol Hepatol 2012;18:368–374.[53]; Kato T, Uematsu T, Nishigaki Y, et al. Therapeutic effects of BRTO on portal-systemic encephalopathy in patients with liver cirrhosis. Intern Med 2001;40:688–691.[54]; and Saad WE, Wagner C, Al-Osaimi A, et al. The effect of balloon-occluded transvenous obliteration of gastric varices and gastrorenal shunts on the hepatic synthetic function: a comparison between Child-Pugh and model for end-stage liver disease scores. Vasc Endovascular Surg 2013;47(4):281–287.[55]

defined. Doppler ultrasonography can reliably evaluate PV and renal vein patency after the procedure.

Lack of gastric variceal opacification and decreased size of the gastric varices is the expected anatomic outcome of BRTO. A non-contrast and contrast-enhanced portal venous phase CT clearly depicts this and will show the patency and anatomy of the PV and tributaries. At the authors' institution, CT imaging follow-up is done 3 to 4 months after the BRTO procedure. In the setting of unexpected fever, drop in hemoglobin, and so on, a more urgent CT is obtained. Whereas varices obliterated using sclerosant mixed with contrast will appear isodense on precontrast CT, lipiodol-filled varices are hyperdense. Contrast-enhanced magnetic resonance imaging is similarly useful in this cross-sectional follow-up.

Clinical Outcomes

The effectiveness of BRTO in controlling gastric variceal bleeding is well documented. Rebleeding rates are generally reported at lower than 5%.[46] When considering as an intent-to-treat basis including technical failures, the gastric variceal rebleed rate ranges from 0% to 31.6%.[4,7,9–13,19–23,31,34,36,46,48] These studies do not clearly note whether rebleeding occurs from gastric varices versus from esophageal and duodenal varices or from portal hypertensive gastropathy. Three studies evaluating a combined 141 patients looked specifically at rates of gastric variceal recurrent bleed (3.2%–8.7%) versus global variceal recurrent bleed (19%–31%) after BRTO. These studies showed an intent-to-treat gastric variceal recurrent bleed rate of 10% to 20%.[7,10,11]

The higher global variceal recurrent bleed rates reflect the increase in PHT after BRTO. Four large studies surveying 160 patients with repeated endoscopy over a 3-year period after BRTO reported 1-, 2-, and 3-year aggravation of esophageal varices rates of 27% to 35%, 45% to 66%, and 45% to 91%, respectively.[9,13,23,32] This worsening of esophageal varices is more likely to occur in patients with preexisting varices at the time of BRTO. A large retrospective study involving 177 patients undergoing BRTO found that new esophageal varices appeared in more than 50% of patients who had no esophageal varices before BRTO. In addition, aggravation of esophageal varices was noted in approximately one third of patients with preexisting esophageal varices.[53] Routine upper endoscopy is encouraged in regular intervals after BRTO at which time band ligation may be required. Two studies evaluating 117 patients found that bleeding from esophageal varices occurred in 36% to 57% of patients who developed aggravation of esophageal varices after BRTO.[10,46]

In recent years, BRTO has become a reliable method for treating encephalopathy refractory to medical management. Complete obliteration of spontaneous gastrorenal shunt in these patients with portosystemic encephalopathy results in enhanced ammonia detoxification from the liver. Several studies have shown immediate reduction or complete resolution of encephalopathy in patients with portosystemic shunt encephalopathy.[4,13,24,34,50,54] Even with partial BRTO obliteration, the plasma ammonia levels significantly decrease after 24 to 48 hours. Six of seven patients with West Haven Criteria hepatic encephalopathy grades II and III were shown in one study to be completely resolved of symptoms at 1 and 4 months after BRTO.[54]

Kaplan-Meier survival rates after BRTO range from 83% to 98% at 1 year, 76% to 79% at 2 years, 66% to 85% at 3 years, and 36% to 69% at 5 years, respectively.[4,19,23,27,32–34] Hepatic synthetic reserve is thought to be the most important prognostic factor for survival after BRTO. The presence of HCC is considered to be the second most important prognostic factor.

Ascites and hepatic hydrothorax have been reported after BRTO despite transient improvement or preservation of hepatic function. Several studies report these transudative complications occurring within 30 to 60 days after BRTO in up to 8% of patients.[30,35,43] Massive or medically refractory ascites develops in up to 2.6% of patients, and up to 5.8 % of patients develop refractory hydrothorax. These complications may be related to worsening of PHT after obliteration of the low-pressure gastrorenal shunt or might be caused by worsening hepatic synthetic function. Saad et al have described evaluating the effect of BRTO on the model for end-stage liver disease (MELD) rather than relying on the Child-Pugh (C-P) score, which considers ascites as a means of differentiating complications that are oncotic driven from those related to hepatic synthetic dysfunction.[55] The MELD score may be a more sensitive indicator of hepatic reserve after BRTO.[55]

The MELD score was originally developed as a predictor of mortality in cirrhotic patients about to undergo TIPS procedures.[56] The MELD score increases after TIPS because of diversion of blood from the hepatocytes. Most publications suggest that based on C-P scores, hepatic function initially improves for 6 to 9 months after BRTO and then returns to baseline.[13,41] This is likely caused by BRTO-induced increased flow to liver parenchyma. Miyamoto et al have described an average about 50% more flow toward the liver after BRTO.[27]

The clear disadvantage of this increased portal flow in a patient with PHT has already been described with the worsening of nongastric varices, portal hypertensive gastropathy, ascites, and hepatic hydrothorax. Of course, not all patients experience these events despite increases in hepatic portal blood flow. Some patients continue to develop other collateral pathways to decompress the increase in portal blood flow; others may simply not respond to augmented flow.

In the Saad et al retrospective study, 26 patients with technically successful BRTO procedures were evaluated for changes in MELD, C-P, and MELD/C-P component contribution. The study found a positive effect on hepatic reserve from 1.5 to 4 months after BRTO. Specifically, serum bilirubin and international normalized ratio were found to drop significantly below baseline levels. No significant changes in serum creatinine were observed in the 4-month study period. These improved markers of hepatic synthetic function decreased MELD scores. C-P scores did not improve despite significant increases in serum albumin levels during the 1- to 4-month study period because of the onset of ascites in 8 of 26 patients. Overall, in the majority of patients, the improvement in hepatic function may be transient with return to baseline pre-BRTO hepatic function within 9 months.[13,27,43]

It is fair to say that not all gastrorenal shunts have the same volume of flow; therefore, the effect of portal venous diversion toward the liver or resulting decompression through new portosystemic collaterals is not the same in all patients. A study by Kumamoto et al showed that BRTO protects hepatic function in patients with gastrorenal shunts. This group found that patients with gastrorenal shunts treated with BRTO had stable hepatic function in up to 3-year follow-up similar to control group C-P class A or B cirrhotic patients without gastrorenal shunts. The BRTO group also experienced a transient improvement in hepatic synthetic function by C-P score for 6 to 12 months after BRTO. In their study, hepatic function progressively deteriorated by C-P score in patients with untreated gastrorenal shunts.[13]

Patients with both TIPS and BRTO pose a unique hemodynamic scenario. In theory, the increased portal pressure burden to the liver and the remaining portal venous circuit could be buffered by the TIPS. In theory, this might be an ideal situation. The typical Western approach of managing PHT using decompression via TIPS creation can worsen hepatic function, be complicated by encephalopathy, and result in significant mortality in patients with MELD scores above 17. A recent study by Saad et al aimed to evaluate the protective value of this TIPS buffer against the development of ascites and/or bleeding after BRTO.[57] In this retrospective study, patients were placed into two groups, BRTO alone and BRTO plus TIPS. Thirty-six patients had successful BRTO procedures. Of these 36 procedures, 9 patients were included in the BRTO plus TIPS group. Two patients in this group had combined procedures; the other four had BRTO in the setting of preexisting TIPS (average, 4.9 months; range, 0–14 months). One-year survival rates in both groups were similar. No patients in the BRTO plus TIPS group experienced recurrent variceal bleeding. Recurrent bleeding for the BRTO-only group at 3, 6, 12, and 24 months was 5%.

Similarly, whereas ascites and hydrothorax did not occur in the BRTO plus TIPS group of patients, the ascites- and hydrothorax-free rate for BRTO alone at 3, 6, 12, and 24 months were 87%, 58%, 43%, and 29%, respectively. Three patients developed symptomatic ascites requiring paracentesis ($n = 2$) or TIPS ($n = 1$). For the BRTO-only group, this is a symptomatic ascites rate of 11% (N = 3/27). This seems to establish a protective role for TIPS against the development of ascites and hydrothorax after BRTO and suggests that if refractory ascites or hydrothorax develops after BRTO, a TIPS may prove to be beneficial.

Conclusion

The conventional BRTO procedure can successfully achieve first- or second-line definitive therapy for gastric variceal bleeding. The procedure is technically feasible in 79% to 100% of patients with few significant procedure-related complications. Obliteration of the gastrorenal shunt that functions to decompress the portal venous circuit may lead to an aggravation of esophageal varices. It appears, however, that the risk of recurrent variceal hemorrhage is not significantly affected. Routine endoscopic surveillance is warranted in these patients. The transient early increase in clinically symptomatic transudative fluid is likely oncotically driven and, if refractory to standard therapies, it can be successfully treated with TIPS. Early experience combining TIPS and BRTO procedures for the management of variceal bleeding has shown encouraging results (decreased bleeding from all sources and fewer instances of ascites). These improved outcomes are superior to results from each procedure alone.

Clinical Pearls

- Gastric variceal bleeding is less common than esophageal variceal bleeding yet is associated with both higher mortality rate and less effective endoscopic treatment options.

- BRTO and or BRTO–BATO have emerged as a clinically advantageous option to treat variceal bleeds associated with gastrorenal shunts.
- BRTO is a reliable method for treating splenorenal shunt–related encephalopathy refractory to medical management.
- Rebleeding rates after successful BRTO are generally reported at lower than 5%.
- Patients with a large (>5 cm) hepatocellular carcinoma or large-volume intractable ascites are not candidates for BRTO.
- Despite a relatively straightforward procedure, BRTO technical failure may occur for a variety of reasons described.
- Transient ascites and hepatic hydrothorax have been reported after BRTO despite some preservation of hepatic function.
- The MELD score may be a more sensitive indicator of hepatic reserve after BRTO.
- Emerging data on TIPS and BRTO combined procedures is encouraging with decreased bleeding from all sources and fewer instances of ascites compared with results from the individual procedures alone.

References

1. Sarin SK, Lahoti D, Saxena SP, et al. Prevalence, classification and natural history of gastric varices: a long term follow-up study in 568 portal hypertension patients. Hepatology 1992;16:1343–1349.
2. Ryan BM, Stockbrugger RW, Ryan JM. A pathophysiologic, gastroenterologic, and radiologic approach to the management of gastric varices. Gastroenterology 2004;126:1175–1189.
3. Sarin SK, Agarwal SR. Gastric varices and portal hypertensive gastropathy. Clin Liver Dis 2001;5:727–767.
4. Hirota S, Matsumoto S, Tomita M, et al. Retrograde transvenous obliteration of gastric varices. Radiology 1999;211(2):349–356.
5. Kiyosue H, Mori H, Matumoto S, et al. Transcatheter obliteration of gastric varices. Part 1. Anatomic classification. Radiographics 2003;23(4):911–920.
6. Kiyosue H, Mori H, Matsumoto S, et al. Transcatheter obliteration of gastric varices. Part 2. Strategy and techniques based on hemodynamic features. Radiographics 2003;23(4):921–937.
7. Kitamoto M, Imamura M, Kamada K, et al. Balloon-occluded retrograde transvenous obliteration of gastric fundal varices with hemorrhage. AJR Am J Roentgenol 2002;178(5):1167–1174.
8. Sarin SK, Lahoti D, Saxena SP, et al. Prevalence, classification and natural history of gastric vaices: a long term follow-up study in 568 portal hypertension patients. Hepatology 1992;16(6):1343–1349.
9. Ibukuro K, Sugihara T, Tanaka R, et al. Balloon-occluded retrograde transvenous obliteration (BRTO) for a direct shunt between the inferior mesenteric vein and the inferior vena cava in a patient with hepatic encephalopathy. J Vasc Interv Radiol 2007;18(1 pt 1):121–125.
10. Ninoi T, Nishida N, Kaminou T, et al. Balloon-occluded retrograde transvenous obliteration of gastric varices with gastrorenal shunt: long-term follow-up in 78 patients. AJR Am J Roentgenol 2005;184(4):1340–1346.
11. Akahoshi T, Hashizume M, Tomikawa M, et al. Long-term results of balloon-occluded retrograde transvenous obliteration for gastric variceal bleeding and risky gastric varices: a 10-year experience. J Gastroenterol Hepatol 2008;23(11):1702–1709.
12. Cho SK, Shin SW, Lee IH, et al. Balloon-occluded retrograde transvenous obliteration of gastric varices: outcomes and complications in 49 patients. AJR Am J Roentgenol 2007;189(6):W365–W372.
13. Kumamoto M, Toyonaga A, Inoue H, et al. Long-term results of balloon-occluded retrograde transvenous obliteration for gastric fundal varices: hepatic deterioration links to portosystemic shunt syndrome. J Gastroenterol Hepatol 2010;25(6):1129–1135.
14. de Franchis R, Primignani M. Natural history of portal hypertension in patients with cirrhosis. Clin Liver Dis 2001;5(3):645–663.
15. Hayashi S, Saeki S, Hosoi H, et al. A clinical and portal hemodynamic analysis for obliteration of gastric-renal shunt communicated with gastric fundic varices. Nippon Shokakibyo Gakkai Zasshi 1998;95(7):755–763.
16. Tanihata H, Minamiguchi H, Sato M, et al. Changes in portal systemic pressure gradient after balloon-occluded retrograde transvenous obliteration of gastric varices and aggravation of esophageal varices. Cardiovasc Intervent Radiol 2009;32(6):1209–1216.

17. Choi YS, Lee JH, Sinn DH, et al. Effect of balloon-occluded retrograde transvenous obliteration on the natural history of coexisting esophageal varices. J Clin Gastroenterol 2008;42(9):974–979.

18. Nakamura S, Torii N, Yatsuji S, et al. Long-term follow up of esophageal varices after balloon-occluded retrograde transvenous obliteration for gastric varices. Hepatol Res 2008;38(4):340–347.

19. Yamagami T, Kato T, Hirota T, et al. Infusion of 50% glucose solution before injection of ethanolamine oleate during balloon-occluded retrograde transvenous obliteration. Australas Radiol 2007;51(4):334–338.

20. Ninoi T, Nakamura K, Kaminou T, et al. TIPS versus transcatheter sclerotherapy for gastric varices. AJR Am J Roentgenol 2004;183(2):369–376.

21. Sonomura T, Sato M, Kishi K, et al. Balloon-occluded retrograde transvenous obliteration for gastric varices: a feasibility study. Cardiovasc Intervent Radiol 1998;21(1):27–30.

22. Kiyosue H, Matsumoto S, Onishi R, et al. Balloon-occluded retrograde transvenous obliteration (B-RTO) for gastric varices: therapeutic results and problems. Nippon Igaku Hoshasen Gakkai Zasshi 1999;59(1):12–19.

23. Koito K, Namieno T, Nagakawa T, Morita K. Balloon-occluded retrograde transvenous obliteration for gastric varices with gastrorenal or gastrocaval collaterals. AJR Am J Roentgenol 1996;167(5):1317–1320.

24. Chikamori F, Kuniyoshi N, Kawashima T, Takase Y. Gastric varices with gastrorenal shunt: combined therapy using transjugular retrograde obliteration and partial splenic embolization. AJR Am J Roentgenol 2008;191(2):555–559.

25. Chikamori F, Kuniyoshi N, Shibuya S, Takase Y. Transjugular retrograde obliteration for chronic portosystemic encephalopathy. Abdom Imaging 2000;25(6):567–571.

26. Chikamori F, Kuniyoshi N, Shibuya S, Takase Y. Combination treatment of transjugular retrograde obliteration and endoscopic embolization for portosystemic encephalopathy with esophageal varices. Hepatogastroenterology 2004;51(59):1379–1381.

27. Miyamoto Y, Oho K, Kumamoto M, et al. Balloon-occluded retrograde transvenous obliteration improves liver function in patients with cirrhosis and portal hypertension. J Gastroenterol Hepatol 2003;18(8):934–942.

28. Sugimori K, Morimoto M, Shirato K, et al. Retrograde transvenous obliteration of gastric varices associated with large collateral veins or a large gastrorenal shunt. J Vasc Interv Radiol 2005;16(1):113–118.

29. Fukuda T, Hirota S, Matsumoto S, et al. Application of balloon-occluded retrograde transvenous obliteration to gastric varices complicating refractory ascites. Cardiovasc Intervent Radiol 2004;27(1):64–67.

30. Shimoda R, Horiuchi K, Hagiwara S, et al. Short-term complications of retrograde transvenous obliteration of gastric varices in patients with portal hypertension: effects of obliteration of major portosystemic shunts. Abdom Imaging 2005;30(3):306–313.

31. Takuma Y, Nouso K, Makino Y, et al. Prophylactic balloon-occluded retrograde transvenous obliteration for gastric varices in compensated cirrhosis. Clin Gastroenterol Hepatol 2005;3(12):1245–1252.

32. Arai H, Abe T, Takagi H, Mori M. Efficacy of balloon-occluded retrograde transvenous obliteration, percutaneous transhepatic obliteration and combined techniques for the management of gastric fundal varices. World J Gastroenterol 2006;12(24):3866–3873.

33. Arai H, Abe T, Shimoda R, et al. Emergency balloon-occluded retrograde transvenous obliteration for gastric varices. J Gastroenterol 2005;40(10):964–971.

34. Choi YH, Yoon CJ, Park JH, et al. Balloon-occluded retrograde transvenous obliteration for gastric variceal bleeding: its feasibility compared with transjugular intrahepatic portosystemic shunt. Korean J Radiol 2003;4(2):109–116.

35. Park KS, Kim YH, Choi JS, et al. Therapeutic efficacy of balloon-occluded retrograde transvenous obliteration in patients with gastric variceal bleeding. Korean J Gastroenterol 2006;47(5):370–378.

36. Kim ES, Park SY, Kwon KT, et al. The clinical usefulness of balloon occluded retrograde transvenous obliteration in gastric variceal bleeding. Taehan Kan Hakhoe Chi 2003;9(4):315–323.

37. Matsumoto A, Hamamoto N, Nomura T, et al. Balloon-occluded retrograde transvenous obliteration of high risk gastric fundal varices. Am J Gastroenterol 1999;94(3):643–649.

38. Hirota S, Matsumoto S, Tomita M, et al. Retrograde transvenous obliteration of gastric varices. Radiology 1999;211(2):349–356.

39. Koito K, Namieno T, Nagakawa T, Morita K. Balloon-occluded retrograde transvenous obliteration for gastric varices with gastrorenal or gastrocaval collaterals. AJR Am J Roentgenol 1996;167(5):1317–1320.

40. Kanagawa H, Mima S, Kouyama H, et al. Treatment of gastric fundal varices by balloon-occluded retrograde transvenous obliteration. J Gastroenterol Hepatol 1996;11(1):51.

41. Fukuda T, Hirota S, Sugimura K. Long-term results of balloon-occluded retrograde transvenous obliteration for the treatment of gastric varices and hepatic encephalopathy. J Vasc Interv Radiol 2001;12(3):327–336.

42. Akahane T, Iwasaki T, Kobayashi N, et al. Changes in liver function parameters after occlusion of gastrorenal shunts with balloon-occluded retrograde transvenous obliteration. Am J Gastroenterol 1997;92(6):1026–1030.

43. Chikamori F, Kuniyoshi N, Shibuya S, Takase Y. Eight years of experience with transjugular retrograde obliteration for gastric varices with gastrorenal shunts. Surgery 2001;129(4):414–420.

44. Kitamoto M, Imamura M, Kamada K, et al. Balloon-occluded retrograde transvenous obliteration of gastric fundal varices with hemorrhage. AJR Am J Roentgenol 2002;178(5):1167–1674.

45. Saad WE, Sabri SS. Balloon-occluded retrograde transvenous obliteration (BRTO): technical results and outcomes. Semin Intervent Radiol 2011;28:333–338.

46. Hong C H, Kim H J, Park J H, et al. Treatment of patients with gastric variceal hemorrhage: endoscopic N-butyl-2–cyanoacrylate injection versus balloon-occluded retrograde transvenous obliteration. J Gastroenterol Hepatol 2009;24(3):372–378.

47. Kanagawa H, Mima S, Kouyama H, et al. Treatment of gastric fundal varices by balloon-occluded retrograde transvenous obliteration. J Gastroenterol Hepatol 1996;11(1):51–58.

48. Fukuda T, Hirota S, Sugimura K. Long-term results of balloon-occluded retrograde transvenous obliteration for the treatment of gastric varices and hepatic encephalopathy. J Vasc Interv Radiol 2001;12(3):327–336.

49. Patel A, Fischamn A, Saad WE. Balloon-occluded obliteration of gastric varices. Am J Roentgenol 2012;199:721–729.

50. Araki T, Hori M, Motosugi U, et al. Can balloon-occluded retrograde transvenous obliteration be performed for gastric varices without gastrorenal shunts? J Vasc Interv Radiol 2010;21(5):663–670.

51. Park SJ, Chung JW, Kim H-C, et al. The prevalence, risk factors, and clinical outcome of balloon rupture in balloon–occluded retrograde transvenous obliteration of gastric varices. J Vasc Intervent Radiol 2010;21(4):503–507.

52. Saad WE, Nicholson D, Lippert A, et al. Balloon-occlusion catheter rupture during balloon-occluded retrograde transvenous obliteration of gastric varices utilizing sodium tetradecyl sulfate: incidence and consequences. Vasc Endovascular Surg 2012;46(8):664–670.

53. Jang SY, Kim GH, Park SY, et al. Clinical outcomes of balloon-occluded retrograde transvenous obliteration for the treatment of gastric variceal hemorrhage in Korean patients with liver cirrhosis : a retrospective multicenter study. Clin Mol Hepatol 2012;18:368–374.

54. Kato T, Uematsu T, Nishigaki Y, et al. Therapeutic effects of BRTO on portal-systemic encephalopathy in patients with liver cirrhosis. Intern Med 2001;40:688–691.

55. Saad WE, Wagner C, Al-Osaimi A, et al. The effect of balloon-occluded transvenous obliteration of gastric varices and gastrorenal shunts on the hepatic synthetic function: a comparison between Child-Pugh and model for end-stage liver disease scores. Vasc Endovascular Surg 2013;47(4): 281–287.

56. Salerno F, Merti M, Cazzaniga M, et al. MELD score is better than Child-Pugh score in predicting 3–month survival of patients undergoing transjugular intrahepatic portosystemic shunt J Hepatol 2002;36(4):494–500.

57. Saad WE, Wagner C, Lippert A, et al. Protective value of TIPS against the development of ascites and/or bleeding after balloon-occluded retrograde transvenous obliteration of gastric varices. Am J Gastroenterol 2013;108(10):1612–1619.

58. Watanabe M, Shiozawa K, Ikehara T, et al. Short term effects and early complication of balloon occluded retrograde transvenous obliteration for gastric varices. ISRN Gastroenterol 2012;2012:919371.

Chapter 32: Management of Duodenal Varices

Ravi N. Srinivasa, Jeffrey Forris Beecham Chick, and Wael E.A. Saad

Introduction

Duodenal varices (DVs) are an uncommon manifestation of portal hypertension or mesenteric/portal vein thrombosis, representing approximately 17% of ectopic varices.[1,2] Pathologically they represent dilated mesoportal varicosities and portosystemic collaterals in the duodenal wall.[3] Despite their infrequency, they may be potentially life threatening as they carry a fourfold risk of bleeding compared with esophageal varices and a mortality rate approaching 40% secondary to unrelenting hemorrhage.[3–6]

The most commonly encountered varices are esophageal and gastric, which are amenable to medical and endoscopic interventions.[4–12] Due to the anatomic location and hemodynamics, however, the medical and endoscopic management of DVs is limited.[1,3,4,6,13] In addition to surgical resection, endovascular management with decompressive transjugular intrahepatic portosystemic shunt (TIPS)[14,22,23] or transvenous obliteration remains a potential treatment option. In the limited data in the literature, the rebleed rate after TIPS is approximately 21% to 37% and approximately 13% following transvenous obliteration.[2,29]

The chapter discusses specifically duodenal varices (DVs). However, with the exception of anatomical location specific to DVs,

the general classification and management approach applies to all ectopic mesenteric varices, whether in the small bowel or large bowel.

Anatomy and Pathophysiology and Hemodynamic Classification

DVs are considered "true veins" when compared with esophageal varices. DVs, however, have thinner walls and larger diameters, resulting in greater wall tension and increased rates of bleeding.[3] DVs are portoportal or portosystemic retroperitoneal collateral vessels (▶ Fig. 32.1).[3] The portal venous supply of DVs includes pancreaticoduodenal veins, cystic branches from the superior mesenteric veins, gastroduodenal veins, and pyloric veins.[3,7] The systemic venous drainage of DVs is commonly via the gonadal veins, particularly the right gonadal vein, and the capsular renal veins, all of which drain into the inferior vena cava.[3,7] The left gonadal vein may be involved in DVs and is typically associated with DVs in the third and fourth portions of the duodenum. In rare instances, DVs may drain directly into the inferior vena cava or right renal vein.[3]

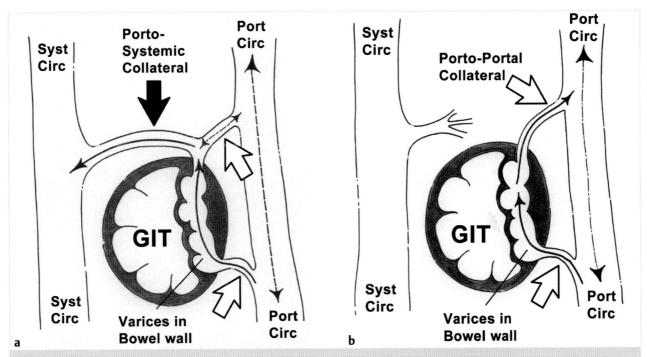

Fig. 32.1 Classification of ectopic varices. (**a,b**) Baseline anatomy images to help interpret the images of the classification system. The image demonstrates a representative portal or mesenteric vein branch (Port Circ) on the right and a representative systemic vein branch (Syst Circ) on the left of a cross-section through a bowel loop, which is representative of the gastrointestinal tract (GIT). Typical portal venous (splanchnic veins) branches would include the portal vein proper, the mesenteric vein, and the splenic vein. Typical systemic veins include the inferior vena cava, the gonadal veins, renal veins, and retroperitoneal and paravertebral veins. Varices are seen in the wall of the bowel. (**a**) Ectopic varices are supplied and drained by portal collaterals (*hollow black arrows*) and drained (efferent collateral) by a portosystemic collateral (*solid black arrow*). (**b**) Ectopic varices are supplied and drained by portal collaterals (*hollow black arrows*) and not drained by a portosystemic collateral. The efferent collateral drainage is portal and not systemic. In both (**a**) and (**b**), there is no portal venous occlusion. (*Reprinted with permission from Saad WE, Lippert A, Saad NE. Ectopic varices: Anatomical classification, hemodynamic classification, and hemodynamic-based management. Tech Vasc Interv Radiol 2013;16(2):158–175.*)

Table 32.1 Typical Locations for Duodenal Varices with Various Locoregional Pathologies

Etiologies	Location
Generalized or global portal hypertension of all etiologies	D1[a] and D2[b]
Status after gastrectomy	D2
Status after balloon-occluded retrograde transvenous obliteration of gastric varices	D1 and D2
Mesenteric carcinoid	D3[c]–D4[d]>D2
Chronic pancreatitis	D1 + D2>D3
Splenoportal thrombosis	D1 + D2>D3
Mesoportal thrombosis	D2 + D3
Focal mesenteric occlusion	D3 or D4

[a]D1: first part of the duodenum (duodenal bulb)
[b]D2: second part of duodenum (duodenal sweep or descending part)
[c]D3: third part of the duodenum (transverse retroperitoneal part)
[d]D4: ascending part to the ligament of Treitz.
Reprinted with permission from Saad WE, Lippert A, Saad NE. Ectopic varices: Anatomical classification, hemodynamic classification, and hemodynamic-based management. Tech Vasc Interv Radiol 2013; 16(2):158–175.

Location of DVs is due to locoregional pathology including splanchnic vein (splenic, splenoportal, mesenteric, mesoportal, or portal) stenosis, thrombosis, or occlusion, adhesions and scarring from prior surgeries, or inflammatory processes (▶ Table 32.1). The most common site for DVs is in the duodenal sweep in the first portion (D1: Duodenal bulb), the second portion (D2), and the proximal portion of the third portion of the duodenum (D3). DVs in the distal duodenum (D3 and D4) are usually associated with splenic vein thrombosis with or without portal vein thrombosis.

There are two classifications for DVs (as in all ectopic varices): the nonocclusive, or oncotic type (secondary to portal hypertension), and the occlusive type (due to mesenteric or portal vein thrombosis) (▶ Table 32.2; ▶ Fig. 32.2).[3]

Endoscopy and Imaging

Standard imaging evaluation for DVs has not been established. Endoscopy, however, is the initial modality of choice to diagnose and localize the ectopic DVs.[5] Contrast-enhanced computed tomography (CT) and magnetic resonance imaging (MRI) are important for the evaluation and management of DVs as these modalities determine if portal hypertension is present and identify portal vein and mesenteric thrombosis. Secondary signs of portal hypertension include splenomegaly, ascites, hepatic hydrothorax, and development of portosystemic collaterals.[3] CT and MRI may also identify DVs that were not appreciated on endoscopy. The use of ultrasound is limited to evaluating the patency of the intrahepatic and extrahepatic portal vein, and the distal splenic and mesenteric veins at their confluence. Ultrasound may also determine the direction of mesoportal blood flow, specifically whether flow is hepatofugal (away from the liver), hepatopetal (toward the liver), or fluctuating.[3]

In the setting of splanchnic vein thrombosis (thrombosis of the portal vein, mesenteric vein, and/or splenic vein), it is important to identify if the DVs occur along the "spleno-portal axis" versus "meso-portal varices" or both axes. This is important to help the management approach of duodenal varices.

Management of Duodenal Varices

Medical management of ectopic DVs includes supportive care with fluid resuscitation and, if necessary, administration of octreotide and systemic vasopressin.[1] Endoscopic-guided management includes banding, sclerotherapy, or injection of thrombin, N-butyl cyanoacrylate, or histoacryl.[15] Sclerosants typically include ethanolamine oleate, sodium tetradecyl sulfate, and polidocanol.[9,21] These endoscopic options are suitable for short-term hemostasis, but long-term hemostasis is difficult to achieve by endoscopic means alone. Bleeding after endoscopic management of DVs is common.

Surgical management of DVs includes resection of varices, duodenectomy, and suture ligation. Surgical portosystemic shunts may also be created, but carry an increased morbidity when compared with the percutaneous approaches including TIPS creation.[4,6,17]

Endovascular management included TIPS decompression with or without sclerosis[16] for nonocclusive (Type-a) DVs and recanalization with or without sclerosis for occlusive (Type-b) DVs (▶ Fig. 32.3). In the setting of splanchnic thrombosis along the spleno-portal axis, partial splenic artery embolization is another option. On the other hand, recanalization is needed if the thrombosis is along the meso-portal axis.

Table 32.2 Classification System for Ectopic Varices

Type	Portoportal Collaterals Only	Both Portoportal and Portosystemic Collaterals	
		Predominantly Portoportal Collaterals with Minimal, if any, Portosystemic Shunting	Predominantly Portosystemic Collaterals with Significant Portosystemic Shunting
Nonocclusive (a)	Type-1a	Type-2a	Type-3a
Occlusive Type (b)	Type-1b	Type-2b	Type-3b

Note: The nonocclusive type is in the setting of a patent portal system and the occlusive type is in the setting of splanchnic thrombosis. The various collaterals may be portoportal or a combination of portosystemic and portoportal.
Reprinted with permission from Saad WE, Lippert A, Saad NE. Ectopic varices: Anatomical classification, hemodynamic classification, and hemodynamic-based management. Tech Vasc Interv Radiol 2013;16(2):158–175.

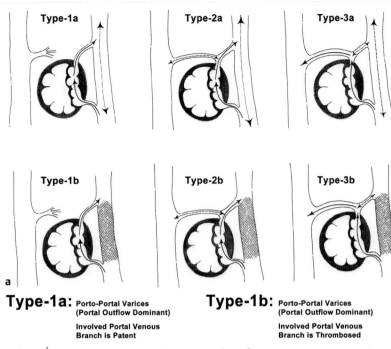

Type-1a: Porto-Portal Varices
(Portal Outflow Dominant)

Involved Portal Venous
Branch is Patent

Type-1b: Porto-Portal Varices
(Portal Outflow Dominant)

Involved Portal Venous
Branch is Thrombosed

a

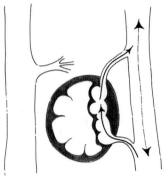

Not common in Mesenteric Varices,
especially in the presence of
Generalized Portal-HTN

Most common type in Duodenal &
Mesenteric Varices, especially in the
absence of Generalized Portal-HTN

Typical of GV in Segmental Portal-HTN
(splenic vein thrombosis) without GRS

b

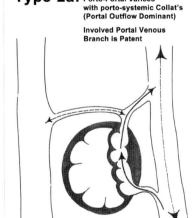

Type-2a: Porto-Portal Varices
with porto-systemic Collat's
(Portal Outflow Dominant)

Involved Portal Venous
Branch is Patent

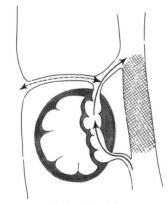

Type-2b: Porto-Systemic Varices
(Systemic Outflow Dominant)

Involved Portal Venous
Branch is Thrombosed

Can be seen in Mesenteric Varices,
especially in the presence of
Generalized Portal-HTN

Can be seen in Duodenal &
Mesenteric Varices, especially in the
absence of Generalized Portal-HTN

c

Fig. 32.2 (**a**) Overview of the classification system. Type-a is nonocclusive and is pressure driven. Type-a usually has some element of portosystemic collaterals (type-a2 and type-a3) to decompress the higher portal pressure. Type-b is the occlusive type and may have no portosystemic collaterals; the varices may simply be part of a portal-to-portal bypass of a focal occlusion (type-b1); however, portosystemic collaterals may exist (type-b2 and type-b3). (**b**) Type-1 ectopic varices without portal venous branch occlusion (type-1a) and with portal venous branch occlusion (type-1b). The portal venous branch may be any vein in the portal circulation. This includes mesenteric vein and tributaries and portal vein tributaries as well as the main portal, mesenteric, and splenic veins. (**c**) Type-2 ectopic varices without portal venous branch occlusion (type-2a) and with portal venous branch occlusion (type-2b). The portal venous branch may be any vein (location or size) in the portal circulation. The main efferent outflow of the ectopic varices in type-2 is portal and not portosystemic. Flow in the existing portosystemic collaterals may be minimal and may even fluctuate. (*continued*)

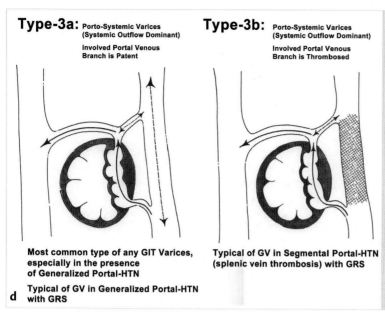

Type-3a: Porto-Systemic Varices (Systemic Outflow Dominant)

Involved Portal Venous Branch is Patent

Type-3b: Porto-Systemic Varices (Systemic Outflow Dominant)

Involved Portal Venous Branch is Thrombosed

Fig. 32.2 (*Continued*) (**d**) Type-3 ectopic varices without portal venous branch occlusion (type-3a) and with portal venous branch occlusion (type-3b). The portal venous branch may be any vein (location or size) in the portal circulation. The main efferent outflow of the ectopic varices in type-3 is portosystemic and not portoportal. GV: gastric varices; HTN: hypertension. (*Reprinted with permission from Saad WE, Lippert A, Saad NE. Ectopic varices: Anatomical classification, hemodynamic classification, and hemodynamic-based management. Tech Vasc Interv Radiol 2013;16(2):158–175.*)

Most common type of any GIT Varices, especially in the presence of Generalized Portal-HTN

Typical of GV in Segmental Portal-HTN (splenic vein thrombosis) with GRS

d Typical of GV in Generalized Portal-HTN with GRS

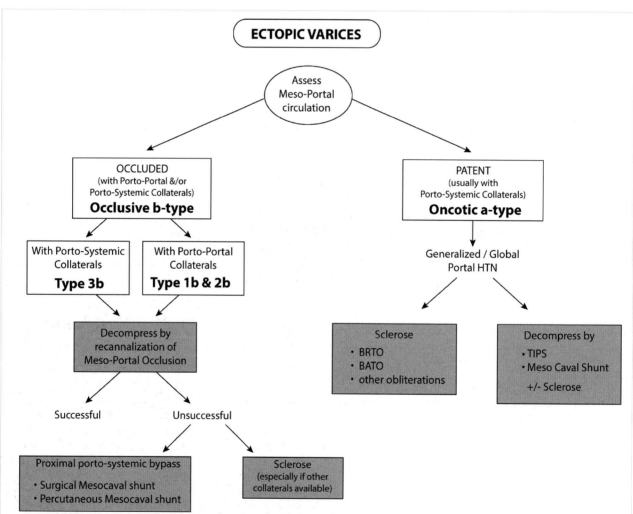

Fig. 32.3 Management approach to duodenal varices. The management approach is simple: if there is no occlusion, decompress with portosystemic shunt with or without sclerosis; if there is an occlusion, recannulate or bypass with or without sclerosis. BATO: balloon-occluded antegrade transvenous obliteration, BRTO: balloon-occluded retrograde transvenous obliteration, HTN: hypertension, TIPS: transjugular intrahepatic portosystemic shunt. (*Reprinted with permission from Saad WE, Lippert A, Saad NE. Ectopic varices: Anatomical classification, hemodynamic classification, and hemodynamic-based management. Tech Vasc Interv Radiol 2013;16(2):158–175.*)

TIPS Decompression with or without Recanalization

Endovascular management of nonocclusive DVs involves the creation of TIPS to decompress the portal circulation (▶ Fig. 32.4). This is then followed by transvenous sclerotherapy using various agents including ethanolamine oleate, 50% glucose and absolute alcohol, or 3% sodium tetradecyl sulfate (STS) foam.[4] STS is mixed in standard fashion with a 1:2:3 ratio of 1 part lipiodol, 2 parts 3% STS, and 3 parts air.

TIPS is ineffective for decompressing DVs caused by thrombosis or occlusion of the splanchnic veins.[3] In these situations, recanalization of the occluded splanchnic veins is an appropriate solution to decompress the varices (▶ Fig. 32.5; ▶ Fig. 32.6). If splanchnic venous occlusion involves the confluence of the splenic and mesenteric veins, recanalization and stent placement should be performed from the mesenteric vein to the portal vein in conjunction with partial splenic artery embolization. If the intrahepatic portal vein is thrombosed, the recanalized portal vein should be extended by a TIPS in order to preserve outflow and maintain patency of the system. If the primary contributor to DVs is the splenic outflow occlusion, then splenic artery embolization may be considered. Splenic artery embolization with or without portal vein recanalization is highly effective.[3]

Transvenous Obliteration

Transvenous obliteration should be performed with a balloon-occluded antegrade transvenous obliteration (BATO)[32,33] approach or a balloon-occluded retrograde transvenous obliteration approach (BRTO).[18–20,24–28,30,31] A BATO approach is used in order to avoid reflux of sclerosant into the portomesenteric circulation and to maximize dwell of the sclerosant within the DVs.[3] Balloon occlusion may be performed using standard occlusion balloons. Alternately, sclerosis may be performed without balloon occlusion and with the placement of 0.035-inch coils, or Amplatzer vascular plugs instead.

Transvenous obliteration may be performed concomitantly at the time of TIPS placement to obliterate the DVs and to occlude the portosystemic shunting. It is important when combining TIPS-decompression and transvenous sclerosis (obliteration) without balloon-occlusion to perform the sclerosis first, and then the TIPS subsequently, so that the portal pressure-head and resultant preferential flow into the varices is capitalized on. If the decompressive TIPS is performed first and is effective, the flow is reversed in the afferent limb and the sclerosant would not impregnate and dwell in the varices, rendering the sclerosis less effective. This principal applies to all varices, ectopic or otherwise.

Transvenous obliteration may also be performed without TIPS placement if the patient is not a TIPS candidate due to profound hepatic encephalopathy, hepatic failure, or right heart failure. This is performed via a transhepatic portal approach with transvenous sclerosis of the DVs with balloon occlusion.

Conclusion

A standard endovascular management protocol for DVs has yet to be established.[4,5] As they are relatively uncommon, the literature consists mostly of case reports and small case series. Due to the

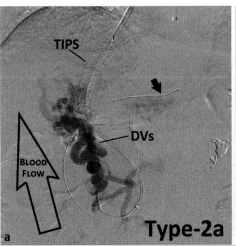
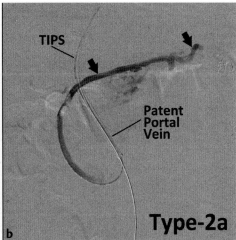

Fig. 32.4 Type-2a ectopic varices with patent portal vein, predominant portoportal collaterals, and diminutive portosystemic collaterals. **(a)** Venogram through a patent transjugular intrahepatic portosystemic shunt (TIPS) and patent portal vein. The selective venogram demonstrates portoportal collaterals, which run parallel to the patent portal vein and through the second portion of the duodenum. Duodenal varices (DVs) in the submucosa of the duodenum are actually the portoportal collaterals themselves. In essence, despite the patency of the portal vein, these collaterals represent a "partial cavernosis" effect of the portal vein. The predominant blood flow hemodynamics are porto-to-portal in a hepatopetal direction. There is lesser portosystemic flow **(b)** via a portosystemic collateral. **(b)** Venogram through a patent transjugular intrahepatic portosystemic shunt (TIPS) and patent portal vein. The selective venogram is of the lesser portosystemic collateral (*solid black arrows*), which connects to systemic retroperitoneal veins. This makes this a type-2a ectopic varices. (*Reprinted with permission from Saad WE, Lippert A, Saad NE. Ectopic varices: Anatomical classification, hemodynamic classification, and hemodynamic-based management. Tech Vasc Interv Radiol 2013;16(2):158–175.*)

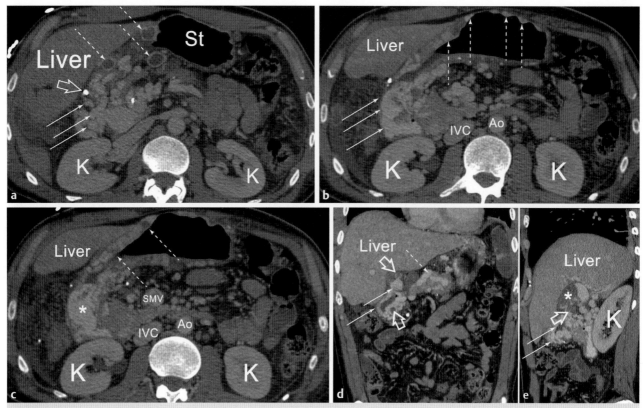

Fig. 32.5 Type-1b ectopic varices due to portal vein thrombosis involving the confluence of the splenic and mesenteric veins. **(a-c)** Contrast-enhanced axial CT images demonstrating varices in the gastric outlet (**b,c**; *dashed white arrows*) and first and second portion of the duodenum (*solid white arrows* and *asterisk*). It is caused by portal vein thrombosis. The varices exhibit partial thrombosis (**a**; *dashed white arrows*) and phleboliths (*hollow white arrow*). Contrast-enhanced CT coronal (**d**) and sagittal (**e**) reformats again demonstrating varices in the gastric outlet (*dashed white arrow*) and first and second portion of the duodenum (*solid white arrows*). Again noted are the partly thrombosed varices (*hollow white arrows*). The portal vein is partly thrombosed (*asterisk*) within the liver. It is completely thrombosed outside the liver. Ao: abdominal aorta; St: stomach; IVC: inferior vena cava; K: kidneys; SMV: superior mesenteric vein. (*Reprinted with permission from Saad WE, Lippert A, Saad NE. Ectopic varices: Anatomical classification, hemodynamic classification, and hemodynamic-based management. Tech Vasc Interv Radiol 2013;16(2):158–175.*)

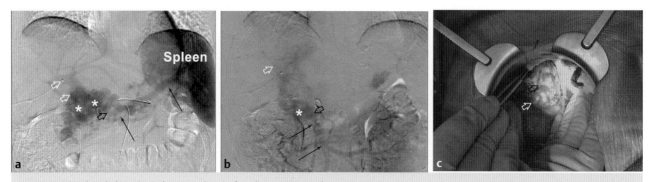

Fig. 32.6 **(a)** Delayed phase (portal venous phase) of a celiac angiogram demonstrating a patent splenic vein along the majority of its course (*between black arrows*). The splenic vein occludes abruptly (*hollow black arrow*) at its confluence with the mesenteric vein(s) (not visualized). The extrahepatic portal vein is completely occluded and is replaced by significant varices and portoportal collaterals (*asterisks*), which run outside the gastrointestinal tract as well as within the wall of the gastric outlet, and first and second parts of the duodenum. The portal vein reconstitutes at the hepatic hilum and continues into the liver (*hollow white arrows*). **(b)** Delayed phase (portal venous phase) of a superior mesenteric angiogram demonstrating a patent mesenteric vein along the majority of its course (*between black arrows*). The mesenteric vein occludes abruptly (*hollow black arrow*) at its confluence with the splenic vein (**a**). The extrahepatic portal vein is completely occluded and is replaced by significant varices and portoportal collaterals (*asterisk*), which reconstitute the portal vein intrahepatically (*hollow white arrow*). **(c)** Photograph of the same patient with a mini laparotomy over the duodenum demonstrating the periportal and duodenal varices (*hollow arrows*), which look like grapes. (*Reprinted with permission from Saad WE, Lippert A, Saad NE. Ectopic varices: Anatomical classification, hemodynamic classification, and hemodynamic-based management. Tech Vasc Interv Radiol 2013;16(2):158–175.*)

varying degrees and etiologic possibilities with DVs, a classification system proposed by Saad et al helps characterize, categorize, and triage the management of DVs (▶ Table 32.1; ▶ Table 32.2). Based on this classification system, a management protocol has been proposed that is directed toward addressing the primary cause of DVs. The nonocclusive type may be treated with portal decompression (with or without obliteration) using a TIPS. The occlusive type requires recanalization of the portal thrombosis or portosystemic decompression proximal to the occlusion.

References

1. Tanaka O, Ohno K, Ohno T, et al. Should balloon-occluded retrograde transvenous obliteration be the first-line interventional radiologic treatment for bleeding duodenal varices? A case report and review of the literature. Acta Radiol 2008;49:32–36.
2. Hashimoto N, Akahoshi T, Yoshida D, et al. The efficacy of balloon-occluded retrograde transvenous obliteration on small intestinal variceal bleeding. Surgery 2010;148:145–150.
3. Saad WE, Lippert A, Saad NE, Caldwell S. Ectopic varices: Anatomical classification, hemodynamic classification, and hemodynamic-based management. Tech Vasc Interv Radiol 2013;16:158–175.
4. Onozato Y, Kakizaki S, Iizuka H, et al. Ectopic varices rupture in the gastroduodenal anastomosis successfully treated with N-butyl-2-cyanoacrylate injection. Acta Med Okayama 2007;61:361–365.
5. Fleming RJ, Seaman WB. Roentgenographic demonstration of unusual extra-esophageal varices. Am J Roentgenol Radium er Nucl Med 1968;103:281–90.
6. Hotta M, Yoshida H, Mamada Y, Taniai N, Bando K, Mizuguchi Y, et al. Successful management of duodenal varices by balloon-occluded retrograde transvenous obliteration. J Nippon Med Sch 2008;75:36–40.
7. Tominaga K, Montani A, Kuga T, et al. Combined balloon-occluded embolization for treatment of concurrent duodenal, gastric, and esophageal varices: A case report. Gastrointest Endosc 2001;53:665–668.
8. Vangeli M, Patch D, Terreni N, et al. Bleeding ectopic varices–treatment with transjugular intrahepatic porto-systemic shunt (TIPS) and embolisation. J Hepatol 2004;41:560–566.
9. Takamura K, Miyake H, Mori H, et al. Balloon occluded retrograde transvenous obliteration and percutaneous transhepatic obliteration for ruptured duodenal varices after operation for rectal cancer with multiple liver metastasis: A report of a case. J Med Invest 2005;52:212–217.
10. Buhler L, Tamigneaux I, Giostra E, et al. Ectopic varices: A rare cause of digestive hemorrhage. Schweiz Med Wochenschr 1996;Suppl 79:70S-72S.
11. Cutler CS, Rex DK, Lehman GA. Enteroscopic identification of ectopic small bowel varices. Gastrointest Endosc 1995;41:605–608.
12. Miller LS, Kim JK, Dai Q, et al. Mechanics and hemodynamics of esophageal varices during peristaltic contraction. Am J Physiol Gastrointest Liver Physiol 2004;287:G830–G835.
13. Arakawa M, Masuzaki T, Okuda K. Pathomorphology of esophageal and gastric varices. Semin Liver Dis 2002;22:73–82.
14. Almeida JR, Trevisan L, Guerrazzi F, et al. Bleeding duodenal varices successfully treated with TIPS. Dig Dis Sci 2006;51:1738–1741.
15. Yoshida Y, Imai Y, Nisjikawa M, et al. Successful endoscopic sclerotherapy with N-butyl-2-cyanoacrylate following the recurrence of bleeding soon after endoscopic ligation for ruptured duodenal varices. Am J Gastroenterol 1997;92:1227–1228.
16. Illuminati G, Smail A, Azoulay D, et al. Association of transjugular intrahepatic portosystemic shunt with embolization in the treatment of bleeding duodenal varix refractory to sclerotherapy. Dig Surg 2000;17:398–400.
17. Jonnalagadda SS, Quison S, Smith OJ. Successful therapy of bleeding duodenal varices by TIPS after failure of sclerotherapy. Am J Gastroenterol 1998;93:272–274.
18. Tsurusaki M, Sugimoto K, Matsumoto S, et al. Bleeding duodenal varices successfully treated with balloon-occluded retrograde transvenous obliteration (BRTO) assisted by CT during arterial portography. Cardiovasc Intervent Radiol 2006;29:1148–1151.
19. Ono S, Irie T, Kuramochi M, et al. Successful treatment of mesenteric varices with balloon-occluded retrograde transvenous obliteration via an abdominal wall vein. J Vasc Interv Radiol 2007;18:1033–1035.
20. Haruta I, Isobe Y, Ueno E, et al. Balloon-occluded retrograde transvenous obliteration (BRTO), a promising nonsurgical therapy for ectopic varices: A case report of successful treatment of duodenal varices by BRTO. Am J Gastroenetrol 1996;91:2594–2597.
21. Ota K, Okazaki M, Higashihara H, et al. Combination of transileocolic vein obliteration and balloon-occluded retrograde transvenous obliteration is effective for ruptured duodenal varices. J Gastroenterol 1999;34:694–699.
22. Tripathi D, Helmy A, Macbeth K, et al. Ten years' follow up of 472 patients following transjugular intrahepatic portosystemic shunt insertion at a single center. Eur J Gastroenterol 2004;16:9–18.
23. Shibata D, Brophy DP, Gordon FD, et al. Transjugular intrahepatic portosystemic shunt for treatment of bleeding ectopic varices with portal hypertension. Dis Colon Rectum 42:1581–1585.
24. Ohta M, Yasumori K, Saku M. Successful treatment of bleeding duodenal varices by balloon-occluded retrograde transvenous obliteration: A transjugular venous approach. Surgery 1999;126:581–583.
25. Somomura T, Horihata K, Yamahara K, et al. Ruptured duodenal varices successfully treated with balloon-occluded retrograde transvenous obliteration: Usefulness of microcatheters. Am J Roentgenol 2003;181:725–727.
26. Soga K, Tomikashi K, Fukamoto K, et al. Successful endoscopic hemostasis for ruptured duodenal varices after balloon-occluded retrograde transvenous obliteration. Dig Endosc 2010;22:329–333.
27. Kim MJ, Jang BK, Chung WJ, et al. Duodenal variceal bleeding after balloon-occluded retrograde transvenous obliteration: Treatment with transjugular intrahepatic portosystemic shunt. World J Gastroenterol 2012;18:2877–2880.
28. Minami S, Okada K, Matsuo M, et al. Treatment of bleeding stomal varices by balloon-occluded retrograde transvenous obliteration. J Gastroenterol 2007;42:91–95.
29. Vidal V, Joly L, Perreault P, et al. Usefulness of transjugular intrahepatic portosystemic shunt in the management of bleeding ectopic varices in cirrhotic patients. Cardiovasc Intervent Radiol 2006;29:216–219.
30. Saad WEA, Darcy MD. Transjugular intrahepatic portosystemic shunt (TIPS) versus balloon-occluded retrograde transvenous obliteration (BRTO) for the management of gastric varices. Semin Interv Radiol 2011;28:339–349.
31. Saad WEA, Al-Ossaimi AM, Caldwell S. Pre- and post-BRTO imaging & clinical evaluation: Indications, management protocols & follow-up. Tech Vasc Interv Radiol 2012;15:165–202.
32. Saad WEA, Saad NE, Koizumi J. Stomal varices: Management with decompression TIPS and transvenous obliteration or sclerosis. Tech Vasc Interv Radiol 2013;16:126–134.
33. Saad WEA, Lippert A, Schwaner S, Al-Osaimi A, Sabri S, Saad N. Management of bleeding duodenal varices with combined TIPS decompression and trans-TIPS transvenous obliteration utilizing 3% sodium tetradecyl sulfate foam sclerosis. J Clin Imaging Sci 2014,4:67.

Chapter 33: Management of Stomal Varices

Ravi N. Srinivasa, Jeffrey Forris Beecham Chick, and Wael E.A. Saad

Introduction

Portal hypertension is associated with the formation of varices in various locations, the most common being the esophagus and stomach. Varices, however, may also occur more distally within the gastrointestinal tract, including within the small bowel, colon, rectum, and in association with intestinal stomas; these are referred to as ectopic varices.

Stomal varices (also called parastomal varices) are extraperitoneal ectopic mesenteric vessels thought to arise secondary to portal hypertension and venous obstruction from surgical scarring related to stomal creation.[1] Stomal varices may also be seen, although less commonly, in association with mesenteric venous thrombosis.[1] The presence of stomal varices may be associated with considerable bleeding, which, although rare, may be life threatening. They are usually not life threatening because manual/digital compression is enough to stop the bleeding until medical attention is sought.[1] This chapter will discuss the anatomy, clinical presentation, classification, imaging findings, management, and outcomes of stomal varices.

Anatomy

Stomal varices may not be related to portal hypertension. The surgical creation of the intestinal stoma itself may result in focal adhesions or segmental scarring, causing constrictive effects on the adjacent venous vasculature and resulting in dilated varices.[1] The afferent feeding vessels of stomal varices are typically tributaries (misnomer is *branches*) of the superior mesenteric vein that drain the bowel segment supplying the stoma.[1] These branches exit the peritoneal cavity, take a sharp turn, and surface in the abdominal wall adjacent to the stoma.[1] Nearly all stomal varices are associated with systemic venous drainage in the anterior abdominal wall; however, the degree of involvement is variable. In the majority of cases there is indirect systemic venous drainage via numerous small venous anastomoses in the subcutaneous tissues of the anterior abdominal wall. These efferent veins aggregate and empty into the ipsilateral iliofemoral vein.[1]

Classification

Saad et al formulated a classification system for stomal varices (▶ Fig. 33.1).[2] Most stomal varices may be classified as type-1a and type-2a. Chronic stomal varices may progress to type-3a with a portosystemic hemodynamic component. Type-1 stomal varices have no physical portosystemic collateral connection, type-2 have a portosystemic connection with minimal flow, and type-3 have a portosystemic connection with hemodynamic shunting (▶ Table 33.1).[13] The "a" and "b" denote the presence of mesoportal occlusion, the nonocclusive or occlusive type, respectively.[13]

A second classification system for stomal varices is based on the type of ostomy. The two most common types are bowel diverting

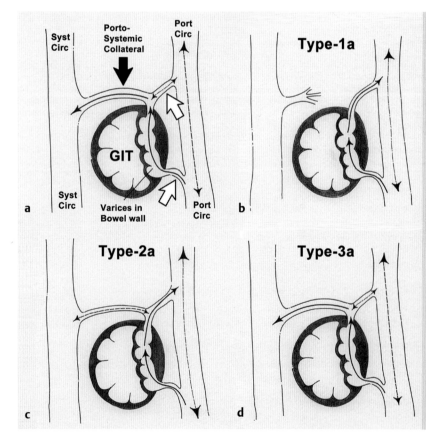

Fig. 33.1 Classification of stomal varices. **(a)** Is a baseline-labeled anatomy image to help interpret the images of the classification system **(b-d)**. **(a)** Demonstrates a representative portal or mesenteric vein branch (Port Circ) on the right and a representative systemic vein branch (Syst Circ) on the left of a cross section through a bowel loop which is a representative of the gastrointestinal tract or stomal bowel loop. Typical systemic veins are anterior abdominal wall veins (usually in subcutaneous tissue) that usually lead to the ipsilateral iliofemoral vein junction. In **(a)**, the "ectopic varices" in this depicted instance are supplied and drained by portal collaterals (*white arrows with black outline*) as well as being drained by a portosystemic collateral. The efferent collateral drainage is portal and not systemic. Varices (ectopic varices) are seen in the wall of the bowel. **(b-d)** This is an overview of the classification system given in ▶ Table 33.1. In short, type-a is nonocclusive and is pressure driven. Type-a is usually with some element of portosystemic collaterals (type-a2 and type-a3) to decompress the higher portal pressure. Type-b varices are not shown because most stomal varices are not of the occlusive type. Most stomal varices fall in the type-1a and type-2a category. Chronic stomal varices may develop portosystemic collaterals to such an extent that they become categorized a type-3a. (*continued*)

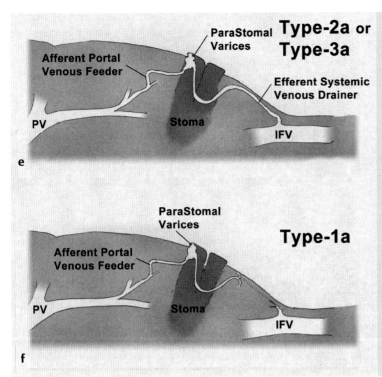

Fig. 33.1 *(Continued)* **(e,f)** Sagittal-labeled anatomy images showing a patient with parastomal varices. Stomal varices are supplied by a mesenteric branch (afferent portal venous feeder), which typically has a sharp turn in its extrahepatic course. **(e)** Demonstrates type-2a or -3a stomal varices (having a degree of portosystemic collateral or shunt component). The efferent draining vein is depicted as connected to the iliofemoral venous junction. **(f)** Demonstrates type-1a parastomal varices (having negligible portosystemic collateral component). IFV: iliofemoral venous; PV: portal vein. *(Reprinted with permission from Saad WE, Saad NE, Koizumi J. Stomal varices: management with decompression TIPS and transvenous obliteration or sclerosis. Tech Vasc Interv Radiol 2013;16(2):176–184.)*

ileostomy or colostomy. Urine diverting ileostomies may also be associated with stomal varices but much less commonly. In theory, colostomies are less vascular and, therefore, sclerotherapy should be performed with more caution due to the increased susceptibility to ischemic complications.[1]

Stomal varices may also be classified based on their bleeding patterns, focal or diffuse.[5] The focal-type is linked to the so called "venous spurt," related to a localized tuft of ectopic varices. In the focal type, the stoma has relatively normal mucosa and the bleeding sites tend to respond to focal single digit compressive therapy prior to definitive treatment.[1] The physical examination in patients with focal type bleeding stomal varices is critical. Localizing the portal or mesenteric venous feeder associated with bleeding is important as it directs percutaneous sclerotherapy. The diffuse type, on the other hand, is associated with congestion and diffuse venous oozing. The diffuse-type is typically managed with transjugular intrahepatic portosystemic shunt (TIPS) decompression.[1]

Endoscopy and Imaging

Endoscopy is not typically utilized as a first-line diagnostic tool in the management of stomal varices because stomal varices are visible to the naked eye on physical examination. If varices are deeper within the stoma, however, endoscopic localization may be necessary.

Preprocedural computed tomographic or magnetic resonance imaging is crucial for treatment planning to exclude portal venous or mesenteric venous thrombosis as the cause for the bleeding varices. In cases of mesoportal occlusion, attempts at recanalization of the occluded vessels should be attempted first as TIPS with decompression is fruitless without a patent portomesenteric circulation. Thrombectomy may be performed via mechanical, or combination mechanical and pharmacologic, means. The pharmacologic approach may be performed with trans-superior mesenteric arterial infusion of tissue plasminogen activator, which is preferred over direct stick percutaneous transhepatic portal access secondary to increased risks of bleeding.

Cross-sectional imaging is important for pretreatment planning in order to identify the systemic venous drainage pattern in the anterior abdominal wall and iliofemoral venous system.

Doppler and grayscale ultrasound are important in the treatment algorithm. This is important as flow dynamics and directionality may be assessed.[1] Ultrasound may be performed with the patient directing the operator to the site of bleeding and the operator may then identify the portal and systemic venous sides of the varices. In stomal varices associated with portal hypertension, the mesenteric venous feeder leading into the stoma

Table 33.1. Hemodynamic Classification of Ectopic Varices

	Portoportal Collaterals Only	Predominantly Portoportal Collaterals with Minimal, if any, Portosystemic Shunting	Predominantly Portosystemic Collaterals with Significant Portosystemic Shunting
Nonocclusive type	Type-1a	Type-2a	Type-3a
Occlusive type	Type-1b	Type-2b	Type-3b

Reprinted with permission from Saad WE, Lippert A, Saad NE. Ectopic varices: anatomical classification, hemodynamic classification, and hemodynamic-based management. Tech Vasc Interv Radiol 2013;16(2):158–175.

demonstrates hepatofugal flow (toward the stoma). The systemic venous end should be evaluated with grayscale ultrasound to assess its compressibility. This will help ascertain the site and degree of compression necessary during sclerotherapy to avoid non-target delivery of sclerosant to the systemic circulation.

Management

Various approaches have been described for the treatment of stomal varices, including creation of surgical shunts or liver transplantation.[4-9] The most definitive treatment of stomal varices is reversal of the ostomy if it is medically and surgically feasible.[1]

There is currently no gold standard on the endovascular management of stomal varices. Endovascular management strategies include creation of TIPS, balloon-occluded retrograde transvenous obliteration (BRTO), and balloon-occluded antegrade transvenous obliteration (BATO).[4,6,7] Patient-specific factors may dictate management. Patients with profound hepatic encephalopathy, metastatic disease to the liver, portal venous thrombosis, heart failure, or high model for end-stage liver disease scores may not be ideal candidates for TIPS creation,[11] and in those cases direct portal puncture, or direct access to the mesenteric circulation with BRTO, BATO,[3] or direct stick percutaneous sclerotherapy approaches may be the best options.

TIPS Decompression

TIPS is the most commonly described method for decompressing the portal circulation and reducing variceal bleeding.[4,6,7,12] TIPS, however, is not beneficial in the setting of portomesenteric venous thrombosis. The diffuse bleeding type of stomal varices is best managed with TIPS creation with or without venous obliteration (▶ Fig. 33.2).

Stomal variceal bleeding may resolve quickly after the creation of a TIPS. TIPS without venous obliteration has a high rebleed rate, up to 21% to 37% in some case series.[4,5,10,11] Due to the fragility of stomal varices, coil embolization is not advised due to the potential erosion of the coils through the walls of the varices. Venous obliteration with sclerosants, such as sotradecol, is preferred. Coils, however, may be used to eliminate collateral vessels in order to create stasis within stomal varices and allow sclerotherapy agents longer dwells. This is particularly helpful when a small occlusion balloon cannot be advanced to the site where venous obliteration is being performed.[1] An alternative to coiling collaterals may include the use of small quantities of N-butyl cyanoacrylate or Onyx to occlude collaterals and generate static flow.[9] Due to their higher viscosity and controlled delivery, they may occlude flow in adjacent draining collaterals and generate static flow within stomal varices prior to delivery of sclerosant.

Transvenous Obliteration

Transvenous obliteration may be performed as a stand-alone procedure or in combination with creation of a TIPS. As described, there are different approaches to transvenous obliteration of stomal varices including: BRTO from a systemic venous approach, BATO from a portal venous approach, and direct stick percutaneous sclerotherapy with systemic venous compression.[1]

A BRTO approach requires, at a minimum, type-2a varices but preferably type-3 ectopic stomal varices (▶ Fig. 33.3). Low-profile balloon occlusion catheters are not readily available in the United States and this approach generally requires use of coils sandwiched with sclerosant, which may be cumbersome.

The BATO approach to venous obliteration is another option that may be performed in conjunction with a TIPS, through an existing TIPS that has failed to relieve variceal bleeding, or via a

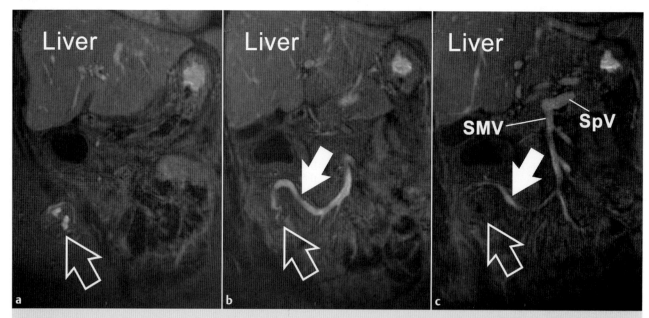

Fig. 33.2 Management of stomal varices with transjugular intrahepatic portosystemic shunt (TIPS) decompression. This is a patient with a diffusely congested ileal stoma and diffuse venous bleeding. (**a-c**) Contrast-enhanced coronal magnetic resonance images demonstrating a right lower quadrant stoma (*hollow arrow*). A mesenteric venous tributary (*solid arrows*) is seen leading to the stoma and its enlarged mesenteric varices (*hollow arrows*). (*continued*)

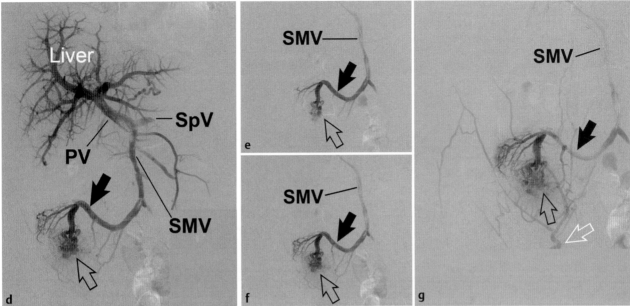

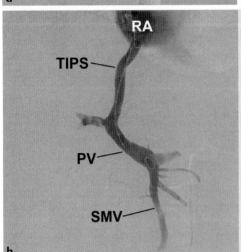

Fig. 33.2 (*Continued*) (**d**) Composite image of a digitally subtracted portogram after TIPS access in the same patient as (**a-c**). There is hepatofugal flow, away from the liver and toward the engorged stoma (*hollow arrow*), via the mesenteric vein branch (*solid arrow*). (**e-g**) Sequential images of a digitally subtracted portogram (mesenteric venogram) demonstrating hepatofugal flow, away from the liver and toward the engorged stoma (*hollow black arrow*), via the mesenteric vein branch (*solid arrow*). There is systemic venous drainage (*hollow white arrow*) via portosystemic anastomoses in the stoma. (**h**) Digitally subtracted TIPS portogram demonstrating a patent transjugular intrahepatic portosystemic shunt (TIPS) with decompression of the mesenteric veins and stoma . The superior mesenteric vein that had hepatofugal flow away from the liver now has antegrade flow toward the liver via the main portal vein. PV: portal vein; RA: right atrium; SMV: superior mesenteric vein; SpV: splenic vein; TIPS: transjugular intrahepatic portosystemic shunt. (*Reprinted with permission from Saad WE, Saad NE, Koizumi J. Stomal varices: management with decompression TIPS and transvenous obliteration or sclerosis. Tech Vasc Interv Radiol 2013;16(2):176–184.*)

transhepatic portal approach (▶ Fig. 33.4; ▶ Fig. 33.5; ▶ Fig. 33.6). Small occlusion balloons may be used in this setting to keep the sclerosant from refluxing into the portomesenteric circulation. Alternately, portal pressure may keep the sclerosant in the stomal varices provided there is no significant systemic venous outflow.[1]

It is important when combining TIPS-decompression and transvenous sclerosis (obliteration) without balloon-occlusion to perform the sclerosis first and then the TIPS subsequently so that the portal pressure-head and resultant preferential flow into the varices is capitalized on. If the decompressive TIPS is performed first and is effective, the flow is reversed in the afferent limb and the sclerosant would not impregnate and dwell in the varices, rendering the sclerosis less effective. This principal applies to all varices, ectopic or otherwise.

In experienced hands, the direct-stick percutaneous sclerotherapy approach is the least invasive and most reliable method for achieving venous obliteration of stomal varices (▶ Fig. 33.7; ▶ Fig. 33.8; ▶ Fig. 33.9; ▶ Fig. 33.10; ▶ Fig. 33.11; ▶ Fig. 33.12; ▶ Fig. 33.13).[1,13] The direct-stick method is a form of antegrade transvenous obliteration. As mentioned previously, the focal bleeding

type of varices is an optimal candidate for this procedure. In addition, the afferent feeder(s) ideally should be large and singular and not small and/or numerous. The likelihood of a technically successful direct-stick sclerosis in the setting of small and/or numerous afferent feeders is low. The mesenteric venous feeder is identified with the assistance of the patient and ultrasound. If flow is fluctuant or hepatopedal then other approaches to treatment should be considered as regulated delivery of the sclerosant cannot be guaranteed. The systemic venous feeder should be identified and is typically inferior or inferomedial relative to the stoma.[13] Identification of the systemic venous feeder may be facilitated by tracing it back from the iliofemoral venous system in the ipsilateral groin. An appropriate point where complete compression of the systemic venous feeder may be achieved should be found using grayscale ultrasound imaging and should be marked. The mesenteric venous feeder is accessed using a 21-gauge micropuncture needle directed toward the stoma. Over-the-wire the needle is exchanged for a micropuncture sheath (3 or 5 French) and venography is performed with and without systemic venous compression. Once flow dynamics confirm that the mesenteric

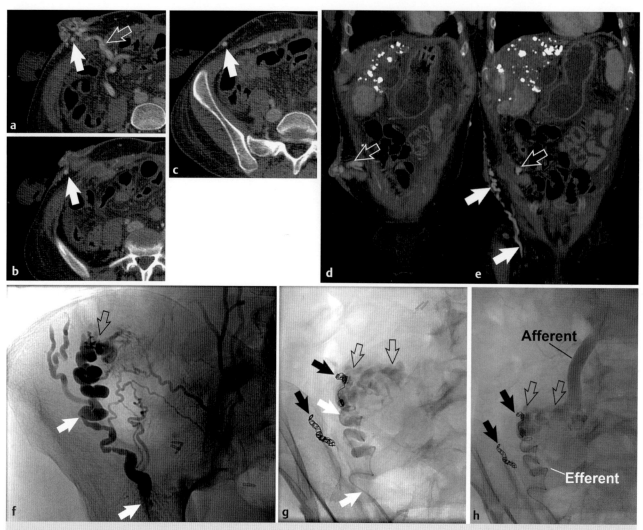

Fig. 33.3 Management of stomal varices with transvenous obliteration via a "balloon-occluded retrograde transvenous obliteration (BRTO)" approach. This is a patient with focal variceal bleeding from an ileal stoma. (**a-c**) Contrast-enhanced axial tomography (CT) images demonstrating a right lower quadrant ileal stoma. A mesenteric venous tributary (*hollow arrow*) is seen leading to the stoma and its enlarged mesenteric varices. A prominent systemic venous draining vein (*solid arrows*) is seen in the subcutaneous tissue of the anterior abdominal wall. (**d,e**) Contrast-enhanced coronal CT reformats again demonstrating the right lower quadrant ileal stoma. The mesenteric venous tributary (*hollow arrows*) is again seen leading to the stoma and its enlarged mesenteric varices. The prominent systemic venous draining vein (*solid arrows*) is seen in the subcutaneous tissue of the anterior abdominal wall heading toward the ipsilateral (right-sided) groin to the right iliofemoral venous junction. (**f**) Retrograde transvenous venogram from the systemic venous side of the system ("BRT approach") is seen demonstrating the systemic venous draining vein (*solid white arrows*) that ends (rather starts from a blood flow standpoint) at the iliostomy (*hollow black arrow*). Numerous systemic venous collaterals are also seen throughout the anterior abdominal wall. In general, these collaterals need to be coil embolized to achieve enough "trapping" to reflux obliterate up the systemic vein and into the stomal varices. (**g,h**) Two venograms taken near the end of the "BRTO approach" transvenous obliteration of the stomal varices. Microcoil embolization was used to occlude two systemic venous collaterals (*solid black arrows*). Foam sclerosant is instilled and refluxed back from the microcatheter (*between solid white arrows*) and into the parastomal varices (*hollow black arrows*). The foam sclerosant is formed from 1 part lipiodol, 2 parts 1% sodium tetradecylsulfate, and 3 parts air. (**h**) Demonstrates a contrast column in the afferent portal (mesenteric) venous feeder with the microcatheter in the efferent systemic draining vein. (*Reprinted with permission from Saad WE, Saad NE, Koizumi J. Stomal varices: management with decompression TIPS and transvenous obliteration or sclerosis. Tech Vasc Interv Radiol 2013;16(2):176–184.*)

venous feeder has hepatofugal flow toward the stoma and that systemic venous compression may be adequately achieved, 1% STS sclerosant is injected through the micropuncture sheath. The sclerosant is mixed in a 1-2-3 ratio of 1 part lipiodol (Lipiodol UltraFluide, Guerbet, Cedex, France), 2 parts 1% sodium tetradecyl sulfate, and 3 parts air.[1,13] After delivery of this mixture through the mesenteric venous feeder, systemic venous outflow compression is maintained for approximately 10 to 15 minutes to ensure adequate dwell of the sclerosant within the varices. It is preferable

to use 1% STS over the more concentrated 3% STS, specifically in the setting of direct puncture of stomal varices, in order to minimize infarction to the adjacent healthy stomal mucosa.

Direct-stick percutaneous sclerotherapy may be performed in less than 30 minutes with minimal fluoroscopy time. The risks are low as it does not require transhepatic or TIPS access and it is a suitable option for patients who are not candidates for TIPS. Furthermore, it does not require delivery of a balloon to occlude the systemic vein, as this may be achieved with ultrasound

(*Text continued on page 314*)

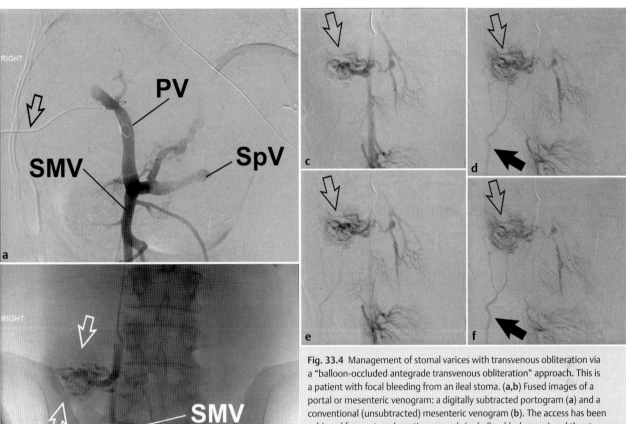

Fig. 33.4 Management of stomal varices with transvenous obliteration via a "balloon-occluded antegrade transvenous obliteration" approach. This is a patient with focal bleeding from an ileal stoma. (**a,b**) Fused images of a portal or mesenteric venogram: a digitally subtracted portogram (**a**) and a conventional (unsubtracted) mesenteric venogram (**b**). The access has been achieved from a transhepatic approach (**a**; *hollow black arrow*) and the stoma shadow is seen *between hollow white arrows* in (**b**). (**c-f**) Sequential images from a digitally subtracted mesenteric venogram showing an engorged stoma with varices in the right lower abdominal quadrant (*hollow black arrows*). A systemic draining vein is seen (*solid black arrows*). PV: portal vein; SMV: superior mesenteric vein; SpV: splenic vein. (*Reprinted with permission from Saad WE, Saad NE, Koizumi J. Stomal varices: management with decompression TIPS and transvenous obliteration or sclerosis. Tech Vasc Interv Radiol 2013;16(2):176–184.*)

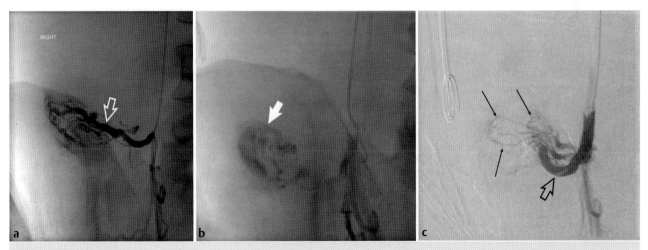

Fig. 33.5 (**a,b**) Selective venogram of the mesenteric vein (*hollow white arrow*) leading to the stomal varices. Foam sclerosant is instilled from the catheter from the pressurized portal venous side (from the afferent mesenteric feeding vein) and into the stomal varices (*solid white arrow*). The foam sclerosant is formed from 1 part lipiodol, 2 parts 1% sodium tetradecyl sulfate, and 3 parts air. The sclerosant foam is kept within the stomal varices by the portal pressure and by the abnormal hepatofugal flow in the mesenteric vein. This is why there is no need for balloon occlusion and that the presclerosant venogram (*hollow white arrow*) is essential to confirm the abnormal hepatofugal flow in the feeding mesenteric vein. (**c**) Selective venogram of the mesenteric vein (*hollow black arrow*) leading to the stomal varices after the foam sclerosant is instilled and has dwelled for 10 to 15 minutes. The venogram is from a 5-French catheter in the mesenteric branch leading to the ileostomy. There is sclerosis of the dilated varices (non-visualized) with residual normal-looking mesenteric venous tributaries (*solid black arrows*). (*Reprinted with permission from Saad WE, Saad NE, Koizumi J. Stomal varices: management with decompression TIPS and transvenous obliteration or sclerosis. Tech Vasc Interv Radiol 2013;16(2):176–184.*)

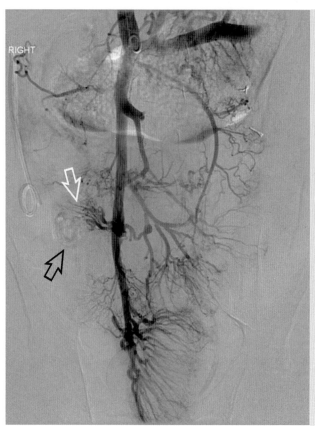

Fig. 33.6 Global mesenteric venogram after the foam sclerosant is instilled and has dwelled for 10 to 15 minutes. The venogram is from a 5-French pigtail catheter in the main portal vein. There is sclerosis of the dilated varices (non-visualized) (*hollow black arrow*) with residual normal-looking mesenteric venous tributaries (*hollow white arrow*). Notice that the entire mesenteric venous system is visualized, which reflects a pressurized portal system (portal pressure exceeds 25 mm Hg in this patient) with continued hepatofugal flow. The transvenous obliteration has not resolved the underlying problem (high portal pressure), but has temporized and focused on the particular problem of bleeding stomal varices. A transjugular intrahepatic portosystemic shunt was not performed because the hepatic reserve was poor. The patient underwent a liver transplant within 8 weeks from the transvenous obliteration, which was considered a temporizing measure bridging to liver transplantation. (*Reprinted with permission from Saad WE, Saad NE, Koizumi J. Stomal varices: management with decompression TIPS and transvenous obliteration or sclerosis. Tech Vasc Interv Radiol 2013; 16(2):176–184.*)

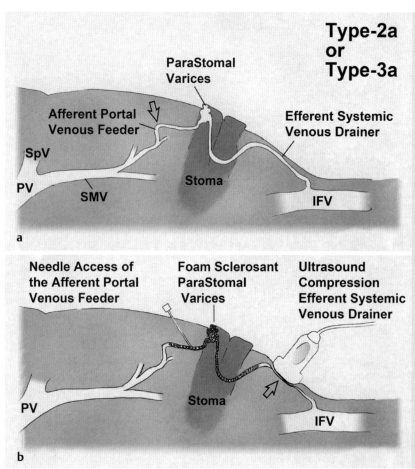

Fig. 33.7 Management of stomal varices with transvenous obliteration via a direct mesenteric venous puncture access with external pressure occlusion of the draining systemic vein. This is a patient with focal bleeding from an ileal stoma. The patient refused any procedure multiple times but continued to bleed. He finally accepted the most minimal of invasive procedures. (**a**) Sagittal anatomy illustration showing a patient with stomal varices. The varices are supplied by a mesenteric branch (afferent portal venous feeder), which typically has a sharp turn in its extrahepatic course. The illustration demonstrates type-2a or -3a stomal varices. The afferent portal venous feeder has a typical sharp turn in its extraperitoneal course (*hollow arrow*). The efferent draining vein is depicted as connected to the iliofemoral venous junction. (**b**) Sagittal anatomy illustration showing the direct mesenteric puncture technique with external systemic venous pressure (exerted by ultrasound transducer; *hollow black arrow*). As can be seen in the illustration, the sclerosant is confined in the afferent mesenteric or portal venous feeder and the stomal varices. The foam sclerosant is "trapped" between the ultrasound transducer compression (on the systemic venous side) and the portal pressure with the hepatofugal flow in the afferent mesenteric or portal venous feeder. IFV: iliofemoral venous; PV: portal vein; SMV: superior mesenteric vein; SpV: splenic vein. (*Reprinted with permission from Saad WE, Saad NE, Koizumi J. Stomal varices: management with decompression TIPS and transvenous obliteration or sclerosis. Tech Vasc Interv Radiol 2013;16(2):176–178.*)

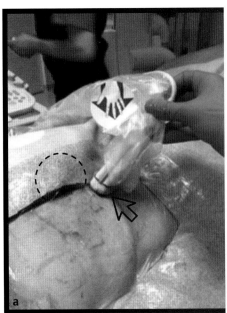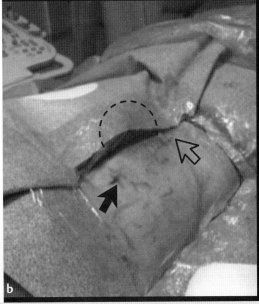

Fig. 33.8 (a,b) Two photographs demonstrating the layout, sterile preparation, draping, and ultrasound planning of the technique. An instrumental part of this layout and planning is based on Doppler and grayscale ultrasound examination. Doppler ultrasound evaluation was performed on the mesenteric venous branch contributing to the stomal varices. The exact location of the contributing mesenteric venous branch is predicted by preprocedural cross-sectional imaging as well as examining and asking the patient. The site of digital compression that stops the bleeding by the patient is almost always where the mesenteric branch approaches the stoma. The Doppler evaluation must identify that the mesenteric branch leading to the stoma is patent and shows hepatofugal flow (blood flow away from the liver and toward the stoma) in the presence of a patent main mesenteric and portal vein. If flow is not hepatofugal, then additional compression may be required over the mesenteric vein proximal to the percutaneous mesenteric venous access site. Doppler and grayscale ultrasound examination of the systemic venous outflow should also be performed with testing for sites of compressibility. If there are numerous systemic venous collaterals, the operators should start at the iliofemoral venous junction where most of these veins aggregate and become a single main compressible vein. As can be seen in the photographs, the mesenteric venous access site is marked (*solid black arrow*) and the systemic venous outflow compression site is marked (*hollow black arrows*) above and below the stoma (draped and depicted by the *dashed arcs* in **a,b**). The ideal mesenteric venous access site is its most superficial extraperitoneal segment before it branches into the stoma. (*Reprinted with permission from Saad WE, Saad NE, Koizumi J. Stomal varices: management with decompression TIPS and transvenous obliteration or sclerosis. Tech Vasc Interv Radiol 2013;16(2):176–184.*)

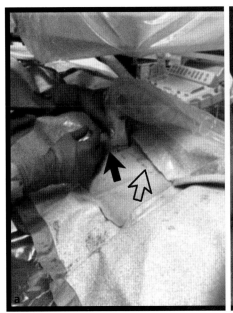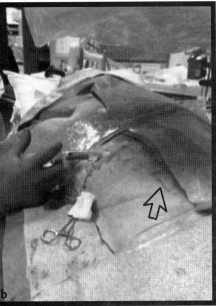

Fig. 33.9 (a,b) Two photographs demonstrating the mesenteric venous access, first with a 21-gauge micropuncture needle (*solid black arrow*). By the Seldinger technique, the 21-gauge needle is exchanged over the wire for a 3-French inner sheath (**b**). The 3-French inner micropuncture sheath is usually enough for venography and subsequent sclerosant administration. Again noted is the planned ultrasound transducer compression site (*hollow black arrows*). (*Reprinted with permission from Saad WE, Saad NE, Koizumi J. Stomal varices: management with decompression TIPS and transvenous obliteration or sclerosis. Tech Vasc Interv Radiol 2013;16(2):176–184.*)

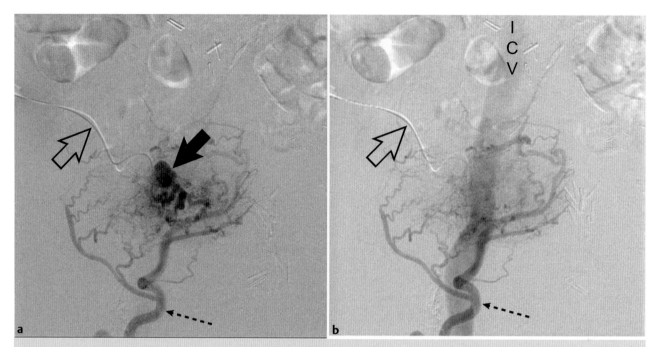

Fig. 33.10 (a,b) Sequential images from a digitally subtracted mesenteric venogram after direct percutaneous access through a 3-French micropuncture sheath (*hollow black arrows*). Significant stomal varices (*solid black arrow*) with shunting and collateralization is seen with systemic venous branches that culminate and aggregate into a single draining systemic vein (*dashed black arrow*), which heads inferiorly to the vicinity of the iliofemoral venous junction (not shown). Contrast is then seen as emptying from the ipsilateral (right-sided) iliofemoral vein and into the inferior vena cava. This is stomal varices with significant portosystemic shunting (type-3a). The venogram is performed without exerting external compression by the ultrasound transducer. (*Reprinted with permission from Saad WE, Saad NE, Koizumi J. Stomal varices: management with decompression TIPS and transvenous obliteration or sclerosis. Tech Vasc Interv Radiol 2013;16(2):176–184.*)

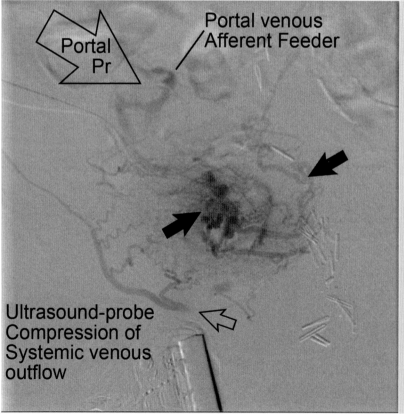

Fig. 33.11 Digitally subtracted mesenteric venogram from the direct percutaneous access through a 3-French micropuncture sheath with exerting external compression by the ultrasound transducer (compare with venogram in ▶ Fig. 33.10). The significant shunting and collateralization with the systemic venous branches is stopped (*hollow black arrow*). Shunting is no longer taking place (IVC not visualized) and the contrast is static in the stomal varices and is kept "trapped" and static in the stomal varices (*between solid black arrows*) by the forward portal pressure (Portal Pr) exerted by the hepatofugal flow in the contributing mesenteric venous branch. This is the ideal presclerosant diagnostic endpoint. At this point, the sclerosant foam should be instilled under the same conditions (exerting the same pressure on the same spot by the ultrasound transducer). (*Reprinted with permission from Saad WE, Saad NE, Koizumi J. Stomal varices: management with decompression TIPS and transvenous obliteration or sclerosis. Tech Vasc Interv Radiol 2013; 16(2):176–184.*)

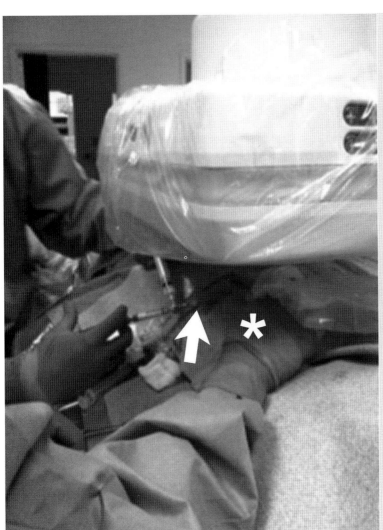

Fig. 33.12 A photograph demonstrating sclerosant foam administration through the 3-French micropuncture sheath at the mesenteric venous access site (*solid white arrow*) while ultrasound transducer compression is held (*asterisk*). The foam sclerosant is formed from 1 part lipiodol, 2 parts 1% sodium tetradecyl sulfate (can be diluted 3% sodium tetradecyl sulfate), and 3 parts air. The sclerosant foam is kept within the stomal varices by the portal pressure and by the abnormal hepatofugal flow in the mesenteric vein. This is why there is no need for balloon occlusion and that the presclerosant venogram is essential to confirm the abnormal hepatofugal flow in the feeding mesenteric vein. (*Reprinted with permission from Saad WE, Saad NE, Koizumi J. Stomal varices: management with decompression TIPS and transvenous obliteration or sclerosis. Tech Vasc Interv Radiol 2013;16(2):176–184.*)

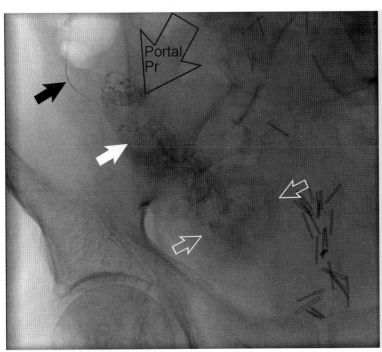

Fig. 33.13 Completion fluoroscopic spot image after the sclerosant administration showing the foam sclerosant (double contrast appearance) filling the afferent mesenteric venous branch (*solid white arrow*) and the stomal varices (*between hollow white arrows*) and sparing the systemic venous outflow (efferent systemic vein) that is not opacified (not shown). The sclerosant is kept "trapped" in place in the mesenteric afferent branch and the stoma by the portal pressure (Portal Pr) exerted by the hepatofugal flow in the portal circulation. At this point, the 3-French percutaneous sheath (*solid black arrow*) is removed and hemostasis is usually achieved easily because the sclerosant is in the access vein proximal and distal to the percutaneous access point (this position of sclerosant proximal and distal to the mesenteric venous access should be intentionally achieved; in other words, this should be a desired procedural endpoint). Dermabond (typical histoacryl) also helps obtain procedural hemostasis. (*Reprinted with permission from Saad WE, Saad NE, Koizumi J. Stomal varices: management with decompression TIPS and transvenous obliteration or sclerosis. Tech Vasc Interv Radiol 2013;16(2):176–184.*)

compression.[1,13] This applies only to type-2 and type-3 stomal varices as type-1a do not have a systemic venous outflow.[1] The key exclusion criteria for this approach are patients who have hepatopedal flow in the mesenteric venous feeder or those with diffuse bleeding-type varices; these patients may benefit from the other endovascular approaches described above.

Pabon-Ramos et al reported a case series of 8 patients undergoing sclerosis and embolization with an 88% technical success rate and a 42.8% rebleed rate in a series of 7 patients, 3 of which had rebleeding with the median time to rebleeding being 45 days. The remaining 4 patients did not have rebleeding during the follow-up period, with a median bleeding-free interval of 131 days.[11] Saad et al published a case series in 2014 of four patients with ileostomy-associated stomal varices who underwent venous obliteration with 1% sodium tetradecyl sulfate (1% STS), one of whom had the diffuse type and required a BRTO approach, and three of whom had focal type and underwent antegrade approaches (one percutaneous transhepatic and two direct stick), all with complete remission of bleeding post-treatment ranging from 8 to 33.9 months (mean 17 months). No complications in the form of necrosis or ulceration of the stomal mucosa occurred. Notably the transhepatic approach patient had intercostal pain post procedure lasting three weeks.[13]

Conclusion

Stomal varices are uncommon but may be particularly bothersome. Repeated bleeding episodes may not only be frustrating but also life threatening. Fortunately, there are a number of endovascular treatments. While a gold standard therapeutic approach has not been identified, classifying the type of stomal varices is important in guiding its management algorithm. Generally speaking, those with focal bleeding type benefit from venous obliteration with or without TIPS, BRTO, and BATO, while those with diffuse bleeding type may benefit from TIPS decompression with or without sclerosis. In appropriately selected patients, however, contingent on the portomesenteric venous flow and systemic venous flow dynamics, a direct stick venous approach with systemic venous outflow occlusion is perhaps the least invasive and most effective initial approach to treatment, reserving more invasive procedures as a second-line treatment.

Clinical Pearls

- Stomal or parastomal varices are types of ectopic varices.
- Stomal variceal bleeding can be diffuse (engorged oozing) or focal (localized as numbers on a clock).
- Stomal varices are more common in ilostomies than colostomies.
- Colostomies are more susceptible to ischemia and ischemic injury after sclerosis compared to ileostomies.
- There are types of stomal (parastomal) varices depending on the degree, of any, of portosystemic shunting and presence

and absence of portal vein/mestentiric vein thrombosis. This hemodynamic classification system (Saad et al) applies for all ectopic and nonectopic varices.
- Due to the scaricity of stomal varices and the variations in types, techniques and reporting, there is no clear data as to the best approach to managing them.
- TIPS is the traditional management approach and is probably the best approach for diffuse bleeding if the patient is a TIPS candidate and is acceptant to its higher morbidity.
- Transvenous obliteration is the least invasive approach with the least morbidity and is showing promising initial longevity results with a rebleed rate of less than 10% at 6 to 12 months compared to TIPS, which has a rebleed rate at 6 to 12 months of 20% to 35%.
- The direct-stick technique seems to be the lest invasive, least expensive, and least time-consuming transvenous approach but is for selected cases with singular large afferent limbs and focal bleeding.

References

1. Saad WE, Saad NE, Koizumi J. Stomal varices: management with decompression TIPS and transvenous obliteration or sclerosis. Tech Vasc Interv Radiol. 2013; 16(2):176–84.
2. Saad WE, Lippert A, Saad NE. Ectopic varices: anatomical classification, hemodynamic classification, and hemodynamic-based management. Tech Vasc Interv Radiol 2013;16(2):158–75.
3. Saad WE, Kitanosono T, Koizumi J. Balloon-occluded antegrade transvenous obliteration with or without balloon-occluded retrograde transvenous obliteration for the management of gastric varices: concept and technical applications. Tech Vasc Interv Radiol. 2012;15(3):203–25.
4. Kocher N, Tripathy D, McAvoy NC, et al. Bleeding ectopic varices in cirrhosis: the role of transjugular intra-hepatic portosystemic stent shunts. Aliment Pharmacol Ther 2008;28:294–303.
5. Hashimoto N, Akhoshi T, Yoshida D, et al. The efficacy of balloon-occluded retrograde transvenous obliteration on small intestinal variceal bleeding. Surgery 2010;148:145–150.
6. Zamora CA, Sugimoto K, Tsurusaki M, et al. Endovascular obliteration of bleeding duodenal varices in patients with liver cirrhosis. Eur Radiol 2006;16:73–79.
7. Vangeli M, Patch D, Terrini N, et al. Bleeding ectopic varices: Treatment with transjugular intrahepatic porto-systemic shunts (TIPS) and embolization. J Hepatol 2004;41:560–566.
8. Minami S, Okada K, Matsuo M, et al. Treatment of bleeding stomal varices by balloon-occluded retrograde transvenous obliteration. J Gastroenterol 2007; 42:91–95.
9. Thouveny F, Aube C, Konate A, et al. Direct percutaneous approach for endoluminal glue embolization of stomal varices. J Vasc Intervent Radiol 2008; 19:774–777.
10. Vidal V, Joly L, Perreault P, et al. Usefulness of transjugular intrahepatic portosystemic shunt in the management of bleeding ectopic varices in cirrhotic patients. Cardiovasc Intervent Radiol 2006;29:216–219.
11. Pabon-Ramos W, Niemeyer M, Dasika N. Alternative treatment for bleeding peristomal varices: percutaneous parastomal embolization. Cardiovasc Intervent Radiol 2013;36:1399–1404.
12. Shreiner A, Dasika N, Sharma P. Lower GI bleeding in a patient with cirrhosis and history of colorectal cancer. Gastroenterology 2013 September;145(3):e3–e4.
13. Saad WE, Schwaner S, Lippert A, Sabri SS, Al-Osaimi A, Matsumoto A, Angle J, Caldwell S. Management of stomal varices with transvenous obliteration utilizing sodium tetradecyl sulfate foam sclerosis. Cardiovasc Intervent Radiol 2014; 37:1625–1630.

Index

Note: Page number followed by *f* and *t* indicates figure and table respectively.